# Returning Home from Iraq and Afghanistan: Assessment of Readjustment Needs of Veterans, Service Members, and Their Families

**Committee on the Assessment of Readjustment Needs of Military Personnel, Veterans, and Their Families**

**Board on the Health of Select Populations**

INSTITUTE OF MEDICINE
*OF THE NATIONAL ACADEMIES*

THE NATIONAL ACADEMIES PRESS
Washington, D.C.
**www.nap.edu**

**THE NATIONAL ACADEMIES PRESS 500 Fifth Street, NW Washington, DC 20001**

NOTICE: The project that is the subject of this report was approved by the Governing Board of the National Research Council, whose members are drawn from the councils of the National Academy of Sciences, the National Academy of Engineering, and the Institute of Medicine. The members of the committee responsible for the report were chosen for their special competences and with regard for appropriate balance.

This study was supported by Contract HHSP23320042509XI between the National Academy of Sciences and the Department of Defense. Any opinions, findings, conclusions, or recommendations expressed in this publication are those of the authors and do not necessarily reflect the views of the organizations or agencies that provided support for this project.

International Standard Book Number-13: 978-0-309-26427-3
International Standard Book Number-10: 0-309-26427-8

Additional copies of this report are available from the National Academies Press, 500 Fifth Street NW, Keck 360, Washington, DC 20001; (800) 624-6242 or (202) 334-3313 http://www.nap.edu.

For more information about the Institute of Medicine, visit the IOM home page at: **www.iom.edu**.



Printed in the United States of America

The serpent has been a symbol of long life, healing, and knowledge among almost all cultures and religions since the beginning of recorded history. The serpent adopted as a logotype by the Institute of Medicine is a relief carving from ancient Greece, now held by the Staatliche Museen in Berlin.

IOM (Institute of Medicine). 2013. *Returning home from Iraq and Afghanistan: Assessment of readjustment needs of veterans, service members, and their families*. Washington, DC: The National Academies Press.

*"Knowing is not enough; we must apply.*
*Willing is not enough; we must do."*

—Goethe

INSTITUTE OF MEDICINE

*OF THE NATIONAL ACADEMIES*

**Advising the Nation. Improving Health.**

THE NATIONAL ACADEMIES

*Advisers to the Nation on Science, Engineering, and Medicine*

The **National Academy of Sciences** is a private, nonprofit, self-perpetuating society of distinguished scholars engaged in scientific and engineering research, dedicated to the furtherance of science and technology and to their use for the general welfare. Upon the authority of the charter granted to it by the Congress in 1863, the Academy has a mandate that requires it to advise the federal government on scientific and technical matters. Dr. Ralph J. Cicerone is president of the National Academy of Sciences.

The **National Academy of Engineering** was established in 1964, under the charter of the National Academy of Sciences, as a parallel organization of outstanding engineers. It is autonomous in its administration and in the selection of its members, sharing with the National Academy of Sciences the responsibility for advising the federal government. The National Academy of Engineering also sponsors engineering programs aimed at meeting national needs, encourages education and research, and recognizes the superior achievements of engineers. Dr. Charles M. Vest is president of the National Academy of Engineering.

The **Institute of Medicine** was established in 1970 by the National Academy of Sciences to secure the services of eminent members of appropriate professions in the examination of policy matters pertaining to the health of the public. The Institute acts under the responsibility given to the National Academy of Sciences by its congressional charter to be an adviser to the federal government and, upon its own initiative, to identify issues of medical care, research, and education. Dr. Harvey V. Fineberg is president of the Institute of Medicine.

The **National Research Council** was organized by the National Academy of Sciences in 1916 to associate the broad community of science and technology with the Academy's purposes of furthering knowledge and advising the federal government. Functioning in accordance with general policies determined by the Academy, the Council has become the principal operating agency of both the National Academy of Sciences and the National Academy of Engineering in providing services to the government, the public, and the scientific and engineering communities. The Council is administered jointly by both Academies and the Institute of Medicine. Dr. Ralph J. Cicerone and Dr. Charles M. Vest are chair and vice chair, respectively, of the National Research Council.

**www.national-academies.org**

## COMMITTEE ON THE ASSESSMENT OF READJUSTMENT NEEDS OF MILITARY PERSONNEL, VETERANS, AND THEIR FAMILIES

**GEORGE W. RUTHERFORD, MD, AM** (*Chair*), Salvatore Pablo Lucia Professor and Vice Chair, Department of Epidemiology and Biostatistics; Director, Prevention and Public Health Group, Global Health Sciences, University of California, San Francisco

**MARGARITA ALEGRÍA, PhD,** Professor, Department of Psychiatry, Harvard Medical School; Director, Center for Multicultural Mental Health Research, Cambridge Health Alliance

**JEFFREY J. BAZARIAN, MD, MPH,** Associate Professor, University of Rochester Medical Center

**DAN G. BLAZER, MD, PhD,** J.P. Gibbons Professor of Psychiatry, Duke University Medical Center

**KATHLEEN M. CARROLL, PhD,** Professor of Psychiatry, Department of Psychiatry, Division of Substance Abuse, Yale University

**IBOLJA CERNAK, MD, PhD, ME, MHS,** Chair, Canadian Military and Veterans' Clinical Rehabilitation Medicine, Faculty of Rehabilitation Medicine, University of Alberta, Edmonton, Canada

**JOHN D. CORRIGAN, PhD,** Professor and Director, Division of Rehabilitation Psychology, Department of Physical Medicine and Rehabilitation, Ohio State University

**E. JANE COSTELLO, PhD,** Professor, Department of Psychiatry and Behavioral Sciences, Duke University School of Medicine

**SUREYYA S. DIKMEN, PhD,** Professor, Department of Rehabilitation Medicine, University of Washington

**NAIHUA DUAN, PhD,** Professor of Biostatistics (in Psychiatry), Department of Psychiatry, Columbia University

**RYAN D. EDWARDS, PhD,** Associate Professor of Economics, Queens College and the Graduate Center, City University of New York; Research Associate, National Bureau of Economic Research, Cambridge, MA

**CHRISTINE EIBNER, PhD,** Economist, RAND Corporation

**NORAH C. FEENY, PhD,** Professor, Department of Psychological Sciences, Case Western Reserve University

**SANDRO GALEA, MD, DrPH,** Gelman Professor and Chair, Department of Epidemiology, Columbia University Mailman School of Public Health

**GREGORY C. GRAY, MD, MPH,** Professor and Chair, Department of Environmental and Global Health, College of Public Health and Health Professions; Director, Global Pathogens Laboratory, University of Florida

**KENNETH W. KIZER, MD, MPH,** Distinguished Professor, University of California, Davis, School of Medicine and Betty Irene Moore School of Nursing; Director, Institute for Population Health Improvement, University of California, Davis, Health System

**MEREDITH A. KLEYKAMP, PhD,** Assistant Professor of Sociology, University of Maryland

**JANICE L. KRUPNICK, PhD,** Professor of Psychiatry and Director, Trauma and Loss Program, Department of Psychiatry, Georgetown University School of Medicine

**RICHARD A. KULKA, PhD,** Consultant, Statistical, Survey and Social Research

**BENNETT L. LEVENTHAL, MD,** Deputy Director, Nathan Kline Institute for Psychiatric Research; Professor, Department of Disability and Human Development, University of Illinois at Chicago; Irving B. Harris Professor, Emeritus, The University of Chicago

**ALAIR MACLEAN, PhD,** Associate Professor, Department of Sociology, Washington State University, Vancouver

**FRANCES MURPHY, MD, MPH,** Health Care Independent Consultant, Silver Spring, MD

**SAMUEL J. POTOLICCHIO, MD,** Professor of Neurology, Department of Neurology, George Washington University Medical Center

**SCOTT L. RAUCH, MD,** Chair, Partners Psychiatry and Mental Health; President and Psychiatrist in Chief, McLean Hospital; Professor of Psychiatry, Harvard Medical School

**WILLIAM E. SCHLENGER, PhD,** Principal Scientist, Abt Associates Inc.

**TYLER SMITH, MS, PhD**, Associate Professor, Department of Community Health, School of Health and Human Services, National University Technology and Health Sciences Center

**S.V. SUBRAMANIAN, PhD**, Professor of Population Health and Geography, Department of Society, Human Development, and Health, Harvard School of Public Health

**SHELLEY MACDERMID WADSWORTH, PhD,** Professor of Human Development and Family Studies; Director, Center for Families; Director, Military Family Research Institute, Purdue University

**ALBERT W. WU, MD, MPH**, Professor and Director, Center for Health Services and Outcomes Research, Department of Health Policy and Management, Johns Hopkins Bloomberg School of Public Health

## STUDY STAFF

**CAROLYN FULCO,** Scholar
**LAURA AIUPPA DENNING,** Senior Program Officer
**HARRIET CRAWFORD,** IT Project Manager
**CARY HAVER,** Senior Program Associate
**RENÉE WLODARCZYK,** Senior Program Associate
**DWAYNE BELL,** Programmer/Analyst
**MARC MEISNERE,** Research Associate
**JOE GOODMAN,** Senior Program Assistant
**JONATHAN SCHMELZER,** Senior Progam Assistant
**NORMAN GROSSBLATT,** Senior Editor
**CATHERINE A. GRUBER,** Editor
**CHRISTIE BELL,** Financial Officer (until January 2012)
**GARY WALKER,** Senior Financial Officer (until November 2012)
**DORIS ROMERO,** Financial Associate
**FREDRICK ERDTMANN,** Director, Board on the Health of Select Populations

**ANALYSTS, CONSULTANTS, AND WRITERS**

**MARK BREWSTER,** Columbia University
**CONNIE CITRO,** National Research Council
**GREG COHEN,** Columbia University
**RUTH CROSSGROVE,** Independent Editor
**MIRIAM DAVIS,** Independent Consultant
**PETER JAMES,** Harvard University
**JOAN MACHAMER,** University of Washington
**ELLEN MANTUS,** National Research Council
**SUE MARCUS,** Columbia University
**MARTHA PRESCOTT,** Columbia University
**THERESA SCHWARTZ,** Research Foundation for Mental Hygiene
**ANDREA SOLARZ,** Independent Consultant
**JAMES WEAVER,** Research Foundation for Mental Hygiene
**WESTAT Staff:** Stephanie Beauvais, Jennifer Berktold, Diane Boyd, Mary Butler, Karla Eisen, Martha Franklin, Rachel Gaddes, Carol Hagen, Wayne Hintze, Teresa Koenig, Chris Manglitz, Shelley Perry, Cynthia Robins, and Eden Segal
**HEATHER YOUNG,** George Washington University

# REVIEWERS

This report has been reviewed in draft form by persons chosen for their diverse perspectives and technical expertise in accordance with procedures approved by the National Research Council's Report Review Committee. The purpose of this independent review is to provide candid and critical comments that will assist the institution in making its published report as sound as possible and to ensure that the report meets institutional standards of objectivity, evidence, and responsiveness to the study charge. The review comments and draft manuscript remain confidential to protect the integrity of the deliberative process. We thank the following for their review of this report:

**Kathleen Brady,** Medical University of South Carolina
**Alicia L. Carriquiry,** Iowa State University
**Kenneth A. Dodge,** Duke University Sanford School of Public Policy
**Jason Hockenberry,** Emory University Rollins School of Public Health
**Kerry Knox,** University of Rochester School of Medicine and Dentistry
**Thomas Kosten,** VA National Substance Use Disorders Program, Quality Enhancement Research Initiative (QUERI)
**Captain (Retired) William P. Nash**
**Colonel (Retired) Elspeth Cameron Ritchie,** Uniformed Services University of the Health Sciences, Washington D.C. Department of Mental Health
**Jennifer J. Vasterling,** VA Boston Healthcare System, Boston University School of Medicine
**Colonel (Retired) Kelly A. Wolgast,** Vanderbilt University School of Nursing

Although the reviewers listed above have provided many constructive comments and suggestions, they were not asked to endorse the conclusions or recommendations, nor did they see the final draft of the report before its release. The review of the report was overseen by **John C. Bailar III** and **Harold C. Sox,** Dartmouth Medical School. Appointed by the National Research Council and the Institute of Medicine, they were responsible for making certain that an independent examination of the report was carried out in accordance with institutional procedures and that all review comments were carefully considered. Responsibility for the final content of the report rests entirely with the authoring committee and the institution.

# CONTENTS



## Appendixes*



* Appendixes A-F are not printed in this book but are available on the CD in the back of the book and online at http://www.iom.edu/Reports/2013/Returning-Home-from-Iraq-and-Afghanistan.aspx.

# PREFACE

In 2008, with the passage of the National Defense Authorization Act for fiscal year 2008 (PL 110-181), the National Academy of Sciences was asked to examine the readjustment needs of Operation Enduring Freedom and Operation Iraqi Freedom service members, their families, and affected communities. The Institute of Medicine assembled a committee to address the tasks in the legislation; the committee has worked for over 4 years to produce a preliminary report in 2010 and this final report. The legislation is broad and required the committee to look at many disparate issues.

As the committee considered the various issues, it became apparent that it would not be able to cover all of them in depth, inasmuch as each could fill a volume. The committee had to decide which issues to focus on and which to leave for future study. It used the legislation as its guide and focused on issues related to traumatic brain injuries, posttraumatic stress disorder, and other mental-health outcomes, although pain, polytrauma, burns, and amputations are also important.

The committee faced additional challenges as it approached its task. In its desire to address all aspects of its charge carefully, as required by the legislation, the committee initially tried to conduct original data analyses by linking various federal administrative datasets. There were, however, substantial organizational hurdles, and much additional time would have been required to obtain the data and conduct the analyses. The committee eventually abandoned that approach with some exceptions.

To say that this study is important understates the great needs of our military men and women and their families. As we traveled the country in Phase 1 of our study, we heard from active-duty personnel, veterans, and family members and we were humbled by the sacrifices made by all of them. As we continued to read the literature, we saw that much more study would be needed, but we recognized that military personnel, veterans, and family members need answers and help now.

We have all read the articles in the popular press, heard the radio broadcasts, and watched the news programs that highlight the troubling statistics regarding brain injuries, posttraumatic stress disorder, and other mental-health outcomes in our military personnel and veterans. We have read and heard about increasing marital stress, suicide, and substance abuse. We have read and heard about long wait times for appointments for treatment and disability examinations. Clearly, the nation, government agencies, communities, and families and friends need to respond. In many cases, there is a growing response, but more needs to be done to assist our active-duty military men and women, our National Guard and reserve members, our veterans, and their families. More coordination among programs is needed, more mental-health professionals are needed, and more treatments for wounds, seen and unseen, are needed. It is also necessary to reduce the stigma associated with mental illness and to reduce wait times for treatment. The Department of Defense and the Department of Veterans Affairs have made great progress in all those matters, but more will be needed—the issues will continue to plague our country for the indefinite future.

I deeply appreciate the work of my fellow committee members and their dedication and commitment to this project, which has been in progress for several years. We extend our appreciation to the many people who helped us along the way and to the numerous consultants whom we relied on for information and data analyses. We also thank the Institute of Medicine staff directed by Carolyn Fulco for their expert assistance, in particular Harriet Crawford for her patience and for generating numerous data files for our analyses, Laura Aiuppa for her work with the family and treatment groups, Renee Wlodarczyk for leading the access and barriers group, Marc Meisnere for his work with the community group, Cary Haver for her assistance with the economics group, Jonathan Schmelzer for his willingness to help out whenever needed, and Joe Goodman for his excellent attention to detail in getting us through 10 meetings. Finally, we thank Carolyn Fulco for her overall guidance and orchestration of the multiple pieces of the study.

The committee hopes that the findings in this report will result in improved outcomes for active-duty personnel, veterans, and their family members. We honor their commitment to the country, and it is for them that we persevered.

George W. Rutherford, MD, AM, *Chair*
Committee on the Assessment of Readjustment Needs of Military Personnel, Veterans, and Their Families

# ABBREVIATIONS

| | |
|---|---|
| AF | Afghanistan |
| AFQT | Armed Forces Qualifying Test |
| BAI | Beck Anxiety Inventory |
| BDI | Beck Depression Inventory |
| BIRLS | Beneficiary Identification records Locator System |
| BMI | body mass index |
| BSI | Brief Symptom Inventory |
| CAPS | Clinician Administered PSTD Scale |
| CBO | Congressional Budget Office |
| CCEP | Comprehensive Clinical Evaluation Program |
| CDC | Centers for Disease Control and Prevention |
| CES | Combat Exposure Scale |
| CHCS | Composite Health Care System |
| CI | confidence interval |
| CIDI | Composite International Diagnostic Interview |
| CMI | chronic multisymptom illness |
| CNS | central nervous system |
| COD | cause of death |
| COSHPD | California Office of Statewide Health Planning and Development |
| CPG | Clinical Practice Guidelines |
| CVLT | California Verbal Learning Test |
| DCOE | Defense Centers of Excellence |
| DEERS | Defense Enrollment Eligibility Reporting System |
| DIBRS | Defense Incident-Based Reporting System |
| DMDC | Defense Manpower Data Center |
| DOD | Department of Defense |
| *DSM* | *Diagnostic and Statistical Manual of Mental Disorders* |
| DTAS | Defense Theater Accountability System |
| FY | fiscal year |
| GAO | Government Accountability Office |
| GWOT | Global War on Terror |
| *ICD* | *International Statistical Classification of Diseases* |
| IOM | Institute of Medicine |
| IZ | Iraq |

| | |
|---|---|
| MCS | Millennium Cohort Study |
| MDD | major depressive disorder |
| MDP | Medical SAS® Datasets |
| MDR | Military Health System Data Repository |
| mTBI | mild traumatic brain injury |
| N | number of study subjects |
| NAS | National Academy of Sciences |
| NCIC | National Crime Information Center |
| NDE | National Data Extract |
| NDI | National Death Index |
| NIH | National Institutes of Health |
| NIMH | National Institute of Mental Health |
| NPCD | National Patient Care Database |
| OED | Outpatient Encounter Database |
| OEF | Operation Enduring Freedom |
| OIF | Operation Iraqi Freedom |
| OND | Operation New Dawn |
| OR | odds ratio |
| PCL | Patient Checklist |
| PCL-C | Patient Checklist–Civilian |
| PCL-M | Patient Checklist–Military |
| PCS | permanent change of station |
| PDHA | Post-Deployment Health Assessment |
| PDHRA | Post-Deployment Health Re-Assessment |
| PHQ | Patient Health Questionnaire |
| PTF | Patient Treatment File |
| PTSD | posttraumatic stress disorder |
| SADR | Standard Ambulatory Data Record |
| SCID | Structured Clinical Interview for *DSM-II-R* |
| SF-12 | 12-Item Short Form Health Survey |
| SF-36 | 36-Item Short Form Health Survey |
| SIDR | Standard Inpatient Data Record |
| SMR | standardized mortality ratio |
| SSA | Social Security Administration |
| SUD | substance-use disorder |
| TBI | traumatic brain injury |
| VA | Department of Veterans Affairs |

| | |
|---|---|
| VAMC | VA Medical Center |
| VBA | Veterans Benefits Administration |
| VETSNET | Veterans Service Network |
| VHA | Veterans Health Administration |
| VISN | Veterans Integrated Service Network |
| VSA | Veterans Service Area |

# SUMMARY

As of December 2012, Operation Enduring Freedom (OEF) in Afghanistan and Operation Iraqi Freedom (OIF) in Iraq have resulted in the deployment of about 2.2 million troops; there have been 2,222 US fatalities in OEF and Operation New Dawn (OND)[1] and 4,422 in OIF. The numbers of wounded US troops exceed 16,000 in Afghanistan and 32,000 in Iraq. In addition to deaths and morbidity, the operations have unforeseen consequences that are yet to be fully understood.

In contrast with previous conflicts, the all-volunteer military has experienced numerous deployments of individual service members; has seen increased deployments of women, parents of young children, and reserve and National Guard troops; and in some cases has been subject to longer deployments and shorter times at home between deployments. Numerous reports in the popular press have made the public aware of issues that have pointed to the difficulty of military personnel in readjusting after returning from Iraq and Afghanistan. Many of those who have served in OEF and OIF readjust with few difficulties, but others have problems in readjusting to home, reconnecting with family members, finding employment, and returning to school.

## BACKGROUND

In response to the return of large numbers of veterans from Iraq and Afghanistan with physical-health and mental-health problems and to the growing readjustment needs of active-duty service members, veterans, and their family members, Congress included Section 1661 of the National Defense Authorization Act for fiscal year 2008. That section required the secretary of defense, in consultation with the secretary of veterans affairs, to enter into an agreement with the National Academies for a study of the physical-health, mental-health, and other readjustment needs of members and former members of the armed forces who were deployed in OIF or OEF, their families, and their communities as a result of such deployment. The study was assigned to the Institute of Medicine (IOM).

The study consisted of two phases. The Phase 1 task was to conduct a *preliminary* assessment. The Phase 2 task was to provide a *comprehensive* assessment of the physical, psychologic, social, and economic effects of deployment on and identification of gaps in care for members and former members, their families, and their communities. The Phase 1 report was completed in March 2010 and delivered to the Department of Defense (DOD), the Department of Veterans Affairs (VA), and the relevant committees of the House of Representatives and the

[1]Operation Enduring Freedom (OEF) is the name for the war in Afghanistan. Operation Iraqi Freedom (OIF) is the name of the conflict in Iraq that began on March 20, 2003, and ended on December 15, 2011. On September 1, 2010, Operation New Dawn (OND) became the new name of OIF. The committee's focus has been on OEF and OIF, inasmuch as no or few data on the OND deployed were available.

Senate. The secretaries of DOD and VA responded to the Phase 1 report in September 2010. The present report fulfills the requirement for Phase 2.

## COMMITTEE'S APPROACH TO ITS TASK

IOM appointed a committee of 29 experts to carry out the Phase 2 study. The committee approached its task by identifying and reviewing data in the peer-reviewed literature; reviewing government reports and testimony before Congress; reviewing recent IOM reports on posttraumatic stress disorder (PTSD), traumatic brain injury (TBI), and physiologic, psychologic, and psychosocial effects of deployment-related stress; obtaining information directly from DOD and VA; and inviting DOD and VA researchers and officials to present data. The committee also sought input from community leaders to determine effects at the community level; it conducted data analyses and examined data in administrative datasets. Those data-gathering efforts provided the committee with a broad overview of possible readjustment needs and possible solutions related to the effects of deployment in OEF and OIF. Chapter 2 describes in detail the committee's approach to its task.

## KEY FINDINGS

The readjustment needs of service members, veterans, and families that have experienced deployment to OEF or OIF encompass a complex set of health, economic, and social issues. Below are the committee's key findings, which to a large extent are the focus of its recommendations.

- Many veterans return from deployment relatively unscathed by their experience, but others return from deployment with a multitude of complex health outcomes that present life-long challenges and hinder readjustment.
- Not all veterans who need treatment receive it despite the offering of evidence-based treatments by the VA and DOD health systems, because systemwide challenges exist.
- Military families often endure the adverse consequences of deployments, for example, health effects, family violence, and economic burdens.
- Numerous programs exist to respond to the needs of returning OEF and OIF active-duty personnel, veterans, and family members, but there is little evidence regarding their effectiveness.
- Unemployment and underemployment are acute problems for military veterans.
- Published data on the effects of deployment on military communities are sparse.
- DOD, VA, and other federal agencies have data that can answer many of the questions posed in the legislation; however, numerous barriers must be overcome to facilitate sharing and linking of data.

The federal government, in particular DOD and VA, is actively seeking to understand the scope of readjustment challenges, implement appropriate policies, and provide programs and services. In many cases, however, the response does not match the magnitude of the problems, and many readjustment needs are unmet or unknown. The urgency of addressing those issues is heightened by the sheer number of people affected, the rapid drawdown of personnel from Afghanistan and Iraq, and the long-term effects that many of the issues might have not only on military personnel and veterans and their families but on the country as a whole. Previous wars have demonstrated that veterans' needs peak several decades after the war in which they served, and that highlights the need for managing current problems and planning future resources.

## RECOMMENDATIONS

To inform its work during the second phase of its study, the committee read the literature, collected data and attempted data analyses, oversaw ethnographic research, and tabulated current research in the OEF and OIF populations. The committee's recommendations are presented below.

## OUTCOMES

The literature on the outcomes of military deployment has grown dramatically over the last two decades. Although discrepant findings do emerge, there is a clear consensus in the literature that the stressors of deployment, from exposure to combat to multiple deployments away from home and family, can lead to a number of adverse conditions. The committee concentrated on deployment-related outcomes—such as TBI, PTSD, depression, substance use, and suicidal ideation—but the list could be expanded to many additional psychiatric conditions and a host of physical conditions. The data on short-term outcomes (outcomes in 6 months or less) is extensive, but data on long-term outcomes (over years) is less extensive and both can be challenged on methodologic grounds. To capture the true long-term outcomes of deployment to war zones and plan services to address them, more data will be essential.

**The committee recommends that the Department of Defense and the Department of Veterans Affairs sponsor longitudinal studies to answer many of the questions regarding long-term effects of traumatic brain injury, posttraumatic stress disorder, and other mental-health disorders. Such studies should strive to improve the validity of exposure measurements, identification and use of biomarkers, and recruitment and retention of subjects. Attention should be paid to whether the outcomes of traumatic brain injuries depend on the severity and number of such injuries, on the presence of comorbid conditions, and on sex and ethnicity.**

Current studies might be the most appropriate platform for developing a strategy for long-term followup, such as the Millennium Cohort Study and the Longitudinal Health Study of Gulf War Era Veterans. Those studies can be augmented with supplementary samples of OEF, OIF, and OND veterans. Other factors that should define such studies include the ability to collect biologic specimens, oversampling of OEF, OIF, and OND female and minority-group populations, and planning for add-on studies to address new needs as they are identified.

Many health consequences of service in OEF, OIF, and OND are related to the inherently dangerous nature of the wartime environment or resulting trauma. However, one major exposure, military sexual trauma (MST), is unrelated to war but rather is due to noncombat violent assault. Studies show that MST has been occurring at high rates in the US military, including during OEF, OIF, and OND. Research demonstrates that MST is associated with poor readjustment and adverse mental-health and physical outcomes. The burden of physical- and mental-health consequences for the victims and their family members is high. Increased efforts by DOD are necessary, and a zero-tolerance approach should be implemented.

**The committee recommends that the Department of Defense develop policies to eliminate military sexual trauma as research demonstrates that it is associated with poor readjustment and mental-health and physical-health outcomes. The committee further recommends that the department reinforce existing policies on military sexual trauma by adding specific mandatory evaluation criteria regarding how well military leaders address the issue, for example, in the formal performance-appraisal and promotion systems.**

The breadth and depth of the challenges faced by military service members and veterans who served in Iraq and Afghanistan result from the complex interaction of issues that must be addressed by primary prevention, diagnostics, treatment, rehabilitation, education and outreach, and community support programs if readjustment after combat service is to be successful.

## TREATMENT

Screening, assessment, and treatment approaches for brain injuries and psychologic health problems are not always implemented between and within DOD and VA in a consistent manner or aligned with the evidence base. DOD and VA use different thresholds for some of the same mental-health screening and assessment instruments, such as the Primary-Care PTSD screen and the PTSD Checklist for PTSD and the Patient Health Questionnaire for depression. Parts of VA and DOD clinical guidance lack recommendations for a specific assessment instrument and leave the selection of instrument to the clinician, for example, for suicide-risk assessments and TBI neurocognitive assessments.

The committee identified topics on which VA and DOD policies are out of step with the evidence base. There is a lack of clear scientific evidence supporting the effectiveness of the neurocognitive assessment tool (Automated Neuropsychological Assessment Metrics) used by DOD to assess cognitive function after a head injury. With respect to suicide prevention, DOD policy prohibits restricting access to privately owned weapons for those who might be at risk for suicide, but research shows that restricting access to lethal means prevents suicides. VA has included Acceptance and Commitment Therapy for depression in its national rollout of evidenced-based treatments; however, there is not sufficient evidence to support its use as a first-line intervention. Moreover, the limited data that are available suggest that patients in need of evidence-based care might not be receiving it. The committee has serious concerns about inadequate and untimely clinical followup and low rates of delivery of evidence-based treatments, particularly psychotherapies to treat PTSD and depression and approved pharmacotherapies for substance use disorder.

**The committee recommends that the Department of Defense and the Department of Veterans Affairs select instruments and their thresholds for mental health screening and assessment in a standardized way on the basis of the best available evidence. The committee also recommends that the two departments ensure that treatment offerings are aligned with the evidence base, particularly before national rollouts, and that all patients consistently receive first-line treatments as indicated.**

Unwarranted variability in clinical practices and deviations from the evidence base present threats to high-quality patient care. Such variability also hampers opportunities to make research comparisons that can inform and improve the effectiveness of screening, assessment, and treatment practices. The committee notes that the emphasis on promoting evidence-based practices should not discourage the use of new or experimental interventions where there is reason to believe that they might lead to better outcomes than standard interventions.

In many ways, DOD and VA clinicians are at the forefront of providing evidence-based care for service members and veterans who have brain injuries and psychologic-health problems. But there are opportunities to improve processes of training and evaluating clinicians. DOD does not have a standardized process for assessing clinicians' competence to administer the Military Acute Concussion Evaluation for TBI. VA is implementing a robust clinician-training program to disseminate evidence-based psychotherapies, but the program appears to lack periodic clinician assessments beyond the 6-month training period to ensure that continued treatment fidelity is maintained. Current approaches for training clinicians on the management of comorbid conditions (by disseminating clinician resources, for example) are not adequate.

**The committee recommends that the Department of Defense and the Department of Veterans Affairs incorporate continuing supervision and education into programs that train clinicians in the use of selected assessment instruments and evidence-based treatments. Once clinicians are trained, the two departments should systematically and periodically evaluate them to assess the degree to which therapeutic interventions are accurately implemented according to a manual, protocol, or model as supported by evidence. The committee also recommends that the two departments place greater focus on coordinated, interdisciplinary care to ensure optimal treatment for service members and veterans.**

The committee determined that there are few data on whether screening, assessment, and treatment interventions in DOD and VA are being implemented according to clinical guidelines and VA and DOD policy. Minimal data are readily available on the numbers of people who have been screened and the extent to which followup is appropriate and timely for those who screen positive. There is a dearth of data on which treatments patients receive and whether the treatments were appropriate, timely, and delivered at the recommended intensity level (for example, individual vs group format and frequency and duration of sessions).

**The committee recommends that the Department of Defense and the Department of Veterans Affairs conduct systematic assessments to determine whether screening and treatment interventions are being implemented according to clinical guidelines and department policy. Data systems should be developed to assess treatment outcomes, variations among treatment facilities, and barriers to the use of evidence-based treatment.**

## MILITARY FAMILIES

The committee found that DOD has many programs and policies to support families. However, DOD policies, programs, and practices typically do not take into consideration the full spectrum of military families. By focusing almost exclusively on traditional families (married heterosexual spouses and their children), DOD is missing critical opportunities to support the readjustment needs of many service members' nontraditional families. To be able to support all families, DOD will need data on the full constellation of service members' family.

**The committee recommends that the Department of Defense ensure that policies, programs, and practices aim to support and strengthen all military families, including nontraditional ones.**

Healthy families help service members to do their jobs effectively and readjust after deployment. The demands placed on military family members call for support in the areas of relationship building, family and individual function, and reduction of risk of psychologic and physical-health problems. The committee found that little information is available on the potential effectiveness of broad-based, universal prevention efforts aimed at military children and their families. In addition, most treatment interventions for family members have been developed and tested in civilian communities and lack evidence of their effectiveness for military families. The committee concludes that military families would benefit from increased efforts to identify, develop, and test new prevention and treatment interventions targeted toward military families, including interventions directed at children and adolescents.

**The committee recommends that the Department of Defense use evidence-based primary prevention programs and treatments that have been specifically evaluated in service members and their families and that are focused on preventing and treating mental-health and relationship problems.**

The committee concludes that there are substantial gaps in knowledge about the effects of deployment on military families that hinder DOD's ability to meet the needs of military service members and their families effectively. The committee found that—although some important large-scale, well-designed studies are under way—much of the research heretofore has been methodologically flawed, suffering, for example, from the use of small convenience samples, use of cross-sectional designs, and the like. The committee concludes that well-designed studies that use rigorous and diverse methods (both qualitative and quantitative) are needed to increase understanding of the challenges faced by military service members and their families.

**The committee recommends that the Department of Defense and other relevant federal agencies fund methodologically rigorous research on the social,**

**psychologic, and economic effects of deployments on families, including nontraditional families.**

Studies of families of service members deployed to OEF and OIF have documented a rise in domestic violence (typically including abuse of spouses or neglect of children). In the FY 2000 National Defense Authorization Act (PL 106-65, Section 591), Congress directed the secretary of defense to establish a Defense Task Force on Domestic Violence to make recommendations for reducing the prevalence of domestic violence in military families. The task force submitted a report in 2003 that identified multiple shortcomings in the current systems and recommended many improvements. The Government Accountability Office, in 2006 and 2010, issued reports concerning progress in implementing the nearly 200 recommendations made by the task force. Both reports described progress on some recommendations but little on others, including a recommendation for reliable documentation of violent events.

**The committee recommends that the Department of Defense place high priority on reducing domestic violence because it degrades force readiness and the well-being of military family members.**

## COMMUNITY

There has been too little research on community effects of deployments to OEF and OIF. To supplement the published research, the committee completed ethnographic assessments in six communities that are near large military installations or that have recently deployed National Guard populations. Those efforts provided some insight, but the lack of communitywide assessments of the effects of OEF and OIF deployments on communities made it difficult to respond to this aspect of the committee's charge.

**The committee recommends that the Department of Defense, the Department of Veterans Affairs, and other relevant federal agencies fund research on the effects of Operation Enduring Freedom and Operation Iraqi Freedom deployments on communities. Such research should include current indicators of community well-being, such as measures of economic performance, availability of social and support services, law-enforcement activity, and school and educational functioning.**

Relevant data are available, but data linkages are needed to allow specific analyses that can more clearly illuminate opportunities to mitigate potential adverse community consequences after service members deploy, return, and separate.

## SOCIOECONOMIC IMPACTS

Problems of unemployment and underemployment, which are broadly felt by the US civilian population today, appear to be more acute for veterans of the post-9/11 era, particularly young veterans. In 2011, the unemployment rate among all post-9/11 veterans 18 years old and older was more than one-third higher than that among equivalent nonveterans—12.1% compared with 8.7%. Among veterans 18–24 years old, the rate was almost twice as high—30.2% compared with 16.1%. The sources of those disparities remain unclear and could include skills mismatch, impeded ability to maintain or obtain employment because of physical- or mental-health trauma, stigma or discrimination, or some combination of those factors or other elements. Successful readjustment depends on reentry into the civilian workforce, and the available evidence suggests that this is an important gap for policy to address. The committee found that the literature assessing the effectiveness of DOD's and VA's transition-assistance programs is relatively thin, even though reentry into the labor force is one of the most important readjustment challenges. One study suggests that recent expansions of hiring tax credits might have been effective in raising rates of employment of older veterans who have disabilities. But OEF, OIF, and OND veterans did not appear to benefit from the expansions.

**The committee recommends that the Department of Defense and the Department of Veterans Affairs evaluate the effectiveness of transition-assistance programs to ensure that they are effective in reducing unemployment among returning veterans of Operation Enduring Freedom, Operation Iraqi Freedom, and Operation New Dawn.**

Evaluation of the effectiveness of transition-assistance programs, with research that examines employment patterns after separation from the military over time, will provide data to ensure that scarce resources can be allocated to effective programs. Further study might focus on whether employment tax credits are a cost-effective means of expanding employment for Operation Enduring Freedom and Operation Iraqi Freedom veterans and whether programs to counsel and prepare service members for long-term postservice careers are effectively implemented.

The Post-9/11 GI Bill is one of the largest expansions of educational subsidies to veterans and their families on record, but its effectiveness is difficult to gauge. The committee is aware of no studies that have explicitly evaluated the effects of deployment to OEF and OIF on the use of the Post-9/11 GI Bill or the effects of the Post-9/11 GI Bill.

**The committee recommends a comprehensive evaluation of the effects of the Post-9/11 GI Bill on the educational attainment of veterans and eligible family members.**

The committee views the current evidence on the costs of caring for injured veterans as an overwhelming challenge. There is a need to assess the costs of caring for injured veterans systematically and publicly. The Congressional Budget Office publicly assesses short-term and medium-term costs, and, as the VA stated in response to the committee's Phase 1 report, it already produces some forecasts of health and disability spending. But the committee continues to believe that long-term planning for veterans' care requires public long-term cost forecasts in the same way that Social Security and Medicare require them, and these forecasts should take a similar form to be internally and externally useful.

**The committee reiterates its call for comprehensive long-term forecasts of the costs of the Veterans Health Administration's medical care and the Veterans Benefits Administration's disability benefits associated with combat deployments; these forecasts should be conducted annually and should be released publicly by the Department of Veterans Affairs and confirmed by an independent external authority.**

## ACCESS AND BARRIERS TO CARE

Transitioning from the DOD health care system to the VA health care system presents challenges for OEF and OIF service men and women. There are numerous difficulties in navigating services because of the complexities of both systems. Although DOD and VA are making administrative changes to alleviate some of the problems, information sharing between the two agencies remains a problem.

**The committee recommends improved coordination of care and services between the Department of Defense and the Department of Veterans Affairs medical treatment facilities, including the completion of an interoperable or single combined electronic health record for all care that begins with entry into military service and continues throughout care in the Department of Veterans Affairs system after transition.**

Stigma is still a problem for military personnel in care or seeking care for mental-health or substance-abuse problems. Active-duty military fear that visits to a mental-health provider will jeopardize their careers because of the military's long-standing policy of reporting mental-health and substance-abuse problems to the chain of command. Mixed messages about seeking treatment and concerns about health-information privacy remain disincentives to seeking care.

**The committee recommends that the Department of Defense continue to promote an environment that reduces stigma and encourages treatment for mental-health and substance-use disorders. The committee recommends that the department undertake a systematic review of its policies regarding mental-health and substance-abuse treatment with regard to issues of confidentiality and the relation between treatment-seeking and military advancement. The committee recommends that the department regularly issue reports describing actions taken with regard to its policies and procedures to determine progress in this area.**

Excessive wait time is a complaint often expressed by both active-duty and veteran service members. Long wait times can compromise health because of delayed use and decreased patient satisfaction. In addition, adverse long-term outcomes, such as death and preventable hospitalizations, are more common for veterans who seek care at facilities that have longer wait times than for veterans at facilities that have shorter wait times.

Poor availability and misdistribution of mental-health specialists in many parts of the United States, especially in rural areas, present substantial barriers to OEF and OIF veterans' access to mental-health care. For active-duty service members, inadequate participating provider networks present a challenge for accessing mental-health care.

**The committee recommends that the Department of Defense and the Department of Veterans Affairs conduct a needs assessment to determine the numbers and types of providers needed to address the long-term health needs of Operation Enduring Freedom, Operation Iraqi Freedom, and Operation New Dawn active-duty service members and veterans. The Department of Defense and the Department of Veterans Affairs should determine the optimal team composition—for example, MDs, PhDs, RNs, master's-trained professionals, and peer counselors—needed to ensure that providers function efficiently and perform at the upper level of their credentials and privileges.**

There is evidence of cultural insensitivity to nonwhite service members, who might have different or more severe physical-health and mental-health problems from their white counterparts. For example, black personnel are less likely than white personnel to use mental-health services and quicker to drop out of treatment. Issues related to types of diagnoses and potential misdiagnoses have also been raised. Whether clinicians who have ethnic characteristics similar to those of their patients would alleviate those problems is unknown.

**The committee recommends that the Department of Defense, the Department of Veterans Affairs, and other federal agencies fund research to determine whether culturally sensitive clinicians and treatment approaches improve retention in care and improve clinical outcomes.**

Women now constitute 14% of deployed forces in the US military, and an unprecedented number of female soldiers are deployed to combat areas. Although all service members are exposed to high levels of workplace stress, women in the military face some unique stressors, such as MST, which may affect their mental health and emotional well-being. Female veterans report a higher burden of medical illness and worse quality-of-life outcomes than do men who are exposed to the same levels of trauma. MST appears to be an important risk factor for the development of PTSD.

**The committee recommends that the Department of Defense and the Department of Veterans Affairs consider ways to remove barriers and improve women's access to and use of health care in their systems. The two departments should examine issues related to women's circumstances and stressors—such as military workplace stress, sexual harassment and assault, posttraumatic stress disorder, and premilitary trauma—in an effort to reduce disparities and to provide health care that is sensitive to their needs and preferences.**

## PROPOSED DATA ANALYSES

There has been little quantitative characterization of the issues described in the legislation, but the committee identified a wide array of data and databases available in DOD, VA, and other federal agencies that could be used to address many of the questions posed by the legislation that motivated its work. On the basis of available data, the committee developed a comprehensive data-analysis plan. The committee notes that in addition to its recommendation for comprehensive data analyses, privacy experts will need to be involved with data owners before data are linked and made accessible to researchers. The committee believes that privacy and confidentiality are essential alongside issues of coordination and synchronization of data sources.

**The committee recommends that the Department of Defense and the Department of Veterans Affairs support comprehensive analyses of relevant data that reside in the two departments and other agencies of the federal government. Their databases should be linked and integrated so that they can be used effectively to address questions regarding readjustment that are not answered in the peer-reviewed literature.**

The committee's preliminary work in this area has provided a clear rationale, justification, and roadmap for comprehensive data analyses. Comprehensive data analyses will require establishment of systematic, timely processes for using available government data and linking them in such a way as to improve the characterization of issues of interest. No databases or files fully integrate basic deployment and demographic data with data on health outcomes, treatment or transition-of-care files, data on access to care, records of employment before and after deployment, and data on other processes and outcomes. A comprehensive analytic database will have to be created and maintained.

**The committee recommends that the secretary of defense and the secretary of veterans affairs establish an interagency work group to identify and examine the feasibility of linking data that exist in Executive Branch departments and agencies throughout the federal government. The work group should be tasked to explore issues related to coordination among agencies, for example, defining common goals, establishing common policies and procedures, creating mechanisms for data sharing, establishing records systems, and overcoming legal impediments and meeting legal requirements. The work group should provide the secretaries with options and recommendations for establishment of a sustainable program for long-term cooperation and data sharing to improve understanding of the outcomes of military service and readjustment after combat deployment.**

The committee believes that many of the issues examined in this study can be addressed through analyses of data already maintained by numerous federal agencies. The committee tried to gain access to the data files so that it could begin such analyses, but it faced numerous obstacles in its attempts to access them. In light of those difficulties, the committee recommends the following actions to address many of the problems that it faced.

**The committee recommends that clear procedures be developed for accessing data held by the Department of Defense, the Department of Veterans Affairs, and other federal agencies. The procedures should appear on each agency's website with access to its data dictionaries. That would enable researchers and others wishing to access data to understand all the requirements before they begin their data-gathering efforts and would provide information about the types of data that are available and how to access them.**

The questions posed to the committee are complex and critical to the well-being of US veterans, their families, and the communities in which they live. A major finding of the committee is that there is no way to provide data-based answers to those questions. All agencies that collect, store, and manage information relevant to veterans and their families should give high priority to coordination of those efforts throughout the federal statistical system so that informed decisions about veterans' readjustment needs can be made in the near future.

The committee believes that such coordination will greatly enhance the ability of researchers and the government to link data held by multiple agencies to allow the types of analyses recommended above.

# 1

# INTRODUCTION

The wars in Afghanistan and Iraq have been the longest sustained US military operations since the Vietnam War, although the war in Iraq formally ended on December 15, 2011. As of December 2012, Operation Enduring Freedom (OEF) in Afghanistan and Operation Iraqi Freedom (OIF) in Iraq have resulted in deployment of about 2.2 million troops; there have been 2,222 US fatalities in OEF and Operation New Dawn (OND)[1] and 4,422 in OIF. The numbers of wounded US troops exceed 16,000 in Afghanistan and 32,000 in Iraq (DOD, 2012). In addition to deaths and morbidity, the operations have unforeseen consequences for military personnel that are yet to be fully understood.

In contrast with previous conflicts, the all-volunteer military has experienced numerous deployments of individual service members; has seen increased deployments of women, parents of young children, and reserve and National Guard troops; and in some cases has been subject to longer deployments and shorter times at home between deployments. Numerous reports in the popular press have made the public aware of issues that have pointed to the difficulty of military personnel in readjusting after returning from Iraq and Afghanistan. Many of those who have served in OEF and OIF readjust with few difficulties, but others have problems in readjusting to home, reconnecting with family members, finding employment, and returning to school. A recent study by the Pew Research Center (2011) notes that veterans who have major injuries resulting from their service are more than twice as likely as their noninjured counterparts to say that they have had difficulties in readjusting to civilian life. Lingering health problems related to injuries that were sustained overseas probably contribute to those readjustment difficulties. Combat-related traumatic brain injury (TBI) and posttraumatic stress disorder (PTSD) and their potential long-term consequences also hinder readjustment.

Although the vast majority of OEF and OIF veterans believe that their military service was rewarding and had favorable outcomes (such as learning how to work with others and building self-confidence), 44% report readjustment difficulties, 48% strains on family life, 47% outbursts of anger, 49% posttraumatic stress, and 32% an occasional loss of interest in daily activities (Pew Research Center, 2011).

---

[1]Operation Enduring Freedom (OEF) is the name for the war in Afghanistan. Operation Iraqi Freedom (OIF) is the name of the conflict in Iraq that began on March 20, 2003, and ended on December 15, 2011. On September 1, 2010, Operation New Dawn (OND) became the new name of OIF (Secretary of Defense Memorandum, February 17, 2010). The committee's focus has been on OEF and OIF, inasmuch as no or few data on the OND deployed were available.

As early as 2004, it was estimated that over one-fourth of troops returning from OEF and OIF were suffering from mental-health disorders (Hoge et al., 2004). Later estimates suggested that one-fifth of the troops reported symptoms of PTSD or depression and about the same fraction a probable TBI during deployment (Tanielian and Jaycox, 2008). Recent RAND reports note that a full one-third of returning OEF and OIF service members reported symptoms of mental-health or cognitive problems (Hosek, 2011; Tanielian and Jaycox, 2008). RAND reports that 18.5% of a representative sample of returning service members met the diagnostic criteria for PTSD or depression, 19.5% reported a probable TBI during deployment, and 7% met the criteria for a mental-health problem and TBI (Tanielian and Jaycox, 2008).

PTSD is often comorbid with depression and anxiety disorders, substance-use disorders, sleep disturbances, and increased risk of suicide. Marital problems, parenting difficulties, and family-adjustment issues have also been associated with PTSD (IOM, 2008). TBI is associated with numerous long-term outcomes, including unprovoked seizures, dementia, decline in neurocognitive function, such adverse outcomes related to social function as unemployment and diminished social relationships, and depression (IOM, 2009).

## BACKGROUND

In response to the return of large numbers of veterans from Iraq and Afghanistan with physical- and mental-health needs and to the growing readjustment needs of active-duty service members, veterans, and their family members, Congress passed Section 1661 of the National Defense Authorization Act for FY 2008 (see Appendix A). That section required the secretary of defense, in consultation with the secretary of veterans affairs, to enter into an agreement with the National Academies for a study of the physical and mental health and other readjustment needs of members and former members of the armed forces who were deployed in OIF or OEF, their families, and their communities as a result of such deployment. The study was assigned to the Institute of Medicine (IOM).

The study consisted of two phases. Phase 1 was a preliminary assessment to identify findings on the physical and mental health and other readjustment needs of and on gaps in care for the members and former members of the armed forces who were deployed in OIF or OEF and their families as described in the legislation and to provide a roadmap for Phase 2. Phase 2 was to provide a comprehensive assessment of the physical, psychologic, social, and economic effects of deployment on and identification of gaps in care for members and former members, their families, and their communities. Phase 1 was completed in March 2010, and the report on it was delivered to the Department of Defense (DOD), the Department of Veterans Affairs (VA), and the relevant committees of the House of Representatives and the Senate (IOM, 2010); Appendix B is the executive summary of the Phase 1 report. The secretaries of DOD and VA responded to the Phase 1 report in September 2010 (DOD and VA, 2010); Appendix C contains their response. The present report fulfills the requirement for Phase 2.

## STATEMENT OF TASK

The statement of task for this study evolved out of discussions among DOD, VA, and IOM. Specifically, it was determined that in Phase 1 the IOM committee would identify preliminary findings regarding the physical and mental health and other readjustment needs of members and former members of the armed forces who were deployed in OEF or OIF and their families. The committee was also tasked with determining the goals of Phase 2 of the study. The Phase 2 task was to provide a comprehensive assessment of the physical, mental, social, and economic effects of deployment and to identify gaps in care for members and former members of the armed forces who were deployed in OIF or OEF, their families, and their communities. The committee was directed to consider the following in its assessment:

- The psychologic, social, and economic effects of deployment and of multiple deployments in OEF and OIF on service members and former members and their families.
- The full scope of the neurologic, psychiatric, and psychologic effects of TBI on the members and former members of the Armed Forces and their families.
- The effects of failure to diagnose such conditions as PTSD and TBI.
- The long-term costs associated with TBI and PTSD and the efficacy of screening and treatment approaches for TBI, PTSD, and other mental-health conditions in DOD and VA.
- The sex-specific and ethnicity-specific needs and concerns of members of the armed forces and veterans.
- The particular needs and concerns of children of members of the armed forces, taking into account different age groups, effects on development and education, and mental and emotional well-being.
- The particular educational and vocational needs of members and former members of the armed forces and their families and the efficacy of existing educational and vocational programs to address such needs.
- The effects of deployments associated with OIF and OEF on communities that have high populations of military families, including military housing communities and townships that have deployed members of the National Guard and reserves, and the efficacy of programs that address community outreach and education concerning military deployments of community residents.
- The effects of increasing numbers of older and married members of the armed forces on readjustment requirements.
- Recommendations, based on such assessments, for programs, treatments, or policy remedies targeted at preventing, minimizing, or addressing the effects, gaps, and needs identified.
- Recommendations, as appropriate, for additional research on such needs.

## COMMITTEE'S APPROACH TO ITS TASK

IOM appointed a committee of 29 experts to carry out the Phase 2 study. The committee members have expertise in sociology, psychiatry, rehabilitation, neurology, economics, epidemiology, survey research, statistics, and health policy and management. A number of them also have knowledge of the workings of DOD and VA, and some are former active-duty military members. The committee divided itself into several work groups to focus on specific elements of its task: health outcomes, treatment, community effects, family issues, economics, access and barriers to care, and methods.

The committee's approach to gathering information included identifying and reviewing data in the peer-reviewed literature; reviewing government reports and testimony before

Congress; reviewing recent IOM reports on PTSD, TBI, and physiologic, psychologic, and psychosocial effects of deployment-related stress; gathering information directly from DOD and VA; and inviting DOD and VA researchers and officials to present data. The committee also sought input from community leaders to determine effects at the community level, conducted limited descriptive data analyses, and examined data in preexisting administrative datasets.[2] Those data-gathering efforts provided the committee with a broad overview of possible readjustment needs and possible solutions related to the effects of deployment in OEF and OIF. Chapter 2 describes in more detail the committee's approach to its task.

In its attempts to understand readjustment needs, the committee conducted extensive searches of the peer-reviewed literature and considered about 3,000 articles (see Chapter 2). It also relied on the gray literature, for example, publications produced by government, business, and industry; conference proceedings; and abstracts presented at conferences. Specifically, the committee members reviewed numerous reports of the Government Accountability Office, the Congressional Budget Office, the inspectors general of VA and DOD, and the Congressional Research Service.

The committee examined the basic demographic data that the Defense Manpower Data Center provided on active-duty forces, the reserve components of the military, and the National Guard, such as numbers of troops deployed, numbers of deployments, marital status, sex, and ethnicity (see Chapter 3). Those data gave the committee a basic understanding of the demographic characteristics of the deployed.

The committee conducted a review of ongoing federal research efforts (Appendix D) in the areas of concern to the committee (as outlined in the legislation) to identify gaps in research. Under subcontract with Westat (a research corporation that consults on statistical design, data collection and management, and analysis), the committee conducted ethnographic research in communities affected by deployments (see Chapters 2 and 7 and Appendix E). Westat sponsored focus-group meetings with community leaders to determine the effects of returning troops on the community and to examine the effects of deployments and redeployments of reserve and National Guard units on the community. The ethnographic research provided the committee with qualitative information about short-term and long-term effects of deployments on communities.

Finally, on the basis of the legislation and the committee's discussions, its members decided to focus their findings on readjustment needs and gaps related to the conditions that are most frequently diagnosed in returning OEF and OIF active-duty personnel and veterans, such as TBI, PTSD, and other mental-health conditions, including depression, substance-use disorders, and suicidal ideation.

## ORGANIZATION OF THE REPORT

This report is organized into 10 chapters and 6 appendixes. Chapter 2 describes the committee's methods for gathering information, including its literature-search strategy and its ethnographic research. Chapter 3 provides information on the characteristics of the deployed and the nature of deployments on the basis of an analysis of the data that the committee obtained.

---

[2]Administrative data collection is the set of activities involved in the collection, processing, storage, and dissemination of statistical data from one or more administrative sources; the source of data is administrative records rather than direct contact with respondents (http://stats.oecd.org/glossary/detail.asp?ID=6; accessed June 18, 2012).

Chapter 4 summarizes long-term outcomes related to TBI, PTSD, and other mental-health conditions. Chapter 5 examines the efficacy of approaches to screening for, assessment of, and treatment for TBI, PSTD, depression, substance-use disorder, suicidal ideation, and comorbid conditions. The committee reviews the clinical-practice guidelines for those conditions and reviews the scientific literature to identify current evidence-based practices. The chapter also discusses the implementation of evidence-based practices for those conditions and identifies available data for assessing quality of care. Chapter 6 explores the effects of deployment on the emotional, mental, and social well-being of family members and identifies the readjustment needs of family members (including spouses, children, and caregivers); it also discusses the availability and use of services for families. Chapter 7 addresses the effects of such deployments on communities on the basis of the literature search and rapid ethnographic assessments of selected communities. Chapter 8 examines the social and economic effects of OEF and OIF deployments on active-duty personnel, veterans, and their family members. Chapter 9 continues the discussion of treatment, focusing on access and barriers to care. Finally, Chapter 10 describes the comprehensive data analyses that the committee believes should be carried out to address unanswered questions about readjustment needs. Chapters 4 through 10 contain the committee's recommendations as well as providing areas for future research. The committee did not prioritize the areas for future research as it hopes that the responsible agencies will carefully consider all the future research directions. This report contains several appendixes that are included in the CD inside the back cover of the report:

- Appendix A—legislation outlining the committee's tasks.
- Appendix B—the executive summary of the Phase 1 report.
- Appendix C—the VA and DOD secretaries' response to the Phase 1 report.
- Appendix D—summary of federal research on OEF and OIF.
- Appendix E—individual ethnographic assessments.
- Appendix F—database descriptions.

## REFERENCES

DOD (Department of Defense). 2012. *OEF/OIF/OND Casualty Status.* http://www.defense.gov/news/casualty.pdf (accessed July 30, 2012).

DOD and VA (Department of Veterans Affairs). 2010. *Report to Congress Section 1661, NDAA FY2008, Phase 1 Supporting Adjustment and Readjustment of Active Military, Veterans, and Family Members: IOM's March 31, 2010 Returning Home from Iraq and Afghanistan: Preliminary Assessment of Readjustment Needs of Veterans, Service Members, and Their Families.* Washington, DC: Department of Defense and Department of Veterans Affairs.

Hoge, C. W., C. A. Castro, S. C. Messer, D. McGurk, D. I. Cotting, and R. L. Koffman. 2004. Combat duty in Iraq and Afghanistan, mental health problems, and barriers to care. *New England Journal of Medicine* 351(1):13-22.

Hosek, J. 2011. *How Is Deployment to Iraq and Afghanistan Affecting US Service Members and Their Families? An Overview of Early RAND Research on the Topic.* Santa Monica, CA: RAND Corporation.

IOM (Institute of Medicine). 2008. *Gulf War and Health, Volume 6: Physiologic, Psychologic, and Psychosocial Effects of Deployment-Related Stress.* Washington, DC: The National Academies Press.

———. 2009. *Gulf War and Health, Volume 7: Long-Term Consequences of Traumatic Brain Injury*. Washington, DC: The National Academies Press.

———. 2010. *Returning Home from Iraq and Afghanistan: Preliminary Assessment of Readjustment Needs of Veterans, Service Members, and Their Families.* Washington, DC: The National Academies Press.

Pew Research Center. 2011. *The Military-Civilian Gap: War and Sacrifice in the Post-9/11 Era.* Washington, DC: Pew Social and Demographic Trends.

Tanielian, T., and L. H. Jaycox. 2008. *Invisible Wounds of War: Psychological and Cognitive Injuries, Their Consequences, and Services to Assist Recovery*. Santa Monica, CA: RAND Corporation.

# 2

# METHODS

This chapter provides an overview of the committee's data-gathering efforts. The committee approached its task by organizing itself into work groups. Each group consisted of four or five members who had expertise in a particular topic, such as family, treatment, outcomes, economics, community, access and barriers to care, and methods. The methods group supervised the limited descriptive data analyses that the committee conducted to ensure uniformity in definitions and approach.

First, the committee directed the overall search of the literature. In an effort to stay current, searches were updated three times over the course of the Phase 2 study period. The literature was provided to the committee members, who read the articles and summarized them for the report. The literature focused primarily on Operation Iraqi Freedom (OIF) and Operation Enduring Freedom (OEF) populations—and Operation New Dawn (OND) as available—but if the literature was sparse or nonexistent, the committee members included studies of other military or civilian populations. Second, the committee inventoried current federal research efforts (Appendix D) in the areas of concern to the committee (as outlined in the legislation) to identify research gaps and to recommend additional research to address them. Chapters 4–9 provide research recommendations, under the heading of Future Research Directions, based on the lack of literature or gaps in funded research, which federal agencies should consider as a way of improving knowledge about readjustment problems. Third, in an effort to understand the characteristics of the all-volunteer military force deployed in support of OEF and OIF, the committee requested data from the Department of Defense (DOD) Defense Manpower Data Center (DMDC). Those data were examined and frequencies or counts of the variables of interest were tabulated so that the committee could have an appreciation of the characteristics of the people deployed (Chapter 3). Fourth, the committee explored other methods of supplementing information on subjects on which the literature was sparse, such as overseeing rapid ethnographic assessments of communities that might have been affected by deployments and repeat deployments (Chapter 7 and Appendix E).

## LITERATURE REVIEW

The committee began its work by overseeing extensive searches of the peer-reviewed medical and scientific literature, including published articles, other peer-reviewed reports, government reports, congressional testimony, and dissertations. The searches retrieved over 7,000 potentially useful studies, and their titles and abstracts were reviewed. The committee focused its attention on studies of OEF and OIF populations and their families. Overall, the committee decided to not use comparisons to civilian populations because military members are likely to differ from civilians in both observable and unobservable dimensions (the military is a highly selected population; applicants meet a range of eligibility criteria and have a desire to take on the duties of military service). To the extent that these differences may themselves be associated with an outcome, direct comparisons between military and civilian populations will be misleading. That said, some civilian studies are included where they are useful for interpreting key findings in the military data. For example, military divorce rates are discussed in the context of civilian divorce rates in the family chapter (see Chapter 6).

The review excluded case reports, case series that involved few participants, and studies of acute outcomes that resolved themselves within days to a few months for the outcomes chapter. After its assessment of the titles and abstracts, the committee members identified about 3,000 studies for further review. The committee conducted three major searches over the Phase 2 study period (in August 2010, May 2011, and February 2012) with MEDLINE and PsycINFO. It also searched the National Technical Information Service database for various government reports, such as those of the Government Accountability Office, the Congressional Budget Office, and the Office of Management and Budget; for congressional testimony; and for annual reports to Congress from DOD and the Department of Veterans Affairs (VA) on issues related to OEF and OIF. In addition to those overall searches, the staff and committee members conducted numerous smaller searches on topics related to the task. All searches were entered into the committee's EndNote database, and titles, abstracts, and papers were made available for the committee members' review.

All searches were run against MEDLINE and PsycINFO by using the OvidSP platform. Results were limited to the English language and articles published from 2000 to the present. All result sets were de-duplicated to eliminate occurrence of the same reference two or more times in the two databases, and all results were exported to an EndNote library.

The strategy for the searches was to establish a "base set" that identified OEF and OIF populations of interest: troops on active duty in the military, National Guard troops, reservists, and veterans; and families, spouses, relatives, and caregivers associated with veterans or with those on active duty. That base set was then combined with four broad categories of terms grouped according to issues of concern to or affecting returning veterans, such as reintegration, debt, and unemployment; programs and resources, such as education, employment, and loan-repayment programs; health outcomes, such as traumatic brain injury, depression, and substance use; and additional health care, social, and psychosocial issues.

## GAP ANALYSIS

The committee directed Institute of Medicine (IOM) staff to assemble a table that would include a list of current federally funded research in the subjects of concern to its task, specifically, studies related to OEF, OIF, and OND service members, veterans, and families (see Appendix D). Searches used the following databases and Web sites: National Institutes of Health (NIH) RePORT (NIH Research Portfolio Online Reporting Tools), a portfolio of NIH research activities; ClinicalTrials.gov, an NIH registry and results database of clinical studies; Congressionally Directed Medical Research Programs, which emphasizes subcategories of Defense Women's Health Research and Deployment Related Medical Research; and VA Health

Services Research & Development Service (HSR&D) and Quality Enhancement Research Initiative (QUERI) projects.

Those sources were first searched in May and June 2010, and a final update was conducted in September 2012. The committee also received updates on the research being conducted by the RAND Corporation (personal communications, Terri Tanielian and Rajeev Ramchand, June 2010 and September 2012). The table of current research was sent to VA in February 2011 and September 2012 for review of its accuracy.

The committee members carefully examined the table and in concert with its literature review conducted a gap analysis so that subjects on which research was lacking would be highlighted and future research recommended. The committee highlights future directions and makes specific research recommendations on the basis of its assessment of the literature and its review of the table of funded research (see "Future Directions" in Chapters 4-9).

## DEMOGRAPHIC ANALYSIS OF DEPLOYED PERSONNEL

Since 1974, the DMDC has maintained the largest archive of DOD data, including all branches and components (regular, reserve, National Guard, and civilian) of military personnel, on manpower, training, and financial matter. Data have been collected on over 42 million people connected to DOD who have been followed through their military careers (accession, service, separation, and retirement). The DMDC accesses, receives, and combines data from many sources, programs, databases, and personnel files—on active-duty, reserve, National Guard, and retired military personnel and contractors and civilians—and data from VA, the Social Security Administration, Medicare, and other sources to allow for reporting of entitlements, benefits, and readiness; personnel identification, validation, and authentication; and decision-support purposes. The committee has accessed and referred to the DMDC for various purposes and at various times throughout its study.

The committee wanted to understand basic information about who was deployed, and members requested and received demographic data from the DMDC on all those who were deployed anywhere in support of OEF, OIF, and OND[1] from September 11, 2001, through December 31, 2010. We received a total of 2,147,398 records, including a file of those on active duty (1,450,004), a file of those in the reserves and National Guard (697,394), and a file that contained the deployment histories of all service members in those two groups.[2] The DOD instruction files that contained the documents that we used to select the variables of interest were

- Active-duty personnel—DODI 1336.5.
- Reserve and National Guard personnel—DODI 7730.54.
- Deployment—DODI 6490.3.

The variables received from DMDC for the deployed active-duty service members and for the deployed reserve active-duty members are listed below in Table 2.1.

---

[1]OND officially began in September 2010. The committee's file ends on December 31, 2010, so it contains few records on the OND population.

[2]IOM staff produced files for committee members that were stripped of all personal identifiers so that committee members did not have access to personal information. Case numbers were assigned to each record.

**TABLE 2.1** DMDC Variables

| | |
|---|---|
| Deployed Active-Duty Variables | |
| Service | Primary service occupation |
| Component | Armed Forces Qualification Test percentile |
| Social Security number | Duty-service occupation |
| Last name | Duty-unit location, state |
| First name | Duty-unit location, country |
| Middle name | Duty-unit location, ZIP |
| Cadency | Transaction effective date |
| Date of birth | Place of birth, state |
| Sex | Place of birth, country |
| Marital status | Home of record, state |
| Race | Service deployment |
| Ethnicity | Component deployment |
| Education level | Deployment start date |
| Residence ZIP | Deployment end date |
| Spouse Social Security number | Location begin date |
| Dependents quantity | Location end date |
| Prior Social Security number | Location, country |
| Active federal military service base calendar date | Active-duty involuntary retention reason code |
| Military Accession Program source code | Pay grade |
| Enlisted career status code | Military career category code (for Army only) |
| Reserve Active-Duty Variables | |
| Service | Date of initial entry into reserve forces |
| Component | Active-duty start date |
| Reserve category code | Active-duty end date |
| Reserve subcategory | Pay grade |
| Social Security number | Active federal military service months quantity |
| Social Security number verification | Service occupation |
| Last name | Armed Forces Qualification Test percentile |
| First name | Duty-service occupation |
| Middle name | Separation incentive benefits and/or pay indicator |
| Cadency | Assigned unit, state |
| Date of birth | Assigned unit, country |
| Sex | Assigned unit, ZIP |
| Marital status | Reserve service bonus incentive type code |
| Race | Reserve service education incentive type code |
| Ethnicity | Service deployment |
| Education level | Component deployment |
| Home mailing state | Deployment start date |
| Home mailing ZIP | Deployment end date |

| | |
|---|---|
| Spouse Social Security number | Location begin date |
| Dependents quantity | Location end date |
| Date of initial entry into uniformed service | Location, country |

The deployment data provided with those two files were for the most recent deployment identified at the time of the file creation. They did not provide the complete deployment history. Therefore, a later file of all deployments with the following data elements was requested: Social Security number, date of birth, deployment start date, deployment end date, location begin date, location end date, and location country. The deployments provided by the DMDC included all deployments to any location considered by DOD to be in support of OIF, OEF, or the Global War on Terror. Each deployment start and end date identified a unique deployment episode that was counted as one deployment.

By using those data, the committee was able to understand some characteristics of the all-volunteer military force that served in support of OEF and OIF during that period. The details of the demographic characteristics are presented in the discussion, tables, and figures in Chapter 3. The following paragraphs describe how the variables selected for use in Chapter 3 were coded.

*Branch of service.* The standard service codes were used: Army, Air Force, Coast Guard, Marine Corps, and Navy.

*Component.* The three components used were regular (active), National Guard, and reserves, although for some analyses the National Guard and reserves were described together as the reserve components. For several analyses, branch and component were crossed as follows: regular and reserves (all five services) and Army and Air Force National Guard.

*Pay grade.* On the basis of the pay-grade or pay-rate variables, pay grades ranged from E1 to E9 for enlisted personnel, from O1 to O10 for commissioned officers, and from W1 to W5 for warrant officers. Those were further collapsed for some analyses to junior enlisted (E1–E4), senior enlisted (E5–E9), junior officers (O1–O3), senior officers (O4–O10), and warrant officers.

*Sex.* Male or female.

*Age.* Age as of December 31, 2010, was calculated by using the date-of-birth variable. For some analyses, the distribution was collapsed in 5-year intervals: less than 20 years old, 20–24, 25–29, 30–34, 35–39, 40–44, 45–49, 50–54, and 55 or older.

*Education.* The variable was created by collapsing the detailed education-attainment variable to less than a high-school education, high-school degree or equivalent (for example, a GED), some college, college degree, or at least some postgraduate education.

*Race.* Coding rules established by the National Center for Health Statistics were used to code race. *White* was coded for those who identified themselves only as white with no other race identified. *Black* was coded for those who identified themselves as black or African American only or as primarily black but with additional race groups. *Asian/Pacific Islander* was coded for those who identified themselves as Asian, Native Hawaiian, or other Pacific Islander only or as primarily Asian, Native Hawaiian, or other Pacific Islander but with additional race groups. *American Indian/Alaskan Native* was coded for those who identified themselves as American Indian or Alaskan Native only or as primarily American Indian or Alaskan Native but with additional race groups. People with missing or unknown race codes were categorized as of *unknown* race.

*Ethnicity.* This was coded as *Hispanic* if a service member identified himself or herself as Mexican, Puerto Rican, Cuban, Latin American, or of other Hispanic descent. Those who indicated no ethnicity or another coded ethnicity were identified as *non-Hispanic*. People with missing or unknown ethnicity codes were categorized as of *unknown* ethnicity.

*Marital status.* Marital status was categorized as never married, married, divorced or legally separated, and other (widowed or interlocutory decree) as of the end date of the file. Those with missing or unknown marital status codes were categorized as of *unknown* marital status. Percentage married was most often used.

*Children.* The proportions of service members who had children and the numbers of children are based on the "dependent" variable that includes only dependent children rather than all dependents.

*Deployment.* Although there are different ways to define deployment, the committee chose to use the DOD definition as provided by the DMDC. In this context, deployment count or *number of deployments* was based on a count of deployment records in the deployment file with discrete (nonoverlapping) start and end dates for each service member. The *length of deployment* was based on the start and end dates of each deployment for both single and multiple deployers; the *cumulative number* of months for multiple deployers was based on summing the length of all their deployments on the basis of their start and end dates. *Dwell time* (the time between deployments) was calculated by taking the end date of a given deployment and subtracting it from the begin date of the next deployment for those who had two or more deployments. *Location of deployment* was more complicated to determine. The DMDC Contingency Tracking System contains data fields for specifying the location of each deployment designated as in direct support of the OEF, OIF, or OND mission, but some individual records do not have movements in and out of country. In particular, before 2005, although the DMDC tracked deployments to Iraq and Afghanistan, the location codes were mostly unknown or based on the embarkation country of the service member (for example, Bahrain, Kuwait, or Qatar). In 2005, the Defense Theater Accountability System increased the level of detail to include each change in country during a given service member's deployment. Thus, use of the Afghanistan and Iraq country codes to identify those who served in these areas of responsibility would underestimate the numbers of service members who actually served there from September 11, 2001, through 2010.

In recognition of the possibility that the deployments of many of those who served in Iraq or Afghanistan were not assigned location codes or were assigned codes based on embarkation countries, each deployment location on the file was classified as

- *Afghanistan* or *Iraq*.
- *Middle East* locations designated as eligible for combat-zone pay or benefits (Djibouti, Israel, Jordan, Kyrgyzstan, Kuwait, Pakistan, Saudi Arabia, Somalia, Turkey, Uzbekistan, and Yemen).
- Other known countries or locations (for example, *Germany* or *Republic of Korea*).
- *Unknown* (location data missing).

On the basis of the codes, it was possible to categorize all those deployed (1) at least one deployment to Afghanistan or Iraq; (2) at least one Middle East country and all other deployment countries/locations are known; (3) Middle East and/or other countries, with at least one unknown location; (4) only countries other than Afghanistan, Iraq, or the Middle East; and (5) none of the deployment locations are known (all are missing). Chapter 3 details all the demographic characteristics of those deployed and provides information on the nature of the deployments and dwell time.

## ETHNOGRAPHIC ASSESSMENTS

In its efforts to gain some understanding of the effects of deployment on communities, the committee reviewed the literature that was available. The committee also contracted with Westat to conduct ethnographic assessments with the committee's oversight and input. (The individual ethnographic assessments may be found in Appendix E, and a summary of findings appears in Chapter 7.)

Ethnography is an approach to understanding communities that involves an array of data-collection strategies, including document review, participant observation, in-depth interviews of key community members, and less formal interviews with persons throughout a community as the opportunity arises. Although ethnographers have traditionally emphasized the importance of spending an extended period (at least 1 year) in the community of interest, there is agreement that under some circumstances valuable and accurate findings can be obtained through a substantially shorter period of field work.

Two-person ethnographic teams from Westat visited six sites to understand the effects of multiple deployments on targeted domains in each of the selected locations. The following paragraphs describe the methods used by the ethnographic teams; they describe the eligibility and selection criteria for study sites and the training of project-team members. The training aimed to ensure a consistent approach to data collection and reporting in the six sites.

### Site Selection

The project team and IOM worked closely together to identify possible study sites and to decide which ones to select. The presence of a large Army or Marine Corps base where service members have been deployed multiple times was the primary criterion for site selection. Mindful of the potential importance of geographic diversity, the project team and IOM agreed on

- Jacksonville, North Carolina
- Watertown, New York
- El Paso, Texas
- Olympia-Tacoma, Washington

IOM requested two additional sites that had National Guard units and suggested that the project team look for communities in states that had a history of a strong National Guard—such as Florida, Indiana, Michigan, Ohio, and Pennsylvania—and from which the local Guard unit had deployed more than once. Because IOM was interested in community-level effects of deployments, the project team added the criterion that units have large numbers of *local* Guard members, as opposed to, for example, members from four neighboring states and Guam.

Research assistants on the project team set about locating several such units and quickly found that, although there are websites for the National Guard in each state, they vary substantially in quality, currency, level of detail (for example, where unit members were from), and even Web domain name (for instance, some have the ".mil" domain name, others use ".org"). Because there was no way to "drill down" to the local units within all the suggested states and thus no ready means of identifying which units had seen more than one deployment to OIF or OEF, the research assistants expanded their search to include other states that had a noted National Guard history. By reviewing various states' National Guard websites, they were able to navigate via hotlinks to more detailed information about the units, including information about their deployment histories; the percentage of unit members who had deployed once, twice, or three times or more; and how many members come from towns near the location of the unit headquarters. The research assistants also accessed newspaper archives to identify the extent to which communities were paying attention to the comings and goings of their Guard members. Feature articles and letters to the editor, for example, offered important insights into a Guard unit's local "presence."

Using those search techniques, the project team identified two National Guard locations that seemed appropriate for the IOM study's objectives: Georgetown, South Carolina, whose armory serves as the headquarters for the 1/178th Field Artillery Battalion; and the town of Little Falls, Minnesota, which hosts Camp Ripley, the training facility for the Minnesota National Guard, and has a long history of its residents' joining the National Guard. Those communities and the rationale for their selection were presented to and approved by IOM for study inclusion.

## Staff Training

IOM and Westat staff participated in training. The training emphasized the objectives of the community assessment and provided an opportunity for team members to review planned data-collection procedures. Interview protocols were also reviewed and discussed.

## Westat Data-Collection Procedures

### Research on Community Background

An ethnographic study can begin before a researcher goes to the field. Project team members conducted Internet-based environmental scans to collect important background information relevant to the site visit and to shape their understanding of the community. They also uncovered important social networks through initial calls to key informants (such as city-council members and the director of a mental-health clinic) and by asking them for additional referrals in the community. Those steps set the foundation for the development of each site-visit plan.

### Ethnographic Data Collection

Study teams used a variety of data-collection approaches that went beyond the initial community scan, including semistructured small-group discussions, in-depth interviews, and on-site materials review (for example, of local daily newspapers). Perhaps the hallmark of ethnography is participant observation, in which the researcher engages with the community "as though" she or he were a regular community member. Observations made during such engagements and personal experiences can offer valuable insights into community dynamics. In a rapid appraisal, venues for participant observation must be chosen with efficiency in mind—that is, selection of events or venues that will provide the best information relevant to the study.

For the present study, community fairs proved to be an excellent venue for team members to observe the degree to which military members and their families interacted with the civilian community. Such fairs also often have dedicated areas where community-based organizations can advertise their services. That is one way in which social-service organizations may conduct outreach to the community, and observing which organizations were present—or absent—was telling during team members' attendance at the fairs.

### Question Matrix Review

The Westat study team created a "working" data matrix (see Table 2.2) that crossed the critical research questions with key categories of interviewees. Team members placed a check mark in the appropriate box each time an interview involved a particular topic. That approach helped to ensure cross-site consistency in data-collection procedures. It also provided the study team with a quick way to ensure that information was being collected on all topics of interest and that interviews were taking place with members of key sectors of the community, such as emergency-services personnel and school faculty and staff.

**TABLE 2.2** Question Matrix for Site-Visit Interviews

| | Respondent Categories | | | | | | |
|---|---|---|---|---|---|---|---|
| **Questions by Domain** | Business Leaders | Social Service Providers | School Personnel | Clergy | Civilian Community Members | Military Families | Civic Leaders |
| **Economic Development** | | | | | | | |
| How has the deployment situation affected overall commerce in the community? How has it affected the labor supply? What impact has it had on consumer demand? (Increased? Decreased?) | ✓ | | | | | | ✓ |
| How has it affected the unemployment rates within the community? What, if any, stores have gone out of business or left town? Conversely, what, if any, new stores have come into town? | ✓ | ✓ | | | ✓ | ✓ | ✓ |
| How have the deployments affected the housing market? Increase in population? People have moved away? Change in foreclosure rates? Change in home ownership vs. rentals? | ✓ | ✓ | ✓ | | ✓ | ✓ | ✓ |

| | | | | | | | |
|---|---|---|---|---|---|---|---|
| **Information and Communication** | | | | | | | |
| To what extent are the issues around deployment being openly discussed within the community, e.g., through news media? How are these issues being discussed? (As challenges? Opportunities?) How are residents finding out about any needed resources? | ✓ | ✓ | ✓ | ✓ | ✓ | ✓ | ✓ |
| **Community Health** | | | | | | | |
| How are children in the community handling the deployments? What, if any, challenges are you seeing? What, if any, differences are you seeing between young children, adolescents, and teenagers? How is the community attempting to address their needs? | | ✓ | ✓ | ✓ | ✓ | ✓ | ✓ |
| In general, what behavioral health issues are you seeing? Increased depression? Anxiety? Alcohol use? Illegal drug use? (What evidence do you have, e.g., increase in substance-related hospitalizations, arrests?) What steps is the community taking to address these issues? | | ✓ | ✓ | ✓ | ✓ | ✓ | ✓ |
| **Community Competence** | | | | | | | |
| What services are available to help residents cope with the potential stresses associated with multiple deployments? What are the eligibility requirements? Who helps link individuals to these services? What resources (e.g., self-help groups) are available for individuals who may not have enough money to pay for certain services? | | ✓ | ✓ | ✓ | ✓ | ✓ | |
| **Social Capital** | | | | | | | |
| What are some of the informal support networks that are available in the community to help with deployments? How well do they work? How has their effectiveness changed over time, if at all (e.g., more effective because more experience? Less effective because of burnout?) | | ✓ | ✓ | ✓ | ✓ | ✓ | |

### Data Management and Security

Team members collected two forms of data: field notes on observations or interviews and audio recordings of formal interviews. Each evening, to enhance data security, site-visit staff uploaded audio recordings to a secure file transfer protocol (SFTP) site and informed an assigned staff member on Westat's Rockville, Maryland, campus of the number of files to expect. Rockville-based staff then downloaded the files to a secure network drive. After being notified that the files had transferred correctly, site-visit staff members deleted the files on their recording devices. Files that had been uploaded to the SFTP were also deleted at this time.

### Data Analysis

Using the data matrix, team members reviewed appropriate audio files and field notes for patterns regarding each key question. For example, to address the effects of multiple deployments on the local economy, analysts reviewed relevant sections of interviews with city leaders and members of the Chamber of Commerce. Staff sometimes also examined notes from less formal discussions with local business leaders (such as the owner of a storage facility or coffee shop). In conducting the analysis, the researchers did not search solely for consensus; often, because interviewees occupied different positions in a community, their perspectives on an issue could be quite different. When possible, analysts relied on other data gathered during the site visit and social theory to try to explain why differences might exist.

**Case-Study Reports**

Each site-visit team conducted its own data analysis and submitted a 12- to 15-page report shortly after each visit. The case-study outline was structured to match the question matrix, so it created a straightforward framework for conveying findings. Each report was reviewed by one or more senior members of the project team before it was submitted to IOM for review. (See Appendix E for the individual site summaries.) The summary of findings from the ethnographic assessments is presented in Chapter 7.

# 3

# CHARACTERISTICS OF THE DEPLOYED

The focus of this chapter is on the demographic characteristics of US military personnel deployed to Operation Enduring Freedom (OEF) and/or Operation Iraqi Freedom (OIF), and it is based on data from the Department of Defense (DOD) Defense Manpower Data Center (DMDC) Contingency Tracking System (CTS). A CTS "deployment" for OEF and OIF is defined as "a DOD service member who is or has been *physically located* within the OEF and/or OIF combat zones or areas of operation (AOR), or has been *specifically identified* by his/her service as 'directly supporting' the OEF and/or OIF mission outside the designated combat zone (e.g., US Air Force aircrew or support personnel located at an airbase outside the combat zone)" (Bonds et al., 2010). The DMDC CTS includes all US military personnel who have been deployed to OEF, OIF, and OND in support of the Global War on Terror from September 11, 2001, to the present time. The committee, however, only has records through December 31, 2010. The file the committee received with the variables requested represents a snapshot in time, that is, the status of the deployed at the time the file was created. Thus, all descriptive analyses in the chapter reflect the characteristics of the deployed at one point in time. The committee did not use the descriptive analyses in this chapter to link with any other data in the report.

## DEMOGRAPHICS

The following analyses are based on the 2.1 million service members who had been deployed to OEF, OIF, and/or OND by the end of 2010 (Table 3.1).[1] Over half those deployed were in the Army, including all components; 28% were in the Regular Army alone. The proportion of those deployed by branch in the Regular components ranged from 56% in the Army to 84% in the Navy and Marine Corps. In turn, those in the National Guard and reserves (combined across all services) constituted one-third of all those deployed.

---

[1]Although these descriptive analyses would ideally have included data and reference comparisons with the nondeployed or the total force during this period, providing comparable data would have required access to identifiable data on all the nondeployed as well as all those deployed. The committee was not able to obtain full identifiable information on all the nondeployed to conduct the descriptive analyses.

**TABLE 3.1** Service Members Deployed, by Branch of Service and Component[a] as of 2010

| Component | Army | Navy | Air Force | Marine Corps | Coast Guard | TOTAL |
|---|---|---|---|---|---|---|
| Regular | 608,634 | 323,701 | 280,182 | 219,335 | 4,813 | 1,436,665 |
| National Guard | 298,728 | N/A | 79,777 | N/A | N/A | 378,505 |
| Reserves | 173,825 | 60,161 | 54,632 | 42,316 | 1,271 | 332,205 |
| TOTAL | 1,081,187 | 383,862 | 414,591 | 261,651 | 6,084 | 2,147,375 |

[a]In contrast with the Army and Air Force, the Navy and Marine Corps do not have National Guard components. Entire file contained 2,147,398, but 23 had an unknown component.
SOURCE: Defense Manpower Data Center.

## Pay Grade

As shown in Table 3.2, over 85% of those deployed in all components and service branches were enlisted, with nearly 6 in 10 of the enlisted in the senior enlisted grades (E5–E9). The proportion of total enlisted personnel (E1–E9) supporting the operations ranged from about 78% in the Coast Guard to about 90% in the Marine Corps. The proportion of senior enlisted personnel in those deployed ranged from 40% in the Marine Corps to about 62% in the Air Force.

**TABLE 3.2** Service Members Deployed, by Branch of Service and Pay Grade, as of 2010

| Pay Grade | Army, N (column %) | Navy, N (column %) | Air Force, N (column %) | Marine Corps, N (column %) | Coast Guard, N (column %) | TOTAL, N (column %) |
|---|---|---|---|---|---|---|
| E1–E4 | 405,014 (37.5) | 121,159 (31.6) | 83,832 (20.2) | 132,049 (50.5) | 1,388 (22.8) | 743,442 (34.6) |
| E5–E9 | 514,722 (47.6) | 210,208 (54.8) | 258,234 (62.3) | 104,225 (39.8) | 3,367 (55.3) | 1,090,756 (50.8) |
| O1–3 | 69,312 (6.4) | 23,012 (6.0) | 27,905 (6.7) | 11,260 (4.3) | 638 (10.5) | 132,127 (6.2) |
| O4–O10 | 63,789 (5.9) | 27,197 (7.1) | 44,639 (10.8) | 11,402 (4.4) | 440 (7.2) | 147,467 (6.9) |
| Warrant Officer | 28,350 (2.6) | 2,275 (0.6) | 0 (0) | 2,716 (1.0) | 251 (4.1) | 33,592 (1.6) |
| TOTAL (row %) | 1,081,187 (50.3) | 383,851 (17.9) | 414,610 (19.3) | 261,652 (12.2) | 6,084 (0.3) | 2,147,384 (100) |

NOTE: Entire file contained 2,147,398, but 11 Navy and three Air Force personnel had missing pay grade.
SOURCE: Defense Manpower Data Center.

## Sex

Of the military personnel serving in OEF and/or OIF through 2010, about 88% were men and about 12% women (Table 3.3); the proportion of women deployed (across all components) ranged from about 3% in the Marine Corps to over 17% in the Air Force. By pay grade, the proportion of women among those deployed ranged from about 8% of the warrant officers to about 16% of the junior officers (O1–O3). The proportion of women deployed by branch and pay grade ranged from about 3% of junior enlisted marines to over 20% of junior officers in the Air Force.

**TABLE 3.3** Proportion of Women Deployed, by Branch of Service and Pay Grade, as of 2010

| Pay Grade | Army, N (%) | Navy, N (%) | Air Force, N (%) | Marine Corps, N (%) | Coast Guard, N (%) | TOTAL, N (%) |
|---|---|---|---|---|---|---|
| E1–E4 | 46,458 (11.5) | 18,163 (15.0) | 14,651 (17.4) | 4,254 (3.2) | 115 (8.3) | 83,641 (11.3) |
| E5–E9 | 56,673 (11.0) | 26,163 (12.4) | 39,545 (15.3) | 4,534 (4.3) | 205 (6.1) | 127,120 (11.7) |
| O1–O3 | 11,265 (16.3) | 3,928 (17.1) | 5,727 (20.5) | 848 (7.5) | 80 (12.5) | 21,848 (16.5) |
| O4–O10 | 7,108 (11.1) | 2,741 (10.1) | 5,568 (12.5) | 378 (3.3) | 36 (8.2) | 15,831 (10.7) |
| Warrant officer | 2,351 (8.3) | 113 (5.0) | 0 (0) | 117 (4.3) | 10 (4.0) | 2,591 (7.7) |
| TOTAL women (% of total deployed) | 123,855 (11.5) | 51,108 (13.3) | 65,491 (15.8) | 10,131 (3.9) | 446 (7.3) | 251,031 (11.7) |

NOTE: N, number of women in each group; %, percentage based on denominators in Table 3.2. Entire file contained 251,033 women, but two Navy women had missing pay grade, and 24 Army personnel had missing sex.
SOURCE: Defense Manpower Data Center.

## Age

As shown in Table 3.4, the average age of those deployed was 33.4 years. Half the deployed were 25–34 years old at the end of 2010 (about 72% were 25–44 years old), with approximately equal proportions either under 25 years old or 45 years old or older. The proportions of those 25–34 years old by branch ranged from about 45% in the Air Force to about 60% in the Marine Corps. In addition, about 25% of marines were less than 25 years old (about 84% less than 35 years old). Marine Corps deployed had the lowest mean age, 29.5 years, and Air Force deployed had the highest mean age, 35.8 years.

**TABLE 3.4** Age Distributions and Mean Ages of Deployed Service Members, by Service Branch, as of 2010

| Age (years) | Army, N (column %) | Navy, N (column %) | Air Force, N (column %) | Marine Corps, N (column %) | Coast Guard, N (column %) | TOTAL, N (column %) |
|---|---|---|---|---|---|---|
| <20 | 4,084 (0.4) | 650 (0.2) | 222 (0.05) | 827 (0.3) | 1 (0.02) | 5,784 (0.3) |
| 20–24 | 164,904 (15.3) | 48,364 (12.6) | 39,222 (9.5) | 63,490 (24.3) | 456 (7.5) | 316, 436 (14.7) |
| 25–29 | 316,570 (29.3) | 111,897 (29.2) | 101,310 (24.4) | 107,262 (41.0) | 1,801 (29.6) | 638,840 (29.8) |
| 30–34 | 212,293 (19.6) | 83,773 (21.8) | 84,739 (20.4) | 48,460 (18.5) | 1,619 (26.6) | 430,884 (20.1) |

| Age (years) | Army, N (column %) | Navy, N (column %) | Air Force, N (column %) | Marine Corps, N (column %) | Coast Guard, N (column %) | TOTAL, N (column %) |
|---|---|---|---|---|---|---|
| 35–39 | 134,686 (12.5) | 51,049 (13.3) | 56,220 (13.6) | 19,789 (7.6) | 888 (14.6) | 262,632 (12.2) |
| 40–44 | 113,491 (10.5) | 43,574 (11.4) | 52,842 (12.7) | 11,973 (4.6) | 632 (10.4) | 222,512 (10.4) |
| 45–49 | 76,570 (7.1) | 28,988 (7.6) | 45,493 (11.0) | 6,606 (2.5) | 400 (6.6) | 158,057 (7.4) |
| 50–54 | 35,050 (3.2) | 11,025 (2.9) | 20,322 (4.9) | 2,435 (0.9) | 174 (2.9) | 69,006 (3.2) |
| ≥55 | 23,466 (2.2) | 4,537 (1.2) | 14,243 (3.4) | 810 (0.3) | 113 (1.9) | 43,169 (2.0) |
| TOTAL | 1,081,114 | 383,857 | 414,613 | 261,652 | 6,084 | 2,147,320 |
| Mean age | 33.4 | 33.6 | 35.8 | 29.5 | 34.1 | 33.4 |

NOTE: Entire file contained 2,147,398, but 73 Army and 5 Navy personnel had missing age.
SOURCE: Defense Manpower Data Center.

The numbers of regular component and National Guard and reserve component officers and enlisted members by age are summarized in Table 3.5. On the average, those deployed from the National Guard and reserves were older than service members in the regular component, 36 vs 32 years old, respectively. Among National Guard and reserve component officers, 75% were 35 years old or older compared with 59% of regular component officers, primarily because of differences between junior officers (grades O1–O3), 47% vs 26%. Forty percent of the National Guard and reserve component enlisted members were under 30 years old compared with 55% of the regular component enlisted members; the magnitudes of the differences were consistent in the junior and senior enlisted.

### Race and Ethnicity

The percentage of missing or unknown data in the DMDC database is especially high for race and ethnicity, particularly for Hispanic origin. Of service members with known race (92%) serving in OEF and/or OIF, about 77% were white, 17% black, 4% Asian, and 2% other races. Of those with reported ethnicity (59%), about 18% were of Hispanic origin.[2]

[2] Because the proportions with missing data on race and ethnicity are significantly higher than the other characteristics in this chapter, we were concerned about providing additional descriptive analyses based on these variables.

**TABLE 3.5** Age Distributions and Mean Age of Deployed Service Members, by Component and Pay Grade, as of 2010

| | Regular | | | | | | Reserve/National Guard | | | | | |
|---|---|---|---|---|---|---|---|---|---|---|---|---|
| Age (years) | E1–E4, N (column %) | E5–E9, N (column %) | O1–O3, N (column %) | O4–O10, N (column %) | Warrant Officer, N (column %) | TOTAL, N (column %) | E1–E4, N (column %) | E5–E9, N (column %) | O1–O3, N (column %) | O4–O10, N (column %) | Warrant Officer, N (column %) | TOTAL, N (column %) |
| <20 | 5,057 (0.9) | 0 (0) | 0 (0) | 0 (0) | 0 (0) | 5,057 (0.4) | 727 (0.4) | 0 (0) | 0 (0) | 0 (0) | 0 (0) | 727 (0.1) |
| 20–24 | 204,874 (38.3) | 41,790 (6.0) | 2,710 (3.1) | 0 (0) | 38 (0.2) | 249,412 (17.4) | 53,298 (26.0) | 12,653 (3.3) | 344 (0.8) | 0 (0) | 99 (0.8) | 67,024 (9.4) |
| 25–29 | 225,939 (42.2) | 201,384 (28.7) | 31,666 (36.0) | 0 (0) | 980 (4.8) | 459,971 (32.0) | 85,207 (41.0) | 84,847 (21.8) | 7,483 (17.0) | 0 (0) | 1,329 (10.0) | 178,867 (25.2) |
| 30–34 | 77,491 (14.5) | 175,745 (25.1) | 31,161 (35.4) | 8,026 (8.8) | 3,870 (19.0) | 296,298 (20.6) | 40,184 (19.3) | 74,663 (19.2) | 15,650 (35.5) | 1,746 (3.1) | 2,329 (17.6) | 134,573 (18.9) |
| 35–39 | 16,339 (3.1) | 115,165 (16.4) | 14,252 (16.2) | 22,378 (24.6) | 5,121 (25.2) | 173,258 (12.1) | 14,101 (6.8) | 54,996 (14.1) | 10,753 (24.4) | 7,554 (13.4) | 1,967 (14.8) | 89,372 (12.6) |
| 40–44 | 5,123 (1.0) | 90,994 (13.0) | 6,311 (7.2) | 25,825 (28.4) | 4,818 (23.7) | 133,071 (9.3) | 7,991 (3.9) | 58,381 (15.0) | 6,739 (15.3) | 14,144 (25.1) | 2,186 (16.5) | 89,441 (12.6) |
| 45–49 | 716 (0.1) | 57,620 (8.2) | 1,541 (1.8) | 20,237 (22.2) | 3,611 (17.8) | 83,725 (5.8) | 3,704 (1.8) | 50,647 (13.0) | 2,249 (5.1) | 15,451 (27.4) | 2,278 (17.2) | 74,329 (10.5) |
| 50–54 | 78 (0.01) | 15,943 (2.3) | 353 (0.4) | 9,903 (10.9) | 1,401 (6.9) | 27,679 (1.9) | 1,423 (0.7) | 28,343 (7.3) | 629 (1.4) | 9,574 (17.0) | 1,356 (10.2) | 41,325 (5.8) |
| ≥55 | 5 (0) | 2,917 (0.4) | 70 (0.08) | 4,669 (5.1) | 483 (2.4) | 8,144 (0.6) | 534 (0.3) | 24,626 (6.3) | 211 (0.5) | 7,944 (14.1) | 1,709 (12.9) | 35,024 (4.9) |
| TOTAL | 535,622 | 701,558 | 88,064 | 91,038 | 20,322 | 1,436,615 | 207,799 | 389,156 | 44,058 | 56,413 | 13,253 | 710,682 |
| Mean age | 26.7 | 34.4 | 32.2 | 43.4 | 40.5 | 32.0 | 29.0 | 38.4 | 35.5 | 47.0 | 42.6 | 36.2 |

NOTE: Entire file contained 2,147,398, but 78 had missing age, and 14 had missing pay grade.
SOURCE: Defense Manpower Data Center.

## Education

Of those deployed to OEF and/or OIF in all service branches and components, less than 1% had less than a high-school education (see Table 3.6). Over two-thirds had a high-school degree or equivalent (GED), and over 30% had at least some college education. Of junior officers (O1–O3), 88% had at least a college degree, and over 70% of those who had advanced degrees were senior officers (O4–O10). High-school degrees and GEDs were most common among junior and senior enlisted, but over 75% of those who had some college education but no college degree were senior enlisted service members.

**TABLE 3.6** Education Status of Deployed Service Members, by Pay Grade, as of 2010

| | Enlisted | | Commissioned Officers | | | |
|---|---|---|---|---|---|---|
| Education Status | E1–E4, N (column %) | E5–E9, N (column %) | O1–O3, N (column %) | O4–O10, N (column %) | Warrant Officer, N (column %) | TOTAL, N (column %) |
| Less than high school | 10,722 (1.4) | 6,935 (0.6) | 55 (0.04) | 28 (0.02) | 15 (0.04) | 17,755 (0.8) |
| GED | 82,194 (11.1) | 47,382 (4.3) | 82 (0.06) | 159 (0.1) | 363 (1.1) | 130,181 (6.1) |
| High school | 588,084 (79.1) | 713,615 (65.4) | 1,141 (0.9) | 451 (0.3) | 5,599 (16.7) | 1,308,896 (61.0) |
| Some college | 40,515 (5.5) | 218,999 (20.1) | 4,837 (3.7) | 1,243 (0.8) | 16,072 (47.8) | 281,669 (13.1) |
| College graduate | 10,978 (1.5) | 77,383 (7.1) | 94,387 (71.4) | 54,328 (36.8) | 8,254 (24.6) | 245,332 (11.4) |
| Postcollege | 622 (0.1) | 10,973 (1.0) | 21,675 (16.4) | 88,152 (59.8) | 1,982 (5.9) | 123,406 (5.6) |
| Unknown | 10,327 (1.4) | 15,469 (1.4) | 9,950 (7.5) | 3,106 (2.1) | 1,307 (3.9) | 40,159 (1.9) |
| TOTAL | 743,442 | 1,090,756 | 132,127 | 147,467 | 33,592 | 2,147,384 |

NOTE: Entire file contained 2,147,398, but 14 had unknown pay grade.
SOURCE: Defense Manpower Data Center.

## Marital Status

As shown in Table 3.7, about 59% of those deployed in all services and components were married—from about 40% of the junior enlisted (E1–E4) to 85% of the senior officers (O4–O10). Marital status differed somewhat by branch of service and component. In all components, the proportions of service members married ranged from about 53% in the Marine Corps to about 65% in the Air Force (see Table 3.8). In the regular component, 61% were married—from about 55% in the Marine Corps to about 66% in the Air Force. Among the two reserve components, 55% of the reserves and 58% of the National Guard were married, and the proportion of members married ranged from 44% in the Marine Corps reserves to 65% in the Air National Guard.

**TABLE 3.7** Proportion of Deployed Service Members Married, by Branch of Service and Pay Grade, as of 2010

| Pay Grade | Army, N (%)[a] | Navy, N (%)[a] | Air Force, N (%)[a] | Marine Corps, N (%)[a] | Coast Guard, N (%)[a] | TOTAL, N (%)[a] |
|---|---|---|---|---|---|---|
| E1–E4 | 167,678 (41.1) | 48,528 (40.1) | 31,687 (37.8) | 52,113 (39.5) | 545 (39.3) | 300,551 (40.4) |
| E5–E9 | 347,800 (67.6) | 141,121 (67.1) | 181,933 (70.5) | 68,257 (65.5) | 2,194 (65.2) | 741,305 (68.0) |
| O1–O3 | 41,765 (60.3) | 14,233 (61.9) | 18,362 (65.8) | 6,817 (60.5) | 416 (65.2) | 81,593 (61.8) |
| O4–O10 | 53,889 (84.5) | 22,947 (84.3) | 38,189 (85.6) | 9,934 (87.1) | 386 (87.7) | 125,345 (85.0) |
| Warrant officer | 23,062 (81.4) | 1,968 (86.5) | 0 (0) | 2,379 (87.6) | 222 (88.5) | 27,631 (82.3) |
| TOTAL | 634,194 (58.7) | 228,800 (59.6) | 270,174 (65.2) | 139,500 (53.3) | 3,763 (61.9) | 1,276,431 (59.4) |

NOTE: Entire file contained 1,276,431 married, but three Navy and three Air Force personnel had missing pay grade.
[a]N, number married in each group; % are cell percentages representing the percentage married in each group based on denominators in Table 3.2.
SOURCE: Defense Manpower Data Center.

**TABLE 3.8** Proportion of Deployed Service Members Married, by Branch of Service and Component[a] as of 2010

| Component | Army, N (%)[b] | Navy, N (%)[b] | Air Force, N (%)[b] | Marine Corps, N (%)[b] | Coast Guard, N (%)[b] | TOTAL, N (%)[b] |
|---|---|---|---|---|---|---|
| Regular | 374,939 (61.6) | 193,350 (59.7) | 183,950 (65.7) | 121,090 (55.2) | 3,095 (64.3) | 876,424 (61.0) |
| National Guard | 166,605 (55.8) | NA | 51,564 (64.6) | NA | NA | 218,169 (57.6) |
| Reserves | 92,650 (53.3) | 35,450 (58.9) | 34,650 (63.4) | 18,409 (43.5) | 668 (52.6) | 181,827 (54.7) |
| TOTAL | 634,194 (58.7) | 228,800 (59.6) | 270,174 (65.2) | 139,500 (53.3) | 3,763 (61.9) | 1,276,431 (59.4) |

NOTE: Entire file contained 2,147,398, but 10 Air Force and 1 Marine Corps personnel had an unknown component.
[a]In contrast with the Army and Air Force, the Navy and Marine Corps do not have National Guard components.
[b]N, number married in each group; % are cell percentages representing the percentage married in each group based on denominators in Table 3.1.
SOURCE: Defense Manpower Data Center.

### Dependent Children

The proportion of deployed service members in all service branches and components who had dependent children was 49%—from 35% in the Marine Corps to 52% in the Air Force (Table 3.9). Half those in the regular component and National Guard had dependent children compared with 44% in the reserves. The proportion in all branches and components who had dependent children ranged from a low of 28% and 35% among Marine Corps and Coast Guard reserves, respectively, to 53% in the regular Army and Air Force. In all services and components, 69% of those currently married and 11% of those who had never married had dependent children. The number of children of those who had children ranged from 1 to 14; the mean was just under 2 (1.97), with a narrow range of 1.8 in the Marine Corp Reserves to 2.02 in the regular Army.

**TABLE 3.9** Proportion of Deployed Service Members with Children,[a] by Branch of Service and Component,[b] as of 2010

| Component | Army, N (%)[c] | Navy, N (%)[c] | Air Force, N (%)[c] | Marine Corps, N (%)[c] | Coast Guard, N (%)[c] | TOTAL, N (%)[c] |
|---|---|---|---|---|---|---|
| Regular | 324,857 (53.4) | 156,179 (48.3) | 148,786 (53.1) | 80,564 (36.7) | 2,364 (49.1) | 712,750 (49.6) |
| National Guard | 147,663 (49.4) | N/A | 40,279 (50.5) | N/A | N/A | 187,942 (49.7) |
| Reserves | 77,055 (44.3) | 29,563 (49.1) | 27,150 (49.7) | 11,957 (28.3) | 442 (34.8) | 146,167 (44.0) |
| Total | 549,575 (50.8) | 185,742 (48.4) | 216,222 (52.2) | 92,521 (35.4) | 2,806 (46.1) | 1,046,866 (48.8) |

NOTE: Entire file contained 2,147,398, but 23 had an unknown component.
[a]Children were defined as dependents under 21 years old.
[b]In contrast with the Army and Air Force, the Navy and Marine Corps do not have National Guard components.
[c]N, number in each group with children; % are cell percentages representing the percentage with children in each group based on denominators in Table 3.1.
SOURCE: Defense Manpower Data Center.

## DEPLOYMENT

Military deployments in support of the operations in Iraq and Afghanistan have varied in duration, frequency, combat intensity, geography, service branch, and service component. Sudden and prolonged deployment and separation from family or home may be enough to warrant implication of deployment as the main exposure, though this approach lacks the understanding of the complex environmental factors that service members may encounter in theater. To begin to understand any lasting health impact of this complex exposure, we must first understand the nature of deployments.

## Number of Deployments

By the end of 2010, 2,147,398 service members had deployed a total of 3,683,746 deployments in support of the operations in Iraq and Afghanistan—an average of 1.72 each and a range in frequency from 1 to 47. Of those who deployed, 57% deployed only once and 43% multiple times. Of those who deployed more than once, nearly two-thirds deployed twice (27% of the total number of deployers), one-fourth deployed three times (10% of the total number of deployers), and about 15% (6% of the total number of deployers) deployed four or more times.

As shown in Tables 3.10 and 3.11, the number of deployments varied substantially among service branches and components. The average number of deployments by service ranged from 1.3 in the Coast Guard and 1.6 in the Army and Marine Corps to 2.1 in the Air Force. Likewise, the proportions of multiple deployers ranged from 19% in the Coast Guard to over half in the Air Force. The proportion having four or more deployments ranged from less than 2% in the Coast Guard and 3% in the Marine Corps to 13% in the Air Force.

The proportion of deployers who had multiple deployments in the National Guard and reserves (35%) was appreciably less than that in the regular component (47%); the average number ranged from 1.56 in the National Guard to 1.77 in the regular component. When one examines the numbers by branch and component, those with the lowest average numbers of deployments were the Coast Guard and Marine Corps reserves (1.22 and 1.29, respectively) and those in the regular Coast Guard (1.28). Those with the highest average numbers of deployments were the Air Force Guard and reserves (2.24 and 2.58, respectively). Over 80% of the two Coast Guard components and over 75% of the Marine Corps reserves had only one deployment compared with fewer than half those in the Air Force Guard and reserve components.

**TABLE 3.10** Proportion of Deployed Service Members Deployed Multiple Times, by Branch of Service and Component,[a] as of 2010

| Component | Army, N (%)[b] | Navy, N (%)[b] | Air Force, N (%)[b] | Marine Corps, N (%)[b] | Coast Guard, N (%)[b] | TOTAL N (%)[b] |
|---|---|---|---|---|---|---|
| Regular | 287,938 (47.3) | 145,043 (44.8) | 137,760 (49.2) | 107,462 (48.9) | 920 (19.1) | 679,123 (47.3) |
| National Guard | 88,291 (29.6) | N/A | 42,935 (53.8) | N/A | N/A | 131,226 (34.7) |
| Reserves | 57,201 (32.9) | 20,876 (34.7) | 28,164 (51.5) | 9,943 (23.5) | 203 (16.0) | 116,387 (35.3) |
| TOTAL | 433,430 (40.1) | 165,919 (43.2) | 208,859 (50.4) | 117,405 (44.9) | 1123 (18.5) | 926,736 (43.2) |

NOTE: Entire file contained 2,147,398, but 10 Air Force and one Marine Corps personnel had an unknown component.

[a]In contrast with the Army and Air Force, the Navy and Marine Corps do not have National Guard components.

[b]N, number with multiple deployments within each group; % are cell percentages representing the percentage with multiple deployments in each group based on denominators in Table 3.1.

SOURCE: Defense Manpower Data Center.

**TABLE 3.11** Mean Number of Deployments,[a] by Branch of Service and Component,[b] as of 2010

| Component | Army | Navy | Air Force | Marine Corps | Coast Guard | TOTAL |
|---|---|---|---|---|---|---|
| Regular | 1.76 | 1.71 | 1.94 | 1.69 | 1.28 | 1.77 |
| National Guard | 1.38 | N/A | 2.24 | N/A | N/A | 1.56 |
| Reserves | 1.45 | 1.59 | 2.58 | 1.29 | 1.22 | 1.64 |
| TOTAL | 1.61 | 1.69 | 2.08 | 1.63 | 1.27 | 1.72 |

[a]The distributions of average length of deployment, average length of dwell time, and number of deployments were symmetric, and the medians were very similar to the means. Thus, the committee elected to report the means.
[b]In contrast with the Army and Air Force, the Navy and Marine Corps do not have National Guard components.

## Length of Deployment

Duration of deployment has varied among service branches and service components and has varied temporally over the decade of deployments (see Table 3.12). The committee has presented the range of average deployment durations per service branch. The average length of deployments (total number of months divided by number of deployments) in all branches and components was 7.7 months—8.3 months for single deployers and 6.8 months for multiple deployers. When stratified by branch of service, deployment length ranged from 4.5 months in the Air Force to 9.4 months in the Army, both appreciably higher among single than among multiple deployers. By component, for single and multiple deployers combined, the range of average deployment length was fairly narrow, ranging from 7.5 months in the regular component to 8.0 in the National Guard and reserves. The higher average among the two reserve components is driven largely by single deployers; among those who had multiple deployments, the average length was actually higher in the regular components. By branch and component, average deployment length ranged from 3.5 months in the Air Force National Guard to 11.9 months in the Marine Corps reserves.

**TABLE 3.12** Mean Length of Deployment in Months, by Branch of Service and Component,[a] as of 2010

| Component | Army | Navy | Air Force | Marine Corps | Coast Guard | TOTAL |
|---|---|---|---|---|---|---|
| Regular | 9.66 | 6.00 | 4.89 | 7.21 | 5.29 | 7.52 |
| National Guard | 9.21 | N/A | 3.46 | N/A | N/A | 8.00 |
| Reserves | 8.96 | 6.13 | 3.85 | 11.96 | 5.29 | 7.96 |
| TOTAL | 9.42 | 6.02 | 4.48 | 7.97 | 6.00 | 7.67 |

[a]In contrast with the Army and Air Force, the Navy and Marine Corps do not have National Guard components.

Considering deployment length over time, Figure 3.1 displays a consistent pattern for Air Force and Navy personnel who maintained the lowest average length of deployments over the decade of operations. The Army and Marine Corps maintained higher average length of deployments that, as one may expect, spiked during times of heavy combat early in the operations and during the 2006 and 2007 heavy combat periods.

If deployment itself is considered an exposure, the "dose" may impact health, so more deployment time would theoretically be worse for subsequent health outcomes. Therefore, another way to examine duration of deployment is to compare the *cumulative* deployment length for multiple deployers. Overall, as shown in Table 3.13, those with two or more deployments averaged 16.9 months across all deployments combined. By branch of service, cumulative average length of deployment among multiple deployers ranged from 9.7 months in the Coast Guard to 20.9 months in the Army. By component, the range was much narrower, but it was higher, 14.6 months in the National Guard to 17.6 months in the regular component. Comparisons by branch and component, however, showed significantly greater variability: from 8.9 and 9.3 months in the Air Force National Guard and Coast Guard reserves, respectively, to 21.1 months in the Marine Corps reserves and 22.7 months in the regular Army.

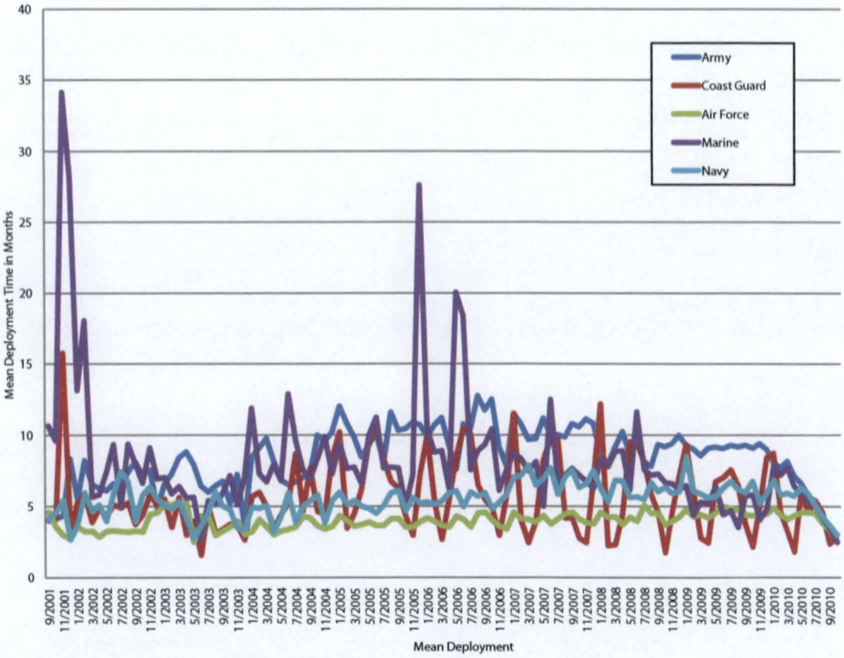


**FIGURE 3.1** Average months deployed, by deployment start date and branch.

**TABLE 3.13** Cumulative Deployment Length in Months of Multiple Deployers, by Branch of Service and Component,[a] as of 2010

| Component | Army | Navy | Air Force | Marine Corps | Coast Guard | TOTAL |
|---|---|---|---|---|---|---|
| Regular | 22.66 | 13.30 | 13.08 | 15.94 | 9.94 | 17.63 |
| National Guard | 17.35 | N/A | 8.89 | N/A | N/A | 14.58 |
| Reserves | 17.37 | 12.08 | 11.19 | 21.06 | 9.32 | 15.23 |
| TOTAL | 20.88 | 13.14 | 11.95 | 16.38 | 9.65 | 16.90 |

[a]In contrast with the Army and Air Force, the Navy and Marine Corps do not have National Guard components.

Potentially as impactful on health and other outcomes as the length and frequency of deployment is the time between deployments during which a military member can "reset" before going back into theater. That has become such a focus of concern that in 2011 the Army initiated a 2-year dwell cycle for deploying units that was contingent on demand for personnel in theater. Over the last decade, however, in all services and components, the average dwell time of those deployed two or more times was 21 months, from 16 months in the Marine Corps to about 22 months in the Army and Navy (Table 3.14). By component, the average dwell time was about 24 months for those in the National Guard compared with about 20 months in the reserves and regular component. Average dwell time ranged from less than 16 months in the regular Marine Corps and Coast Guard to over 26 months in the Army National Guard.

There was also a notable downward trend in the length of dwell time over the decade of operations as seen in dwell times of the regular and reserve National Guard components stratified by service branch (Figures 3.2 and 3.3). Independently, the three components indicate the same trends, although reserve and National Guard components had a substantial decrease in average length of deployment early in 2003, potentially indicating the redeployment of reserve and National Guard back into theater as the operations in Iraq were about to begin (Figure 3.3).

**TABLE 3.14** Mean Dwell Time of Multiple Deployers, in Months, by Branch of Service and Component,[a] as of 2010

| Component | Army | Navy | Air Force | Marine Corps | Coast Guard | TOTAL |
|---|---|---|---|---|---|---|
| Regular | 20.37 | 22.46 | 21.95 | 15.76 | 15.86 | 20.40 |
| National Guard | 26.21 | N/A | 21.08 | N/A | N/A | 25.53 |
| Reserves | 21.85 | 21.31 | 17.74 | 18.69 | 19.62 | 20.48 |
| TOTAL | 21.75 | 22.32 | 21.20 | 16.00 | 16.54 | 21.00 |

[a]In contrast with the Army and Air Force, the Navy and Marine Corps do not have National Guard components.

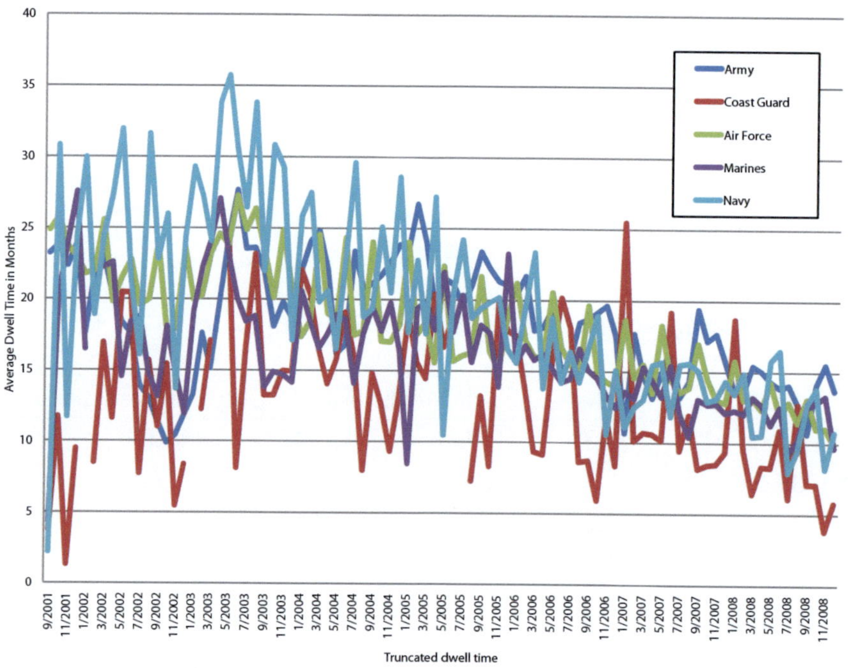


**FIGURE 3.2** Average dwell time, by deployment end date and branch, regular component only.

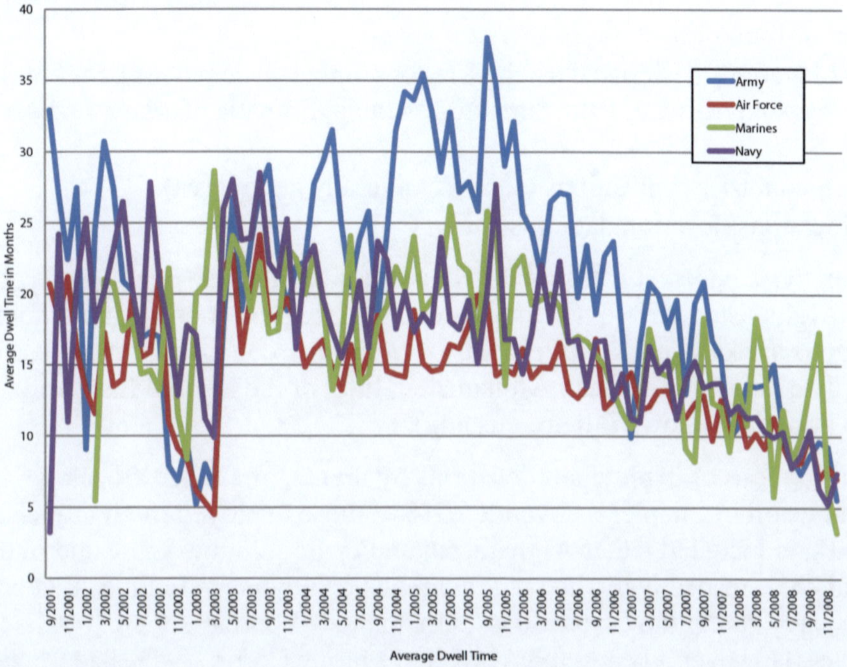


**FIGURE 3.3** Average dwell time, by deployment end date and branch, reserve and Guard components only.

## Location of Deployment

Understanding where military members deployed can be just as important as understanding how long and how often they deployed. The statement of task and the focus of this report is on *all those deployed to OEF and OIF*, including (a) those *physically located* within the OEF and OIF combat zones or areas of operation (AORs) and (b) those *specifically identified* by their service as "directly supporting" the OEF and/or OIF mission outside the designated combat zone. For many purposes, a more refined analysis would focus on deployed members who specifically served in the combat areas of operation in Afghanistan, Iraq, or both. While the DOD DMDC Contingency Tracking System contains data fields for specifying the location of each deployment designated as in direct support of the OEF, OIF, or OND mission, some individual records do not have movements in and out of country. In particular, before 2005, while DMDC did track deployments to Iraq and Afghanistan, the location codes were mostly unknown or based on the embarkation country for the service members (such as Bahrain, Kuwait, and Qatar). In 2005, the Defense Theater Accountability System increased the level of detail to include each change in country during a given service member's deployment. Thus, use of only the Afghanistan and Iraq country codes to identify those who served in these AORs would underestimate the numbers of service members who actually served there from September 11, 2001, through 2010.

Because that distinction is likely to be raised in many discussions on the impact of deployment on service members, veterans, and their families in the years ahead, we sought to explore the data further. Specifically, using the country codes, each deployment location in the file was service-classified as

- Afghanistan or Iraq.
- Middle East locations designated as eligible for combat-zone pay or benefits (Djibouti, Israel, Jordan, Kyrgyzstan, Kuwait, Pakistan, Saudi Arabia, Somalia, Turkey, Uzbekistan, and Yemen).
- Other known countries or locations (such as Germany and Korea).
- Unknown locations (location data missing).

Based on those codes, it was possible to categorize all those deployed as (1) at least one deployment to Afghanistan or Iraq; (2) at least one Middle East country and all other deployment countries/locations are known; (3) Middle East and/or other countries, with at least one unknown location; (4) only countries other than Afghanistan, Iraq, or the Middle East; and (5) none of the deployment locations are known (all are missing).

The distributions of deployment locations by branch of service are shown in Table 3.15 and described in detail in Chapter 2. Overall, 62% of those deployed in all branches had at least one deployment that included either Afghanistan and/or Iraq. In the Army and in the Marine Corps, 82% and 75%, respectively, had unambiguous deployments to those two countries. In contrast, in the Navy and in the Coast Guard, less than 20% and less than 10% had deployments to those countries. However, even in the Army and Marine Corps, 2–5% had no location coded for their deployments, and 15–17% had deployments to designated Middle East countries, some of which could well have been points of embarkation for Afghanistan or Iraq. Nearly 57% of those deployed in the Navy had no location specified, and over half those in the Coast Guard were deployed to other known countries and locations. Distributions by component show less variation in deployments by location in the regular and two reserve components. When they are examined by branch and component (Table 3.16), the differences described by branch on the average tended to be greater among the regular components (for example, 88% of those in the regular Army were deployed to Afghanistan or Iraq, and 62% of the regular Navy had no location specified).

**TABLE 3.15** Distribution of Deployment Location of Deployed Service Members, by Service Branch, as of 2010

| Deployment Location | Army, N (column %) | Navy, N (column %) | Air Force, N (column %) | Marine Corps, N (column %) | Coast Guard, N (column %) | TOTAL, N (column %) |
|---|---|---|---|---|---|---|
| Afghanistan or Iraq known | 881,444 (81.5) | 67,138 (17.5) | 179,146 (43.2) | 196,295 (75.0) | 564 (9.3) | 1,324,587 (61.9) |
| Middle East only or Middle East and other known location | 154,407 (14.3) | 31,452 (8.2) | 72,852 (17.6) | 42,604 (16.3) | 1,531 (25.2) | 302,846 (14.1) |
| Middle East only or Middle East and other known location and unknown other location | 10,936 (1.0) | 31,575 (8.2) | 31,609 (7.6) | 4,534 (1.7) | 31,609 (7.6) | 78,774 (3.7) |
| Known other location | 8,872 (0.8) | 35,220 (9.2) | 65,770 (15.9) | 4,064 (1.6) | 3,282 (53.9) | 117,208 (5.5) |

| Deployment Location | Army, N (column %) | Navy, N (column %) | Air Force, N (column %) | Marine Corps, N (column %) | Coast Guard, N (column %) | TOTAL, N (column %) |
|---|---|---|---|---|---|---|
| Unknown location | 25,528 (2.4) | 218,477 (56.9) | 65,236 (15.7) | 14,155 (5.4) | 587 (9.7) | 323,983 (15.1) |
| TOTAL | 1,081,187 | 383,862 | 414,613 | 261,652 | 6,084 | 2,147,398 |

SOURCE: Defense Manpower Data Center.

**TABLE 3.16** Distribution of Deployment Location of Deployed Service Members, by Component, as of 2010

| Deployment Location | Regular, N (column %) | National Guard, N (column %) | Reserves, N (column %) | TOTAL, N (column %) |
|---|---|---|---|---|
| Afghanistan or Iraq known | 882,603 (61.4) | 254,865 (67.3) | 187,119 (56.3) | 1,324,587 (61.7) |
| Middle East only or Middle East and other known location | 175,727 (12.2) | 56,926 (15.0) | 70,175 (21.1) | 302,846 (14.1) |
| Middle East only or Middle East and/or other known location and unknown other location | 50,965 (3.6) | 13,598 (3.6) | 14,211 (4.3) | 78,774 (3.7) |
| Known other location | 94,752 (6.6) | 9,168 (2.4) | 13,286 (4.0) | 117,208 (5.5) |
| Unknown location | 232,618 (16.2) | 43,948 (11.6) | 47,414 (14.3) | 323,986 (15.1) |
| TOTAL | 1,436,665 | 378,805 | 332,205 | 2,147,375 |

NOTE: Entire file contained 2,147,398, but 23 had an unknown component.
SOURCE: Defense Manpower Data Center.

## SUMMARY

The chapter describes the basic characteristics of all those deployed in support of OEF and/or OIF between September 11, 2001, and December 31, 2010. Of the 2.15 million who were deployed during that period, over half were in the Army—nearly one-third in the regular Army alone—and those in the National Guard and reserves combined constituted one-third of those deployed. Over 85% of those deployed were enlisted, and 12% were women, including 20% of the junior officers in the Air Force. The average age of those deployed was 33.4 years—from an average of 29.5 years in the Marine Corps to an average of 35.8 years in the Air Force. Those deployed from the reserves and National Guard were older. Over two-thirds had a high-school degree or equivalent, and over 30% had at least some college education. Nearly 60% of those deployed were married, and nearly half had dependent children, 1.97 on average. By the end of 2010, the 2.15 million service members had been deployed an average of 1.7 times: 57% once, 27% twice, 10% three times, and 6% four or more times. Those in the National Guard and reserves had fewer multiple deployments than those in the regular component. The average length of deployments was 7.7 months—from an average of 4.5 months in the Air Force to an average of 9.4 months in the Army. The average cumulative length of deployments of multiple deployers was 16.9 months. The average dwell time between deployments was 21 months.

## REFERENCE

Bonds, T. M., D. Baiocchi, and L. L. McDonald. 2010. *Army Deployments of OIF and OEF*. Santa Monica, CA: RAND Corporation.

# 4

# LONG-TERM OUTCOMES

This chapter explores long-term outcomes associated with diagnoses of mild traumatic brain injury (TBI), posttraumatic stress disorder (PTSD), or other mental-health disorders, such as depression, substance-use disorders (SUDs), and suicidal ideation. The committee focused on those outcomes as TBI and mental-health disorders were highlighted in the legislation directing its task. Not everyone who receives a diagnosis of any of those conditions will necessarily experience the sequelae discussed. Many active-duty personnel and veterans will return home and not have any adverse effects, however, others will suffer the consequences of deployment. Many of those who receive diagnoses of the outcomes discussed in this chapter will need support from family members and friends, treatment, and programs to assist them.

The committee has defined long-term outcomes as those lasting more than 6 months from the time of diagnosis. The committee did not conduct an exhaustive evidence-based review of the literature (see Chapter 2). It reviewed studies that focused on mild TBI, PTSD, and other mental-health disorders and possible outcomes in Operation Enduring Freedom (OEF) and Operation Iraqi Freedom (OIF) active-duty and veterans. If studies of OEF and OIF personnel were not available, studies of other combat veterans and civilians were included. The committee did not attempt to describe every study in detail but rather highlighted studies and reviews that demonstrated an outcome associated with the conditions of interest. The committee notes that there are difficulties in untangling long-term outcomes from preexisting disease, from diseases that have similar symptoms, and from various comorbid conditions that might occur with the conditions of interest. In its review of the literature, the committee also has summarized and included in this chapter relevant sections of recent Institute of Medicine (IOM) reports: *Gulf War and Health, Volume 6: Physiologic, Psychologic, and Psychosocial Effects of Deployment-Related Stress* (IOM, 2008a), *Gulf War and Health, Volume 7: Long-Term Consequences of Traumatic Brain Injury* (IOM, 2009), and *Returning Home from Iraq and Afghanistan: Preliminary Assessment of Readjustment Needs of Veterans, Service Members, and Their Families* (IOM, 2010).

Since the committee's Phase 1 report, a large volume of government-sponsored research, statistics, reports, and peer-reviewed studies have been published and a significant portfolio of research has been funded. Despite the focused efforts of DOD and VA to increase understanding of the risk and resiliency factors, military occupational exposures, health consequences, and readjustment challenges of those who had wartime service in Iraq and Afghanistan, the committee finds that the efforts to date do not provide definitive answers sought nor do they adequately address the major concerns faced by combat veterans. Although the last decade has seen much advancement in the empirical documentation of combat exposures and postwar outcomes in military service members, there is still a need for further elucidation of key research questions and improvement in study design. For example, Tanielian and Jaycox (2008) reviewed 22 epidemiologic studies of returnees from deployment to OEF and OIF and found that only one included clinical diagnostic assessment for PTSD and other psychiatric disorders. The other 21 studies identified "cases" solely on the basis of brief, self-report screening scales or from medical record reviews. Although screening scales and medical records are useful for many purposes, Tanielian and Jaycox note that using either as the sole basis of estimating the prevalence of PTSD and other psychiatric disorders is fraught with hazard—a finding echoed by an earlier IOM report (2006).

Our understanding of the health consequences of service in Iraq and Afghanistan remains incomplete; even simple questions such as prevalence rates of physical and psychologic morbidity after military service in Iraq or Afghanistan continue to lack precision. For example, the literature reviewed by the committee reported PTSD prevalence rates that ranged from approximately 1% to 30% in different studies. Those wide-ranging prevalence estimates have added to the public's confusion, have not been informative for health care planning, and fail to assist in projecting long term readjustment needs. As noted previously by the committee, these differences might be explained by variations in study design factors including, population sampling strategy (e.g., random versus nonrandom samples; deployed population versus individuals seeking health care); use of different screening instruments or the same instrument with different cutoff values; self-reports versus medical record reviews versus clinician examinations; levels of combat exposure; length, number, and time elapsed after deployment; demographic and service-related characteristics including military component (Reserve/National Guard versus active); military training and occupation (combat versus combat support); and Service (Air Force, Army, Marines versus Navy). Accounting for, understanding, and reconciling those differences to provide the insights and answers needed for effective public policy, prevention, treatment and readjustment purposes has proved difficult.

## ORGANIZATION OF THE CHAPTER

This chapter is organized into six main sections: mild TBI, PTSD, depression, substance-use disorders, suicide and suicidal ideation, and women's health outcomes. The TBI section begins with a definition of TBI and how its severity is measured; discusses what we have learned about TBI (of all levels of severity) from previous wars and in civilian populations (primarily summarized from *Gulf War and Health, Volume 7: Long-Term Consequences of Traumatic Brain Injury* [IOM, 2009]); includes a rationale for the committee's focus on mild TBI; presents the methodologic difficulties in studying mild TBI in the OEF and OIF populations; and discusses outcomes and conditions that are often comorbid with mild TBI. It also includes a subsection that focuses on the complexity in separating the effects of TBI from those due to co-morbid conditions such as PTSD, depression, and other mental-health disorders.

The remaining sections of the chapter include a discussion of PTSD, associated outcomes, and comorbidities, followed by discussions of depression, substance-use disorders, and suicidal ideation and associated outcomes, comorbidities, and risk or protective factors. The final major section focuses on women's health outcomes in active-duty and veteran populations.

The issue of comorbidity is a recurring theme in this chapter and adds complexity to a study of outcomes. The committee found that in many cases it was difficult or impossible to separate sequelae from comorbid conditions and often could not make the distinction accurately. In fact, the construct of comorbidity does not do justice to the complexity that clinicians and service members encounter when attempting to understand symptoms. From the perspective of an individual patient, an event that is experienced is coupled with the biopsychosocial response to the event and might lead to a constellation of symptoms that express the particular circumstances. Our diagnostic systems cannot capture that level of complexity adequately, so we apply multiple diagnoses (such as depression, PTSD, and TBI) in our attempts to capture what is observed in the individual patient. From the perspective of the population, we divide people who experience symptoms and signs of various classes (such as cognitive, mood, and anxiety) into discrete categories for a host of purposes (such as case counting and assignment to standard protocols of diagnosis and treatment); but the categorization does not do justice to the reality of the distribution of symptoms among individuals in the population.

## TRAUMATIC BRAIN INJURY

TBI is a common injury of the wars in Iraq and Afghanistan. The Department of Defense (DOD) and Veterans Brain Injury Center estimate that brain injuries account for 22% of all OEF and OIF combat casualties, whereas in Vietnam only 12% of combat casualties were attributed to brain injuries (Summerall, 2012). Several organizations, such as the American Congress of Rehabilitation Medicine and the Brain Injury Association of America, and government agencies, such as the National Institutes of Health and the Centers for Disease Control and Prevention (CDC), have developed definitions of TBI, but the committee will focus on the definition developed by DOD and the Department of Veterans Affairs (VA) as it focuses on service members and veterans.

The DOD–VA common definition of TBI is

> A traumatically induced structural injury and/or physiological disruption of brain function as a result of an external force that is indicated by new onset or worsening of at least one of the following clinical signs, immediately following the event (DOD, 2009a), such as
> - Any period of loss of or a decreased level of consciousness;
> - Any loss of memory for events immediately before or after the injury;
> - Any alteration in mental state at the time of the injury (confusion, disorientation, slowed thinking, etc.);
> - Neurological deficits (weakness, loss of balance, change in vision, praxis, paresis/plegia, sensory loss, aphasia, etc.) that may or may not be transient;
> - Intracranial lesion.

The DOD–VA guidance notes that external forces may include any of the following events: the head being struck by an object, the head striking an object, the brain undergoing an acceleration/deceleration movement without direct external trauma to the head, a foreign body penetrating the brain, forces generated from events such as a blast or explosion, or other force yet to be defined. Not all individuals exposed to an external force will sustain a TBI.

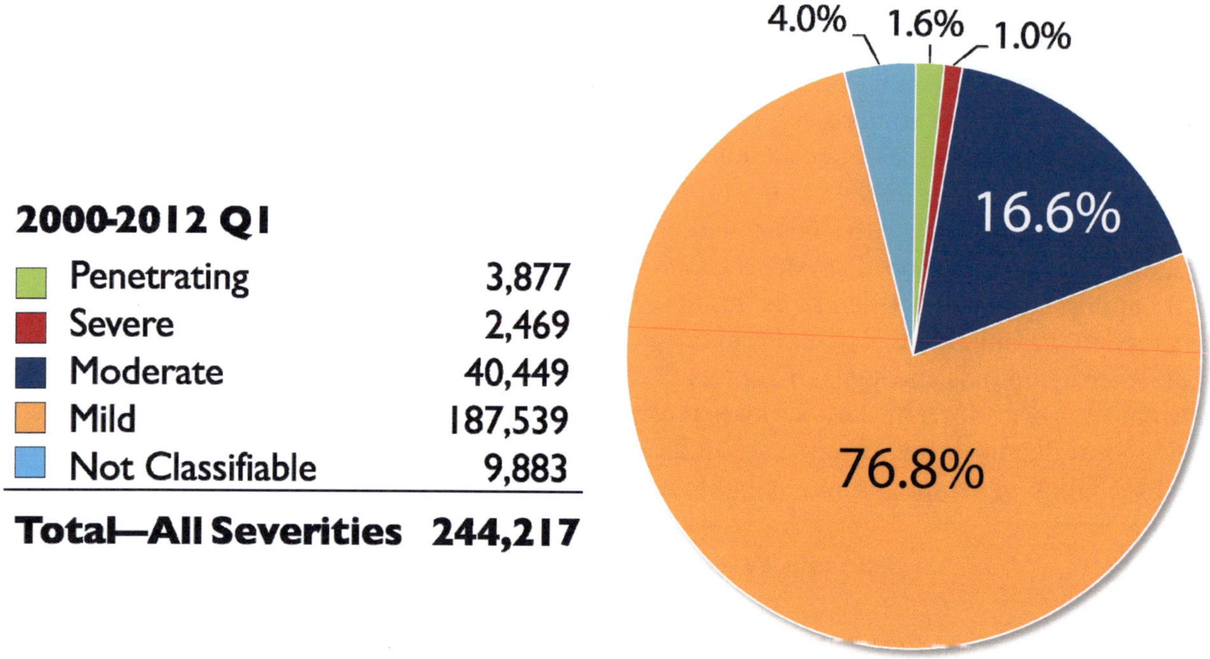


**FIGURE 4.1** TBI by severity in all armed forces, 2000–2011, as of May 16, 2012.
SOURCE: DVBIC, 2012.

A TBI may be closed or penetrating. TBI is often classified according to severity: mild, moderate, or severe. A mild TBI is typically referred to as a concussion, and the two terms are often used interchangeably. In a review of TBI incidence by severity, the number of mild TBIs suffered by all the armed forces far exceeds the numbers of penetrating, severe, or moderate TBIs; in fact, mild TBI accounts for 76.8% of all brain injures (see Figure 4.1).

## Severity

TBI, as noted above, is categorized as mild, moderate, or severe. TBIs can also be penetrating or closed head injuries. Severity is typically based on measures of loss of consciousness (LOC) and posttraumatic amnesia; alteration of consciousness and structural imaging are also used to determine acute severity (see Table 4.1).

**TABLE 4.1** Criteria for Assessing Severity of TBI

| Measuring Severity | Mild | Moderate | Severe |
|---|---|---|---|
| Structural imaging | Normal | Normal or abnormal | Normal or abnormal |
| Loss of consciousness | Up to 30 minutes | 30 minutes–24 hours | Over 24 hours |
| Alteration of consciousness | Up to 24 hours | Over 24 hours | Over 24 hours |
| Posttraumatic amnesia | Up to 1 day | 1–7 days | Over 7 days |
| Glasgow Coma Scale rating | 13–15 | 9–12 | 3–8 |

SOURCE: Adapted from VA and DOD, 2009.

**TABLE 4.2** Glasgow Coma Scale

| Type of Response and Score | | Type of Response and Score | | Type of Response and Score | |
|---|---|---|---|---|---|
| Eye Opening: | | Motor: | | Verbal: | |
| Spontaneous | 4 | Obeys commands | 6 | Alert and oriented | 5 |
| To speech | 3 | Localizes pain | 5 | Confused, yet coherent | 4 |
| To pain | 2 | Withdraws from pain | 5 | Inappropriate words | 3 |
| No eye-opening | 1 | Abnormal flexion | 4 | Incomprehensible sounds | 2 |
| | | Extensor response- | 3 | No sounds | 1 |
| | | No response | 2 | | |

NOTE: Overall score is the sum of all scores.
SOURCE: Adapted from IOM, 2009; adapted from Teasdale and Jennett, 1974.

Although the above definitions, except the Glasgow Coma Scale (GCS), rely on length of impaired consciousness, depth of impaired consciousness as measured with the GCS is another method used to classify acute severity of the injury (see Table 4.2) (Teasdale and Jennett, 1974). The GCS is useful in diagnosing moderate and severe TBI, but most civilian and combat TBIs are in the mild range (GCS 13–15) with little differentiation in outcomes.

## TRAUMATIC BRAIN INJURY OUTCOMES FROM PREVIOUS WARS AND THE CIVILIAN POPULATION

### Traumatic Brain Injury and Cognition in Active-Duty Personnel and Veterans of Previous Wars and in Civilians

Over the last 30 years, much has been learned about the nature of impairments, disabilities, and participation problems that occur in the survivors of civilian closed TBI. Numerous neuropsychologic difficulties—such as problems with memory, attention, executive functions, and speed of information processing—are frequent consequences of TBI (Dikmen et al., 1990, 1995; Levin et al., 1990). Research has also determined that neuropsychologic outcome after TBI is significantly related to the severity of the brain injury (that is, whether it is penetrating or closed and whether it is mild, moderate, or severe). On the basis of review of available literature, a recent IOM report (2009) concluded that the presence, degree, and nature of cognitive impairments depend on the severity of the brain injury.

The results of research on the cognitive effects of penetrating brain injuries in military populations in previous wars clearly and consistently show a decline in cognitive functioning as a result of brain injury (Corkin et al., 1989; Grafman et al., 1986, 1988, 1990; Raymont et al., 2008; Salazar et al., 1986; Teuber and Weinstein, 1954; Weinstein and Teuber, 1957). Research also indicates that the decline is related to the volume of brain tissue lost (Grafman et al., 1988) and the affected region of the brain (Corkin et al., 1989). And there is evidence from long-term longitudinal studies that over many years intellectual ability continues to decline at a greater rate in veterans who have penetrating brain injuries than in veterans who do not (Corkin et al., 1989; Raymont et al., 2008).

Most studies of civilians who have mild TBI have found early neuropsychologic deficits that resolve by 1–3 months after injury in most cases (McCrea et al., 2009). Belanger et al.

(2005) performed a meta-analysis of 39 studies of 1,463 adults who had non-sports-related mild TBI and 1,191 control cases. They excluded sports-related injuries from their meta-analysis and included only those who sought medical attention for mild TBI. Their results indicate that the overall size of the effect of mild TBI on neuropsychologic functioning was moderate. However, the results varied by type of cognition affected, time since injury, patient characteristics, and sampling methods. Delayed memory and fluency were the types of cognition most affected by mild TBI when measured less than 3 months after injury. There were no neuropsychologic effects of mild TBI by 3 months after injury in unselected or representative, prospectively studied samples of subjects. However, clinic-based samples or groups involved in litigation showed greater cognitive sequelae of mild TBI at 3 months or more after injury. Moreover, litigation was associated with stable or worsening neuropsychologic performance. Belanger and Vanderploeg (2005) performed a separate meta-analysis of the neuropsychologic effects of sports-related concussion. They examined 21 studies that included 790 cases of sports-related concussion and 2,014 control cases. The results indicated that the overall effect size of concussion ($d = 0.49$) was similar to that found with mild TBI. Effect size was greater in studies that included subjects who had additional prior head injury than in studies that excluded subjects who had prior head injury. Neuropsychologic impairments were no longer found when testing occurred later than 7–10 days after injury. Such impairments are measured by psychometric testing and do not necessarily pertain to subjective neuropsychologic complaints.

On the basis of the literature, TBI clearly has an effect on cognitive functions with a clear dose–response relationship. However, the findings regarding mild TBI indicate that there is insufficient evidence that a single, mild civilian TBI has long-term effects on cognition (Dikmen et al., 2009; IOM, 2009). There may be differences between civilian and military exposures, including "blast" due to improvised explosive devises and other explosive munitions.

### Traumatic Brain Injury and Postconcussive Symptoms in Active-Duty Personnel and Veterans of Previous Wars and in Civilians

IOM recently reviewed studies that evaluated the relationship between TBI and self-reported symptoms (2009). The results of studies of mild TBI (Gerber and Schraa, 1995; Heitger et al., 2007; Mickeviciene et al., 2002, 2004; Stulemeijer et al., 2006) varied, but the majority of evidence indicated that those who had mild TBI reported significantly more symptoms than those whose injuries did not involve the head. Dikmen et al. (2010) examined rates of new or worse symptoms 1 month and 1 year after civilian TBI in a large, representative series of cases and compared symptom reports with those of people whose injuries spared the head. The TBI group reported significantly more symptoms than the control group at 1 month and 1 year after injury. Symptom reports declined from 1 month to 1 year after injury, but 53% of the TBI group and 24% of the control group continued to report three or more symptoms at 1 year after injury. The most frequently reported symptoms at 1 year were problems with memory, concentration, fatigue, anxiety, and irritability. People who had severe TBI reported significantly more problems with memory, temper, and irritability and had three or more symptoms compared with controls at 1 year after injury. There were no significant differences between the most mildly injured TBI group and controls, possibly because the TBI group was small. However, those in the mild TBI group did endorse the majority of symptoms at least 50% more often than the controls at 1 year after injury. In fact, 44% of the mild TBI group reported three or more symptoms at 1 year after injury. Similar rates were reported in a very mild TBI sample 6 months after injury (Bell et al., 2008) and in a nonhospitalized population-based sample of very mild TBI 3 months after injury (Lannsjo et al., 2009). The rates are much higher than the common belief that the occurrence of three or more symptoms for more than a month after a mild TBI is rare and occurs in less than 5% of the population (McCrea et al., 2009).

### Traumatic Brain Injury and Depression in Active-Duty Personnel and Veterans of Previous Wars and in Civilians

The recent IOM review of this literature (2009) found strong evidence of an association between TBI and depression. Regardless of the severity of the TBI (mild, moderate, or severe), the rates of major depression 6 months or more after injury are higher than in control groups. The association could not be totally explained by depression before injury (Fann et al., 2004; Jorge et al., 2004; Vanderploeg et al., 2007). In addition, there is some evidence that prior mood disorder may predispose to TBI (Fann et al., 2002; Vassallo et al., 2007), and depression after TBI is more frequent in those who had depression before the injury than in those who did not (Bombardier et al., 2010; Fann et al., 2004). For instance, Bombardier et al. (2010) found that although about 70% of the cases with preinjury depression showed major depressive disorder by 1 year after injury, only 41% of the cases with no prior history did so.

The strong association between depression and TBI has also been reported in studies of World War II and Vietnam veterans. Holsinger et al. (2002) found that the odds of lifetime and current major depression were significantly higher in World War II veterans who had TBI than in controls. In addition, the odds of lifetime depression were highest in those who sustained severe TBI. The odds of depression also increased as the veterans aged. There is some evidence that depression is associated with mild TBI in veterans. A study of postdischarge Vietnam veterans found that those who reported mild TBI had a significantly higher frequency of depression than the control group (Vanderploeg et al., 2007).

### Traumatic Brain Injury and Social Functioning in Active-Duty Personnel and Veterans of Previous Wars and in Civilians

A recent review by IOM (2009) concluded that TBI can have adverse effects on all aspects of social functioning, including employment, social relationships, independent living, functional status, and leisure activities. Research in civilians has shown that the severity of TBI decreases the probability of employment after injury and lengthens the time to return to work (Dikmen et al., 1993, 1994; Doctor et al., 2005; Oddy et al., 1978). There is evidence of an association between penetrating TBI and long-term unemployment in the military (Schwab et al., 1993), and return to work has been associated with computed-tomography findings in veterans who had penetrating head injury (Groswasser et al., 2002). For more comprehensive information about the effects of TBI on employment and other aspects of social functioning, see IOM (2009).

### Traumatic Brain Injury in the Operation Enduring Freedom and Operation Iraqi Freedom Populations and the Committee's Focus on Mild Traumatic Brain Injury

TBI is a common injury of the wars in Iraq (OIF) and Afghanistan (OEF). A recent report on US army soldiers deployed in 2001–2007 found that 0.14% (207 of 145,505) of those deployed to Afghanistan and 0.31% (2,241 of 722,474) of those deployed to Iraq had one or more TBI-related hospitalizations. Almost all those had moderate or severe brain injuries

(Wojcik et al., 2010). However, the estimated number of cases of mild TBI outweighs all the other types of brain injury. As noted early in this chapter, 76.8% of all brain injuries in OEF and OIF are considered mild TBI.

The committee decided to focus its attention on mild TBI because the vast majority of TBI in OEF and OIF is considered mild, it is difficult to identify and diagnose mild TBI, and long-term outcomes of mild TBI are much less understood than those of moderate and severe TBI (see IOM, 2009). In fact, many veterans returning from OEF and OIF have presented to the VA with symptoms of mild TBI, although they had not received the diagnosis while on active duty (Elder and Cristian, 2009). In an attempt at earlier diagnosis, DOD began screening all soldiers for mild TBI on their return from deployment by using the Post-Deployment Health Assessment (PDHA) and the Post-Deployment Health Reassessment (PDHRA).[1] In addition, DOD began to assess soldiers with the Military Acute Concussion Evaluation while they were still on active duty, and VA began to screen all OEF and OIF veterans for mild TBI when they were seen by VA medical care providers.

The prevalence of mild TBI in the OEF- and OIF-deployed is based on a few large studies that have reported estimates of probable TBI of around 20%. For example, RAND conducted a telephone survey of 1,938 soldiers who had been deployed in OEF and OIF to determine probable TBI and other mental-health issues. Probable TBI was determined by the Brief Traumatic Brain Injury Screen, which was considered positive for probable TBI if a soldier reported being injured during deployment and experienced "being dazed, confused or seeing stars," "not remembering the injury," or "losing consciousness." Results were weighted to improve the representativeness of the sample. The results of the study indicate that 19.5% had probable TBI (Tanielian and Jaycox, 2008).

Finally, all 3,973 members of a brigade combat team returning to Fort Carson from a 1-year deployment to Iraq were screened with the Warrior Administered Retrospective Casualty Assessment Tool (WARCAT). The WARCAT is a self-administered tool for ascertaining detailed information regarding injury; it enables soldiers to indicate whether they were injured through mechanisms commonly associated with TBI while deployed, whether any of their injuries resulted in an altered mental state, and whether symptoms often associated with mild TBI occurred after their injury. After completing the WARCAT, all soldiers were interviewed by a clinician, all available medical records were reviewed, and information was obtained from witnesses. The results indicate that 22.8% of the brigade had sustained a probable deployment-related mild TBI (Terrio et al., 2009).

A recent longitudinal study of a National Guard brigade combat team found much lower rates of mild TBI in theater than previous studies (Polusny et al., 2011). The authors administered an adapted version of the Defense and Veterans Brain Injury Center screening tool to determine probable mild TBI in a large group of soldiers still in Iraq who would be returning from deployment in about 1 month and then again 1 year after their return from deployment. Soldiers were determined to have a history of in-theater mild TBI if they endorsed an injury with altered mental status or loss of consciousness. The initial assessment, while the soldiers were still deployed, resulted in self-reporting of mild TBI in 9% of the cases. That percentage more than

[1]The PDHA is given immediately on return from deployment. The PDHRA, mandated by the assistant secretary of defense for health affairs, has been used since March 2005; it provides a second health assessment and is meant to be completed 90–180 days after return to home station from deployment.

doubled to 22% a year after return from deployment. It is not clear whether those results are due to recall bias, to soldiers' minimizing their reports of mild TBI so that they might remain with their units, to soldiers' wanting to ensure that health concerns did not delay their return home, to poor reliability of the questionnaire, or to other issues associated with attribution of current psychosocial difficulties to mild TBI.

**Methodologic Problems in Studies of Mild Traumatic Brain Injury in Operation Enduring Freedom and Operation Iraqi Freedom Populations**

Most epidemiologic studies have methodologic problems, but the outcomes being studied are often easier to identify or measure than those associated with mild TBI. The methodologic problems in the existing studies of mild TBI sustained during OEF and OIF conflicts add to the complexity of understanding the outcomes. The problems include the use of convenience samples of soldiers recently returned from deployment or convenience samples of soldiers receiving clinical care many months after sustaining mild TBI. The use of convenience samples makes it difficult to generalize study results to the entire military population engaged in OEF and OIF. Furthermore, many of the studies of mild TBI have involved small groups of subjects receiving clinical services typically in the VA health care system (Belanger et al., 2009; Campbell et al., 2009; Cooper et al., 2011). Many of the groups studied have substantially different demographic features, differ in the amount of time that has passed since the mild TBI, and often comprise people who had more complex outcomes; all those factors might affect the results of the studies.

In addition, many studies have low enrollment rates. For example, although Wilk et al. (2010b) studied outcomes in 3,952 soldiers after their return from Iraq, participants made up only 52% of the sample population surveyed. Similarly, the Hoge et al. (2008) study represented 59% of the sample, and Brenner et al. (2010b) approached 399 soldiers back from their second deployment to Iraq but had only a 12% enrollment rate. The effects of low enrollment rates are unknown, but one must seriously consider participation bias as having a potentially important effect on study results.

Many studies of mild TBI do not include a control group. A control group is essential to rule out the effect of other factors—such as physical, emotional, and preinjury characteristics—to determine whether an outcome is due to the TBI. Some studies have compared service members returning from OEF and OIF who have no injuries (control group) with those who self-report a mild TBI and a subset of the mild-TBI group who also self-report postconcussion symptoms (Roebuck-Spencer et al., 2012) or with those who report injuries to the body but not to the head (Hoge et al., 2008). Those strategies attempt to compare people drawn from the same population (such as deployed service members), but it is unclear whether the groups are similar with respect to other relevant characteristics that might influence outcomes.

The determination of probable mild TBI in an active-duty soldier is by necessity through self-reporting with little or no acute-injury information from the field to accompany or substantiate the diagnosis. And a report of mild TBI is typically related to distant events that could have occurred at any time during deployment. Retrospective recall of events is likely to introduce bias. Another complicating factor is a determination of the number of possible TBIs and when they were sustained.

The questions used in screening subjects for mild TBI vary among researchers, and the psychometric properties of the measures are often unknown. Other methodologic problems include lack of information about baseline neuropsychologic functioning and other information about the individual, including demographic information and preexisting psychiatric or neurologic conditions or substance-use disorders; all these can complicate the effects of mild TBI on outcomes.

## Traumatic Brain Injury Outcomes and Comorbidities in Operation Enduring Freedom and Operation Iraqi Freedom Populations

The presence of conditions that present as comorbid with mild TBI, such as PTSD or depression, makes it difficult to separate the outcomes related to mild TBI from the outcomes related to the comorbid conditions. This issue is the subject of current research. The subsections below discuss outcomes associated with mild TBI and outcomes of conditions that appear to be comorbid with mild TBI. The overall subject of comorbidities and the difficulties presented in diagnosis and treatment is discussed in detail in the section "Mild Traumatic Brain Injury, Comorbidities, and Complicated Issues of Causality in Operation Enduring Freedom and Operation Iraqi Freedom Populations."

### Mild Traumatic Brain Injury and Cognition in Operation Enduring Freedom and Operation Iraqi Freedom Populations

There has been a paucity of research on the cognitive effects of mild TBI sustained during the current conflicts and assessed with formal performance measures. Most studies suffer from the methodologic problems described above. There is some evidence that mild TBI has cognitive effects soon after injury. Luethcke et al. (2011) examined 82 active-duty military personnel and a few civilian contractors referred to an outpatient TBI clinic at a combat support hospital in Iraq within 72 hours of mild TBI; they were assessed on measures of cognitive performance with the Automated Neuropsychological Assessment Metrics (ANAM).[2] Subjects were divided into those who had blast injuries and those who had nonblast injuries on the basis of clinical interviews. The authors examined the magnitude of change in ANAM from baseline (before deployment) to after injury in a subsample of 53 who completed the ANAM before deployment. The results indicated significantly worse reaction time from baseline to after injury. Differences were not found between those injured by blast and those injured who had nonblast injuries. Accuracy was also significantly related to duration of loss of consciousness rather than to type of injury.

Conflicting results with respect to the cognitive effects of mild TBI have been reported when cognition was evaluated months after mild TBI, that is, once the service members had returned from deployment. Brailey (2009) conducted a prospective and longitudinal study that examined the effects of mild TBI on postdeployment cognitive performance. The author examined 780 active-duty soldiers who had been deployed to Iraq before deployment (Time 1) and after deployment (Time 2) and collected data on cognitive measures by using a series of hierarchic regressions. The cognitive measures administered before and after deployment

[2]The ANAM is a neurocognitive assessment tool designed to detect speed and accuracy of attention, memory, and thinking ability. It records a service member's performance through responses provided on a computer.

included several tests of neuropsychologic functioning, including the Trail Making Test, Wechsler Memory Scale Verbal Paired Associates and Visual Reproduction subtests (Wechsler, 2009), and the Neurobehavioral Evaluation System Continuous Performance Test (Letz, 1990) and measures from the ANAM (Reeves et al., 1992). The cognitive functions evaluated included attention, executive functioning, learning and memory, psychomotor problems, and self-reported health and cognitive problems. In the sample, 70 soldiers reported deployment-related TBI with LOC, and 87 soldiers screened positive for deployment-related PTSD. Predictors of postdeployment cognitive outcome were entered into the regression in steps starting with the relevant predeployment cognitive function; then demographics, mild TBI, and emotional status (such as PTSD or depression or deployment risk and resilience inventory); and finally interactions between mild TBI and emotional status. The results indicated that PTSD was a reliable predictor of postdeployment cognitive outcome. The pattern of results was similar when self-reported depression was substituted for PTSD. However, self-reported mild TBI was not a significant predictor of cognitive outcome.

Roebuck-Spencer et al. (2012) found cognitive decline in a sample of people who reported mild TBI as a result of their most recent deployment. The authors obtained deidentified data on 10,869 service members who were deployed to OIF and OEF and who had been evaluated with the ANAM version 4 TBI battery before and less than 1 week after return from deployment. The average test–retest interval was 398 days. The 1,609 service members who reported having sustained one or more TBIs in the 4 years before deployment were excluded. The remaining subjects were divided into four groups on the basis of their responses to the TBI questionnaire. Mild TBI was defined as an injury with alteration of consciousness. Those who reported no TBI or other important injury during their most recent deployment formed the control group of 8,002. A sample of 400 of the controls was randomly selected for use in the analysis. Those who reported one or more TBIs in their most recent deployment were divided into those reporting current symptoms (197) and those who had no current symptoms (305) at the postdeployment evaluation. A small fourth group (28) consisted of those who reported an injury but not TBI during their most recent deployment and who had current symptoms. Cognitive performance was evaluated by using a composite score that covered all the ANAM tests.

The results showed that there were no significant differences between the groups in predeployment ANAM performance. However, there were significant differences between the groups in postdeployment ANAM performance: the TBI group who had active symptoms performed significantly worse than controls ($p < 0.0001$) and worse than those who had TBI but no current symptoms ($p < 0.0001$). The control group and the TBI group who had no current symptoms were not significantly different in postdeployment ANAM performance. In addition, the control group showed significant predeployment–postdeployment improvement, the TBI group who had no current symptoms showed no predeployment–postdeployment change, and the TBI group who had current symptoms showed a significant predeployment–postdeployment decline in ANAM performance. Another analysis of the small group who were injured and had current symptoms but did not sustain TBI showed similar predeployment–postdeployment improvement in ANAM performance. In an analysis of reliable change using a 90% confidence interval (CI), 4.3% of the control group, 10.8% of the group who had TBI but no current symptoms, 10.7% of the non-TBI group, and 30.5% of the TBI group who had current symptoms had a clinically significant predeployment–postdeployment reduction in ANAM performance.

The authors note that 70% of those who reported TBI had no reduction in cognitive performance; this finding is consistent with the civilian literature. However, the authors did not have information on such comorbid conditions as PTSD, depression, or pain, so the results could not be taken into account as was possible in the study by Brailey (2009). Still, it is important to note that Brailey (2009) did not find a significant association between mild TBI and neuropsychologic performance even before adjusting for other factors, such as PTSD (Vasterling et al., 2012).[3] The evidence in the best literature suggests cognitive decline within days of mild TBI, but the evidence is mixed with respect to longer-term outcomes and the factors (mild TBI vs PTSD) that might be responsible for the decline in cognition.

**Mild Traumatic Brain Injury and Chronic Traumatic Encephalopathy in Operation Enduring Freedom and Operation Iraqi Freedom Populations**

As study of the effects of a single mild TBI has been generating information about time-limited cognitive problems or inconsistent findings, the construct of chronic traumatic encephalopathy (CTE) has been drawing increased attention. CTE is a long-term consequence of repetitive mild trauma to the brain. It is marked by progressive decline of memory and cognition and is often accompanied by suicidal behavior, poor impulse control, parkinsonism, and, in advanced cases, dementia.

With current methods, the diagnosis of CTE can be confirmed only at autopsy on the basis of the pathologic appearance of neurodegeneration, inflammation, and staining for the protein tau found in insoluble deposits of two types—neurofibrillary tangles and neuritic threads (Saulle and Greenwald, 2012; Shively et al., 2012; Stern et al., 2011). Previously called dementia pugilistica, CTE was first diagnosed in the 1920s in boxers (Martland, 1928), but it is now recognized as possibly occurring in several contact sports in which repetitive mild head injuries occur, namely, soccer, field hockey, boxing, and football. More recently, the diagnosis has been extended to combat veterans.

CTE has been studied most intensively in boxers. Several studies revealed consistently poorer performance on neuropsychologic tests, according to a previous IOM report on TBI (IOM, 2009). Boxers were found to have deficits in memory, information processing and speed, finger-tapping speed, attention and concentration, sequencing, and other characteristics in a standard neuropsychologic test battery (Drew et al., 1986; Porter, 2003; Porter and Fricker, 1996). The largest pathology study involved 15 retired boxers. Their autopsies revealed cerebellar damage, cortical damage, substantia nigra degeneration, and neurofibrillary tangles in the cerebral cortex and temporal areas (Corsellis et al., 1973).

Those findings were extended to football players and other athletes in professional contact sports, such as soccer, wrestling, and field hockey. The first autopsy study appeared in 2005 and included findings in a professional football player 12 years after retirement. There was no cortical atrophy, but CTE was evident in sparse neurofibrillary tangles and neuritic threads in neocortical areas but not in the hippocampus or entorhinal cortex (Omalu et al., 2005). A year later, the same investigators reported on a second autopsy case of a football player (Omalu et al., 2006), and that was followed by larger case series that showed the hallmark pathologic evidence of CTE: neurofibrillary tangles and neuritic threads in the cerebral cortex, neurodegeneration,

---

[3] Vasterling et al. (2012) used the same data as Brailey (2009).

and neuroinflammation (Omalu et al., 2010, 2011a). Pathologic findings were similar in two other case series of professional athletes (McKee et al., 2009, 2010).

The first postmortem case in blast-exposed veterans was reported in 2011 (Omalu et al., 2011b). The investigators reported degeneration characteristic of CTE: multifocal, neocortical, and subcortical neurofibrillary tangles and neuritic threads and mild fibrillary astrogliosis. The next published study was a controlled case series of four veterans who had a history of multiple blast or concussive injuries (Goldstein et al., 2012). The investigators had similar pathologic findings, including neurofibrillary and glial tangles in frontal, temporal, and parietal cortexes; tau immunoreactivity; myelinated axonopathy; and astrocytosis. The pathologic appearance in veterans was indistinguishable from that in four professional athletes who were studied as a comparator population. None of the features was seen in postmortem brains of age-matched normal subjects who had no history of blast or concussive injuries. The study also produced the first mouse model of blast injury, showing similar memory and cognitive deficits and CTE-like neurodegeneration, including tau immunoreactivity and astrocytosis, starting 2 weeks after a single blast exposure. Memory and cognitive deficits were prevented by head immobilization of the mice during blast exposure (Goldstein et al., 2012). The advent of this study and related studies indicates that this line of evidence is important for monitoring for repeated blast-exposed veterans and has generated increased interest in the neurobiologic basis of PTSD and TBI in combat veterans (Shively et al., 2012). No epidemiologic studies on OEF, OIF or OND active duty or veterans exist at present; the relevance of CTE to blast or concussive brain injuries remains to be studied.

**Mild Traumatic Brain Injury and Postconcussive Symptoms in Operation Enduring Freedom and Operation Iraqi Freedom Populations**

A variety of symptoms associated with mild TBI—including cognitive, somatic, and affective complaints—are collectively referred to as postconcussive symptoms (PCS). Research in service members who have returned from deployment to OEF and OIF has focused on whether mechanism of injury plays an important role in symptom reporting. There is some evidence that service members who report mild TBI with LOC from a blast have significantly higher rates of headaches and tinnitus after injury than those injured by a nonblast mechanism, although both groups report a variety of other posttraumatic symptoms. Wilk et al. (2010b) looked at self-reported concussion in US Army infantry soldiers 3–6 months after returning from a year-long deployment to Iraq. Of the 587 who met the criteria for concussion, 201 reported LOC and 373 reported an alteration of consciousness without LOC; 424 reported being in a blast, 150 did not experience a blast mechanism. Of those who experienced LOC, being in a blast was associated with headaches and tinnitus 3–6 months after deployment at a significantly higher rate than having been subject to a nonblast mechanism. However, in soldiers who had self-reported concussion and no LOC, blast was not associated more highly with physical or mental-health symptoms, absenteeism, or sick-call days than in those who reported a nonblast mechanism.

Studies that have examined other factors in relation to symptom reporting have concluded that symptom reporting is not specific to TBI alone and may be related to other co-occurring conditions or distressing experiences. For example, Hoge et al. (2008) used self-reported screening of 2,525 US Army infantry soldiers 3–4 months after their return from deployment to Iraq and found that 124 (4.9%) reported injuries with LOC, 260 (10.3%) reported injuries with altered mental state, and 435 (17.2%) reported other injuries during their deployment. Of those who had LOC, 43.9% met the criteria for PTSD, 27.3% reported altered mental state, 16.2% reported other injuries, and 9.1% reported no injury. The researchers found that soldiers who had mild TBI and had experienced LOC were more likely to report poor general health, more sick days and doctor visits, and a higher number of symptom complaints, including PCS, than soldiers who had other injuries. However, after adjustment for PTSD and depression, mild TBI was not found to be associated with adverse outcomes, except headache. Wilk et al. (2012) reported that multiple mild TBIs with LOC increased the odds of headache compared with a single mild TBI (odds ratio [OR] = 4.0, CI = 2.4–6.8), although depression also increased the odds of headache (OR = 4.2, CI = 2.6–6.8).

## Mental-Health Disorders Associated with Mild Traumatic Brain Injury

A recent review by IOM (2008a) concluded that service members deployed to a war zone have a greater prevalence of psychiatric disorders—especially PTSD, other anxiety disorders, and major depression—than veterans not deployed to a war zone. Another review notes that psychiatric disorders can contribute to disability in TBI and delay recovery (Silver et al., 2011). Rates of specific disorders in those who have TBI are presented below.

### Depression and Mild Traumatic Brain Injury in Operation Enduring Freedom and Operation Iraqi Freedom Populations

Depression and symptoms of depression are often seen in those who have brain injury. In military populations, the prevalence of depression in OEF and OIF participants has been reported by RAND. Findings of a 2008 study indicate that 13.7% of OEF and OIF veterans who served through October 2007 had a diagnosis of depression (Tanielian and Jaycox, 2008). Of those who received a diagnosis of TBI, 31.8% suffered from major depression. A study by Hoge et al. (2008) evaluated major depression in US soldiers returning from OIF. Depression was associated with brain injury and LOC (22.9%) more than with other system injury. Of soldiers who had brain injury and altered mental state but no LOC, only 8.4% met the criteria for depression.

### Substance-Use Disorders and Mild Traumatic Brain Injury

Whether survivors of mild TBI are at increased risk of substance-use disorders is unclear. Many studies have shown that drug and alcohol use often precede brain injury, but not many studies have examined whether sustaining a TBI, particularly a mild TBI, increases the likelihood of substance use in previous nonusing people. Studies based on civilian injuries that monitor substance use after head injury do not always indicate the severity of brain injury or include brain injury of all severity levels (e.g., Bombardier et al., 2003; Horner et al., 2005; Jorge et al., 2005). Most of the studies and reviews of the civilian population and one study of the military have indicated that there is an overall decline in substance use after TBI (Bombardier et al., 2003; Graham and Cardon, 2008; Heltemes et al., 2011), although a subset may continue heavy alcohol use (Bombardier et al., 2003). A 2009 IOM report on TBI concludes that there is limited but suggestive evidence of an association between TBI (of all severity levels) and *decreased* drug and alcohol use, relative to preinjury use, in the 1–3 years after the TBI. One civilian study of TBI found that the amount of drinking and reported problems with alcohol decreased, relative to the time before the injury, 1 month after injury but then increased at 1 year, although not to preinjury levels (Dikmen et al., 1995). Those who had more severe TBI decreased alcohol use significantly more than those who had milder TBIs.

**Suicidal Ideation and Mild Traumatic Brain Injury**

Suicidal behavior is a serious consequence of mood disorders and may consist of suicidal ideation (thoughts), suicide attempts, or completed suicide. It is often associated with such psychologic conditions as depression or other mental disorders. In a Danish population-based study, Teasdale and Engberg (2001) compared the incidence of suicide in a group of patients who were admitted to a hospital from 1979 to 1993 with a concussion (n = 126,114), a cranial fracture (n = 7,560), or a cerebral contusion or traumatic intracranial hemorrhage (n = 11,766) with the incidence in the general population stratified by age and sex. The results demonstrated an increased incidence of suicide in the TBI groups compared with the general population (standardized mortality ratio = 3.0, 2.7, and 4.1, respectively). The diagnosis of substance misuse was associated with increased suicide rates in all three TBI groups. The authors concluded that concomitant risk factors (such as psychiatric illness and psychosocial disadvantage) might predispose to completed suicide in the mild-TBI group.

A recent study of active-duty soldiers was conducted by Skopp et al. (2012). The study was a retrospective case–control study, and the period of surveillance was 2001–2009. Those who died from suicide (n = 1,764) were compared with a control group (n = 7,018) matched by sex, race, age, service, date of entry into the active military component, and years of service. The two groups were similar regarding frequencies and types of TBI and number of deployments. Results of multivariate analyses demonstrated that there was an increased risk of suicide in those who had mood disorders, partner relationship problems, and family circumstance problems, but not in those who had mild TBI, alcohol dependence, or PTSD. In a separate analysis, an increased risk of suicide was found in those who had psychiatric comorbidities. The differences in results between the Skopp et al. study and that by Teasdale and Engberg (2001) were discussed as possibly reflecting differences between the populations and injury events. Civilian TBI tends to be associated with high-risk behaviors, and it is possible that preexisting personality characteristics increase the risk of suicide in civilians. In contrast, TBI in the military might often occur as the result of unpredictable incidents during training and combat.

**Posttraumatic Stress Disorder and Mild Traumatic Brain Injury**

An extensive literature review of brain injury and long-term outcomes (IOM, 2009) noted that there was limited or suggestive evidence of an association between mild TBI and PTSD in Gulf War military populations. The overlapping symptomatology between mild TBI, PCS, and PTSD complicates the issue. In 2009, VA published a systematic review of evidence on assessment of and treatment for TBI and PTSD. The findings show a wide range of prevalence of TBI and PTSD, depending on the population (military or civilian), the instruments used to diagnose TBI or PTSD (self-reports vs validated diagnostic instruments), and the size and representativeness of the population being studied. Another review of the literature on PTSD and TBI noted that studies varied considerably in their design and that there was not consistent evidence on the frequency of mild TBI and PTSD (Carlson et al., 2011b). There are important contextual distinctions between civilian and combat trauma that might influence the difference in prevalence of the comorbidity of PTSD and TBI.

Numerous studies have shown that OEF and OIF military veterans who had diagnoses of mild TBI had symptoms of PTSD (Carlson et al., 2010; Hill et al., 2009; Hoge et al., 2008; Kennedy et al., 2010; Schneiderman et al., 2008). For example, TBI and PTSD prevalence in OEF and OIF veterans has been reported in a RAND study of 1,965 OEF and OIF participants (Tanielian and Jaycox, 2008): 19.5% had probable TBI, and 13.8% had probable PTSD on the basis of the PTSD Checklist.[4] However, in veterans who had TBI, the prevalence of PTSD was 33.8%. Hoge et al. (2008) examined soldiers 3–4 months after return from a year-long deployment in Iraq. The authors divided the soldiers into four groups: those who reported injury involving LOC, those who reported sustaining an injury with an altered mental state (for example, dazed, confused, "seeing stars," or not remembering the injury) without LOC, those who had another type of injury that did not involve LOC or altered mental state, and those who reported no injury. The rates of PTSD were significantly and systematically different among the four groups: 44% in the group who reported injury with LOC, 27% in the group who reported injury with altered mental state, 16% in the group who had another type of injury, and 9% in the group who had no injury.

## Mild Traumatic Brain Injury, Comorbidities, and Complicated Issues of Causality in Operation Enduring Freedom and Operation Iraqi Freedom Populations

Although estimates of PTSD, depression, PCS, and poor health are reported to be high in OEF and OIF active-duty personnel and veterans who have mild TBI, the relationships among those conditions are complicated and controversial. PTSD is often comorbid with several other mental-health disorders—such as depression, substance abuse, and suicidal behavior—and the conflicts in Iraq and Afghanistan have increased awareness of the relationship between mild TBI and PTSD, although it is confusing. Complicating the picture of PTSD that develops *after* a mild TBI is the issue of the overlapping symptomatology of mild TBI, PCS, and PTSD. In addition, it has been noted that PTSD can impede recovery from mild TBI and make clinical management difficult (Vasterling et al., 2009) and that the co-occurrence of TBI (of all severities) and PTSD increases the risk of self-reported cognitive impairment compared with that in civilians who do not have PTSD (Zatzick et al., 2010).

It is generally accepted that mild TBI, PTSD, and depression co-occur and that the rates of PTSD and depression are much higher after a mild TBI than are found in the general public or in non-TBI-injured soldiers. The controversy centers on whether symptoms and other adverse psychosocial outcomes reported by soldiers who have mild TBI and PTSD are due to the aftermath of the emotional trauma (possible PTSD) or to neurologic consequences of the mild TBI. Hoge et al. (2008) found that soldiers who reported injury with LOC were significantly more likely to report ill health, doctor visits, and missed workdays than soldiers who reported another type of injury that did not involve LOC or altered mental state. In addition, a significantly higher percentage of those reporting LOC also reported symptoms of irritability, sleep disturbance, fatigue, and other symptoms than the percentage of people who had a different type of injury. However, when the effects of PTSD and depression were covaried, all significant findings except headache disappeared. The authors concluded that the high rates of health

[4] The PTSD Checklist (PCL) is a 17-item self-reporting measure of the 17 *DSM-IV* symptoms of PTSD. The PCL has a variety of purposes, including screening for and diagnosis of PTSD and monitoring of symptom change during and after treatment.

problems and symptoms reported by soldiers 3–4 months after return from deployment are associated largely with PTSD or depression rather than TBI.

Polusny et al. (2011) conducted a longitudinal study of National Guard soldiers deployed to Iraq. The soldiers completed a questionnaire evaluating probable mild TBI, PTSD, and depression about 1 month before return from a 16-month deployment to Iraq and again 1 year after return from deployment. The assessment at 1 year evaluated additional outcomes, including problematic drinking, social adjustment, and quality of life. The soldiers were divided into four groups on the basis of their mild TBI status as determined by their responses while they were still in Iraq and their PTSD status as determined by their responses after they returned from deployment. The groups consisted of those who had neither mild TBI nor PTSD (the control group), those who had mild TBI only, those who had PTSD only, and those who had both mild TBI and PTSD. The results showed that report of symptoms 1 year after return from Iraq was least frequent in the group who had neither mild TBI nor PTSD, more frequent in the group who had only mild TBI, and most frequent in the groups who had only PTSD or both mild TBI and PTSD. For example, irritability was reported by 64% of the group who had neither condition, 83% of the mild-TBI group, 99% of the PTSD group, and 100% of the group who had both mild TBI and PTSD. There were a number of significant differences in symptom reporting between the control group and the other groups, but after covarying the effects of PTSD symptoms in the mild-TBI-only group, the authors found no differences between the controls and the mild-TBI group in any outcome. Therefore, they concluded that mild TBI alone does not play a role in long-term impairments and suggested that their findings have policy implications for widespread screening for mild TBI in the military. They argued that the current screening policy may have unintended consequences of misattribution to mild TBI of symptoms that may be more properly attributable to PTSD, pain, sleep problems, or stress.

Other researchers have found different results in their investigation of TBI, PTSD, and PCS. Brenner et al. (2010a) examined separate groups of soldiers who had mild TBI alone, PTSD alone, and both conditions to look for relationships between those conditions and symptoms without trying to control for the effects of one of the conditions. Their focus was on whether having both PTSD and mild TBI resulted in a higher risk of symptoms than either condition alone. They performed a retrospective analysis of 1,247 injured members of a single Army brigade combat team who returned to Fort Carlson, Colorado, after a 1-year deployment to Iraq. The sample comprised the injured portion of the entire team previously reported on by Terrio et al. (2009). On return from Iraq, all members of the team were examined with the WARCAT, which included questions about injuries sustained in Iraq, symptoms experienced at the time of the incidents, and current symptoms. In addition to the questionnaire, each soldier was interviewed by a clinician, all available medical records were reviewed, and information from witnesses was gathered. Some 71% of the sample had at least one clinician-confirmed mild TBI, and the remainder reported an injury history not consistent with mild TBI. PTSD was diagnosed by using four questions from the PDHA, which assessed reexperiencing, numbing, avoidance, and hyperarousal dimensions of the disorder. Positive responses on any two of the four questions indicated PTSD. Symptoms experienced after return from Iraq included headaches, dizziness, memory difficulties, balance problems, and irritability. Symptoms were examined in four groups: mild TBI alone, PTSD alone, both mild TBI and PTSD, and neither condition. The analyses adjusted for age, education, sex, military rank, and military occupational specialty. The results showed that mild TBI alone (adjusted prevalence ratio = 4.03; CI = 2.67–6.07), PTSD alone (adjusted prevalence ratio = 2.74; CI = 1.58–4.74) and both conditions together (adjusted prevalence ratio = 6.27; CI = 4.13–9.43) were significantly associated with having any symptom compared with absence of both mild TBI and PTSD. The combination of the two disorders was more strongly associated with a higher prevalence of each symptom than either condition alone. For example, the adjusted prevalence ratio for memory problems in those who had PTSD only was 4.00. The ratio increased to 6.22 in those who had mild TBI only and increased further to 12.70 in those who had both PTSD and mild TBI. The authors argued that their results support the additive effects of PTSD and mild TBI on symptoms and urged continued screening for both mild TBI and PTSD for early identification and treatment.

It is difficult to reconcile the contrasting results because of the many differences in study methods and design and in conceptualization of the problem. Statistical adjustment has been based on the assumptions that PTSD (or events that cause PTSD) confounds the relationship of mild TBI and that PTSD mimics the effects of mild TBI. In other words, PTSD is correlated with both mild TBI (independent variable) and outcomes (PCS and poor health) but has no causal relationship to mild TBI. That assumption might be questionable on the basis of findings that mild TBI might increase the likelihood of PTSD (Brenner et al., 2010a; Vasterling et al., 2009). If PTSD is indeed in the causal chain, statistical adjustments with covariance or other multivariate methods are inappropriate. What is not clear is whether the same event causes both and there is no causal link between them or whether they are causally related. The available evidence suggests that they are likely to be causally related.

Several authors have tried to address the conceptual issues of comorbidities, the controversy, and the causes for the complexity of the problem (Kennedy et al., 2007; McAllister and Stein, 2010; Stein and McAllister, 2009; Vasterling and Dikmen, 2012). Mild TBI and PTSD are known or hypothesized to share a number of properties. They have common symptoms, hypothesized underlying biologic mechanisms, other comorbid conditions (such as depression and substance abuse), and premorbid risk and resilience factors. Given known and hypothesized common properties, it is difficult to reconcile whether psychologic or neurologic factors are responsible for the high morbidity observed in those who have both conditions. Overlapping symptoms, as seen in Figure 4.2, may include depression, anxiety, insomnia, irritability or anger, trouble in concentrating, fatigue, hyperarousal, avoidance, and others (Stein and McAllister, 2009).

Recent efforts are attempting to find the answer in biologic underpinnings although much of this approach is based on theory rather than empirical support. It is hypothesized that some areas of the brain—including the hippocampus, amygdala, and medial and prefrontal cortex—are typically damaged in TBI and implicated in the development of PTSD; this suggests a common origin of the overlapping symptom profile (Kennedy et al., 2007; Koenigs and Grafman, 2009; McAllister, 2011; McAllister and Stein, 2010; Stein and McAllister, 2009). PTSD and TBI may also have similar risk factors. For example, many studies have reported that lower IQ before trauma is associated with a higher risk of PTSD and other psychologic disorders (Breslau et al., 2006; Gale et al., 2008; Koenen et al., 2007; Kremen et al., 2007). If one considers IQ to be a proxy for cognitive reserve, lower cognitive reserve, either innate or acquired (for example, as a result of mild TBI), could increase the risk of psychologic health problems. Vasterling et al. (2009) suggest that mild TBI may interfere with the development of trauma memories because of cognitive impairment immediately after the TBI and thus influence the development of PTSD.

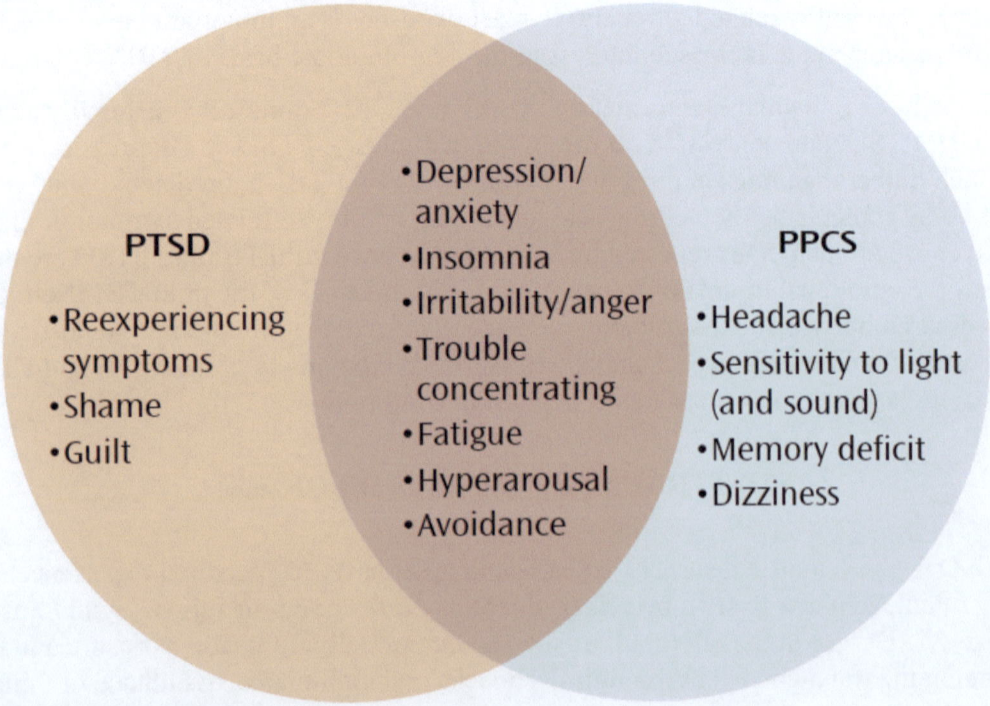


**FIGURE 4.2** Interface of PTSD and persistent postconcussive symptoms following mTBI that involves biomechanical force to the brain with loss of consciousness, amnesia, and/or altered mental state.
SOURCE: Stein and McAllister, 2009, reprinted with permission from the *American Journal of Psychiatry*.

Although the comorbidity of PTSD and TBI has become widely known in recent years as the result of OEF and OIF, the history of this issue dates back to World War I (Jones et al., 2007), and there has been no clear consensus. The same issues have long plagued the study of civilian mild TBI in attempts to explain the lack of recovery. In the current literature related to war injuries, some have concluded that there is sufficient evidence to attribute PCS to TBI. The suggestion is that the PCS might result from stress reactions after TBI rather than from the neurologic trauma itself (Bryant, 2011). Others have cautiously concluded that more research is needed—especially multidisciplinary research in psychiatry, neuropsychology, neurology, and other fields—to examine PTSD, TBI, and their interaction with the use of comprehensive definitions and language that spans different disciplines (Stein and McAllister, 2009).

Disentangling the outcomes related to mild TBI and PTSD is important for understanding the underlying reasons for the symptomatology so that prevention strategies and more precise treatment protocols might be developed.

### Summary

Outcomes associated with TBI that occurred in previous wars and in the civilian population have been well described (IOM, 2008b, 2009), but outcomes associated with mild TBI that has occurred in the current conflicts (OEF and OIF) are not yet well understood. Although there is evidence to suggest cognitive impairment shortly after a mild TBI sustained during OEF and OIF, there is conflicting evidence on the longer-term cognitive outcomes and on the factors that might be associated with cognitive decline if it is observed. The study of chronic traumatic encephalopathy related to repetitive blast exposure is an important new subject of research and has generated increased interest in the neurobiologic basis of TBI.

On the basis of available information on OIF and OEF injuries, it is generally accepted that mild TBI, PTSD, and depression co-occur and that rates of PTSD and depression after mild TBI are much higher than rates in the general public or in non-TBI-injured active duty personnel. The controversy centers on whether physical and emotional health-related symptoms and other adverse psychosocial outcomes reported by soldiers who have mild TBI and PTSD are due to the aftermath of the emotional trauma or to neurologic consequences of the mild TBI itself. Current scientific research has yielded insufficient evidence to answer that important diagnostic question. Better exposure data and objective diagnostic tests for or biomarkers of mild TBI and PTSD will improve our understanding of these highly comorbid conditions.

## POSTTRAUMATIC STRESS DISORDER

PTSD is a psychiatric disorder that can develop after direct, personal experience or witnessing of an event that poses a perceived threat of death or serious injury. Symptoms that characterize PTSD arise in the aftermath of such an emotionally traumatic exposure and include reexperiencing the traumatic event through flashbacks and nightmares, avoidance of things associated with the trauma, and hyperarousal (exaggerated startle and difficulty in sleeping and in concentrating) (IOM, 2006). The *Diagnostic and Statistical Manual of Mental Disorders, 4th Edition* (*DSM-IV*) recognizes that the onset of PTSD may be acute, beginning within 6 months of exposure to the traumatic event, or delayed, beginning more than 6 months after the event. Symptoms typically begin shortly after exposure—even on the same day (North et al., 1999). If the symptoms persist for 2 days to 4 weeks, the diagnosis is acute stress disorder; if the symptoms endure for more than 1 month, the diagnosis is PTSD. The time between exposure and development of enough symptoms to meet the diagnostic criteria (see Box 4.1) is variable and may be years (Bremner et al., 1996; Bryant and Harvey, 2002; Carty et al., 2006; Gray et al., 2004; Green et al., 1990; Op den Velde et al., 1996; Port et al., 2001; Ruzich et al., 2005). It is considered to be chronic PTSD by *DSM-IV-Text Revision* (*DSM-IV-TR*) criteria if symptoms persist for 3 months or longer. PTSD can be chronic and have no remission, or it can be recurrent and have periods of remission and recurrence (Friedman, 2003).

The *DSM-IV* criteria are undergoing revision currently with the upcoming publication of *DSM-5*. At the time of this report, the *DSM-5* criteria for PTSD are not final. Draft criteria of *DSM-5* vary from those of *DSM-IV* in that they are framed to increase the specificity of the diagnosis. Examples include the following: Criterion A (prior exposure to traumatic events) is more specifically stated, and evaluation of a person's emotional response at the time is deleted; Criterion C focuses solely on avoidance of behaviors or of physical or temporal reminders of the traumatic experiences; and new Criterion D focuses on adverse alterations in cognition and mood associated with the traumatic events. Those changes should not adversely affect the case frequency of PTSD or the factors associated with the diagnosis substantially.

It should be noted that before the development of *DSM-5* two interrelated issues have been raised (Rosen et al., 2008). First, some have suggested that, given the overlap of symptoms of PTSD with other diagnoses (such as major depression), mental-health workers have reflexively assumed that PTSD is the expected response to severe traumatic experiences (and some that are not so serious). Second, there are suggestions that the constellation of symptoms that make up the diagnosis of PTSD may occur in the absence of trauma. Neither of those concerns appears to have gained a consensus in the overall scientific community, so in this report we state with confidence that the *DSM-IV* criteria for PTSD, on which the bulk of the reported studies are based, remain current and applicable.

The types of trauma exposure that are of high incidence in military personnel deployed to war zones are those known to be most likely to precipitate PTSD. Wojcik et al. (2009) evaluated data on soldiers deployed to OIF (2001–2004) and OEF (2002–2004) and found that PTSD explained 4.6 hospital admissions per 10,000 soldier-years and accounted for 35–45% of anxiety-disorder hospitalizations.

**BOX 4.1**
***DSM-IV* Criteria for Posttraumatic Stress Disorder (309.81)**

A. The person has been exposed to a traumatic event in which both of the following have been present:
- (1) the person experienced, witnessed, or was confronted with an event or events that involved actual or threatened death or serious injury, or a threat to the physical integrity of self or others
- (2) the person's response involved intense fear, helplessness, or horror. Note: In children, this may be expressed instead by disorganized or agitated behavior.

B. The traumatic event is persistently reexperienced in one (or more) of the following ways:
- (1) recurrent and intrusive distressing recollections of the event, including images, thoughts, or perceptions. Note: In young children, repetitive play may occur in which themes or aspects of the trauma are expressed.
- (2) recurrent distressing dreams of the event. Note: In children, there may be frightening dreams without recognizable content.
- (3) acting or feeling as if the traumatic event were recurring (includes a sense of reliving the experience, illusions, hallucinations, and dissociative flashback episodes, including those that occur upon awakening or when intoxicated). Note: In young children, trauma-specific reenactment may occur.
- (4) intense psychological distress at exposure to internal or external cues that symbolize or resemble an aspect of the traumatic event.
- (5) physiological reactivity on exposure to internal or external cues that symbolize or resemble an aspect of the traumatic event.

C. Persistent avoidance of stimuli associated with the trauma and numbing of general responsiveness (not present before the trauma), as indicated by three (or more) of the following:
- (1) efforts to avoid thoughts, feelings, or conversations associated with the trauma
- (2) efforts to avoid activities, places, or people that arouse recollections of the trauma
- (3) inability to recall an important aspect of the trauma
- (4) markedly diminished interest or participation in significant activities
- (5) feeling of detachment or estrangement from others
- (6) restricted range of affect (e.g., unable to have loving feelings)
- (7) sense of a foreshortened future (e.g., does not expect to have a career, marriage, children, or a normal life span)

D. Persistent symptoms of increased arousal (not present before the trauma), as indicated by two (or more) of the following:
- (1) difficulty falling or staying asleep

(2) irritability or outbursts of anger
(3) difficulty concentrating
(4) hypervigilance
(5) exaggerated startle response
E. Duration of the disturbance (symptoms in Criteria B, C, and D) is more than one month.
F. The disturbance causes clinically significant distress or impairment in social, occupational, or other important areas of functioning.

SOURCE: Reprinted with permission from the *Diagnostic and Statistical Manual of Mental Disorders, Fourth Edition, Text Revision* (Copyright 2000). American Psychiatric Association.

## Prevalence

PTSD is one of the disorders most commonly diagnosed in US combat troops after their deployment to Afganistan and Iraq. A range of estimates have been reported for PTSD prevalence, and the estimates depend on when the evaluation is conducted and the diagnostic method (for example, self-reported symptoms vs diagnosis by a health care professional). The prevalence may also depend on whether the full criteria for PTSD are met as opposed to a positive screen for PTSD. A sample of studies is described below:

- Hoge et al. (2004a) reported the prevalence of PTSD 3–4 months after deployment as 6.2% and 12.9% in Army troops returning from Afghanistan and Iraq, respectively, and 12.2% in marines returning from Iraq. The prevalence of PTSD before deployment was 5.0% in all the military personnel screened with the PTSD Checklist (PCL), a self-reporting instrument.
- Hoge et al. (2007) later reported that 16.6% of US Army combat troops met the screening criteria (not *DSM* diagnosis) for PTSD a year after their return from Iraq.
- DOD conducted a mental-health survey of Army soldiers and marines deployed in Iraq in 2003, 2004, and 2006. In 2003, 16% of the soldiers and marines met the screening criteria for PTSD while deployed; in 2004, 14% met the criteria; and in 2006, 17% of soldiers and 14% of marines met the criteria (MHAT-III, 2006).
- Smith et al. (2008) conducted a prospective cohort analysis of 50,184 participants in the millennium cohort. PTSD was measured by self-reports using the PCL Civilian. New onset of self-reported PTSD was reported in 7.6-8.7% of deployers who reported combat exposures, 1.4–2.1% of deployers who did not report combat exposure, and 2.3–3% of nondeployers.
- Using the PCL, Booth-Kewley (2010) reported the prevalence of PTSD in OIF and OEF marines as 17.1%.
- Thomas et al. (2010) collected 18,305 mental-health surveys from members of four active components and two National Guard brigade combat teams at 3 and 12 months after deployment to Iraq; they analyzed 13,226 surveys. The prevalence of PTSD depended on how PTSD was defined (broad vs strict definition) and ranged from 14.7% to 21.5% at 3 months and from 16.6% to 30.5% at 12 months. Rates were significantly higher at 12 months in both groups; much larger increases were observed in National Guard participants.
- Thomas et al. (2010) also estimated prevalence on the basis of impairment and found that prevalence of PTSD with some functional impairment ranged from 12.6% (3 months) to

29.4% (12 months) and prevalence of PTSD with serious functional impairment ranged from 5.6% (3 months) to 12.4% (12 months).

A review of 22 studies (Tanielian and Jaycox, 2008) found that 5–15% experienced PTSD following deployment to war zones. The review also suggested that the prevalence of PTSD (and depression) increases with time after deployment (that is, in the readjustment period). A critical review by Richardson et al. (2010) yielded a similar result: estimated prevalence of combat-related PTSD of 4–17% in OIF veterans. The authors noted that PTSD prevalence in other Western countries is typically lower than in the United States, and they attributed that finding to differences in combat experience and in methods used to estimate prevalence and to sociopolitical and cultural factors. The difference in PTSD prevalence between the United States and other Western countries is supported by Fear et al. (2010), who estimated PTSD prevalence in UK armed forces who had been deployed to Iraq and Afghanistan at 4%.

Service members who experience combat exposure and are wounded appear to have higher prevalence of PTSD. Hoge et al. (2007) found that 31.8% of soldiers who had physical injuries had PTSD. In a more recent study of over 2,000 postdeployment active-duty service members, those who reported LOC had the highest rate of PTSD (43.9%) compared with those who had altered mental states (27.3%), those who had only physical injuries (16.2%), and those who reported no injury (9.1%) (Hoge et al., 2008). Gaylord et al. (2008) evaluated 76 service members who had sustained a burn and a blast injury for PTSD by using the PCL and excluded those who had moderate or severe TBI; the prevalence was 32%. However, Greiger et al. (2006) evaluated 613 soldiers who were seriously injured in combat in Iraq or Afghanistan for PTSD with the PCL 1, 4, and 7 months after their injury; 243 participated at all three times. At 1 month, 4.2% met the criteria for PTSD; at 4 and 7 months, about 12% met the criteria. The authors noted that 78.8% of people who received a diagnosis of PTSD or depression at 7 months were negative for the conditions at 1 month.

Seal et al. (2009) investigated new mental-health diagnoses in 289,328 OEF or OIF veterans who were new users of VA health care services from April 2002 to March 2008. Diagnoses were based on the *International Classification of Diseases, 9th Revision, Clinical Modification* (*ICD-9-CM*) codes 290.0–319.0. Their investigation found that the 2-year cumulative prevalence increased from 6.4% in 2002 to 36.9% in 2008; PTSD diagnoses showed the greatest change, increasing from 0.2% to 21.8%. Figure 4.3 illustrates the increasing 2-year prevalence of PTSD and other mental-health disorders, particularly after the start of the Iraq War. It is consistent with the increasing trend noted by Seal et al. (2009) that Bagalman (2011) reported the PTSD prevalence in OEF and OIF veterans who used VA health care services in FY 2002–2010 as 27%.

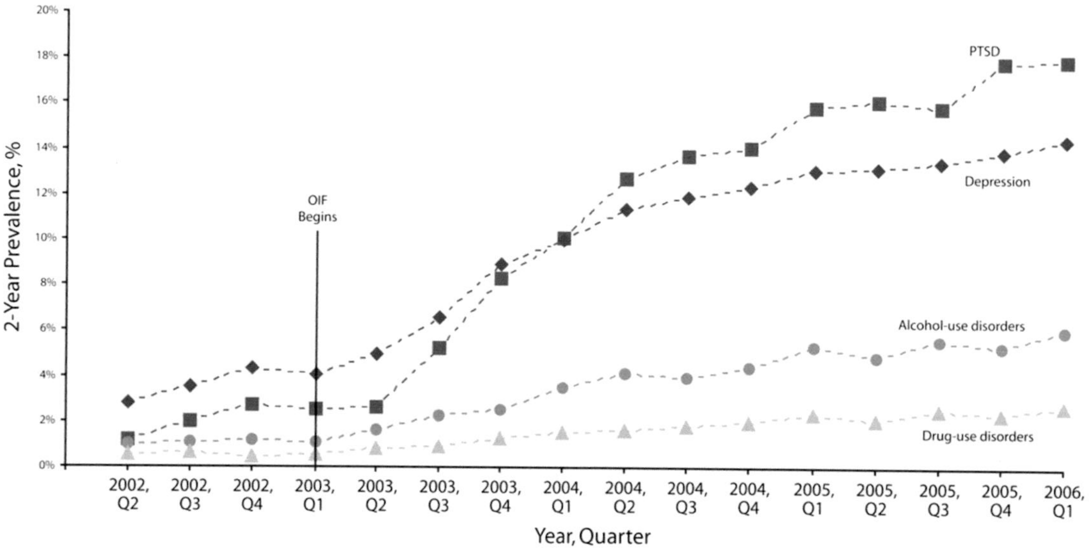


**FIGURE 4.3** Two-year prevalence of PTSD and other mental-health disorders among OEF and OIF veterans entering the Department of Veterans Affairs health care system.
SOURCE: From Seal et al., 2009, with permission.

The studies described above clearly indicate the variability in estimates of PTSD prevalence in the OEF and OIF military populations. Ramchand et al. (2010) reviewed 29 studies of OIF and OEF service members to characterize the variability in PTSD estimates and possible sources of the variability. They found that the studies could be divided into studies of military personnel who were seeking treatment and those who were not seeking treatment. Studies of non-treatment-seeking service members generally provided PTSD prevalence estimates of about 5–20%, and studies of treatment-seeking service members yielded estimates as high as 50% on the basis of screening, although rates were typically lower when actual diagnoses were made. Recent research indicates that 23% of those seeking treatment receive a PTSD diagnosis. The authors found that the variability in PTSD estimates was probably related to representativeness and case definitions. Most studies used convenience samples, which may not be representative of the entire population deployed to war zones, and the studies used different definitions of PTSD. Methodologic differences in outcome measurements in the studies may lead to substantial underestimation of the prevalence of PTSD (and depression) in the postdeployment samples (Tanielian and Jaycox, 2008). Those methodologic issues are similar to the issues discussed above in determining estimates of mild TBI. Regardless, using different definitions most likely contributes to much of the variability observed in the various studies and indicates the need to use a consistent set of criteria for PTSD and a standardized assessment for optimal estimation of prevalence.

## Risk Factors

### Demographic Factors

Many factors have been associated with an increased likelihood of PTSD, although the literature contains some conflicting findings. Age, sex, race or ethnicity, rank, marital status, and educational level have been associated with PTSD. Specifically, studies have shown that a young age (less than 25 years) is associated with increased odds of PTSD in OEF and OIF veterans (Seal et al., 2009), although National Guard and reserve veterans older than 30 years old had significantly higher risks of PTSD than younger National Guard and reserve veterans. Wojcik et al. (2009) found that female soldiers had 3.3 times the risk of hospitalization for PTSD of male soldiers. Black soldiers had half the risk of PTSD hospitalization of white soldiers, and enlisted personnel had 6 times higher risk of PTSD than officers. Lapierre et al. (2007) and Phillips et al. (2010) also found that junior rank was associated with PTSD, but the absence of an association between sex and PTSD is consistent with results of other research (see discussion below in the section "Women's Health Outcomes").

Studies also have shown that being single or divorced is associated with increased risk of PTSD (Booth-Kewley et al., 2010; Lapierre et al., 2007). Higher educational status has been reported to be protective against PTSD (Booth-Kewley et al., 2010; Dedert et al., 2009), but some have found increased PTSD risks with higher educational level (Reger et al., 2009). In a small study of health care workers, Kolkow et al. (2007) found that the only demographic factor related to increased risk of PTSD was nonwhite race. Although Grieger et al. (2006) found some associations of demographic factors with PTSD at 1 month, they did not find any associations with demographic factors at later evaluation times.

### Deployment-Related Stressors

Deployment and deployment-related stressors have been associated with increased risk of PTSD. Booth-Kewley et al. (2010) used the PCL to evaluate 1,569 marines deployed to Iraq or Afghanistan; multivariate analyses indicated that deployment-related stresses—such as concerns back home, lack of privacy, and problems with leadership—were significantly associated with PTSD. Vasterling et al. (2010) used the PCL to evaluate changes in PTSD symptom severity in 774 deployed and 309 nondeployed soldiers. Multiple regression analyses indicated that PTSD symptoms increased with deployment; the greatest positive increase was observed in those who had high combat exposure. Results could not be explained on the basis of preexisting symptoms.

Some investigations have indicated that National Guard soldiers suffer disproportionately from deployment (Milliken et al., 2007; Thomas et al., 2010). Riviere et al. (2011) reviewed self-report data to determine risk factors for PTSD and depression in 4,034 National Guard soldiers who had been deployed to Iraq. Soldiers were evaluated at 3 or 12 months, and the factors evaluated were specific to National Guard soldiers who leave and then return to civilian employment. They included "financial hardship, job loss, [lack of] employer support, and the effect of deployment absence on co-workers." The investigators found that PTSD was associated with all factors at one or both evaluation times. Depression was associated with financial hardship, job loss, and lack of employer support at 3 and 12 months. The authors noted that their results indicated that "National Guard soldiers have unique post-deployment social and material concerns that impair their mental health."

### Combat Exposure

As expected, combat exposure and PTSD are linked. Seal et al. (2009) reported higher combat exposure associated with increased PTSD risk in OEF and OIF veterans but not in National Guard or reserve veterans. Booth-Kewley et al. (2010) also reported a strong association between combat exposure and PTSD in marines deployed to Iraq and Afghanistan. MacGregor et al. (2009) compared mental-health diagnoses in 831 men serving in OIF who had sustained a battle injury with those in 1,137 who had sustained a nonbattle injury; men were evaluated at least 1 month after injury. Men who suffered battle injuries had significantly higher rates of PTSD and other mental-health conditions than men who suffered nonbattle injuries, and mental-health diagnoses were significantly associated with severity of injury. Grieger et al. (2006), however, did not find combat exposure (or long deployments) to be predictive of PTSD at later evaluation points in the severely injured soldiers.

In a small study of 317 Gulf War veterans with the PCL, Maguen et al. (2011c) found that killing someone was a significant predictor of PTSD symptoms (and other mental-health outcomes) after control for other combat-related factors. In their review of 29 studies of OIF and OEF military personnel, Ramchand et al. (2010) found that the only factor that was consistently significantly associated with PTSD was combat exposure and that other factors that often appear to be associated with PTSD may simply be surrogates of combat exposure. For example, those who are younger and of lower rank may be exposed to more combat than those who are older and of higher rank. Assuming that combat exposure is an important risk factor for PTSD, Pietrzak et al. (2011b) evaluated survey data on 285 OIF and OEF National Guard or reserve veterans to identify specific combat experiences as predictors of PTSD. After adjustment for various factors, they found that two combat experiences—"personally witnessing someone from one's unit or an ally unit being seriously wounded or killed" and experiencing "friendly" fire—were associated with PTSD symptom severity and were independent predictors of probable PTSD. Exposure to land mines or traps was also associated with PTSD symptom severity.

Another risk factor related to combat exposure is the threat of personal harm. Kolkow et al. (2007) used the PCL to survey 102 health care providers who had been deployed to a combat setting in Iraq or Afghanistan and found that PTSD was increased in those who experienced "direct and perceived threats of personal harm." They did not observe an association between PTSD and exposure to the dead or wounded. Peterson et al. (2010) compared mental-health outcomes in 4,408 active-duty Air Force noncombatants returning from deployment to a combat zone in Iraq with those in 959 personnel returning from a noncombat zone in Qatar. They used the PDHA to evaluate PTSD and found that those deployed to Iraq were significantly more likely to report combat experiences, such as "feeling in great danger of being killed," and to screen positive for PTSD. Phillips et al. (2010) evaluated self-report data on 706 male marines who had been deployed at least 30 days to Iraq or Afghanistan between baseline and followup assessments. They conducted multivariate logistic regression analyses and found that the most significant predictor of screening positive for PTSD was "feeling in great danger of death." Other significant predictors were being shot or seriously injured and witnessing an injury or death.

**Prior Traumatic Exposure**

Veterans who have experienced prior traumatic stress appear to be more likely to develop PTSD than those who do not have such a history. In addition to the combat-related risk factors noted above, Phillips et al. (2010) found that two or more exposures to violence before entering the military also increased the likelihood of screening positive for PTSD. Dedert et al. (2009) evaluated 356 military veterans who served after September 11, 2001, using the Structured Clinical Interview for *DSM-IV*, and investigated the contribution of lifetime traumatic events[5] to PTSD. Multiple traumatic events, including childhood assault and disasters or accidents, increased the likelihood of PTSD in veterans who had comorbid psychiatric conditions. The only

[5]The author defined a *traumatic stressor* as a "life threatening event to which the person responded with fear, helplessness or horror."

predictors of PTSD in veterans who did not have comorbid psychiatric conditions were combat exposure and adult physical assault.

Fritch et al. (2010) also found an association between childhood physical abuse and PTSD symptoms. They reviewed self-report data on 1,045 OIF and OEF National Guard or reserve veterans who had been referred to a behavioral-health clinic. Multiple regression analyses revealed a significant association between postdeployment psychiatric symptoms—those of PTSD, anxiety, and depression—and childhood physical abuse. An association between psychiatric symptoms and combat-related trauma was also noted. No interactive effects between child abuse and combat were observed.

Cabrera et al. (2007) investigated the relationship between adverse childhood experiences[6] and rates and symptoms of mental-health disorders. They compared self-report data on 2,392 male active-duty soldiers who had recently returned from Iraq (surveyed 3 months after deployment) with data on 4,529 male active-duty soldiers who had not served in Iraq; about 43% of the latter had served in Afghanistan, but their rates of PTSD and depression were similar to those in soldiers who had not been previously deployed. The investigators found that soldiers who reported at least two categories of childhood adversity were significantly more likely to screen positive for PTSD and depression. More important, the authors stated that adverse childhood experiences "independently predicted higher depression and post-traumatic stress symptoms, beyond the expected contribution of combat exposure." Similarly, Gahm et al. (2007) evaluated self-report data on 1,626 active-duty soldiers at an outpatient mental-health clinic and found that adverse childhood experiences were stronger predictors of PTSD and depression than were demographic characteristics. Combat experience was also associated with PTSD, but depression was not.

**Military Sexual Trauma**

Estimates of military sexual trauma (MST) have been reported on the basis of a universal screening program implemented by VA. In 2003, shortly after implementation of the VA program, it was reported that 21.5% of women and 1.1% of men reported MST (Kimerling et al., 2007). It has been noted that those estimates have remained fairly consistent; as of 2008, they translate to 48,106 women and 43,693 men screening positive for MST (Hyun et al., 2009). DOD estimates of MST indicate that the annual prevalence of sexual assault in women and men was 6.8% and 1.8% (Lipari et al., 2008). A study of reservists (Street et al., 2008) examined sexual harassment and assault during military service and found that sexual assault was reported by 13.1% of women and 1.6% of men.

MST appears to be an important risk factor for PTSD. Suris and Lind (2008) reviewed research on health consequences of MST and found higher rates of PTSD, depression, and substance abuse in female veterans who had a history of sexual assault. In fact, female veterans who had a history of MST were nine times more likely to develop PTSD compared to female veterans who had no history of sexual trauma. Recent research on OIF and OEF veterans supports that finding. Kimerling et al. (2010) reviewed medical records of OIF and OEF veterans (17,580 women and 108,149 men) for diagnoses of mental-health disorders and found that those who had a history of MST were significantly more likely to receive a diagnosis of PTSD, other

[6]The authors defined adverse childhood experiences by using six categories: exposure to a mentally ill, alcoholic, or violent person in the home or exposure to physical, sexual, or psychologic abuse.

anxiety disorders, depression, or substance-use disorders than those who did not have a history of abuse. Odds ratios remained significant after adjustment for other significant associations, and effect sizes in women were substantially greater than those in men. The link between MST and PTSD is discussed further below in the section "Women's Health Outcomes."

### History of Mental-Health Condition

Military personnel who have been previously diagnosed with a mental-health condition, particularly PTSD, are at greater risk for a repeat diagnosis in theater (Larson et al., 2011). Using self-report data, Sandweiss et al. (2011) assessed the relationship between postdeployment PTSD and predeployment (baseline) psychiatric conditions and injury severity among 22,630 military personnel who had been deployed to Iraq or Afghanistan. PTSD was significantly associated with baseline psychiatric conditions; service members who had one or more baseline psychiatric conditions were 2.52 times more likely to report PTSD symptoms than those who had no baseline psychiatric conditions.

### Injury Severity and Neurologic Dysfunction

Although injury severity was significantly associated with PTSD symptoms, the observed association was weak. Grieger et al. (2006), however, evaluated seriously injured soldiers and found that severe physical problems were significantly associated with PTSD at all times of evaluation. As noted above, MacGregor et al. (2009) also observed a positive association between injury severity and PTSD and other mental-health diagnoses.

Subtle neurologic dysfunction may predispose people to PTSD. Gurvits et al. (2006) evaluated 25 male Vietnam veterans who had received a diagnosis of PTSD and 24 who had no PTSD diagnosis and compared them with each other and with their combat-unexposed identical twins. Combat veterans who had a diagnosis of PTSD had significantly higher scores on subtle neurologic dysfunction (neurologic soft signs) than combat veterans who did not have PTSD. However, the combat-unexposed twins of the combat veterans who had PTSD also had increased scores. The results suggest that the dysfunction is not a result of PTSD but rather might indicate a vulnerability to PTSD.

**An earlier study by Gilbertson et al. (2002), using a case-control design, examined male monozygotic twin pairs in which one twin was a combat Vietnam veteran and the identical twin had no combat exposure. Hippocampal volume was measured in both twins. Because monozygotic twins are genetically identical, the authors interpreted differences in hippocampal volume to be due to environmental effects. The authors concluded that smaller hippocampal volume was found to constitute a risk factor for the development of PTSD.**

## Protective Factors

Some research has been conducted on factors that might protect soldiers from PTSD and other mental-health disorders. IOM (2008a) reviewed studies of veterans of such past conflicts as World War II, the Gulf War, and the Vietnam War and noted that psychologic resilience—often characterized by hardiness, personal control, and positive coping strategies—is inversely related to the risk of PTSD after traumatic or stressful events. Studies have indicated that strong social support is protective against the onset of PTSD. A recent study of OIF and OEF veterans supports the past research on protective factors. Pietrzak et al. (2009b, 2009c) reviewed self-report data on 272 OIF and OEF veterans; PTSD was assessed with the PCL. They found that the PTSD group had significantly lower total and individual resilience scores than those who did not have PTSD.[7] The only exception was the individual score that measured spiritual influences. They also found that unit support and postdeployment support were inversely related to PTSD and depressive symptoms.

In results that were consistent with findings from Pietrzak and colleagues, Skopp et al. (2011) found that soldiers who had positive appraisals of military service were less likely to screen positive for PTSD after deployment, and Phillips et al. (2010) found that marines who had five or more close confidants were less likely to screen positive for PTSD. MacGregor et al. (2012) investigated the effect of dwell time on new diagnoses of PTSD and other mental-health disorders in male marines deployed to Iraq once (49,328) or twice (16,376).[8] They reviewed military and medical records, conducted logistic regression analyses, and found that longer dwell times were associated with significantly lower odds of new diagnoses of PTSD and other mental-health disorders.

## COMORBID CONDITIONS

PTSD is often comorbid with other psychiatric conditions and substance-use disorders. The 2008 IOM report *Gulf War and Health, Volume 6: Physiologic, Psychologic, and Psychosocial Effects of Deployment-Related Stress* noted that the temporal relationship between PTSD and these other conditions is complex. PTSD increases the likelihood of other psychiatric disorders, and the other disorders increase the likelihood of PTSD. The subsections that follow discuss PTSD and the comorbid conditions in veteran populations. The complex and most important association between PTSD and TBI is described above.

### Depression and Other Psychiatric Disorders

IOM (2008a) reviewed the research on psychiatric disorders in veteran populations and concluded that PTSD is highly comorbid with other psychiatric conditions, especially generalized anxiety disorder (GAD) and major depressive disorder. For example, Kulka et al. (1990) found that 75% of male veterans who had PTSD had a lifetime diagnosis of alcohol abuse or dependence, 44% had GAD, and more than 20% had another psychiatric disorder.

Magruder et al. (2005) conducted clinical interviews via telephone with 746 randomly selected patients who had visited a VA hospital in FY 1999. They found that those who had a diagnosis of PTSD were significantly more likely to have a comorbid mental-health disorder than those who did not have PTSD (87% vs 21%). The most common comorbid psychiatric condition was major depression, which was followed by other anxiety disorders—such as GAD, panic disorder, and agoraphobia—and then substance-use disorders.

Recent studies have confirmed the common occurrence of psychiatric comorbidities in OIF and OEF veteran populations. As discussed above, Seal et al. (2009) investigated mental-health diagnoses in OIF and OEF veterans. They found that 29% of the 106,726 veterans who

---

[7]Individual scores included measures of personal competence, tolerance of negative affect and stress-related growth, acceptance of changes, and personal control.
[8]The authors defined *dwell time* as time at home between deployments.

had mental-health diagnoses had two diagnoses and 33% had three or more. PTSD was the most common mental-health diagnosis (see Figure 4.3, from Seal et al., 2009).

The individual effects of the comorbid psychiatric conditions on mental or physical functioning or quality of life have also been examined. Rauch et al. (2010) evaluated the effects of depression and anxiety on health satisfaction in 249 combat veterans who had and did not have PTSD. PTSD was diagnosed by using clinical interviews. Average scores on self-report questionnaires indicated that the veterans had moderately high levels of anxiety, moderately severe levels of depression, and low levels of health satisfaction. Anxiety and depression were shown to have adverse effects on health satisfaction. However, when the study authors controlled for PTSD severity, combat exposure, and age and examined the conditions simultaneously in the model, only depression had a significant adverse effect on health satisfaction.

Similarly, Pittman et al. (2012) used a self-report questionnaire (SF-36) to evaluate the individual effects of PTSD and depression on mental and physical health-related quality of life in 220 OIF and OEF combat veterans. PTSD was diagnosed in 46% by using structured clinical interviews; all the veterans showed some level of depression, from minimal to severe. The investigators controlled for overlapping symptoms (anhedonia, difficulty concentrating, and insomnia) and found that PTSD and depression both had adverse effects on mental and physical health outcomes. However, the two conditions were significant independent predictors only of mental-health–related quality of life, not physical-health–related quality of life. Depression was the more significant contributor with respect to mental-health–related quality of life.

**Substance-Use Disorders**

IOM (2008a) noted that it is now well accepted that alcohol and drug use are often comorbid with PTSD in veteran populations. Several studies have shown that veterans who have PTSD are at increased risk for alcohol or drug abuse or dependence (O'Toole et al., 1998; Ouimette et al., 1996; Shipherd et al., 2005; Yarvis et al., 2005).

Recent studies support the correlation between PTSD and substance-use disorders. Jakupcak et al. (2010a) investigated the relationship of psychiatric disorders and alcohol misuse in 287 OIF and OEF veterans who had PTSD (37.3%), depression (37.3%), or alcohol misuse (28%). PTSD was identified by using the PCL; 76.6% of veterans who had PTSD screened positive for depression. Several significant independent predictors of alcohol misuse were identified, including PTSD and depression. Veterans who had PTSD or depression were twice as likely to abuse alcohol as those who had neither disorder. Investigation of the PTSD symptom clusters revealed that emotional numbing correlated most significantly with alcohol misuse. The authors suggested that the co-occurrence of these disorders indicates that veterans misuse alcohol to blunt the symptoms of PTSD or depression.

Stecker et al. (2010) reviewed VA data on 293,861 OIF and OEF veterans to determine common medical and psychiatric diagnoses. They found that alcohol misuse, sleep problems, and pain were common co-occurring conditions with PTSD or depression. They noted that pain was diagnosed in about 50% of the sample population. Similarly, Thomas et al. (2010) found that alcohol misuse or aggression was a common comorbidity with PTSD or depression in soldiers who had been deployed to Iraq; they concluded that "the significant overlap between alcohol misuse, aggressive behavior, and mental disorders highlights the high rate of comorbidity in this population."

## Health Outcomes Associated with Posttraumatic Stress Disorder

A variety of health outcomes have been associated with PTSD. The following sections briefly review several health outcomes that have been reported in studies of OIF and OEF veterans who have PTSD.

### Cardiovascular Effects and Risk factors

IOM (2008a) reviewed the relationship between PTSD and cardiovascular effects. As stated in that report, there is strong evidence that resting heart rate is slightly increased in veterans who have PTSD but no clear indication that PTSD leads to hypertension (Buckley and Kaloupek, 2001). Such changes are potentially important for long-term development of heart disease because there is extensive evidence that increased heart rate is a risk factor for hypertension and cardiovascular events (Palatini and Julius, 1997). However, the findings on an association between PTSD and cardiovascular disease were mixed; a few studies indicated a positive association, and one found no association.

Andersen et al. (2010) reviewed medical records of 4,416 OIF and OEF veterans to determine whether there is an association between PTSD and various physical diseases. Enrolled study participants were followed from 2001 to 2007, and physical disease was diagnosed by primary care providers using *ICD-9* codes. The authors adjusted for possible confounders and found that veterans who had a diagnosis of PTSD had significantly increased odds of developing several diseases, including circulatory and hypertensive diseases, compared with veterans who did not have PTSD. Not only was prevalence increased, but survival analyses indicated early onset of several diseases, including circulatory and hypertensive diseases, in veterans who had PTSD (see Figure 4.4).

Trief et al. (2006) investigated whether PTSD and other comorbid psychiatric conditions affect diabetes outcomes. They evaluated male veterans enrolled in a VA primary care database with diabetes and sorted them into four comparison groups: PTSD only (480), depression only (1,696), PTSD and depression (649), and neither PTSD nor depression (11,613). Outcomes evaluated were glycemic control, cholesterol, triglycerides, weight, and body mass index (BMI). The PTSD–depression group had significantly higher cholesterol, low-density lipoprotein, weight, and BMI than one or more of the other groups.

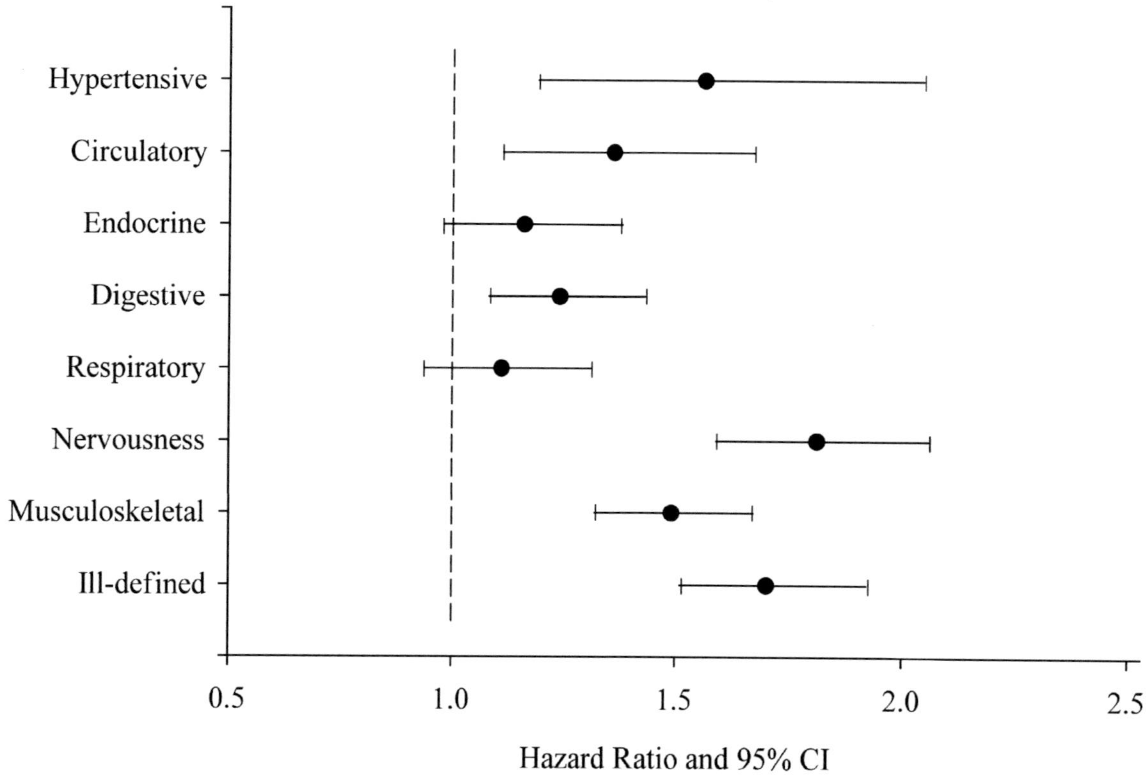


**FIGURE 4.4** Hazard ratio of eight disease categories for veterans with PTSD compared to veterans without PTSD.
SOURCE: Andersen et al., 2010 (with permission).

**Digestive System Disorders**

IOM (2008a) evaluated the relationship between PTSD and gastrointestinal effects and found several studies that reported increased prevalence of gastrointestinal symptoms and disorders in veterans who had PTSD (Barrett et al., 2002; Boscarino, 1997; Dobie et al., 2004; Hoge et al., 2007; Irwin et al., 1996; Schnurr et al., 2000). However, the studies were limited by self-reporting and cross-sectional design. Furthermore, IOM (2008a) noted that the gastrointestinal symptoms are among many somatic symptoms reported by veterans who have PTSD, and this raises the likelihood that PTSD is like other stress-related conditions in which lower sensation thresholds lead to reporting of multiple symptoms.

As described above, Andersen et al. (2010) assessed OIF and OEF veterans for physical disease and found that veterans who had a diagnosis of PTSD had higher odds of developing digestive system diseases and experienced earlier onset of the diseases than veterans who did not have PTSD.

**Endocrine Diseases**

As reviewed in IOM (2008a), veterans who have PTSD do not appear to be at significantly greater risk for diabetes or thyroid disease than veterans who do not have PTSD (Boscarino, 1997; Dobie et al., 2004; Schnurr et al., 2000; Spiro et al., 2006), although one small study did find that Vietnam veterans who had PTSD had a greater risk of hypothyroidism

(Boscarino, 2004). Differences in some serum thyroid-hormone concentrations have been noted in a few small studies (Mason et al., 1994; Wang and Mason, 1999; Wang et al., 1995), but the results did not suggest hyperthyroidism or hypothyroidism. Andersen et al. (2010) did not find a significant association between PTSD and increased risk of endocrine, nutritional, or metabolic diseases, and this was consistent with the conclusions of IOM (2008a).

**Neurocognitive and Neurobehavioral Effects**

IOM (2008a) evaluated the relationship between PTSD and neurocognitive and neurobehavioral effects in veteran populations. (The association of PTSD and TBI is covered elsewhere.) Most of the relevant studies have focused on Vietnam veterans. Overall, no association was found between PTSD alone and deficits on tests of cognition in large, well-controlled studies, using overlapping populations (Barrett et al., 1996; Crowell et al., 2002; Zalewski et al., 1994). However, the studies did not appear to have included specific tests for memory, such as explicit memory. Other studies that compared veterans who had and did not have PTSD had inconsistent findings; however, when test results were positive, the most common findings were deficits in attention and memory (Gilbertson et al., 2001; Koso and Hansen, 2006; Uddo et al., 1993; Vasterling et al., 1998, 2000, 2002; Yehuda et al., 1995).

Samuelson et al. (2006) compared neuropsychologic functioning in veterans who had PTSD (37), who had PTSD and a history of alcohol abuse (30), who had a history of alcohol abuse (30), and who had neither PTSD nor a history of alcohol abuse (31). The study attempted to eliminate the confounding often caused by comorbid alcohol abuse. PTSD was diagnosed on the basis of structured interviews conducted by a clinical psychologist. The authors controlled for confounders—such as alcohol abuse, depression, education, and vocabulary—and found that PTSD was significantly associated with decreases in verbal memory, attention, and processing speed. They stated that "by controlling for alcohol and depression, the authors can more conclusively demonstrate that verbal memory and attention differences are associated with PTSD."

Marx et al. (2009) evaluated neuropsychologic outcomes (verbal learning, visual memory, attention, and retention time) in 268 active-duty soldiers before and after deployment to Iraq. One group was tested a median of 42 days before deployment and a median of 404 days after deployment, and the other group was tested a median of 378 days before deployment and a median of 122 days after deployment. PTSD was assessed with the PCL. Soldiers assessed 1 year after deployment showed reduced attention with greater PTSD symptoms. At either postdeployment assessment, greater combat exposure was related to better reaction time. Depression was not associated with neuropsychologic outcomes.

Yaffe et al. (2010) investigated the relationship between PTSD and dementia in 181,093 veterans who were at least 55 years old and free of dementia in 1997–2000. Followup examinations occurred during 2000–2007, and diagnoses were made according to *ICD-9-CM* codes. Authors compared veterans who had a diagnosis of PTSD (53,155) with veterans who did not (127,938) and found that those who had PTSD had significantly higher rates of dementia. After adjusting for demographic factors and medical and neuropsychiatric comorbidities, the authors found that the veterans who had PTSD still had nearly twice the risk of dementia of veterans who did not have PTSD.

Afari et al. (2009) evaluated the relationship of PTSD, combat-related physical injuries, and headache in 308 OIF and OEF veterans with a battery of questionnaires. They found that PTSD and combat injuries independently predicted headaches. Veterans who had PTSD were 4 times more likely to report headaches than veterans who did not have PTSD or combat injuries. Furthermore, PTSD was significantly associated with tension and migraine headaches, whereas combat injuries were significantly associated only with migraine headaches.

**Sexual Dysfunction**

Few studies have examined the relationship of sexual dysfunction and PTSD. IOM (2008a) reviewed one small study of combat veterans (Cosgrove et al., 2002) that found that 85% of male veterans who had PTSD and only 25% of those who did not have PTSD had erectile dysfunction. PTSD severity was associated with the severity of erectile dysfunction. However, psychotropic drugs may have contributed to the findings, given that more than 50% of veterans who had PTSD used the medications compared with only 17% of veterans who did not have PTSD.

Hirsch (2009) evaluated sexual dysfunction in 53 male OIF and OEF veterans in a PTSD-treatment facility. Study participants were younger and had received a diagnosis of PTSD more recently than in earlier studies. Conditions reported were diminished libido (39), erectile dysfunction (26), and ejaculatory dysfunction (8). However, most participants were abusing alcohol, were depressed, and had suffered multiple TBIs, all of which were serious study limitations.

Nunnink et al. (2010) investigated which PTSD cluster might be associated with sexual dysfunction in 197 OIF and OEF veterans who completed a battery of questionnaires. Sexual problems were reported by 30.5% of veterans and were characterized as "diminished sexual desire/function" (36) or "impotence or other sexual problems" (32). They found that PTSD symptom severity was significantly higher in the veterans who reported sexual problems and that the numbing cluster[9] was the only significant predictor of sexual function. A serious study limitation is that no information was collected on prescription medication, which could have caused or explained the results observed.

**Sleep Disorders**

Sleep disturbances are common complaints of veterans who have PTSD. In fact, nightmares and difficulty in falling or staying asleep are two of the diagnostic criteria for PTSD. Furthermore, as discussed above, PTSD is often comorbid with other psychiatric conditions that are associated with sleep disturbance, such as depression. IOM (2008a) reviewed the relationship between PTSD and sleep disturbances and noted several studies (Engel et al., 2000; Inman et al., 1990; Neylan et al., 1998) that indicated significantly more problems in veterans who had PTSD than in those who did not on the basis of self-reported information. Several small studies have used objective sleep measures to assess sleep quality, but the results have been inconsistent; some reported no differences (Dagan et al., 1991; Dow et al., 1996; Engdahl et al., 2000), and others reported more sleep disturbances in the PTSD groups (Mellman et al., 1995, 1997; Woodward et al., 2000). The IOM report concluded that objective sleep measures have not been

---

[9]The authors noted that the numbing cluster includes such symptoms as "detachment from others, loss of interest, and restricted range of affect."

studied in veteran populations large enough to permit generalizations about the association between PTSD and sleep disturbances.

Recent research indicates that sleep disturbances are common generally in veterans and that other health factors contribute to the sleep disturbances observed. Lewis et al. (2009) evaluated 65 Australian Vietnam veterans who had probable PTSD and 87 who did not meet the PTSD criteria. PTSD was assessed with the PCL. The authors reviewed self-report data and found that significant sleep disturbances were reported by all those who had PTSD and by 90% of those who did not. The data indicated, however, that those who had PTSD had more severe sleep problems than those who did not.

Gellis et al. (2010a) investigated health factors that were associated with sleep disturbance in 201 OIF and OEF veterans who had experienced a psychologic trauma and had been referred for a behavioral assessment. The veterans were assessed with the PCL, and 120 were found to have symptom severity consistent with PTSD. Although waking PTSD-symptom severity was strongly associated with sleep disturbances, multivariate analysis that controlled for demographics and waking PTSD symptoms indicated that head injury with LOC was associated with moderate and severe nightmares, alcohol abuse or dependence was associated with moderate nightmares, and depression was associated with moderate and severe difficulties in initiating and maintaining sleep. The data indicate that other comorbid conditions play a role in the sleep disturbances reportedly associated with PTSD.

New research suggests that sleep disturbances might contribute to the development or maintenance of mental-health conditions, such as PTSD and depression. Picchioni et al. (2010) evaluated 567 Army veterans 3 months after their return from an Iraq deployment. PTSD was identified with the PCL. Having nightmares was evaluated as a possible mediator between combat stressors and PTSD, and insomnia was evaluated as a possible mediator between combat stressors and depression. Modeling results indicated that the sleep disturbances were partial mediators and thus could play a role in the development of the mental-health outcomes observed. Research by McLay et al. (2010) supports that hypothesis in that they found that active-duty military personnel who reported insomnia on return from deployment had significantly higher PTSD scores at a 3-month followup than those who did not report insomnia. Furthermore, Wright et al. (2011b) investigated the relationship between insomnia and mental-health disorders—specifically PTSD and depression—in 659 active-duty soldiers who had been deployed to Iraq. Study participants completed questionnaires at 4 and 12 months after deployment; PTSD was assessed with the PCL. They found that insomnia at 4 months significantly predicted PTSD and depression symptoms observed at 12 months, but not vice versa; that is, psychologic symptoms did not significantly predict insomnia. They concluded that their findings supported the idea that insomnia plays a role in the development of PTSD and depression. Wright et al. (2011a) assessed how insomnia affects the relationship between combat exposure and mental-health disorders, specifically PSTD and "alcohol problems." Study participants—522 military personnel who had been deployed to Iraq—were screened at 12 months before and 3 months after their deployment; PTSD was assessed with the PCL. The authors observed a stronger association between combat exposure and mental-health disorders when insomnia symptoms were more severe than when they were not, and this supported the mediating role of insomnia in the development of these mental-health disorders.

**General Symptoms and Health Status**

Several investigators have examined the relationship between PTSD and general symptoms or health status. IOM (2008a) concluded that PTSD is associated with increased reports of symptoms, medical conditions, and poor physical health in male and female veterans regardless of whether physical health is determined through physical examinations or self-reports. In fact, PTSD appears to be an even stronger predictor of poor health than does combat exposure. Furthermore, veterans, including OIF and OEF veterans, who have PTSD report more nonspecific chronic pain—such as back pain, headaches, and joint pain—than veterans who do not. The co-occurrence of PTSD and pain appears to be equally common in men and women (Asmundson et al., 2004).

Evaluating the relationship of chronic pain and PTSD, Otis et al. (2010) reviewed data from self-report questionnaires on 149 veterans suffering from chronic pain. Almost half (49%) met the criteria for PTSD on the basis of the PCL. Controlling for age, sex, pain duration, and depressive symptom severity, they found that PTSD was a significant predictor of pain and that veterans who had PTSD and chronic pain scored significantly higher on measures of affective distress than veterans who had pain but not PTSD. Seal et al. (2012) evaluated data on 141,029 OIF and OEF veterans and found that veterans who had PTSD were significantly more likely to be prescribed opioids to treat pain than veterans who did not have PTSD or who had another mental-health diagnosis. The findings held for all PTSD groups, including veterans who had PTSD and a substance-use disorder. Furthermore, the opioids were prescribed at higher doses, in combination with other opioids, and more frequently in the veterans who had PTSD. Consequently, the veterans who had PTSD were at greater risk for adverse clinical outcomes.

Using a battery of questionnaires and medical history interviews, Spiro et al. (2006) compared the health status of veterans who had PTSD (456), depression only (351), and neither condition (1,455). Most of the veterans who had PTSD (83%) screened positive for depression. Health status was assessed by using scales related to physical functioning, bodily pain, general health perceptions, vitality, limitations in activities for various reasons, and mental health (SF-36 Health Survey). Veterans who had PTSD scored significantly lower on all measures than veterans who had depression or veterans who had neither condition, and they reported significantly more medical conditions. The authors concluded that PTSD substantially affects health and that the effects are equal to or greater than those of depression. Their results are consistent with those of an earlier study by Magruder et al. (2004) in which the mental and physical functioning of 513 VA patients was evaluated with the PCL and the SF-36 Health Survey. They controlled for potential confounding factors and found that PTSD symptom severity was significantly associated with decreased mental and physical functioning.

Ouimette et al. (2004) evaluated health status in 134 patients in the VA health care system. They reviewed medical records for physician-diagnosed illnesses and self-report questionnaires on quality of life. PTSD was diagnosed in 33 patients on the basis of structured clinical interviews. A variety of traumatic events were noted; only 12% were combat related. The authors controlled for potential confounders and found that PTSD diagnoses and symptoms were significantly associated with an increased risk of circulatory and musculoskeletal disorders. They observed a positive correlation between PTSD symptom severity and total number of medical conditions. PTSD diagnoses and symptoms also were associated with a poorer quality of life as indicated by lower scores on all measures of the questionnaire (physical function, role limitations due to physical health, energy or fatigue, pain, and general health). Similar results were obtained after controlling for comorbid psychiatric conditions, such as depression, GAD, and panic attacks. The results are consistent with those reported by Andersen et al. (2010). In addition to the positive associations noted above, Andersen and co-workers found that PTSD was significantly associated with increased prevalence and onset of nervous system diseases, musculoskeletal diseases, and ill-defined signs and symptoms.

Nazarian et al. (2012) evaluated the relationship between medical comorbidities and PSTD (and substance-use disorders) in 62,496 male and 11,224 female OIF and OEF veterans who had at least two visits to a VA medical center over a 2-year period. They reviewed medical records and conducted separate analyses for men and women in 11 medical categories. Prevalences of PTSD, substance-use disorders, and both were 28.2%, 6.2%, and 3.8%, respectively, in women and 35.7%, 12.5%, and 8.1% in men. After adjusting for sociodemographic factors, they found that PTSD significantly increased the odds of a diagnosis in nine categories in men and women and that substance-use disorders significantly increased the odds of a diagnosis in two categories in women and three in men. The investigators did not observe a significant interaction between PTSD and substance-use disorders and concluded that PTSD was more strongly associated with medical comorbidities than were substance-use disorders.

Carlson et al. (2011a) investigated the relationship between postdeployment injuries and PTSD and other mental-health disorders in 742 OIF and OEF veterans using VA health care. They evaluated self-report data and found that about 50% of veterans reported an injury that had occurred after deployment. Results did not differ between men and women. Multivariate analysis indicated that probable PTSD, depression, and anger problems were significantly associated with increased odds of a postdeployment injury.

## Psychosocial Effects

Many studies have shown an association between PTSD and a variety of psychosocial effects. IOM (2008a) reviewed the research on PTSD and marital and family conflict and noted several studies of Vietnam veterans that found that marital conflict and family adjustment problems were significantly higher in veterans who had combat-related PTSD than in veterans who did not have PTSD and that the problems persisted for years after the war. For example, Jordan et al. (1992) found that veterans who had PTSD reported significantly more marital and relationship problems, more parenting problems, and poorer family adjustment than veterans who did not. Their spouses or partners were significantly more likely to report lower levels of happiness and life satisfaction and to be more demoralized. Furthermore, children of veterans who had PTSD were substantially more likely to have a behavior problem than those of veterans who did not have PTSD.

### *Violence and Aggression*

Closely related to the reports of marital and family conflict and adjustment problems are studies of intimate-partner violence. IOM (2008a) reviewed the research on this topic and noted an association between combat-related PTSD and increased intimate-partner violence and reports of hostility and violence toward other family members. Jordan et al. (1992), for example, found that family violence was significantly more prevalent in families of veterans who had PTSD. The mean numbers of violent acts committed or threatened over a year by veterans who had and did not have PTSD were 4.86 and 1.32, respectively, and the mean numbers of violent acts committed or threatened by spouses or partners of veterans who had and did not have PTSD were 3.03 and 0.96. Furthermore, Glenn et al. (2002) found that PTSD symptoms were associated with reports of hostility and violence toward the children of veterans who had PTSD and that the veterans' violent behavior correlated with their children's violent behavior.

Reports on OIF and OEF veterans support the findings noted in IOM (2008a). Jakupcak et al. (2007) investigated the relationship between PTSD symptoms and measures of anger, hostility, and aggression by comparing responses in self-report questionnaires by OIF and OEF veterans who had PTSD (47), subthreshold PTSD (21), and no PTSD (49). PTSD was identified by using the PCL. After controlling for such factors as problem drinking and combat exposure, the authors found that veterans who had PTSD or subthreshold PTSD reported significantly greater anger, hostility, and aggression than veterans who had no PTSD; and veterans who had PTSD reported significantly greater anger and hostility than veterans who had subthreshold PTSD. No significant difference in aggression was found between veterans who had PTSD and those who had subthreshold PTSD.

Elbogen et al. (2010) evaluated anger and hostility in 676 Iraq and Afghanistan veterans who served since 2001. The outcome measures evaluated were "aggressive impulses or urges, difficulty managing anger, and perceived problems controlling violent behavior." The Davidson Trauma Scale was used to assess PTSD symptoms; structural clinical interviews were conducted in a subset of study participants to verify the diagnostic accuracy of the survey. The authors found that PTSD hyperarousal symptoms were significantly associated with all three measures; other PTSD symptoms were less strongly or inconsistently associated with the measures.

Widome et al. (2011) investigated the relationship between PTSD and health-risk behaviors in 406 OIF and OEF veterans attending college. They evaluated self-report data and found that PTSD was significantly associated with a greater risk of physically fighting. They also found a marginally significant association between PTSD and high-risk drinking, which was defined as having at least five drinks at one time.

Taft et al. (2009) investigated intimate-partner aggression and general aggression in 236 male combat veterans at a PTSD clinic. The cohort comprised primarily Vietnam veterans (63%); only 5% and 1% were OIF and OEF veterans, respectively. The majority (68%) were involved in an intimate relationship in the preceding year. Structured clinical interviews were used to diagnose PTSD; 78% of veterans had diagnoses of PTSD. The data indicated that most veterans who had partners had engaged in some type of aggressive behavior in the preceding year; 33% reported physical aggression toward a partner, and 91% reported psychologic aggression toward a partner. Furthermore, veterans who had and did not have partners reported general physical aggression (32% partnered and 39% nonpartnered) and general psychologic aggression (81% partnered and 87% nonpartnered). The PTSD symptoms that best predicted aggressive behavior were those related to "arousal" and "lack of control."

Teten et al. (2010) compared intimate-partner aggression in male OIF and OEF veterans who had PTSD (27) or did not have PTSD (31) and in Vietnam veterans who had PTSD (28). PTSD was identified at a routine diagnostic screening at a VA medical clinic. The results suggested that OIF and OEF veterans who had PTSD were more likely than the other groups to abuse a female partner but also that OIF and OEF veterans who had PTSD were more likely to sustain abuse by a female partner. In an earlier study of OIF, OEF, and Vietnam veterans, Teten et al. (2009) found that PTSD was not associated with sexual aggression.

*Relationship Problems*

Monson et al. (2009) reviewed the research on intimate-relationship problems and PTSD and found that veteran studies indicated that "PTSD is strongly associated with intimate relationship problems and a number of other indices of family adjustment difficulties." Numbing or avoidance symptoms were most strongly associated with family-relationship problems, and hyperarousal symptoms were most strongly associated with physical and psychologic aggression. Furthermore, comorbid conditions appeared to contribute to the problems observed. The authors noted that few theories have been proposed to explain the association and concluded that "study of the connection between PTSD and intimate relationship functioning is sorely in need of theory development and testing to further understanding of these associations and ultimately advance prevention and treatments."

*Legal Problems*

Producing results consistent with the association between PTSD and anger, hostility, and aggression, Highfill-McRoy et al. (2010) found that PTSD was associated with behavior problems in active-duty marines. They compared 77,998 marines deployed to Iraq, Afghanistan, or Kuwait (war-deployed marines) with 13,944 marines deployed elsewhere outside the United States (non-war-deployed marines) on the basis of information from military records that contained physician-diagnosed conditions. They found that war-deployed marines who had PTSD were more likely to receive demotions and punitive discharges than war-deployed marines who had no psychiatric diagnosis. Both groups of deployed marines who had PTSD were more likely to receive drug-related discharges than were marines who did not have a psychiatric diagnosis. The finding that most troubled the authors was that war-deployed marines who had PTSD were over 11 times more likely than their peers who had no psychiatric diagnosis to commit serious offenses that resulted in punitive discharges. Kulka et al. (1990) found an association between PTSD and arrest and incarceration: 45.7% of Vietnam veterans who had current PTSD had been arrested or jailed more than once in their lives compared with 11.6% of the veterans who did not have PTSD, and 11.5% of the veterans who had PTSD had been convicted of a felony.

*Quality of Life*

Several recent studies have investigated overall well-being among veterans and found that veterans who have PTSD have more psychosocial problems than veterans who do not. Pietrzak et al. (2009a) investigated the psychosocial effects of partial PTSD in 557 OEF and OIF veterans. PTSD was identified by using the PCL, and psychosocial effects were assessed by using a self-report questionnaire. Study authors found that 120 had full PTSD, 124 had partial PTSD, and 313 had no PTSD. Veterans who had partial PTSD exhibited significantly worse health and psychosocial difficulties than veterans who had no PTSD. A severity–response trend was observed; veterans who had full PTSD exhibited the most significant decrements in health and psychosocial scores.

Similarly, Gellis et al. (2010b) investigated the effects of partial PTSD on quality of life in OIF and OEF veterans who had experienced a traumatic event and were referred for behavioral assessment. All study participants were interviewed by telephone; PTSD was identified by using the PCL. Comparison groups were full PTSD (120), partial PTSD (37), and trauma only (44). The study authors found that veterans who had partial PTSD had significantly worse mental-health functioning than the trauma-only group; however, when they controlled for "other psychiatric factors," the two groups did not differ significantly. As in previous studies, those who had full PTSD had the most significant decrements. No differences in physical functioning were found among the groups. The study authors noted that the lack of significant differences between groups could be due to various study limitations, including misclassification (that is, veterans who had partial PTSD might have been assigned to the trauma-only group and those who had full PTSD might have been assigned to the partial-PTSD or trauma-only group).

In a longitudinal study, Shea et al. (2010) investigated the relationship between PTSD and impaired psychosocial functioning in 124 National Guard or reserve veterans who had been deployed to Iraq or Afghanistan. PTSD was diagnosed by using structured clinical interviews at about 6 months after deployment. Controlling for potential confounders, the authors found that PTSD diagnosis and symptoms were significantly associated with poor psychosocial functioning and distress. Numbing or avoidance symptoms adversely affected relationships and strongly predicted impaired interpersonal and social functioning. Hyperarousal symptoms strongly affected overall functioning and predicted overall severity and distress. The authors noted that the results are important because they show that poor function and distress can occur soon after exposure (that is, within months), not necessarily only years after exposure.

Overall, Kehle et al. (2011b) found a negative association between PTSD and social functioning and quality of life in a study of 348 OIF National Guard soldiers. The soldiers were surveyed 1 month before and 3 months after deployment. Structured clinical interviews were conducted 6–12 months after deployment, and self-report responses were collected on social functioning and quality of life. PTSD and subthreshold PTSD were diagnosed in 7% and 9% of the cohort, respectively. Other psychiatric diagnoses—including depression (15%), other anxiety disorders (13%), alcohol-use disorders (13%), and drug-use disorders (1%)—were noted. They found that soldiers who had PTSD or subthreshold PTSD were significantly more likely to have impaired social functioning and decreased quality of life than those who did not have such a diagnosis. Comorbid psychiatric diagnoses were associated with greater impairment in the soldiers who had PTSD. Those general findings are consistent with the adverse psychosocial effects that have been noted in military personnel or veterans who have PTSD.

*Employment*

One factor important for successful reintegration of veterans into civilian life is gainful employment. IOM (2008a) reviewed several studies (Jordan et al., 1992; Savoca and Rosenheck, 2000; Zatzick et al., 1997a, 1997b) that found that veterans who had PTSD were more likely to be unemployed and, if employed, likely to receive lower wages than their counterparts who did not have PTSD. Smith et al. (2005) investigated employment outcomes in 325 Vietnam veterans who had severe or very severe PTSD and found that veterans who had severe symptoms were more likely to be unemployed or to have only part-time employment. They, however, did not find a significant association between earnings and symptom severity in people who had comparable employment.

Adler et al. (2011) recently evaluated work-performance measures in 797 OIF and OEF veterans who were referred for behavioral-health assessment. They reviewed self-report data from standard questionnaires and surveys and found that psychiatric disorders—major depressive disorder, PTSD, and GAD or panic disorder—adversely affected multiple dimensions of work performance, including mental–interpersonal demands, time management, and output.

Substantial decrements in productivity were noted in those veterans compared with nonveteran employees who did not have psychiatric disorders. Similarly, Erbes et al. (2011) investigated the relationship between mental-health disorders and occupational functioning in 262 National Guard or reservists who had been deployed to Iraq. Mental-health disorders—PTSD, subthreshold PTSD, major depressive disorder, and alcohol-use disorder—were diagnosed by using structured clinical interviews about 6 months after deployment, and occupational functioning was assessed at the diagnostic interview and again 1 year later. A high prevalence of comorbidity was found, ranging from 46% in participants who had alcohol-use disorder to 85% for participants who had PTSD. The investigators found that employment status did not differ between those who had mental-health disorders and those who did not; however, "work role functioning" was lower in those who had mental-health disorders, and those who had PSTD had high rates of deterioration in work role functioning.

### *Homelessness*

Homelessness is closely related to employment difficulties, but few studies have investigated the possible association between PTSD and homelessness in veteran populations. IOM (2008a) noted one study (Rosenheck and Fontana, 1994) that did not find a direct relationship between PTSD and homelessness but did find that combat exposure and other psychiatric illnesses were directly related to homelessness.

### *Effects on Caregivers*

Veterans or military personnel who have PTSD are not the only ones to suffer adverse psychosocial effects; their caregivers also appear to be adversely affected. Calhoun et al. (2002) investigated perceived burden and psychologic distress in the partners of 71 Vietnam veterans seeking treatment for PTSD. PTSD was diagnosed by using structured clinical interviews; 51 received a diagnosis of PSTD. The investigators found that partners of those who had PTSD reported greater burden and had worse psychologic adjustment—such as more depression, hostility, and aggression—than partners of those who did not have PTSD. Greater severity of PTSD correlated with greater burden, and caregiver burden was strongly associated with the veterans' psychologic adjustment.

## Summary

Estimates of prevalence of PTSD in service members deployed to OEF and OIF range from 5% to 20%. Some risk factors for PTSD are low age in active duty (higher age in reservists); combat exposure; being single or divorced; prior traumatic exposure, especially childhood physical abuse and other adverse experiences; MST; and a history of mental-health diagnosis. PTSD is often comorbid with several other health and mental-health conditions, such as depression, anxiety disorders, and substance use (particularly alcohol abuse). Numerous psychosocial conditions have been found to be associated with PTSD, for example, violence and aggression, relationship problems, decreased quality of life, legal problems, and homelessness. Research demonstrates that PTSD can cause substantial distress and functional impairment. The various effects and the interconnections of PTSD with other physical, mental, and social outcomes can interfere with readjustment into one's previous life.

## MULTIPLE DEPLOYMENTS AND POSTTRAUMATIC STRESS DISORDER

### Multiple Deployments, Deployment Location, and Dwell Time

Soldiers deployed to Iraq report long deployment as the foremost stressor in theater (MHAT-II, 2005). To study the mental-health impact of deployment length, most researchers measure the number of deployments. The mental-health outcome most commonly diagnosed is PTSD or PTSD in conjunction with other mental disorders, such as depression and anxiety, as measured by validated symptom checklists used for screening purposes. Many studies have found that multiple deployments place soldiers at increased risk for PTSD, but the evidence is more ambiguous with respect to other mental-health outcomes. A few studies, described below, have examined the mental-health impact of dwell time; the data are conflicting as to whether a longer dwell time increases or decreases the risk of mental-health problems.

Phillips and colleagues (2010) studied marines in the Recruitment Assessment Program, of whom 433 were deployed once and 273 twice. Using the PCL, they found that two deployments nearly doubled the risk of PTSD (adjusted OR = 1.91 [1.10–3.33]). However, the cumulative length of deployment was not a significant predictor of PTSD.

Reger and colleagues (2009) studied Army troops in the Soldier Wellness Program, an extension of a standard postdeployment screening program conducted throughout the Army and DOD. They screened 661 who had a single deployment and 661 who had two deployments. They found a higher risk of PTSD in those who had two deployments—an adjusted OR of 1.64 ($p = 0.001$) with a less conservative cutoff and an OR of 1.60 ($p = 0.001$) with a more conservative cutoff. They did not find an association between the number of deployments and major depression, panic, other anxiety, and hazardous alcohol consumption.

To determine the effects of multiple deployments, Kline et al. (2010) reviewed self-report data on 2,543 National Guard troops deployed to Iraq and found that those who had at least one previous deployment to Iraq or Afghanistan were three times more likely than those not previously deployed to screen positive for PTSD and major depression. Alcohol dependence, chronic pain, and worse physical function were also significantly more likely in previously deployed troops. Phillips et al. (2010) also found that multiple deployments significantly increased the odds of screening positive for PTSD in marines who had been deployed to Iraq or Afghanistan. Fear et al. (2010) evaluated the effect of deployment location and multiple deployments on the mental health of UK armed forces and found a significant association between deployment to Iraq or Afghanistan and probable PTSD in reservists (1,712) but not in "regular" armed forces (8,278); PTSD was assessed with a questionnaire. No association was found for multiple deployments, but PTSD was associated with combat exposure. The UK experience may not be comparable with US experience, and the difference may account for the apparently conflicting results that have been observed.

The largest study of multiple deployments was published in the *Medical Surveillance Monthly Report* (AFHSC, 2011). It studied medical records of all 1.35 million active-duty military in 2003–2010 who had served in OIF, OEF, or Operation New Dawn (OND). The study was large enough to enable examination of not only a second deployment but third through fifth deployments. A greater percentage of deployers received a diagnosis of PTSD after the second through fourth deployments than after the first. Anxiety-related disorders, depression, and adjustment reactions were significantly higher after the second or third than after the first deployment; after the third deployment, there was a dropoff in rates of disorders, which was indicative of a "healthy-warrior" effect. Health care workers had the highest rates of disorders—even higher than those of combat troops. There was no association between multiple deployments and alcohol dependence or abuse or between multiples deployments and suicidal ideation or self-inflicted injury.

The same study investigated the effects of dwell time and found that as dwell time lengthened, most mental disorders were increased, including PTSD, major depression, anxiety-related disorders, and suicidal ideation. But there was no association between dwell time and substance abuse. Those findings are at odds with those of MacGregor and colleagues (2012), who studied nearly 16,400 marines deployed to Iraq. Using medical records and deployment databases, they found significantly reduced rates of disorders when dwell time doubled.[10] For PTSD only, the OR was 0.47 (0.32–0.70); for PTSD with other mental health disorders, the OR was 0.56 (0.33–0.94); and for "other mental health disorder," the OR was 0.62 (0.51–0.75). Thus, this study found that longer dwell time had a protective effect.

The Millennium Cohort study is a large, population-based prospective DOD study of military personnel in all branches of service. One of the investigations spawned by this undertaking was a study of multiple vs single deployers in relation to PTSD (Bonanno et al., 2012). The sample contained nearly 3,400 single deployers and 4,400 multiple deployers screened for PTSD before deployment and at two times thereafter spaced 3 years apart. The study was focused on the trajectory of symptoms assessed with the PCL-Civilian. It found moderate to improving PTSD in 8% of single and 8.5% of multiple deployers and a worsening to chronic course in 6.7% of single and 4.5% of multiple deployers. The study concluded that the trajectories were similar. No information was given on the specific number of deployments, on the grounds that this information might influence the outcome, according to a separate study (AFHSC, 2011), which found that PTSD rates declined precipitously at fourth and fifth deployments.

In a program that began in 2003, DOD conducts annual or biennial detailed assessments of soldiers' mental health during deployment in Iraq or Afghanistan. The teams carrying out the assessments are known as mental-health assessment teams. Dispatched by the Army surgeon general, they survey up to 2,300 personnel, typically combat units of the Army and, more recently, marines. They also conduct focus groups, but their data on multiple deployments are based on surveys. Their method varies somewhat from year to year, but the investigators are most likely to use the PCL and other validated surveys to assess mental health. Their reports use the term *acute stress* to denote PTSD symptoms in a combat zone (MHAT-IV, 2006).

Four reports over the last 6 years have analyzed the effects of multiple deployments. The first, of 1,320 service personnel in 2006 (MHAT-IV, 2006), compared one-time with two-time deployers and found that the latter were significantly more likely to screen positive for acute stress (24% vs 15%), depression (10% vs 8%), anxiety (12% vs 7%), and any mental-health problem (27% vs 17%).

The next report compared three groups: first-time, second-time, and third-time deployers. Of a total of 2,163 service members, third-time deployers (27.2%) and second-time deployers (18.5%) were significantly more likely to screen positive for any mental-health problem than

[10]They measured dwell time as the length of time between deployments divided by the length of the first deployment.

were first-time deployers (11.9%). There was no relationship between multiple deployments and individual disorders, suicidal ideation, or marital discord. But there was a significant relationship between multiple deployments and use of alcohol (MHAT-V, 2008). The report did not specify whether personnel screened positive for individual disorders.

The ensuing report, published in 2009, also looked at first-, second-, and third-time deployers. Of a total of 638 service personnel, third-time deployers (31%) and second-time deployers (18%) were significantly more likely to screen positive for any mental-health problem than were first-time deployers (13.6%). Regarding medications, third-time deployers (9.8%) were more likely than second-time deployers (4.5%) and first-time deployers (3.5%) to report taking "any mental health" medication. The study also found that the longer the deployment or the greater the number of deployments, the more likely were multiple deployers to report marital problems. The report did not specify whether personnel screened positive for individual disorders (MHAT-VI, 2009).

The most recently published report, published in 2011, found that third- or second-time deployers were more likely than first-time deployers to report any psychologic problem, any mental-health medication, and considering divorce or separation. The report did not specify findings on individual mental disorders (MHAT-VII, 2011) (see Figure 4.5 below).

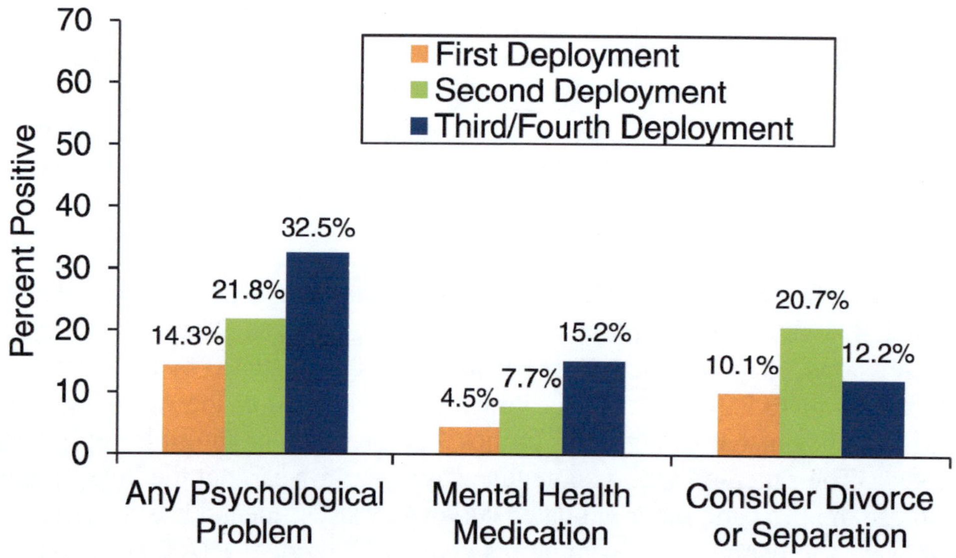


**FIGURE 4.5** Number of deployments and selected outcomes.
SOURCE: MHAT-VII, 2011.

Shen et al. (2010) and Shen and Arkes (2009) examined the relationship between PTSD diagnosis and deployment location and duration in 678,227 active-duty enlisted personnel in all four branches of the armed services. They found that deployment to Iraq or Afghanistan significantly increased the odds of a PTSD diagnosis in all four services; the greatest effect was found in the Navy, and the smallest in the Air Force. Deployments longer than 180 days were associated with increased odds of a PTSD diagnosis. An analogous study of 95,873 officers in all four services yielded similar results, but the deployment effects were smaller and deployment duration appeared to be a risk factor only in Army and Navy officers (Shen and Arkes, 2009). Reger et al. (2009) reviewed routine mental-health screening of 1,322 regular, active-duty soldiers who were evaluated 90–180 days after deployment to Iraq and reported increased odds of PTSD after two deployments.

## MOOD DISORDERS

Mood disorders are signature conditions of the current conflicts. The present report focuses on TBI and PTSD, and depression is frequently comorbid with both. The centrality of depression has been emphasized in previous IOM reports on deployment and postdeployment health, so only a brief discussion of mood disorders, specifically depression, is provided below.

Mood disorders are a cluster of mental disorders that are characterized by mood swings or an abnormally depressed (low) mood or a manic mood or irritability. The most common mood disorder is depression, and the clinically most important form is major depression, which is characterized by persistent feelings of sadness accompanied by several symptoms related to changes in appetite or sleeping patterns, loss of interest in activities, fatigue, inability to concentrate, and hopelessness or suicidal thoughts. As described in *DSM-IV* (APA, 2000), major depressive disorder is characterized by the occurrence of at least one major depressive episode (see Box 4.2). It is the second-most common mental-health diagnosis in veterans after PTSD (Seal et al., 2009).

Like PTSD, depression may be defined by strict criteria, such as the *DSM* criteria for major depression, or by self-assessment of depression symptoms. The RAND (Tanielian and Jaycox, 2008) report reviewed 12 studies that assessed the prevalence of depression in service members who served in OEF or OIF. Estimates of prevalence in active-duty service members ranged from 5% (Hoge et al., 2006; Kolkow et al., 2007; MHAT-II, 2005) to 37% (Lapierre et al., 2007). Thomas et al. (2010), described above, also estimated the prevalence of depression in active-duty and National Guard troops at 3 and 12 months after deployment to Iraq. They used three case definitions of depression, each reflecting a level of functional impairment. At 3 months, the prevalence ranged from 16% (no functional impairment) to 8.3% (serious impairment) in active-duty soldiers and from 11.5% (no impairment) to 5.0% (serious impairment) in National Guard soldiers. At 12 months, the rates were similar to those at 3 months in active-duty soldiers but substantially increased in National Guard soldiers.

Prevalence varies by sex. For example, as in the general population, female veterans have higher rates of major depression and depressive symptoms, whereas male veterans typically have higher rates of substance use disorders. As noted above, a number of studies have documented that various aspects of deployment increase the risk of depression (Fritch et al., 2010; Kline et al., 2010; Riviere et al., 2011). For example, Wells et al. (2010) investigated the relationship between deployment and the risk of depression as defined by the Primary Care Patient Health Questionnaire. They evaluated data on over 30,000 men and 10,000 women in the Millennium Cohort Study who did not have depression at baseline and found that deployed service members who were exposed to combat in Iraq or Afghanistan had the highest rates of new-onset depression (men, 5.7%; women, 15.7%). Those who did not deploy had intermediate rates (men, 3.9%; women, 7.7%), and those who deployed and were not exposed to combat had the lowest rates (men, 2.3%; women, 5.1%).

**BOX 4.2**
**Criteria for Major Depressive Episode**

A. Five (or more) of the following symptoms have been present during the same 2-week period and represent a change from previous functioning; at least one of the symptoms is either (1) depressed mood or (2) loss of interest or pleasure.

Note: Do not include symptoms that are clearly due to a general medical condition, or mood-incongruent delusions or hallucinations.

1. depressed mood most of the day, nearly every day, as indicated by either subjective report (e.g., feels sad or empty) or observation made by others (e.g., appears tearful). Note: In children and adolescents, can be irritable mood.
2. markedly diminished interest or pleasure in all, or almost all, activities most of the day, nearly every day (as indicated by either subjective account or observation made by others)
3. significant weight loss when not dieting or weight gain (e.g., a change of more than 5% of body weight in a month), or decrease or increase in appetite nearly every day. Note: In children, consider failure to make expected weight gains.
4. insomnia or hypersomnia nearly every day
5. psychomotor agitation or retardation nearly every day (observable by others, not merely subjective feelings of restlessness or being slowed down)
6. fatigue or loss of energy nearly every day
7. feelings of worthlessness or excessive or inappropriate guilt (which may be delusional) nearly every day (not merely self-reproach or guilt about being sick)
8. diminished ability to think or concentrate, or indecisiveness, nearly every day (either by subjective account or as observed by others)
9. recurrent thoughts of death (not just fear of dying), recurrent suicidal ideation without a specific plan, or a suicide attempt or a specific plan for committing suicide

B. The symptoms do not meet criteria for a Mixed Episode (see DSM-IV-TR, 2000)

C. The symptoms cause clinically significant distress or impairment in social, occupational, or other important areas of functioning

D. The symptoms are not due to the direct physiological effects of a substance (e.g., a drug of abuse, a medication) or a general medical condition (e.g., hypothyroidism)

E. The symptoms are not better accounted for by Bereavement, i.e., after the loss of a loved one, the symptoms persist for longer than 2 months or are characterized by marked functional impairment, morbid preoccupation with worthlessness, suicidal ideation, psychotic symptoms, or psychomotor retardation

SOURCE: Reprinted with permission from the *Diagnostic and Statistical Manual of Mental Disorders*, Fourth Edition, Text Revision (Copyright 2000). American Psychiatric Association.

Similarly, Shen et al. (2012) evaluated the relationship between deployment and major depression and substance-use disorders in 678,382 active-duty military personnel (Army, 333,548; Marines, 98,524; Navy, 134,015; and Air Force, 112,295). They reviewed military and medical records and found that deployment during Iraq and Afghanistan wars increased the likelihood of major depression and substance-use disorders; the greatest effect was observed in the Army and the Marine Corps. Deployment duration appeared to increase the odds of depression and substance-use disorders only in Army personnel. As noted in the section "Posttraumatic Stress Disorder," other risk factors for depression include MST (Kimerling et al.,

2010; Suris and Lind, 2008), childhood physical abuse (Fritch et al., 2010), and adverse childhood experiences (Cabrera et al., 2007).

There have been no population-based studies of US service members deployed to war zones in which investigators used structured diagnostic interviews, which permit more direct estimation of major depression and have an advantage over the screening instruments that are commonly used in epidemiologic surveys. According to RAND (Tanielian and Jaycox, 2008), the extant studies may substantially underestimate the prevalence of depression in the postdeployment samples. Furthermore, most studies used convenience samples, which may not be representative of the entire population deployed to war zones.

Investigators have shown that depression is a major contributor to health dissatisfaction (Rauch et al., 2010) and to mental-health and physical-health outcomes (Pittman et al., 2012). In fact, Kinder et al. (2008) found a positive association between depression and all-causes mortality. They evaluated self-report data and administrative medical records on 35,715 patients of VA medical centers, who were assigned to four groups—those who had a history of depression (6,876), those who had a history of PTSD (748), those who had a history of depression *and* PTSD (3,762), and those who had no history of either condition (24,329). After adjusting for potential cofounders (age, demographic factors, alcohol and drug use, smoking status, and medical comorbidities), they found that those who had a history of depression were at higher risk for death over a 2-year period than those who had no history of depression or PTSD. Furthermore, those who had a history of depression and PTSD were not at greater risk than those who had only a history of depression; this is consistent with the finding that those who had a history of PTSD were not at greater risk of death. The authors noted that further analyses indicated that current depression symptoms might explain the observed relationship between death and history of depression. Regardless of a precise estimate of prevalence, depression in OIF and OEF veterans remains a serious problem that has increased since initiation of the Iraq War (see Figure 4.3).

## SUBSTANCE-USE DISORDERS

Substance-use disorders include the abuse of and dependence on drugs (including illicit drugs, prescription drugs, alcohol, and other toxic agents). According to *DSM-IV TR* (APA, 2000), substance abuse is a "maladaptive pattern of substance use manifested by recurrent and significant adverse consequences related to the repeated use of substances," whereas substance dependence is defined as "a cluster of cognitive, behavioral, and physiological symptoms indicating that the individual continues use of the substances despite significant substance-related problems. There is a pattern of repeated self-administration that can result in tolerance, withdrawal, and compulsive drug-taking behavior" (APA, 2000).

### Substance-Use Disorders in the General Population

#### Illicit Drugs

According to the results of the 2010 National Survey on Drug Use and Health (NSDUH) (SAMHSA, 2011), 8.9% of the general population of Americans 12 years old or older reported using illicit drugs in the month before the survey. That represents about 22.6 million people and was similar to the 2009 rate of 8.7% and higher than the 2008 rate of 8%. Illicit drugs included marijuana and hashish, cocaine (including crack), heroin, hallucinogens, inhalants, and nonmedical use of prescription drugs.

### Alcohol

With regard to alcohol abuse and dependence, 51.8% of Americans 12 years old or older, 131.3 million people, reported using alcohol, a rate that is similar to the 51.9% of 2009. Binge drinking (having five or more drinks per occasion on 1 day) was reported by 23.1% of the people 12 years old or older in the month before the survey, about 58.6 million people, a rate similar to the 23.7% of 2009.

Heavy drinking (defined as binge drinking on at least 5 days in the preceding 30 days) was reported by 6.7% of the population in 2010. However, among those 18–25 years old, the rate of binge drinking was 40.6% and the rate of heavy drinking 13.6%; both these rates were similar to the rates of 2009.

### Prescription Drugs

According to the National Institute on Drug Abuse, the most commonly abused prescription drugs are opioids, which are often prescribed for pain relief; central nervous system depressants, such as barbiturates and benzodiazepine, often prescribed for anxiety or sleep problems; and stimulants, often prescribed for attention-deficit hyperactivity disorder, the sleep disorder narcolepsy, and obesity.

Abuse of prescription drugs has resulted in overdose deaths. According to CDC, 36,450 overdose deaths resulted from prescription drugs in 2008, and 73.8% of them involved opioid pain relievers (CDC, 2011b).

In 2010, the NSDUH found that about 9.0 million Americans 12 years old or older reported nonmedical use of prescription drugs, including 5.1 million users of pain relievers, 2.2 million users of tranquilizers, 1.1 million users of stimulants, and 374,000 users of sedatives (SAMHSA, 2011).

## Substance Use Disorders in the Military

### Illicit Drugs

The 2008 DOD Health Related Behavior Survey (Bray et al., 2009b), which is conducted in a random sample of active-duty military and questions them about drug use in the previous month, found the rate of illicit-drug use, excluding prescription drugs, to be about 2% and noted that the rate had been unchanged since 2002. However, in the Army, Marine Corps, and Air Force, rates of illicit-drug use (excluding prescription drugs) were significantly higher in personnel deployed to combat theaters other than OEF and OIF than in those deployed to OEF and OIF or those not deployed. Illicit-drug use, including prescription-drug use, increased from 5% in 2005 to 12% in 2008.

*Status of Drug Use in the Department of Defense Personnel: Fiscal Year 2008 Drug Testing Statistical Report* (DOD, 2009b) notes the rates of illicit-drug use in FY 2004–2008. That report indicates that illicit-drug use rates were below 2% in active-duty forces. Rates were also below 2% in reserve personnel not on active duty but exceeded 2% in National Guard personnel not on active duty. Drugs tested included amphetamines, cocaine, ecstasy, marijuana, MDA (methylenedioxyamphetamine), opioids, and phencyclidine.

**Alcohol**

Milliken et al. (2007) found that rates of problem alcohol use—detected with a two-item screen on the PDHRA—in those screened by DOD after deployment ranged from 11.8% (active duty) to 15.0% (National Guard and reserve). They also noted that of the 56,350 active-duty soldiers who endorsed alcohol misuse (6,669, or 11.8%), only 134, or 0.2%, were referred to alcohol services and that only 29 of those referred were seen within 90 days.

The 2008 DOD HRBS (Bray et al., 2009b) found that military rates of alcohol use are higher than in civilians 18–35 years old but lower in those 46–64 years old. The 2008 survey noted that heavy drinking (five or more drinks per occasion at least once a week) remained at about the 2005 level (20% and 19%, respectively). The services that had the most pronounced increases were the Marine Corps, increasing from 25% in 2005 to 29% in 2008, and the Air Force, increasing from 10% in 2005 to 14% in 2008.

In a recent report that examined health and discipline in the Army (Department of the Army, 2012), findings indicated that incidents of drug and alcohol abuse in soldiers had increased from 28,740 offenses in 2006 to 34,586 in 2009 and then decreased by 9.1% to 31,617 offenses in 2010 and by 4% to 29,708 in 2011. Those recent decreases have been coupled with increased rates of referral for drug and alcohol treatment. In FY 2010, there were over 24,000 referrals of soldiers to the Army Substance Abuse Program; about 50% of those referred were enrolled. It has been found that 43% of active-duty Army personnel reported binge drinking within the preceding month. Although 12% of soldiers reported alcohol problems on the PDHRA, only 2% have been referred for further evaluation or treatment. The report also noted that alcohol abuse is associated with several risk factors related to combat service, such as exposure to the threat of death or injury and a diagnosis of PTSD.

Several earlier studies of military populations found similar problems with substance abuse and dependence, particularly alcohol abuse and dependence, when deployed service members returned from service in Iraq or Afghanistan (Hoge et al., 2004b; Jacobson et al., 2008; Lande et al., 2008; Stahre et al., 2009).

**Prescription Drugs**

The 2008 DOD HRBS (Bray et al., 2009b) found that in all services there was no significant difference in the rates of prescription-drug misuse in the preceding 12 months. Findings indicate that rates were significantly higher in combat personnel deployed to theaters other than OEF and OIF than in those deployed to OEF and OIF and those who had not been combat deployed (9% in combat deployed, 5% in OEF and OIF deployed, and 6% in nondeployed).

According to the Office of National Drug Control Policy, the number of active-duty military personnel reporting misuse of prescription drugs (12%) is more than twice that in the civilian population (4.4%) in those 18–65 years old. Similarly, 13.1% of women in the military report prescription-drug abuse compared with 3.2% of civilian women (Office of National Drug Control Policy, 2010).

A recent Army report, *Army 2020 Generating Health and Discipline in the Force Ahead of the Strategic Reset* (Department of the Army, 2012), notes that pain is a leading cause of disability and that 47% of soldiers returning from OEF and OIF report problems associated with pain. About 14% of US soldiers have been prescribed opiate pain medications, and about 25–35% of wounded soldiers are addicted to prescription pain medications or illegal drugs. The report defines polypharmacy as the use of four or more prescription medications of which at least one is a psychotropic drug or a controlled substance, and it notes that the number of soldiers receiving polypharmacy increased in FY 2010–2011 from 141,199 to 160,175.

### Substance-Use Disorders in Veterans: Drugs and Alcohol

Several studies have attempted to determine the prevalence of substance use in OEF and OIF veterans and in all veterans. The present committee has focused its attention on studies of OEF and OIF veterans, but it also presents one study that examined prevalence in all veterans.

Wagner et al. (2007) analyzed the NSDUH data from 2000 to 2003 to estimate the prevalence of substance use and abuse in all veterans. Findings indicated that 22.6% of veterans reported binge drinking, 7.5% heavy alcohol use, and 4.4% illicit-drug use in the preceding month. Veterans reported higher rates of any alcohol use and heavy alcohol use than did comparable nonveterans; binge drinking and illicit-drug use did not differ between veterans and nonveterans. In 2010, Hawkins et al. published findings on alcohol misuse in veterans whose records had been randomly selected from among those of VA outpatients for a standardized medical review for quality-monitoring purposes. Veterans were identified (12,092, including 2,009 women) and screened for alcohol misuse in FY 2007. Alcohol misuse had been assessed with the Alcohol Use Disorders Identification Test (AUDIT);[11] findings indicated that the prevalence of alcohol misuse was 21.8% in OEF and OIF men, 10.5% in non-OEF and non-OIF men, 4.7% in OEF and OIF women, and 2.9% in non-OEF and non-OIF women.

Calhoun et al. (2008) conducted an analysis of data extracted from the VA outpatient Survey of Healthcare Experiences of Patients; the survey included a random sample of OEF and OIF veterans who were using VA clinics from October 1, 2004, to September 30, 2005. Findings indicated that 40% of the sample screened positive for hazardous alcohol use and 22% for possible alcohol-use disorder. The majority of the sample was white, male, and married; most were working or in school and had some college education. About 40% of the sample served in active-duty units, and the remaining 60% in the reserves or National Guard.

Eisen et al. (2012) examined alcohol and drug use in OEF and OIF veterans within a year of returning from deployment; PTSD and other mental-health conditions were also examined. A national sample of 596 OEF and OIF veterans were surveyed with validated screening instruments; surveys were mailed, and the authors allowed up to a year for the completed surveys to be returned. Findings indicated that 13.9% screened positive for probable PTSD, 39% for probable alcohol abuse, and 3% for probable drug abuse; men reported more alcohol and drug abuse than women. When examining health records of OEF and OIF veterans who were using VA health care services, Bagalman (2011) found the prevalence of drug abuse to be 4% and of dependence to be 3% during FY 2002–2010.

---

[11]The Alcohol Use Disorders Identification Test screen is a 10-item instrument that is used to assess alcohol-related problems and hazardous drinking.

The VA produces a quarterly analysis of VA health care service use by OIF and OEF veterans (VA, 2012). The numbers include the 834,463 veterans who separated from active duty service and who obtained care at VA facilities since from FY 2002 to the third quarter of FY 2012. That analysis found that 52,672 veterans had alcohol-dependence syndrome and 28,218 were diagnosed with drug dependence.

A study of 4,270 veterans who were 18–30 years old and were seeking care at the VA Palo Alto Health Care System noted that the prevalence of opioid use had increased from 3% in 2003 to 4.5% in 2007 (Wu et al., 2010). The patients overwhelmingly were male (91%) and white (69.9%) and had a comorbid mental-health diagnosis (29.8% had a mood disorder, 26.8% PTSD, and 20.7% a substance-use disorder). The average veteran had prescriptions from three providers and was exposed to two opioids. The prescriptions were typically written by primary-care providers; less than 1% were written by pain specialists.

In another study of opioid use in OEF and OIF veterans, researchers conducted a retrospective review of VA administrative data (Macey et al., 2011). Findings indicated that prescription opioid use was fairly common in OEF and OIF veterans who had pain and diagnoses of particular medical conditions (for example, lower back pain, migraine headaches, and PTSD). Of the 763 OEF and OIF veterans who had chronic pain (not associated with cancer), about two-thirds were prescribed opioids over a 1-year period, and at least one-third were prescribed opioids on a long-term basis.

### Risk Factors for Substance-Use Disorders in Active-Duty Personnel

Two recent studies examined predictors of alcohol use in National Guard soldiers before deployment (Ferrier-Auerbach et al., 2009) and after deployment (Kehle et al., 2011a). Some 515 members of a National Guard unit completed questionnaires about alcohol use before deployment to OIF. Findings indicated that 2.7% had not consumed any alcohol in the preceding year, but 26.8% of the sample engaged in binge drinking at least once per week. Rates of probable PTSD were 7%, and 6% endorsed symptoms of depression. Being single was associated with drinking more total alcohol over the year and a greater frequency of binge drinking.

In the postdeployment group, 348 National Guard soldiers deployed to Iraq from March 2006 to July 2007 completed self-report measures a month before deployment and 3–6 months after deployment. About 13% had diagnoses of alcohol-use disorder; 38% of these had an alcohol-use disorder that developed after return from deployment and was predicted by higher levels of PTSD symptom severity.

Bray et al. (2009a) compared 2007 rates of substance use in civilians with 2008 rates in military personnel and found that after adjustment for sociodemographic differences, rates of heavy alcohol use were higher in military personnel than in civilians (20% vs 14%). Bray et al. (2010) examined stress, mental health, and substance use in 28,546 US military personnel who completed the 2008 DOD survey. Trends showed reductions in tobacco use and illicit-drug use but increases in prescription-drug misuse, heavy alcohol use, stress, PTSD, and suicide attempts. Deployment exacerbated some of those changes. Heavy alcohol use was higher in personnel who had been deployed to any operational theater than in the nondeployed. There were no differences by theater for any illicit-drug use, including prescription-drug misuse, in the preceding year. Perceived high work stress in the preceding 12 months was significantly higher in personnel in any operational theater than in those who had not been deployed. Rates of experiencing high family stress in the preceding year were significantly higher in those deployed to Afghanistan or Iraq than in those deployed to other operational theaters.

Blume et al. (2010) assessed alcohol use in 876 US Army soldiers who mobilized and demobilized from Iraq during a 9-month period in 2003. HRBS questions were used to evaluate substance use and stress. The soldiers reported a moderate level of general stress at mobilization and demobilization, but only a minority reported substantial combat stress. Lower age, non-active-duty status before mobilization, and more general stress were associated with alcohol use in the 2 weeks before the demobilization evaluation. Male sex was associated with ingesting more drinks per drinking day. The results suggest that younger, non-active-duty men experiencing stress may be at risk for increased drinking after deployment.

Wilk et al. (2010a) found that a high rate of combat exposure involving threatening situations and witnessing of atrocities was associated with alcohol misuse. The authors anonymously surveyed 1,120 US Army infantry soldiers within 3–4 months after their return from deployment to Iraq regarding their experiences in combat and their physical and mental health. Soldiers who had higher rates of exposure to the threat of death or injury were significantly more likely to screen positive for alcohol misuse; exposure to atrocities predicted misuse of alcohol and alcohol-related behavioral problems.

Burnett-Ziegler et al. (2011) studied 585 members of recently returned Michigan National Guard members at a reintegration weekend. Some 36% of the National Guard members who participated met the AUDIT criteria for alcohol misuse. In the multivariate logistic regression analysis, service members who were male, were younger, and reported symptoms of depression and PTSD were at increased risk of meeting criteria for alcohol misuse. Of the National Guard members who met criteria for alcohol misuse, 31% reported receiving mental-health services in the preceding year, but only 2.5% reported receiving specific substance-abuse treatment. Those who reported misusing alcohol were most likely to report receiving services from a general physician at a military facility. National Guard members frequently identified stigma—particularly concerns related to their military career, commanding officers, and peers—as a barrier to treatment.

Spera et al. (2011) surveyed a stratified random sample of 56,137 active-duty Air Force members on 80 bases worldwide to determine the relationship between deployment and SUDs. Logistic regression analysis demonstrated that both higher frequency of deployment and greater cumulative time deployed since September 11, 2001, were associated with a greater likelihood of problem drinking. For each incremental increase in deployment frequency, the risk of being a problem drinker increased by 14%. Moreover, for each additional year that an Air Force member was deployed, the risk increased by 23%.

*Army 2020 Generating Health and Discipline in the Force Ahead of the Strategic Reset* (Department of the Army, 2012) notes that alcohol abuse is associated with several issues related to combat service, such as high rate of exposure to the threat of death or injury and a diagnosis of PTSD. A 2010 study by the Office of the Army Surgeon General (Office of the Army Surgeon General, 2010) identified numerous risk factors that may be associated with misuse of opioids, that is, being 45 years old or older, male sex, family history of prescription drugs, cigarette-smoking, substance disorder, preadolescent sexual abuse in women, major psychiatric disorder, prior legal problems, motor-vehicle accidents, and poor family support.

## Risk Factors for Substance-Use Disorders in Veterans

Numerous studies have examined risk factors for substance-use disorders in veterans. Findings from the studies below indicate the following risk factors: childhood trauma, PTSD and depression, service in the Army or Marine Corps, deployment to OEF or OIF, and pain disorders.

In a study of 60 rural and urban OEF and OIF veterans enrolled at three VA sites in Nebraska, childhood trauma was associated with drug dependence, polysubstance dependence, and four or more attempts at treatment for SUDs (Nash et al., 2011). There were no significant differences in trauma exposure between the rural and urban veterans.

A sample of 287 OEF and OIF veterans assessed at a VA facility in Seattle from 2004 to 2007 were screened for PTSD, depression, and alcohol misuse with validated screening instruments. Findings indicate that 28% of the veterans screened positive for alcohol misuse, 37.3% for PTSD, and 37.3% for depression; 76.6% of the PTSD cases also screened positive for depression. There did not appear to be any significant difference in marital status, race, employment status, or family income as a function of alcohol misuse. However, veterans who screened positive for alcohol misuse were younger, more likely to have served in the Army or Marine Corps than in the Navy or Air Force, and more likely to have reported direct combat experience. Predictors of alcohol misuse included sex, branch of service, PTSD status, and depression; PTSD and depression were associated with a twofold increase in the likelihood of alcohol misuse (Jakupcak et al., 2010a).

A study by Hawkins et al. (2010) compared a national sample of OEF and OIF veterans with a sample of non-OEF and non-OIF veterans who were all seen in the VA health care system in FY 2007. Findings indicated that alcohol misuse was higher in OEF and OIF male veterans than non-OEF and non-OIF male veterans even after adjustment for recognized substance-use and mental-health disorders, such as PTSD. The highest-risk group was OEF- and OIF-deployed men under 30 years old.

Seal et al. (2012) note that opioid analgesic prescriptions have nearly doubled in the United States since 1994 with the recognition of pain treatment. OEF and OIF veterans who have pain and PTSD and are prescribed opioids might be at high risk for misuse of prescription opioid drugs. A national sample of OEF and OIF veterans were studied to look for risks and adverse clinical outcomes associated with prescription opioid use. A retrospective cohort of OEF and OIF veterans identified by using a VA database included veterans who received a new noncancer pain diagnosis within a year of entry into the VA health care system. A total of 141,029 veterans were identified and followed for a year beyond the pain diagnosis. The veterans were overwhelmingly male (88.5%), white (50.6%), and enlisted (93.3%), and most (64.3%) had served in the Army. Most (66%) of the veterans had received two or more pain diagnoses; 51% received at least one mental-health diagnosis—19% a diagnosis of excluding PTSD and the remaining 32% a PTSD diagnosis with or without other mental-health diagnoses.

The 141,029 veterans who received pain diagnoses included 15,676 (11%) who received prescription opioids for 20 or more consecutive days and were in most cases (77%) given prescriptions by VA primary care physicians. Patterns of high-risk opioid use were detected in the 15,676 if they also had a mental-health diagnosis other than PTSD or with PTSD. Compared with veterans who did not have a mental-health diagnosis, veterans who had PTSD were more likely to be in the highest quintile for dose (22.7% vs 15.9%), to receive more than one type of opioid concurrently (19.8% vs 10.7%), to receive concurrent sedative hypnotics (40.7% vs 7.6%), and to obtain opioid refills (33.8% vs 20.4%). Thus, veterans who receive PTSD diagnoses were more likely than those who had other mental-health disorders to be prescribed opioids for longer periods and to receive sedative hypnotics in addition to opioids.

Veterans in all mental-health diagnostic categories who were prescribed opioid medications had a higher prevalence of adverse clinical outcomes than those who were not prescribed opioids (9.5% vs 4.15%). The types of adverse clinical outcomes, in an emergency setting or in inpatient admissions, included accidents resulting in wounds or injuries, opioid-related accidents, overdoses, alcohol and nonopioid drug-related accidents and overdoses, self-inflicted injuries, and violence-related injuries. The absolute risk of all adverse clinical outcomes except wounds and injuries was highest in the PTSD group.

## Substance-Use Disorders and Comorbid Conditions

Numerous studies have documented the epidemiology of the co-occurrence of substance-use disorders and anxiety disorders (e.g., Flynn and Brown, 2008). A review article by Brady et al. (2009) examines comorbidity issues related to PTSD, SUDs, and TBI in veterans and notes that there is symptom overlap among those disorders in addition to a common neurobiology. It has been noted that veterans who have a diagnosis of depression and SUD at the time of entry into the VA system have an increased risk of greater disease burden that remains constant (Possemato et al., 2010). Several studies have examined the co-occurrence of PTSD and SUD in OEF and OIF veterans, and they are discussed briefly below.

Seal et al. (2008) conducted a study of 338 OEF and OIF veterans who participated in postdeployment screening at a VA medical center or associated VA community-based clinics from 2004 to 2006. Their results demonstrated that a substantial number of the veterans met the criteria for co-occurring mental-health outcomes. Of the 338, 69% (233) screened positive for one or more mental-health disorders, and 61% for comorbid mental-health symptoms. In a followup study, Seal et al. (2011), using the VA OEF/OIF Roster of veterans, examined diagnoses in veterans who used VA health care for the first time from October 16, 2001, through September 30, 2009. The study population included 456,502 veterans; 12% were female, median age of 28 years; 36% belonged to nonwhite ethnic minorities; 60% served in the Army; and 37% had multiple deployments. Alcohol-use disorder was found in 9% of the overall sample, and drug-abuse disorder was diagnosed in 4.5%. Substance-use disorder was found in 11%, and the prevalence was higher in male veterans than in female veterans. Veterans who had alcohol-use disorder, drug-use disorder, or both had at least one comorbid mental-health diagnosis (PTSD, depression, anxiety, adjustment disorder, or a combination of these).

Stecker et al. (2010) reviewed VA data on 293,861 OEF and OEF veterans to determine common medical and psychiatric diagnoses. They found that alcohol misuse, sleep problems, and pain commonly co-occurred with PTSD or depression, and they noted that pain was diagnosed in about 50% of the sample population. Similarly, Thomas et al. (2010) found that alcohol misuse or aggression was a common comorbidity with PTSD or depression in soldiers who had been deployed to Iraq.

McDevitt-Murphy et al. (2010) investigated relationships among PTSD, alcohol abuse, and health functioning—assessed with a self-report questionnaire (SF-36)—in 151 OEF and OIF veterans. PTSD was identified in 39.1% by using the PCL and a cutoff score of 50. Alcohol abuse (or hazardous drinking) was identified in 26.5%, and PTSD and alcohol abuse in 15.9%. PTSD was negatively associated with all health measures. Mediation modeling, however, indicated that alcohol abuse was a mediator only for the association of PTSD and mental health, not physical health.

Nazarian et al. (2012) evaluated relationships among medical comorbidities, PSTD, and substance-use disorders in 62,496 male and 11,224 female OEF and OIF veterans who had at least two visits to a VA medical center over a 2-year period. They reviewed medical records and conducted separate analyses of men and women in 11 medical categories. Prevalences of PTSD, substance-use disorders, and comorbid PTSD and substance-use disorders were 28.2%, 6.2%, and 3.8%, respectively, in women and 35.7%, 12.5%, and 8.1% in men. After adjusting for sociodemographic factors, they found that PTSD significantly increased the odds of a diagnosis in nine categories in men and women and that substance-use disorders significantly increased the odds of a diagnosis in two categories in women and three categories for men. The investigators did not observe a significant interaction between PTSD and substance-use disorders and concluded that PTSD was more strongly associated with medical comorbidities than were substance-use disorders.

Shen et al. (2012) evaluated relationships among deployment, depression, and substance-use disorders in 678,382 active-duty military personnel (Army, 333,548; Marines, 98,524; Navy, 134,015; and Air Force, 112,295). They reviewed military and medical records and found that deployment during Iraq and Afghanistan wars increased the likelihood of depression and substance-use disorders; the greatest effect was observed in the Army and Marine Corps. Deployment duration appeared to increase the odds of depression and substance-use disorders only in Army personnel.

## OUTCOMES

The different outcomes associated with substances of abuse have been well documented; for example, cocaine use can precipitate heart attack, respiratory failure, strokes, seizures, abdominal pain, and nausea. Alcohol use has long been associated with damage to the liver and pancreas, fetal alcohol syndrome, changes in the brain, and effects on the heart. Alcohol has also been identified as posing a risk of several types of cancers, such as cancers of the mouth, esophagus, pharynx, larynx, liver, and breast (see http://www.drugabuse.gov; http://www.niaaa.nih.gov).

Studies in active-duty and veteran populations, not necessarily focused on OEF and OIF populations, have revealed additional outcomes associated with substances of abuse; most studies have concentrated on alcohol abuse. In active-duty personnel, the findings focus on spouse abuse, job performance, and alcohol-impaired driving. In veterans, sexual assault, suicide, and increased risk of homelessness have been noted.

Bell et al. (2006) found that alcohol abuse in heavy drinkers (defined as more than 14 drinks per week) and answering "yes" to two or more of six questions on alcohol-related problems was a predictor of domestic violence in whites and Hispanics but not blacks. In 2009, Stahre et al. examined results of the 2005 DOD HRBS (Stahre et al., 2009). Their findings indicated that binge drinkers (defined above) were more likely to report alcohol-related harms, such as poor job performance, alcohol-impaired driving, and criminal-justice problems than nonbinge drinkers. Similarly, Mattiko et al. (2011) examined the 2008 HRBS and noted that there was a dose–response relationship between frequency of drinking and serious consequences and productivity. Heavy drinkers showed three times the rate of self-reported serious consequences and productivity loss. The types of serious consequences noted in binge drinkers include health consequences and injuries, poor academic performance, unsafe sex, drinking and driving, and a higher risk of sexual assault.

Finally, a study by Martin et al. (2010) examined data on soldiers who abused their spouses to determine the prevalence of substance use during abusive incidents. The authors examined the data in the Army Central Registry for 2000–2004 and noted that 1,873 of the 7,424 soldier spouse abuse offenders had been using substances at the time of the abusive incident. On examination of the records, it was found that 96% of the abusers were using alcohol only, 1% were using illicit drugs only, and 3% were using both alcohol and illicit drugs during abuse incidents. It was also found that 3% of the spouse abusers were women. The offenders using substances during a spouse-abuse incident were more likely to be male (97%) than female, and to be non-Hispanic white (51%) or non-Hispanic black (33%). The offenders were also more likely to be enlisted and in the lower pay grades (98%).

Suicides have been increasing in the military and among veterans; Ilgen et al. (2010) examined violent and nonviolent suicides in veterans who had substance-use disorders. Records of VA patients who had SUDs who were alive at the beginning of FY 2002 and died by suicide during FY 2002–2006 were examined (854) and compared with a random sample of SUD patients who did not die by suicide during that period (4,228). Data were obtained from VA medical records and the National Death Index. Findings indicated that 70% (600) of those who died of suicide used violent means. There was no association between the type of SUD and increased risk of violent suicide. The authors noted that psychiatric disorders are often comorbid with SUDs and increase the risk of suicide.

Cucciare et al. (2011) examined sexual assault and substance use in male veterans. Data were collected on male veterans who were receiving VA outpatient mental-health care. The authors found that 9.5% of the sample (880) reported a history of sexual assault and also reported increased alcohol consumption, increased alcohol-related consequences, and increased use of illicit substances (such as cannabis, cocaine, and opiates) in the preceding 90 days.

A study of substance use in veterans and VA service-connected disability benefits with risk of homelessness was conducted by Edens et al. (2011). The authors conducted a case–control study with VA administrative data from FY 2009 (1,120,424) and compared the data with those who had recently been homeless and those who had not been homeless. The authors used an *ICD-10* diagnostic code indicating lack of housing to identify cases. The control group was a population of 1,011,368 veterans who did not receive VA homeless services or a code indicating homelessness. As a result of the analyses, with controlling for demographic and diagnostic factors, illicit-drug use remained the strongest predictor of homelessness, followed by pathologic gambling, alcohol-use disorders, personality disorders, being 40–49 years old, and being black.

## Summary

Recent studies have confirmed evidence of an association between deployment to a war zone and alcohol and drug abuse and dependence. The risk of abuse and dependence increased with greater number of deployments, length of deployment, rate of exposure to the threat of death or injury, and exposure to atrocities. Deployment to OEF or OIF also increased the likelihood of depression and substance-use disorders; the greatest effect was observed in the Army and Marine Corps.

Findings from the 2008 DOD HRBS (Bray et al., 2009b) indicated that military rates of alcohol use are higher than in civilians 18–35 years old but lower than in civilians 46–64 years old. Heavy alcohol use was higher in personnel who had been deployed to any operational theater than in nondeployed personnel. Younger members and members of the Air Force, Marine Corps, and National Guard higher rates of alcohol misuse. Trends show increases in prescription-drug misuse, heavy alcohol use, stress, PTSD, and suicide attempts; deployment exacerbated some of these behavior changes. Findings also indicated that the proportion of active-duty military personnel reporting misuse of prescription drugs (12%) is more than twice that in the civilian population (4.4%) 18–65 years old. Similarly, 13.1% of women in the military report prescription-drug abuse compared with 3.2% of civilian women (Office of National Drug Control Policy, 2010). Many active-duty personnel do not actively seek treatment for substance-use disorders; barriers to reporting and treatment include stigma, concern about effects on military career, and the perceptions of commanders, units, and peers.

Studies of veterans reported higher rates of any alcohol use and heavy alcohol use than in comparable nonveterans. Recent studies of OEF and OIF veterans found that 13.9% screened positive for PTSD, 39% for probable alcohol abuse, and 3% for probable drug abuse (Eisen et al., 2012). Quarterly analysis of OEF and OIF veterans examined in VA health care facilities found that 6.2% had diagnoses of alcohol-dependence syndrome, 4.4% nondependent abuse of drugs, and 3.29% drug dependence.

Risk factors for alcohol abuse include lower age, deployment to OEF or OIF, non-active-duty status before deployment, more general stress, exposure to atrocities, exposure to the threat of death or injury, cumulative length of deployment, and high frequency of deployment.

Numerous studies have documented the epidemiology of comorbid SUDs and other mental-health conditions in OEF and OIF veterans. The comorbid conditions include anxiety disorders, PTSD (McDevitt-Murphy et al., 2010; Nazarian et al., 2012; Seal et al., 2008, 2011; Stecker et al., 2010), and depression (Seal et al., 2011; Shen et al., 2012; Stecker et al., 2010). Studies of suicide in veterans have found that mental-health disorders are often comorbid with SUDs and increase the risk of suicide. Studies of veterans who have used VA health care services have found that veterans who have alcohol-use disorder, drug-use disorder, or both also had at least one comorbid mental-health diagnosis (PTSD, depression, anxiety, or adjustment disorder). Other comorbidities reported were sleep problems and pain.

Alcohol abuse is a predictor of domestic violence (Bell et al., 2006). In Army populations, 96% of abusers were using alcohol during the violent events. Alcohol abuse was also associated with poor job performance, productivity loss, and criminal-justice problems (Stahre et al., 2009). Service members have experienced increased rates of acute anxiety disorders, PTSD, sleep disorders, depression, substance-abuse disorders, and chronic pain. Concerns have been raised about the safety and effectiveness of prescription-medication practices for those disorders. In recent studies, prescription-drug misuse has been identified as an important problem in military personnel and veterans who served in OEF or OIF.

## SUICIDE AND SUICIDAL IDEATION

The committee focused on suicidal ideation because it was directed to examine outcomes and treatments related to the mental health issues of concern. As there are no long-term outcomes of suicide (at least for the decedent) and no treatments for suicide, the committee examined the long-term outcomes and treatments (Chapter 5) for suicidal ideation.

Suicide is a lethal self-inflicted action, a suicide attempt is a nonfatal action, and suicidal ideation consists of suicidal thoughts, such as wishing to commit suicide (see Chapter 5). The suicide literature focuses primarily on studies of risk factors for suicide; long-term outcomes of suicide attempts or suicidal ideation have not been systematically studied. It is difficult to determine the percentage of people who have suicidal ideation that go on to attempt or complete suicide. However, a recent study of suicidal ideation and suicide attempts in a large number (52,780) of active-duty members of the US Air Force found that 3% of the male and 5.2% of the female study participants reported suicidal ideation in the previous year, and 8.7% of those who reported suicidal ideation also reported a recent suicide attempt (Snarr et al., 2010).

CDC has reported that in 2009, the rate of suicide in the general population was 16.25 per 100,000 in people 25–64 years old (CDC, 2012). That recent analysis indicates that there were about 36,500 suicides. In 2009, suicide was the tenth-leading cause of death in the US population. Prevalence estimates of suicidal thoughts and behaviors indicate that during 2008–2009, an estimated 8.3 million adults in the United States reported having suicidal thoughts in the preceding year, and 2.9 million of them were 18–29 years old (CDC, 2011a).

At the beginning of the chapter, the committee notes numerous limitations of the studies it reviewed and makes a recommendation to address its concern. Although the committee has noted those limitations generally, it highlights some of them as they related to studies on suicide and suicidal ideation. Some findings are from studies of self-reported data (e.g., Jakupcak et al., 2010b, Snarr et al., 2010); others are based on VHA data, which only include veterans enrolled in VHA (McCarthy et al., 2012); the Kaplan et al. study (2012) is based on data extracted from the National Violent Death Reporting System (NVDRS). Currently only 16 states contribute data to NVDRS, which might not be representative of the veteran population.

### Suicide Rates in the Military

Historically, suicide rates in the military have been lower than those in the civilian population. However, suicide in US military personnel has recently been of increasing concern. In 2009, the suicide rate in active-duty service members was 18.3 per 100,000, the highest rate since 2008. DOD confirmed about 2,000 suicides from 2003 to 2010, of which 300 occurred during deployment. In 2010, 50% of suicides occurred in active-duty personnel who had deployed to OEF or OIF; higher rates of suicide were found in the Army and Marine Corps than in other branches of the military (CBO, 2012). The Department of Defense Suicide Event Report (DCoE, 2011) summarized suicides and suicide attempts and relied on the Armed Forces Medical Examiner System (AFMES) for its data. In 2010, the AFMES provided data indicating that 295 service members committed suicide. Demographic data indicate that risk factors for suicide include being male, white, under the age of 25 years, junior enlisted or high-school educated, and divorced (the suicide rate in divorced service members was 55% higher than that in married service members). Active-duty service members had a 70% higher risk of suicide than did deployed reserves and National Guard members. Firearms accounted for 62% of all suicides, and drug overdose was the most frequent method of suicide attempts (57%).

Some 57% of suicides were completed by persons who did not have a known history of suicide attempt or suicidal ideation, but 17% were known to have a mood disorder, specifically major depressive disorder (7%), 5% had an anxiety disorder (most frequently PTSD), and about 26% had a history of substance-use disorder (DCoE, 2011).

According to the Armed Forces Health Surveillance Center (AFHSC), suicide was the third-leading cause of death in US service members. The number of suicides in US military deployed to Iraq and Afghanistan has increased, and the estimated suicide rate in the Army almost doubled from 2004 to 2008 (from 10.8 to 20.2 per 100,000) and is now higher than that in the civilian population (Trofimovich et al., 2012). More recently, the AFHSC examined mortality data on 1998–2011 and found that since 2010 suicide has become the second-leading cause of death in service members. There were 2,990 suicides in 1998–2011 in active-duty members. The most common method of suicide in males and females was the use of firearms (AFHSC, 2012).

The AFHSC examined health care experiences that preceded suicide in US service members in January 2001–December 2010 (Trofimovich et al., 2012). Death and medical records maintained in the Defense Medical Surveillance System and the DOD Medical Mortality Registry (MMR) were used to indentify three retrospective cohorts: a suicide cohort, a self-inflicted injury cohort, and a likely self-harm cohort. During 2001–2010, 1,939 service members completed suicide, 19,955 had diagnoses of self-inflicted injuries, and 3,463 were hospitalized for likely self-harm. Among the three cohorts, the type of health care that was accessed in the month before the "event" was primary care. Specifically, 45% of those who died of suicide, 73% of those who had self-inflicted injuries, and 76% of the likely self-harm cohort had outpatient visits within 30 days before their cohort-defining events. The authors speculated that there might be "triggering" events that lead to seeking health care and that people might be screened for suicide risk in primary care (Trofimovich et al., 2012).

### Risk Factors for Suicide in Active-Duty US Military Personnel

A study conducted by Bell et al. (2010) examined death, inpatient, and emergency-room records on 1,873 Army suicides and compared them with records on 5,619 matched controls. Their analysis revealed several risk factors for suicide, including being older, being male, being white, being single, having enlisted with a prior injury, having alcohol abuse, and having had a mental-health hospitalization. The authors noted that the risk was greatest after a mental-health diagnosis but remained high for 5 years or more.

In 2011, RAND completed a study of suicide prevention in the US military. A review of the scientific literature indicated that those at risk for suicide were in several broad categories: prior suicide attempt; mental-health disorders, specifically depression and anxiety disorders, including PTSD; known SUDs; TBI (concussion, cranial fractures, cerebral contusions, or traumatic intracranial hemorrhages); feelings of hopelessness, aggression, and impulsivity; and problem-solving deficits (Ramchand et al., 2011).

A study by Black et al. (2011) examined prevalence and risk factors associated with suicides in the US Army from 2001 to 2009. Data were selected from the Army Behavioral Health Integrated Data Environment, and 874 suicides in Army soldiers were examined. The data included information on sociocultural and military risk factors, psychologic and environmental risk factors, and suicide-event characteristics. The data were compared with available data on Army personnel over the same period. Findings indicated that suicide rates doubled from 9.0 per 100,000 in 2001 to 22 per 100,000 in 2009 in all Army components (active duty, reserves, and National Guard). About 75% of suicides occurred in the United States, 20% occurred in the combat theater of operations, and the remainder occurred elsewhere. An overwhelming increase in suicide rates was observed from 2005 to 2009. The authors speculated that it might be associated with deployments to OEF and OIF. The most common method of suicide involved firearms (a finding common to all studies reviewed). Their findings are also consistent with those of other studies in that the relative risk of committing suicide is higher in men than in women, blacks are at lower risk for suicide than whites, junior enlisted committed suicide more often than senior enlisted and officers, and those deployed to OEF or OIF were at greater risk than those never deployed. In addition, 46% of those who committed suicide had a mental-health diagnosis, and 79% had personal stressors, most commonly involving relationship problems, military or work-related stress, and health issues (Black et al., 2011).

Having examined medical records, mental-health diagnoses, mental-health visits, prescriptions for anxiety and depression, and deployments to OEF and OIF, Hyman et al. (2012) determined risk factors for suicide in active-duty members during 2005 or 2007. The 2005 cohort consisted of 2,064,183, and the 2007 cohort 1,981,810. Study variables other than deployment and suicide were based on events that occurred in 2004 and 2005 for the 2005 cohort and in 2006 and 2007 for the 2007 cohort. The authors found that suicide rates increased in all services from the 2005 cohort to the 2007 cohort. Risk factors included mental-health diagnosis (especially PTSD and depression, previous suicide attempts, and suicidal ideation), prescriptions for selective serotonin reuptake inhibitors (commonly prescribed for depression or anxiety), use of sleep medications, reduction in rank, separation or divorce, and deployment to OEF or OIF. During deployments through 2005, suicide risk factors included being in the Army, particularly the National Guard and the Army reserves; in 2007, increases in suicide were experienced in all the services.

Skopp et al. (2012) conducted a study of active-duty members who served in the US military during 2001–2009. Suicide cases (1,764) according to the DOD MMR maintained by the Office of the Armed Forces Medical Examiner were included if they had been officially declared suicides. Controls (7,018) were randomly selected and matched by service, sex, age, race, entry into active component, and within 1 year of total active-duty service. The number of OEF or OIF deployment was studied as a potential risk factor. Military Health System records were reviewed (according to *ICD-9-CM* codes) for psychiatric diagnoses and partner-relationship and family problems. The standard DOD surveillance case definition was used to determine TBI status. With regard to demographic characteristics of the study population, 96% were male; about 43% were Army, 20% Air Force, and 17% Navy; and 72% were younger than 25 years old. The authors found suicide attempts were associated with mood disorders and partner and family problems. Psychiatric comorbidities were associated with increased risk for suicide.

Logan et al. (2012) obtained data on active-duty Army soldiers who committed suicide during 2005–2007. Using the CDC National Violent Death Reporting System and the DODSER, they were able to characterize the decedents. They found that the decedents were overwhelmingly male, white, less than 30 years old, married, and enlisted personnel. The circumstances preceding the suicides were health-related and stress-related and included intimate-partner problems (45%) and military-related stress (41%), such as job problems and combat experiences. The decedents had shown symptoms of mental-health problems (32% were identified as having a depressed mood). Family members, friends, co-workers, and clinicians described the decedents as sad, depressed, or suicidal (36% had communicated their intent to harm themselves).

There is a great deal of agreement in the numerous studies of risk factors for suicide in the military, particularly in OEF and OIF active-duty personnel. As suicide rates have increased, many researchers have sought to provide information to identify those at risk for suicide so that treatments might be offered and prevention strategies developed.

**Suicide Rates and Risks in Veteran Populations**

A review in the *Annals of the New York Academy of Sciences* examined the available data on risk and rates of suicide in veterans served by VA. Although the review examined all veterans, the report noted that the data were most complete for OEF and OIF veterans. Findings indicated that there was a lower risk of all-causes mortality in veterans than in the general population, but OEF and OIF veterans and the general population were at equal risk for suicide, and the findings varied little with the branch of the military. The author highlighted risk factors for suicide in the OEF and OIF veteran population: higher age, prolonged combat or injury, and having a diagnosis of TBI or a psychiatric disorder, such as PTSD. The author noted that evidence in the reports reviewed suggested that OEF and OIF veterans might have fewer psychologic and social resources that might have served as protective factors (Bruce, 2010). An earlier review by Kang and Bullman (2009) examined suicides in veteran populations and found that being a former OEF or OIF active-duty veteran and having a select mental disorder resulted in a suicide risk higher than that in the general population.

It should be noted, however, that there is a paucity of data on the entire veteran population of the United States. The VA provides data for veterans enrolled in its health care and benefits systems. Those veterans are often older and sicker than the general US population; that is particularly true for veterans seen at the VA for psychosocial and mental-health problems.

Jakupcak et al. (2010b) examined PTSD as a moderating variable in the relationship between social support and suicide risk in treatment-seeking OEF and OIF veterans. Using a self-completed questionnaire, the authors assessed suicide risk in 431 OEF and OIF veterans referred for VA mental-health services. The veterans were mostly men (88.9%) and had an average age of 32.4 years; about 67% were white, and 55.5% were not married. The researchers found that PTSD was related to increased suicide risk and that married veterans and those satisfied with social networks were less likely than unmarried veterans to be at high risk for suicide. The authors noted that the presence of PTSD might diminish the protective effect of social networks.

Studies that included an examination of risk factors for suicide in all populations of veterans found that rural residence (McCarthy et al., 2012); poor mental health, substance abuse, adverse life events (related to financial matters, health, criminal problems, and so on) (Kaplan et al., 2012); and TBI (Brenner et al., 2011) were associated with greater suicide risk.

## Risk Factors for Suicidal Ideation in Active-Duty and Veteran Populations

Several recent studies have evaluated risk factors for suicidal ideation in OEF and OIF active-duty or veteran populations.

### Active-Duty Personnel

Suicidal ideation and suicide attempts were assessed in a sample of US Air Force active-duty members by Snarr et al. (2010). They assessed suicidality during the year before participation in the study at 82 US Air Force sites worldwide. It was not noted in the study whether or what percentage of the sample were deployed to OEF or OIF. The final sample included 52,780 participants who logged on to the survey and completed it. The 1-year prevalence of suicidal ideation in the sample was 3.3% in men and 5.5% in women (according to Substance Abuse and Mental Health Services Administration, comparable 2009 civilian rates were 3.4% in men and 3.9% in women). Risk factors for suicidal ideation in the sample of women included lower rank and being non-Christian; risk factors in men included not being married, being non-Christian, being junior enlisted, and an occupation of medical personnel. The authors noted that suicidal ideation and suicide attempts are more common than completed suicides in the Air Force. They suggested that identifying risk factors would assist public health officials in targeting vulnerable groups with suicide-prevention programs.

Using the same sample as above, Langhinrichsen-Rohling et al. (2011) conducted a study of four factors and their association with suicidal ideation: individual, family, workplace, and community. Active-duty members sampled from 82 Air Force bases worldwide were invited to complete an anonymous survey, the 2006 Community Assessment. The analysis reveals that depression was the strongest predictor of suicidal ideation in both sexes. Additional risk factors in men were personal coping ability, physical well-being, alcohol problems, relationship satisfaction, interpersonal violence, dissatisfaction with the Air Force as a way of life, number of hours worked, community unity, and social support. Additional risk factors in women were financial stress, alcohol problems, relationship satisfaction, interpersonal violence, workplace satisfaction, hours worked, and social support. The authors suggested that the military develop prevention and early-intervention programs.

Using the DOD Survey of Health-Related Behaviors, which collects population-based data from reserve and active-duty forces, Lane et al. (2012) examined stress levels and mental-health status. People who participated in the survey included those who served in OEF or OIF, those who served in a different theater of operations (that is, not OEF or OIF), and those who did not served in theater. Data on the 2006 reserve component and the 2005 active-duty component of the surveys were analyzed and results revealed notable differences between reservists and active-duty personnel. For example, reservists who were deployed were more likely to report suicidal ideation and suicide attempts than those who were not deployed; active-duty personnel showed no differences in reports of suicidal ideation between deployed and nondeployed. Reservists deployed to OEF or OIF were more likely to report suicidal ideation and suicide attempts than reservists who served in other theaters or who were not deployed. Reservists reported mental-health issues related to deployment, especially more severe PTSD symptoms than the other groups, although all deployed personnel (reservists and active-duty) had higher rates of positive screening for PTSD. Deployment was also associated with perceived family and work stress, particularly in active-duty personnel; a greater percentage of deployed active-duty personnel and reservists than of nondeployed personnel reported depression symptoms.

**Veterans**

Jakupcak et al. (2009) examined PTSD as a risk factor for suicidal ideation. A sample of 435 OEF and OIF veterans who were consecutively referred and assessed for mental-health services at a VA facility (VA Puget Sound Health Care System) in 2004–2007 were screened for PTSD symptoms and suicidal ideation with self-report screening methods. Veterans who had suicidal ideation (187) and veterans who did not (220) were compared on sociodemographic variables (such as sex, age, race or ethnicity, years of education, and marital status). PTSD was significantly associated with suicidal ideation (after accounting for age, depression, and substance abuse); in fact, veterans with who screened positive for PTSD were 4 times more likely than veterans who did not to report suicidal ideation, and the likelihood of suicidal ideation was 5.7 times greater in veterans who screened positive for PTSD and two or more comorbid disorders.

In a later study, Jakupcak et al. (2011) examined the association between PTSD symptoms and suicidal ideation in OEF and OIF veterans. Participants included 336 veterans who were assessed at the VA Puget Sound Health Clinic from May 3, 2004, to January 1, 2007. The final sample of 275 veterans was included in the study after removal of those who did not complete the self-report assessments or on whom information on key variables was missing. Analyses indicated that veterans who had subthreshold PTSD were more likely than veterans who did not have PTSD to express hopelessness or suicidal ideation. Those reporting hopelessness or suicidal ideation had poorer social support, higher levels of combat exposure, lower income, depression, and alcohol abuse. Depression, followed by PTSD, was the strongest correlate of hopelessness and suicidal ideation. The authors noted that people who had subthreshold PTSD might not be able to receive mental-health treatment, so there is a need to educate providers to address symptoms of PTSD to mitigate suicide risk.

Pietrzak et al. (2010) analyzed results of a survey of OEF and OIF veterans and found that those veterans contemplating suicide were more likely to screen positive for PTSD, depression, and an alcohol problem and scored lower on measures of resilience and social support. They also scored higher on measures of stigma, barriers to care, and psychosocial difficulties. The study identified 1,050 OEF and OIF veterans from Connecticut, but only 272 veterans returned the survey (a response rate of 26%).

Pietrzak et al. (2011a) studied suicidal ideation in treatment-seeking OEF and OIF veterans. Veterans were recruited from VA primary care and mental-health clinics; 80% of veterans who were approached completed the assessments on site. In all, 167 OEF and OIF veterans who were within a year of returning from their most recent deployment participated. The authors found that almost 22% of treatment-seeking OEF and OIF veterans contemplated suicide; compared with those who did not, those who contemplated suicide were older and more likely to screen positive for depression, PTSD, and deployment-related pain. They were also more likely to score low on measures of psychologic resilience and social support.

In 2011, Kline et al. (2011) examined suicidal ideation in National Guard troops deployed to OIF. Survey data for the study were obtained from 1,665 (of 1,723) New Jersey National Guard soldiers attending a 3-month postdeployment reintegration event after deployment to Iraq in 2008–2009. The group had an average age of 31.3 years, were 89.5% male, and 45.9% white, 29.1% Hispanic, and 16.9% black. About 70% had some college experience; 52.5% had full-time employment, and 47.5% had part-time employment or were unemployed; 43.2% were married, 45.4% had never married, and 11.4% were separated, widowed, or divorced. Screening criteria were met in 5.6% for depression, in 10.8% for PTSD, 12.6% for alcohol dependence, and 13.2% for illicit-drug use. The group of respondents had low combat exposure—specifically, 33% reported no combat exposure, 47.7% low exposure, and 19.2% high exposure. The authors found that readjustment stressors correlated with psychiatric disorders and were more strongly associated with suicidal ideation than were the psychiatric disorders reported. After adjustment for the mental-health disorders, veterans who had readjustment problems were at 5.5 times greater risk for suicidal ideation than were those who did not.

Lemaire and Graham (2011) conducted a retrospective chart review of 1,740 veterans' initial health screens after return from OEF or OIF to determine factors associated with suicidal ideation. The review highlighted 113 (6.5%) who reported suicidal ideation and identified a number of risk factors: physical- or sexual-abuse exposure, prior suicide attempts, female sex, and a diagnosis of a mental-health disorder, such as psychosis, depression, or PTSD. Comorbid PTSD and depression were associated with higher risk than PTSD or depression alone.

Maguen et al. (2011a) examined risk factors for suicidal ideation in 2,854 US soldiers returning from deployment in OIF. Data on the newly returning veterans were collected as part of a postdeployment screen at a large Army medical facility, and 2.8% of them reported suicidal ideation. It was noted that prior suicide attempts, prior psychiatric medication, and killing in combat were risk factors for suicidal ideation. Findings indicated that returning veterans who endorsed depression symptoms were at greatest risk.

Guerra and Calhoun (2011) examined the relationship between PTSD and suicidal ideation in a group of veterans who had been deployed to OEF or OIF. Participants included veterans who had served in the armed forces after September 11, 2001, and were recruited into a registry from June 2005 to August 2008. Participants (393) were administered structural clinical interviews for psychiatric disorders. They were primarily male (322) and were primarily white (186), and their average age was 38.3 years. Results showed that 36% of the sample (143) met the criteria for PTSD, 22% (88) met the criteria for major depressive disorder, 4% (17) met the criteria for alcohol-use disorder, and almost 9% (34) reported a prior suicide attempt. The authors found that prior suicide attempt was positively associated with suicidal ideation; PTSD was related to heightened suicidal ideation even in the absence of major depressive disorder or alcohol-use disorder. The authors advise clinicians treating patients who have PTSD to assess them regularly for suicidality.

## Summary

Suicide in US military personnel is increasingly of concern, and suicidal ideation, suicide attempts, and suicide are increasingly associated with modern military service. In 2010, 50% of suicides in military personnel occurred in active-duty personnel who had been deployed to OEF or OIF; higher rates of suicide were found in the Army and Marine Corps than in other branches of the military (CBO, 2012). The AFHSC examined mortality data for 1998–2011 and found that since 2010 suicide has become the second-leading cause of death in service members. There were 2,990 suicides during 1998–2011 in active-duty members. The most common method of suicide among males and females was through the use of firearms (AFHSC, 2012).

Demographic data highlight risk factors for suicide, including being male, being white, being under 25 years old, being junior enlisted or high-school educated, and being divorced (the suicide rate was 55% higher in divorced service members than in married service members). Active-duty service members had a 70% higher rate of suicide than did deployed reserve and National Guard personnel. Firearms accounted for 62% of all suicides, and drug overdose was the most frequent method for suicide attempts (57%).

Reservists who were deployed were more likely to report suicidal ideation and suicide attempts than those who were not deployed. Reservists deployed to OEF or OIF were more likely to report suicidal ideation and suicide attempts than were reservists who served in other theaters or who were not deployed.

Veterans who screened positive for PTSD were 4 times more likely to report suicidal ideation than veterans who did not, and the likelihood of suicidal ideation was 5.7 times greater in veterans who screened positive for PTSD and two or more comorbid disorders. Those reporting hopelessness or suicidal ideation had poorer social support and higher levels of combat exposure. Additionally, veterans with lower income, depression, and reported alcohol abuse were more likely to endorse feelings of hopelessness and suicidal ideation. Depression was the strongest correlate of hopelessness and suicidal ideation, followed by PTSD.

Some risk factors might be mitigated or prevented, but others, such as deployment and combat exposure, are difficult to prevent in a military population.

In the military population, 57% of the suicides occurred in people who had no known history of suicide attempts or suicidal ideation, but 17% of those who committed suicide were known to have had a mood disorder, specifically major depressive disorder (7%), 5% had an anxiety disorder (most frequently PTSD), and about 26% had a history of substance-use disorder (DCoE, 2011).

## WOMEN'S HEALTH OUTCOMES

Women have served in operational support roles in every US military operation since the Revolutionary War. Mary Edwards Walker, a physician and surgeon, was denied a commission as a medical officer in the Civil War but volunteered and served as the first female surgeon in the US Army. She was the only woman to be awarded the Congressional Medal of Honor for military service. Today, women make up a rapidly growing segment of the military population. They make up about 14% of all active-duty military and 17.6% of National Guard and reserve personnel, and about 12% of women veterans served in OEF, OIF, or OND.[12]

The recent military operations in Iraq and Afghanistan are the most sustained ground combat operations involving American forces since the Vietnam era, and although women are still barred from direct combat roles, they have served in those theaters in expanded roles and in greater numbers (Fontana and Rosenheck, 2008). Women in combat-support roles, like the men they serve beside, experience high-intensity asymmetric warfare and the constant threat of

---

[12]See http://www.womenshealth.va.gov/WOMENSHEALTH/facts.asp.

roadside bombs and other types of improvised explosive devices. For almost a decade, military personnel have been subject to repeated deployments and endured prolonged separation from families and loved ones and exposure to harsh wartime conditions, including witnessing or experiencing traumatic injuries and deaths of civilians and military forces. Asymmetric warfare produces combat exposures that result in continuous stress and a frontless war in which no location or military occupation can be considered without risk. Historically, research on the health of veterans has focused on the health consequences of combat service in men, and there has been little scientific research on or longitudinal study of the health consequences of military service in women who served. Research that has examined sex differences is generally mixed, and a recent review (Street et al., 2009) highlighted the need to conduct studies with larger samples of women to improve understanding of issues relevant specifically to women. This section highlights studies that have investigated sex differences or issues particularly relevant to women.

### Women and Traumatic Brain Injury

TBI has important health implications for readjustment after deployment to Iraq or Afghanistan, but little information is available on whether the outcomes of patients suffering from TBI are affected by sex. One study suggested that sex differences may affect cognitive recovery after TBI. Ratcliff et al. (2007), in a multicenter civilian cohort study of 325 adult patients who had blunt TBI and were admitted to an acute-care facility, found that women performed significantly better than men on tests of attention or working memory and language. However, men outperformed women in visual analytic skills. Sex remained significantly associated with performance in those characteristics even after control for demographic variables, severity of injury, history of drug abuse, and length of acute hospitalization and of inpatient rehabilitation. The authors noted that further studies are needed to control for possible preinjury sex-related differences and to determine the long-term impact and health outcomes.

Slewa-Younan et al. (2008) conducted a systematic qualitative literature review and identified 13 human studies that examined sex differences in functional outcome measures after moderate to severe TBI. Contrary to findings in animal studies, results of human studies do not indicate that women do better than men after moderate to severe TBI. However, the authors noted that the studies examined functional outcomes 3–18 months after injury and that women may do better in the longer term in which psychosocial factors may play a role.

Iverson et al. (2011) investigated sex differences in psychiatric and neurobehavioral outcomes of deployment-related mild TBI in 11,951 male and 654 female OIF and OEF veterans who were using VA health care services. They reviewed records of VA's standardized comprehensive TBI evaluation and found that men had significantly greater odds of receiving diagnoses of PTSD and SUDs but women had significantly greater odds of receiving diagnoses of depression (2 times greater), anxiety disorders other than PTSD (1.3 times greater), and comorbid PTSD and depression (1.5 times greater). Severity of neurobehavioral symptoms in several domains was significantly higher in women than in men; women were more likely to report "severe" or "very severe" cognitive, somatosensory, and vestibular symptoms. Significant sex differences in PTSD disappeared after controlling for blast exposure. Depression in female military personnel or veterans is discussed further below.

## Women and Mental-Health Disorders

Retrospective research studies have indicated that women who serve in the military suffer more mental-health problems than their male counterparts. Rundell (2006) reviewed records of 1,264 military personnel who had been evacuated from Iraq or Afghanistan for psychiatric reasons and found that the evacuees were more likely to be female. Wojcik et al. (2009) reviewed records of 473,964 Army soldiers who had served in Iraq or Afghanistan and found that 1,948 of them were hospitalized for a primary psychiatric diagnosis. Their analysis indicated that women were at significantly higher risk for mental disorders—including mood, adjustment, and anxiety disorders—and that young women (less than 30 years old) made up a group at high risk for attempted suicide or self-inflicted injuries. Zouris et al. (2008) reviewed hospitalization records of OIF Marine Corps and Army personnel and found that a higher percentage of women than of men had diagnoses of mental-health disorders. Gibbons et al. (2012) evaluated data from the 2005 DOD Survey of Health Related Behaviors on 265 male and 180 female active-duty health care providers who had been deployed to OEF or OIF and found that female enlisted personnel and officers were more likely than their male counterparts to screen positive for serious psychologic distress, generalized anxiety disorder, depression, and harmful drinking habits. In a small study of female veterans who used VA health care services, Grubaugh et al. (2006) found that female veterans appeared to suffer worse mental (and physical) health than the general population. Overall, the research raises substantial concerns about the mental-health consequences of combat deployment of women.

The following subsections focus mainly on two mental-health outcomes, PTSD and depression, that are of particular concern for women who are on active duty and for female veterans.

### Posttraumatic Stress Disorder

Regarding sex differences, three questions that are relevant to PTSD arise: Does prevalence differ between women and men? Do the type and frequency of risk factors differ between women and men? Do outcomes as a consequence of combat deployments differ between women and men? Studies of the general population have indicated that women have higher rates or greater prevalence of PTSD than men (Breslau, 2002; Holbrook et al., 2002; Pietrzak et al., 2012; Tolin and Foa, 2006). However, the findings are mixed in OEF and OIF military personnel or veterans. A telephone survey of 1,965 veterans who had been deployed to Iraq or Afghanistan found that female veterans had a significantly higher risk of self-reported PTSD (and depression) than male veterans (Tanielian and Jaycox, 2008). Luxton et al. (2010) evaluated screening data collected on 6,427 male and 516 female active-duty soldiers at a single large Army installation before and after deployment to OEF or OIF and found that women who reported higher levels of combat exposure were more likely to report PTSD (and depression) symptoms than men. The authors concluded that combat exposure was a strong predictor of PTSD and depression in women and that there were sex-based differences in risks.

In contrast, other research has not found that women have a higher risk of PTSD than men. Baker et al. (2009) reviewed self-report data on 302 male and 37 female OEF and OIF veterans or reservists who were enrolled in the VA health care system and did not find any significant relationship between PTSD and sex. Haskell et al. (2009) reviewed VA data on 134,731 male and 18,481 female OEF and OIF veterans to evaluate possible sex differences in the prevalence and characteristics of pain. PTSD was more common in men than in women (11.3% vs 9.9%) whereas depression was more common in women (12.2% vs 7.5%). Later, Haskell et al. (2010) reviewed screening data from electronic medical records of 1,032 male and 197 female OEF and OIF veterans who used VA health care services and found that women were significantly less likely than men to screen positive for PTSD but significantly more likely to screen positive for depression. Maguen et al. (2010) reviewed VA administrative data on 288,348 male and 40,701 female OEF and OIF veterans who were seeking treatment and found that men were older than women and more often diagnosed with PTSD and alcohol abuse whereas women were more likely to be black and were more often diagnosed with depression than men. Women older than 30 years old were significantly more likely to receive diagnoses of PTSD than younger women; an opposite trend was observed in men, that is, younger men had a greater risk of PTSD than older men. Similar research on active-duty service members supports the study findings in the OEF and OIF veteran population. Maguen et al. (2011b) reviewed screening data on 6,697 male and 554 female active-duty soldiers collected before and after deployment to Iraq or Afghanistan. Men were more likely than women to report high-intensity combat exposure, but there were no sex differences in PTSD symptoms. However, the study did find that men were more likely than women to screen positive for alcohol abuse whereas women were more likely to screen positive for depression. Reviewing the literature, Zinzow et al. (2007) concluded that although the PTSD rates in the civilian population appear to be higher in women than in men, findings in the veteran population are mixed, and there is a general indication that the rates may be similar in men and women or higher in men than women.

Another question relevant to the development of PTSD in women is whether they suffered traumatic events before joining the military or have experienced MST, which would place them at higher risk for PTSD. Female military personnel and female veterans have high rates of sexual assault, particularly in comparison with men (Haskell et al., 2010; Maguen et al., 2011b; Murdoch et al., 2007). In a literature review, Zinzow et al. (2007) examined the nature and prevalence of trauma in female veterans, its effect on their physical and mental health, and their use of medical services. The authors found that over 50% of women who enter military service have already experienced physical or sexual abuse. A wide range of estimates of MST have been reported, but the authors estimated a range of 30–45%. The wide range of estimates was attributed to the various ways in which sexual assault was defined in the studies. For example, the authors estimated the lifetime rate of sexual assault as 38–64%, noted that nearly all female veterans report some type of trauma at some point in their lives (81–93% any type of trauma, 38–64% lifetime sexual assault, 27–49% child sexual abuse, 46–51% physical assault, 35% child physical abuse, and 18–19% domestic violence), and note that the rates are much higher in female veterans than in the civilian population.

The high rates of MST are particularly troubling given recent research that has shown strong correlations between MST and PTSD. Suris et al. (2004) conducted a retrospective evaluation of the effect of military, civilian adult, and childhood sexual trauma and the risk of PTSD in 270 female veterans who were using a single VA health care facility. The authors conducted structured interviews and reviewed medical records and found that veterans who reported MST were 9 times more likely than veterans who had no history of sexual assault to receive a diagnosis of PTSD, veterans who reported childhood sexual assault were 7 times more likely, and veterans who reported civilian sexual assault were 5 times more likely to receive a diagnosis of PTSD than veterans who did not have a history of sexual assault. The study suggests a worse PTSD outcome after MST than after civilian assault. Himmelfarb et al. (2006) reviewed responses to questionnaires and interviews of 196 female veterans to evaluate the relationship between sexual trauma and PTSD. The authors found that MST was much more prevalent than sexual trauma before or after military service (41% vs 19% or 24%, respectively) and that women who reported MST had the greatest odds of receiving a diagnosis of PTSD.

As discussed earlier, Kimerling et al. (2010) reviewed electronic medical records of 108,149 male and 17,580 female OEF and OIF veterans who were using VA health care services to evaluate the relationship between MST and mental-health diagnoses.[13] The authors adjusted for demographic factors and other potential confounders and found that victims of MST were significantly more likely to have received a PTSD diagnosis and to have other mental-health disorders, including depression, other anxiety disorders, and SUDs. Because the positive relationship between MST and PTSD was substantially greater in women than in men, the authors suggested that "military sexual trauma may be a particularly relevant gender-specific clinical issue in PTSD treatment settings."

Maguen et al. (2011b) reviewed screening data on 6,697 male and 554 female active-duty soldiers collected before and after deployment to Iraq or Afghanistan and found that women reported MST more frequently than men (12% vs over 1%) and that MST was a significant predictor of PTSD (and depression) symptoms. Coincidentally, the authors also noted that women were experiencing higher rates of combat exposure than expected. In a later study, Maguen et al. (2012) assessed the effects of MST on comorbid mental-health disorders in 7,255 female and 67,238 male OEF and OIF veterans who had PTSD. They reviewed administrative data and medical records and found that MST increased odds of a PTSD diagnosis by 3 and 4 in men and women, respectively; that 31% of women and 1% of men who had PTSD reported MST; and that men and women who had PTSD and a history of MST had significantly more mental-health comorbidities than veterans who had PTSD and no history of MST. Female victims had significantly higher odds of having a diagnosis of depression, anxiety, or eating disorders than male counterparts, whereas male victims had significantly higher odds of SUDs than female counterparts.

Dutra et al. (2011) evaluated the effects of combat experiences and military sexual harassment on PTSD and depression. The authors reviewed screening data collected within 3 months after deployment to Iraq on 54 active-duty female military personnel and found that about 74% reported combat experiences, over 50% reported having experienced sexual harassment during deployment, and 11% screened positive for PTSD; regression analyses indicated that military sexual harassment was a unique predictor of PTSD symptoms. In fact, the authors concluded that MST might be more strongly associated with PTSD in women than combat exposure, a known risk factor for PTSD, and noted that their findings were consistent with those of previous studies that highlighted MST as a "factor of particular clinical importance for the female military population."

The committee notes that although MST is much more common in women and therefore is particularly relevant for female military personnel and veterans, men appear to suffer similarly. Shipherd et al. (2009) investigated the relationship between MST and health and whether posttraumatic stress symptoms mediated the relationship. The authors reviewed self-

---

[13]Kimerling et al. (2010) followed an earlier study (Kimerling et al., 2007) that evaluated the relationship between MST and mental and physical health in a large veteran population (134,894 women and 2,900,106 men) and that had results similar to those of the later study in the OEF and OIF veteran population.

report data on 226 female and 91 male current or former marines who had reported MST in the previous 6 months and found that it was positively associated with increased posttraumatic stress symptoms in women and especially in men. Worse physical health was associated with higher levels of MST in men but with lower levels of MST in women.

Murdoch et al. (2007) reviewed cross-sectional survey questionnaire data on 487 male and 327 female active-duty military personnel to evaluate the relationship between sexual stressors and mental and physical functioning. Sexual stressors were defined as sexual-identity challenges (for example, accusations of homosexuality), sexual harassment, and sexual assault. The authors found that those who reported multiple stressors had more severe PTSD symptoms—and poorer physical, work, role, and social functioning; more sleep disorders; more severe depression; and more severe anxiety symptoms—than those who reported fewer or no stressors. Men and women in similar categories reported similar functioning and psychiatric symptoms.

As noted above, women have experienced higher levels of combat exposure than in previous conflicts (Dutra et al., 2011; Maguen et al., 2011b). That finding is troublesome because combat exposure is a known risk factor for PTSD and some have suggested that women may be more vulnerable to the effects of combat exposure than men. However, Vogt et al. (2011) reviewed survey and questionnaire data on 252 male and 340 female OEF and OIF veterans to determine whether there were significant sex differences in the effects of combat exposure and in mental-health outcomes, such as PTSD, depression, and substance abuse. As expected, men reported more exposure to combat-related stressors than women, and women reported more prior-life trauma and exposure to sexual harassment during deployment. Controlling for prior-life trauma and sexual harassment, the authors found only one statistically significant difference that suggested that men may be more likely to suffer substance abuse after exposure to combat. However, the effect was small and considered clinically insignificant. They concluded that the effects of combat-related stressors "may be more similar than different for female and male US service members" and that female OEF and OIF "service members may be as resilient to combat-related stress as men." A study of UK military men and women (Woodhead et al., 2012) concluded similarly that their investigation showed "little evidence of gender differences in the impact of exposure to combat on mental health."

Regardless of the similarity of response to combat exposure, the adverse effect on women is important to note. Hassija et al. (2012) investigated the differential effect of various types of trauma—combat exposure, childhood neglect and abuse, and adult sexual assault and noncombat physical violence—on mental-health disorders in 115 female veterans of the Persian Gulf, Iraq, and Afghanistan wars who had visited VA health clinics. The authors used regression analyses to evaluate questionnaire data and found that only combat exposure was significantly associated with more severe PTSD symptoms, depression-symptom severity, and alcohol misuse. The authors stated that they did not separate MST from the categories of adult traumatic events evaluated and noted that this distinction might be important given the particularly detrimental effects of MST that have been reported.

The burden of PTSD in women is of concern because, like men, women who have PTSD suffer worse physical and mental health and quality of life than those who do not have PTSD. For example, Frayne et al. (2004) evaluated the contribution of PTSD to poor physical health and functional status in female veterans who were using the VA health care system. They evaluated self-report data on 4,348 women who had PTSD, 7,580 women who had depression, and 18,937 women who had neither condition; 89% of the women who had PTSD also had depression. The authors found that women who had PTSD, regardless of age, had more medical conditions and worse functional status than women who had depression.

Because the research focus in the military setting has traditionally been on outcomes in men, the question arises whether women suffer different outcomes of PTSD than their male active-duty and veteran counterparts. Schnurr and Lunney (2008) evaluated possible sex differences in quality of life of veterans who had PTSD. The sample population consisted of 358 male Vietnam veterans and 203 female Vietnam veterans who were in group therapy or individual psychotherapy in a VA setting. PTSD was determined by using structured interviews, and quality of life was evaluated by using the Quality of Life Inventory, which assesses four domains (achievement, self-expression, relationships, and surroundings). As others had (Magruder et al., 2004; Suris et al., 2007), the authors found that veterans who had PTSD had poorer quality of life than those who did not, and they did not find clear differences between men and women who had PTSD. Although there were a few statistically significant differences, they were small and clinically insignificant. Frayne et al. (2011) investigated sex differences in the burden of medical illnesses by reviewing VA clinical and administrative data on 77,727 male and 12,831 female OEF and OIF veterans. They found that 27,083 men and 3,501 women had received diagnoses of PTSD and that women who had PTSD had a higher burden of diagnosed medical conditions than men. As expected, men and women who had PTSD had more medical conditions than their counterparts who did not. Lumbosacral spine disorders and lower extremity joint disorders were the most frequent conditions diagnosed in women and men who had PTSD. Headaches were also noted in women, and hearing problems in men. The results reported by Frayne et al. are consistent with those of a recent study of a civilian population (Galovski et al., 2011) that investigated sex differences in 45 men and 162 women who had PTSD that developed after sexual or physical assault. They found that men and women exhibited similar PTSD and depression symptoms and experienced similar guilt. However, women had significantly more health complaints, and men reported feeling more anger (as found with the anger-state scale of the State-Trait Anger Expression Inventory). The authors concluded that although civilian men and women may differ in the likelihood of developing PTSD after assaults, there are no differences in PTSD presentation once it is manifested.

**Depression**

Recent research appears to indicate that female OEF and OIF military personnel and veterans have a higher risk or greater prevalence of depression than their male counterparts. Many studies described above that investigated possible sex differences in PTSD also evaluated sex differences in depression. A study of 1,965 OEF and OIF veterans found that female veterans had a significantly higher risk of major depression than male veterans after control for confounding factors (Tanielian and Jaycox, 2008). Similarly, Seal et al. (2009), in their investigation of new mental-health diagnoses in 289,328 OEF and OIF veterans, found that women had a higher risk of depression than men. Haskell et al. (2009, 2010) consistently found that depression was more common in OEF and OIF female veterans than in their male counterparts. In their investigation of 6,943 active-duty soldiers who had been deployed to Iraq or Afghanistan, Luxton et al. (2010) found that women who had high combat exposure were more likely than men to report depression symptoms and concluded that there are sex-based differences in depression risks. Wells et al. (2010) found that women consistently had higher rates of new-onset depression than men in their investigation of the relationship between deployment and the risk of depression. Carter-Visscher et al. (2010) found higher rates of depression in female National Guard soldiers than in their male counterparts on the basis of self-report data collected before deployment to Iraq but did not find that sex moderated the relationship between various risk or resilience factors and baseline mental health. And Maguen et al. (2010, 2011b) found that female OEF and OIF active-duty soldiers and veterans were more likely than their male counterparts to receive a diagnosis of depression or to screen positive for depression. Thus, the evidence indicates that depression is a health issue that is particularly relevant to the female active-duty and veteran populations.

Depression is an especially relevant concern for women given the association of depression with MST and the high reported rates in female active-duty personnel and veterans. Hankin et al. (1999) reviewed questionnaire data on 3,632 female veterans and found that 23% reported military sexual assault. Furthermore, female victims of military sexual assault were significantly more likely than female veterans who had no history of such assault to screen positive for depression (60% vs 33%) and alcohol abuse (7% vs 4%). Suris et al. (2004) found that female veterans who had experienced military sexual assault had significantly higher rates of depressive-disorder diagnoses than veterans who had no history of such assault; the authors also noted that female veterans who had a history of civilian adult but not childhood sexual assault had significantly higher rates of depressive-disorder diagnoses than female veterans who had no history of such assault. Kimerling et al. (2010) found similar results specifically in OEF and OIF veterans; they reviewed electronic medical records of 108,149 male and 17,580 female OEF and OIF veterans and found that victims of MST were significantly more likely to have received diagnoses of depression.

**Substance-Use Disorders**

Few data are available for evaluating SUDs in female active-duty military personnel or veterans, and far fewer data are available specifically on the OEF and OIF female population. Where researchers have investigated sex differences, the results have appeared to indicate that women have significantly lower rates of alcohol abuse than their male counterparts. Bray et al. (1999) investigated the relationship between perceived stress and substance use during peacetime conditions by using questionnaire data on 16,193 active-duty military personnel obtained from the 1995 DOD Survey of Health Related Behaviors.[14] They found that military men and women had similar rates of cigarette and illicit-drug use but that military men had significantly higher rates of heavy alcohol use. "Work" stress and "family" stress were significantly associated with substance use in men, but no such relationship was observed in women. The only significant relationship observed in women was between "stress associated with being a woman in the military" and cigarette and illicit-drug use. Brown et al. (2010) compared alcohol use in military men and women by using questionnaire data on 9,506 male and 3,250 female active-duty military personnel obtained from the 2002 DOD Survey of Health Related Behaviors. The investigators found that men had significantly higher rates of heavy or binge drinking and more alcohol-related problems than women. On the basis of their data, however, they concluded that women might experience alcohol-related problems at lower consumption levels. They appeared to base that conclusion on an analysis that indicated that female officers did not have statistically significant different rates of dependence symptoms, productivity loss, or serious consequences

---

[14]*Substance use* was defined as cigarette smoking, heavy alcohol use, or illicit-drug use.

from their male counterparts who had significantly higher rates of moderate, heavy, and binge drinking.

One issue to consider is whether risk factors for SUDs occur more commonly in women or have a greater effect on women. For example, Federman et al. (2000) investigated the relationship between peacetime deployment and substance use by using the 1995 DOD Survey of Health Related Behaviors. Regression analyses indicated a positive association between deployment and heavy alcohol use in both men and women, but a stronger association was observed in women; the authors noted that deployment was significantly associated with cigarette use, nonheavy alcohol use, and alcohol dependence in men but not in women.

As is the case with the other mental-health outcomes discussed above, the higher rate of military sexual abuse in women is relevant to SUDs. As noted earlier, Hankin et al. (1999) found that female victims of military sexual assault were significantly more likely to screen positive for alcohol abuse (7% vs 4%) than female veterans who had no such history. In their review of administrative data on 2,900,106 male and 134,894 female outpatients at VA health centers, Kimerling et al. (2007) found that alcohol disorders were much more common in women and men who reported MST than in those who did report MST and that the association was stronger in women. In a later study specifically on OEF and OIF veterans, Kimerling et al. (2010) found that MST was significantly associated with SUDs and that the effect again was stronger in women than in men. Booth et al. (2011) conducted a retrospective evaluation of the relationship between sexual assault and SUDs in 1,004 female veterans by using data collected in telephone interviews. The authors found that about 50% had been raped at some point in their lives (31% during childhood, 11% before military service, 25% during military service, and 11% after military service). A strong association between a rape history of any kind and a lifetime SUD was found.

**Suicidal Ideation**

Little information is available about sex differences in the prevalence of suicidal ideation. As in research on the general population, McCarthy et al. (2009) found in their review of data on 4,670,968 patients that female veterans using the VA health care system had a lower suicide rate than male veterans. However, female veterans 40–59 years old had significantly higher suicide rates than women of similar ages in the general population. The authors concluded that "female patients had particularly high relative risks."

Although research indicates that suicide rates are lower in women than in men in the general and military populations, women tend to suffer higher rates of depression, which is a known risk factor for suicidal ideation. Zivin et al. (2007) evaluated demographic and clinical factors in 807,694 patients of the VA health care system who had diagnoses of depression and had been prescribed antidepressants, a group at high risk for suicide. The suicide rate was higher in male veterans than in female veterans, but the difference between the rates was smaller than the difference typically found in the general population (1:3 vs 1:4).

## Summary

Although women are banned from combat, the reality of recent conflicts in OEF and OIF is that women serve in combat-support roles that expose them to high-intensity asymmetric warfare and combat trauma. For more than a decade, female military service members have been subject to repeat deployments, have endured prolonged separation from family, have served side by side with men, and have been exposed to harsh wartime conditions, including witnessing death and destruction.

In contrast with results of animal research, there is little evidence of sex-based differences in TBI outcomes in women, but a study of neuropsychologic outcomes of mild TBI in female veterans did demonstrate that they had significantly higher rates of PTSD, other anxiety disorders, and depression than their male counterparts. Women were also more likely to report "severe" or "very severe" cognitive, somatosensory, and vestibular symptoms.

Research has raised substantial concerns about the mental-health consequences of OEF and OIF combat deployments in women. Women have been found to suffer more mental-health problems than men who served in Iraq or Afghanistan as evidenced by higher rates of medical evacuations and hospitalizations for primary psychiatric conditions. Women have higher rates of self-reported PTSD and depression symptoms in predeployment and postdeployment screenings and are more likely to received diagnoses of depression than their male counterparts. They also suffer from more comorbid mental-health conditions than men.

Exposure to MST has been associated with higher risks of poor mental health, physical health, and quality of life in women than in men. Trends in cross-sectional studies of VA health care user populations suggest that men more often screen positive for PTSD and women more often screen positive for depression. Studies have also identified persistently high rates of MST in OIF and OEF. Military sexual assault has been shown to convey a greater risk of PTSD and other mental-health conditions, such as depression and SUD, than either childhood or civilian adult sexual assault. MST is a stronger predictor of PTSD in women than in men.

Longitudinal studies of women who served in combat theaters and evaluations of the diagnosis of SUDs have not been performed, and far less research is available regarding those who served in Iraq or Afghanistan. Studies of veterans seeking care at VA facilities have not identified significant sex-based differences in PTSD risk. Well-designed longitudinal studies have not been completed to increase our understanding of those issues.

## CONCLUSIONS

Being deployed to a war zone can result in numerous adverse outcomes. The committee focused on TBI, PTSD, depression, suicide and suicidal ideation, and SUDs in its review as specified in the legislation directing its work (see Appendix A). Any one of those outcomes can, in turn, have numerous sequelae and associated outcomes (comorbidities) that can have significant impacts on health, quality of life, functional impairment, and socioeconomic status. Emerging issues regarding multiple deployments, short dwell times, the relationship of multiple concussions to chronic traumatic encephalopathy, risk of suicide, and the importance of comorbidities with TBI, PTSD, and depression await study and clarification. With regard to suicide prevention, increased efforts are needed to train military personnel, health care providers, and family members in recognizing the signs of suicide risk. Increased emphasis on the importance of social networks and health care in reducing that risk is also needed, as is training to reduce the stigma associated with seeking care. It must be understood that occupational stressors associated with military service may continue long after troops leave the theater of conflict. Finally, military sexual trauma continues to occur at high rates in OEF and OIF populations, and increased efforts to eliminate this violence are critically needed.

## FUTURE RESEARCH DIRECTIONS

As the committee reviewed the literature and examined the range of federally funded research on TBI and mental health outcomes in OEF and OIF (Appendix D), it identified a number of unaddressed questions and areas for future study and research. The literature is incomplete and there remain significant challenges in determining the prevalence of physical and psychologic morbidity and comorbidities after military service in Iraq and Afghanistan.

Although the current reports and studies of OEF and OIF have progressively built upon knowledge gained from prior conflicts and have made valuable contributions to the growing understanding of the consequences associated with deployment to OEF and OIF, the have a set of common limitations. The committee noted in its Phase 1 report that most of the literature falls short of meeting the methodological standards it described. Additionally, many studies provide very broad ranges for prevalence estimates of various mental health outcomes making them difficult to use for policy makers. The committee reiterates its recommendation from Phase 1 regarding future studies and the need to be both scientifically sound and comprehensive (see Appendix B and Chapter 11).

Longitudinal studies are needed to answer many of the questions that are not answered by the literature and current studies. Such studies should strive to improve the recruitment and retention of subjects. Current studies might be the most appropriate platform for developing a strategy for long-term followup, such as the Millennium Cohort Study and the Longitudinal Health Study of Gulf War Era Veterans. Those can be augmented with supplementary samples of OEF and OIF veterans. Other characteristics that such studies should have include the ability to collect biologic specimens, oversampling of OEF and OIF female and minority-group populations, and planning for add-on studies to address newly identified needs. Specifically, what are the long-term outcomes of most conditions of concern? Do the outcomes vary by severity, comorbidity, ethnicity, or sex?

The committee provides areas for future research studies below.

- Longitudinal studies are needed to examine long-term outcomes of mild TBI using better exposure data, biological markers, and performance-based cognitive measures as well as measures of emotional health. Examine whether the results vary by number of mild TBIs, and various demographic factors including sex, race, and ethnicity. Do the results vary as a function of type and number of comorbidities?
- Longitudinal studies to examine evidence for accelerated aging and CTE in those with TBI. What are the risk factors for and protective factors against CTE?
- Studies to determine whether biologic markers can help in predicting outcomes?
- Studies with better exposure data, and objective diagnostic tests or biomarkers for mild TBI and PTSD are needed to improve our understanding of those highly comorbid conditions.
- Studies to elucidate how brain imaging can provide information about outcomes?
- Studies to determine if specific symptomatic markers predict the outcome of PTSD? The current array of PTSD symptoms might not be the most clinically relevant for tracking

outcome. For example, a focus on sleep disturbance coupled with troubling dreams as a specific symptom might be of more value.
- Studies to determine how the current distinction between diagnosis and symptoms might predict outcome? The line between a diagnosis of PTSD and PTSD symptoms is not well validated. Can longitudinal studies determine a threshold and a constellation of symptoms that point clearly to a diagnosis?
- Prospective studies of veterans, who present with first reports of suicidal ideation and have no previous mental-health diagnoses, to provide clarity in understanding risk factors for future suicide and future mental-health morbidity?
- Systematic studies on MST delineating where it occurs, the characteristics of perpetrators, the relationship between perpetrators and victims, and what types of sexual trauma are most common. A better understanding of those issues might be important in the design of initiatives to eliminate it.

## RECOMMENDATIONS

The literature on the outcomes of military deployment has grown dramatically over the last two decades. Although discrepant findings do emerge, there is a clear consensus in the literature that the stressors of deployment, from exposure to combat to multiple deployments away from home and family, can lead to a number of adverse conditions. The committee concentrated on deployment-related outcomes—such as TBI, PTSD, depression, substance use, and suicidal ideation—but the list could be expanded to many additional psychiatric conditions and a host of physical conditions. The data on short-term outcomes (outcomes in 6 months or less) is extensive, but data on long-term outcomes (over years) less extensive and both can be challenged on methodologic grounds. To capture the true long-term outcomes of deployment to war zones and plan services to address them, more data will be essential.

**The committee recommends that the Department of Defense and the Department of Veterans Affairs sponsor longitudinal studies to answer many of the questions regarding long-term effects of traumatic brain injury, posttraumatic stress disorder, and other mental-health disorders. Such studies should strive to improve the validity of exposure measurements, identification and use of biomarkers, and recruitment and retention of subjects. Attention should be paid to whether the outcomes of traumatic brain injuries depend on the severity and number of such injuries, on the presence of comorbid conditions, and on sex and ethnicity.**

Current studies might be the most appropriate platform for developing a strategy for long-term followup, such as the Millennium Cohort Study and the Longitudinal Health Study of Gulf War Era Veterans. Those studies can be augmented with supplementary samples of OEF, OIF, and OND veterans. Other factors that should define such studies include the ability to collect biologic specimens, oversampling of OEF, OIF, and OND female and minority-group populations, and planning for add-on studies to address new needs as they are identified.

Many health consequences of service in OEF, OIF, and OND are related to the inherently dangerous nature of the wartime environment or resulting trauma. However, one major exposure, military sexual trauma (MST), is unrelated to war but rather is due to noncombat violent assault.

Studies show that MST has been occurring at high rates in the US military, including during OEF, OIF, and OND. Research demonstrates that MST is associated with poor readjustment and adverse mental-health and physical outcomes. The burden of physical and mental-health consequences for the victims and their family members is high. Increased efforts by DOD are necessary, and a zero-tolerance approach should be implemented.

**The committee recommends that the Department of Defense develop policies to eliminate military sexual trauma as research demonstrates that it is associated with poor readjustment and mental-health and physical-health outcomes. The committee further recommends that the department reinforce existing policies on military sexual trauma by adding specific mandatory evaluation criteria regarding how well military leaders address the issue, for example, in the formal performance-appraisal and promotion systems.**

The breadth and depth of the challenges faced by military service members and veterans who served in Iraq and Afghanistan result from the complex interaction of issues that must be addressed by primary prevention, diagnostics, treatment, rehabilitation, education and outreach, and community support programs if readjustment after combat service is to be successful.

## REFERENCES

Adler, D. A., K. Possemato, S. Mavandadi, D. Lerner, H. Chang, J. Klaus, J. D. Tew, D. Barrett, E. Ingram, and D. W. Oslin. 2011. Psychiatric status and work performance of veterans of Operations Enduring Freedom and Iraqi Freedom. *Psychiatric Services* 62(1):39-46.

Afari, N., L. H. Harder, N. J. Madra, P. S. Heppner, T. Moeller-Bertram, C. King, and D. G. Baker. 2009. PTSD, combat injury, and headache in veterans returning from Iraq/Afghanistan. *Headache: The Journal of Head and Face Pain* 49(9):1267-1276.

AFHSC (Armed Forces Health Surveillance Center). 2011. Associations between repeated deployments to OEF/OIF/OND, October 2001-December 2010, and post-deployment illnesses and injuries, active component, US Armed Forces. *Medical Surveillance Monthly Report* 18(7):2-11.

AFHSC. 2012. Deaths by suicide while on active duty, active and reserve components, US Armed Forces, 1998-2011. *Medical Surveillance Monthly Report* 19(6):7-10.

Andersen, J., M. Wade, K. Possemato, and P. Ouimette. 2010. Association between posttraumatic stress disorder and primary care provider-diagnosed disease among Iraq and Afghanistan veterans. *Psychosomatic Medicine* 72(5):498-504.

APA (American Psychiatric Association). 2000. *Diagnostic and Statistical Manual of Mental Disorders (DSM-IV-TR)*, 4th ed. Washington, DC: American Psychiatric Association.

Asmundson, G. J. G., K. D. Wright, and M. B. Stein. 2004. Pain and PTSD symptoms in female veterans. *European Journal of Pain* 8(4):345-350.

Bagalman, E. 2011. *Suicide, PTSD, and Substance Use Among OEF/OIF Veterans Using VA Health Care: Facts and Figures.* Washington, DC: Congressional Research Service.

Baker, D. G., P. Heppner, N. Afari, S. Nunnink, M. Kilmer, A. Simmons, L. Harder, and B. Bosse. 2009. Trauma exposure, branch of service, and physical injury in relation to mental health among US veterans returning from Iraq and Afghanistan. *Military Medicine* 174(8):773-778.

Barrett, D. H., M. L. Green, R. Morris, W. H. Giles, and J. B. Croft. 1996. Cognitive functioning and posttraumatic stress disorder. *American Journal of Psychiatry* 153(11):1492-1494.

Barrett, D. H., G. C. Gray, B. N. Doebbeling, D. J. Clauw, and W. C. Reeves. 2002. Prevalence of symptoms and symptom-based conditions among Gulf War veterans: Current status of research findings. *Epidemiologic Reviews* 24(2):218-227.

Belanger, H. G., and R. D. Vanderploeg. 2005. The neuropsychological impact of sports-related concussion: A meta-analysis. *Journal of the International Neuropsychological Society* 11(4):345-357.

Belanger, H. G., G. Curtiss, J. A. Demery, B. K. Lebowitz, and R. D. Vanderploeg. 2005. Factors moderating neuropsychological outcomes following mild traumatic brain injury: A meta-analysis. *Journal of the International Neuropsychological Society* 11(3):215-227.

Belanger, H. G., T. Kretzmer, R. Yoash-Gantz, T. Pickett, and L. A. Tupler. 2009. Cognitive sequelae of blast-related versus other mechanisms of brain trauma. *Journal of the International Neuropsychological Society* 15(1):1-8.

Belanger, H. G., and R. D. Vanderploeg. 2005. The neuropsychological impact of sports-related concussion: A meta-analysis. *Journal of the International Neuropsychological Society* 11(4):345-357.

Bell, K. R., J. M. Hoffman, N. R. Temkin, J. M. Powell, R. T. Fraser, P. C. Esselman, J. K. Barber, and S. Dikmen. 2008. The effect of telephone counselling on reducing post-traumatic symptoms after mild traumatic brain injury: A randomised trial. *Journal of Neurology, Neurosurgery, and Psychiatry* 79(11):1275-1281.

Bell, N. S., T. C. Harford, C. H. Fuchs, J. E. McCarroll, and C. E. Schwartz. 2006. Spouse abuse and alcohol problems among white, African American, and Hispanic US Army soldiers. *Alcoholism: Clinical and Experimental Research* 30(10):1721-1733.

Bell, N. S., T. C. Harford, P. J. Amoroso, I. E. Hollander, and A. B. Kay. 2010. Prior health care utilization patterns and suicide among US Army soldiers. *Suicide and Life-Threatening Behavior* 40(4):407-415.

Black, S. A., M. S. Gallaway, M. R. Bell, and E. C. Ritchie. 2011. Prevalence and risk factors associated with suicides of Army soldiers 2001–2009. *Military Psychology* 23(4):433-451.

Blume, A. W., K. B. Schmaling, and M. L. Russell. 2010. Stress and alcohol use among soldiers assessed at mobilization and demobilization. *Military Medicine* 175(6):400-404.

Bombardier, C. H., N. R. Temkin, J. Machamer, and S. S. Dikmen. 2003. The natural history of drinking and alcohol-related problems after traumatic brain injury. *Archives of Physical Medicine and Rehabilitation* 84(2):185-191.

Bombardier, C. H., J. R. Fann, N. R. Temkin, P. C. Esselman, J. Barber, and S. S. Dikmen. 2010. Rates of major depressive disorder and clinical outcomes following traumatic brain injury. *Journal of the American Medical Association* 303(19):1938-1945.

Bonanno, G. A., A. D. Mancini, J. L. Horton, T. M. Powell, C. A. Leardmann, E. J. Boyko, T. S. Wells, T. I. Hooper, G. D. Gackstetter, T. C. Smith, and Millennium Cohort Study Team. 2012. Trajectories of trauma symptoms and resilience in deployed US military service members: Prospective cohort study. *British Journal of Psychiatry* 200(4):317-323.

Booth, B. M., M. Mengeling, J. Torner, and A. G. Sadler. 2011. Rape, sex partnership, and substance use consequences in women veterans. *Journal of Traumatic Stress* 24(3):287-294.

Booth-Kewley, S., G. E. Larson, R. M. Highfill-McRoy, C. F. Garland, and T. A. Gaskin. 2010. Correlates of posttraumatic stress disorder symptoms in Marines back from war. *Journal of Traumatic Stress* 23(1):69-77.

Boscarino, J. A. 1997. Diseases among men 20 years after exposure to severe stress: Implications for clinical research and medical care. *Psychosomatic Medicine* 59(6):605-614.

———. 2004. Posttraumatic stress disorder and physical illness: Results from clinical and epidemiologic studies. *Annals of the New York Academy of Sciences* 1032:141-153.

Brady, K. T., P. Tuerk, S. E. Back, M. E. Saladin, A. E. Waldrop, and H. Myrick. 2009. Combat posttraumatic stress disorder, substance use disorders, and traumatic brain injury. *Journal of Addiction Medicine* 3(4):179-188.

Brailey, K. 2009. *MTBI Effects on Emotion Symptoms, Neurocognitive Performance, and Functional Impairment: A Longitudinal Study of Deployed and Non-Deployed Army Soldiers.* Fort Detrick, MD: Army Medical Research and Materiel Command.

Bray, R. M., J. A. Fairbank, and M. E. Marsden. 1999. Stress and substance use among military women and men. *American Journal of Drug and Alcohol Abuse* 25(2):239-256.

Bray, R. M., M. R. Pemberton, L. L. Hourani, M. Witt, K. L. Olmsted, J. M. Brown, B. Weimer, M. E. Lance, M. E. Marsden, and S. Scheffer. 2009a. *2008 Department of Defense Survey of Health Related Behaviors Among Active Duty Military Personnel.* Research Triangle Park, NC: RTI International.

Bray, R. M., M. R. Pemberton, L. L. Hourani, M. Witt, K. L. Rae Olmsted, J. M. Brown, B. Weimer, M. E. Lane, M. E. Marsden, S. Scheffler, R. Vandermaas-Peeler, K. R. Aspinwall, E. Anderson, K. Spagnola, K. Close, J. L. Gratton, S. Calvin, and M. Bradshaw. 2009b. *Department of Defense Survey of Health Related Behaviors Among Active Duty Military Personnel: A Component of the Defense Lifestyle Assessment Program (DLAP).* Research Triangle Park, NC: RTI International.

Bray, R. M., M. R. Pemberton, M. E. Lane, L. L. Hourani, M. J. Mattiko, and L. A. Babeu. 2010. Substance use and mental health trends among US military active duty personnel: Key findings from the 2008 DOD Health Behavior Survey. *Military Medicine* 175(6):390-399.

Bremner, J. D., S. M. Southwick, A. Darnell, and D. S. Charney. 1996. Chronic PTSD in Vietnam combat veterans: Course of illness and substance abuse. *American Journal of Psychiatry* 153(3):369-375.

Brenner, L. A., B. J. Ivins, K. Schwab, D. Warden, L. A. Nelson, M. Jaffee, and H. Terrio. 2010a. Traumatic brain injury, posttraumatic stress disorder, and postconcussive symptom reporting among troops returning from Iraq. *Journal of Head Trauma Rehabilitation* 25(5):307-312.

Brenner, L. A., H. Terrio, B. Y. Homaifar, P. M. Gutierrez, P. J. Staves, J. E. Harwood, D. Reeves, L. E. Adler, B. J. Ivins, K. Helmick, and D. Warden. 2010b. Neuropsychological test performance in soldiers with blast-related mild TBI. *Neuropsychology* 24(2):160-167.

Brenner, L. A., R. V. Ignacio, and F. C. Blow. 2011. Suicide and traumatic brain injury among individuals seeking veterans health administration services. *Journal of Head Trauma Rehabilitation* 26(4):257-264.

Breslau, N. 2002. Gender differences in trauma and posttraumatic stress disorder. *Journal of Gender-specific Medicine* 5(1):34-40.

Breslau, N., V. C. Lucia, and G. F. Alvarado. 2006. Intelligence and other predisposing factors in exposure to trauma and posttraumatic stress disorder: A follow-up study at age 17 years. *Archives of General Psychiatry* 63(11):1238-1245.

Brown, J. M., R. M. Bray, and M. C. Hartzell. 2010. A comparison of alcohol use and related problems among women and men in the military. *Military Medicine* 175(2):101-107.

Bruce, M. L. 2010. Suicide risk and prevention in veteran populations. *Annals of the New York Academy of Sciences* 1208:98-103.

Bryant, R. 2011. Post-traumatic stress disorder vs traumatic brain injury. *Dialogues in Clinical Neuroscience* 13(3):251-262.

Bryant, R. A., and A. G. Harvey. 2002. Delayed-onset posttraumatic stress disorder: A prospective evaluation. *Australian and New Zealand Journal of Psychiatry* 36(2):205-209.

Buckley, T. C., and D. G. Kaloupek. 2001. A meta-analytic examination of basal cardiovascular activity in posttraumatic stress disorder. *Psychosomatic Medicine* 63(4):585-594.

Burnett-Zeigler, I., M. Ilgen, M. Valenstein, K. Zivin, L. Gorman, A. Blow, S. Duffy, and S. Chermack. 2011. Prevalence and correlates of alcohol misuse among returning Afghanistan and Iraq veterans. *Addictive Behaviors* 36(8):801-806.

Cabrera, O. A., C. W. Hoge, P. D. Bliese, C. A. Castro, and S. C. Messer. 2007. Childhood adversity and combat as predictors of depression and post-traumatic stress in deployed troops. *American Journal of Preventive Medicine* 33(2):77-82.

Calhoun, P. S., J. C. Beckham, and H. B. Bosworth. 2002. Caregiver burden and psychological distress in partners of veterans with chronic posttraumatic stress disorder. *Journal of Traumatic Stress* 15(3):205-212.

Calhoun, P. S., J. R. Elter, E. R. Jones, H. Kudler, and K. Straits-Troster. 2008. Hazardous alcohol use and receipt of risk-reduction counseling among US veterans of the wars in Iraq and Afghanistan. *Journal of Clinical Psychiatry* 69(11):1686-1693.

Campbell, T. A., L. A. Nelson, R. Lumpkin, R. E. Yoash-Gantz, T. C. Pickett, and C. L. McCormick. 2009. Neuropsychological measures of processing speed and executive functioning in combat veterans with PTSD, TBI, and comorbid TBI/PTSD. *Psychiatric Annals* 39(8):796-803.

Carlson, K. F., D. Nelson, R. J. Orazem, S. Nugent, D. X. Cifu, and N. A. Sayer. 2010. Psychiatric diagnoses among Iraq and Afghanistan war veterans screened for deployment-related traumatic brain injury. *Journal of Traumatic Stress* 23(1):17-24.

Carlson, K. F., A. A. Gravely, S. Noorbaloochi, A. B. Simon, A. K. Bangerter, and N. A. Sayer. 2011a. Post-deployment injury among new combat veterans enrolled in Veterans Affairs (VA) healthcare. *Injury Prevention* 17(5):343-347.

Carlson, K. F., S. M. Kehle, L. A. Meis, N. Greer, R. Macdonald, I. Rutks, N. A. Sayer, S. K. Dobscha, and T. J. Wilt. 2011b. Prevalence, assessment, and treatment of mild traumatic brain injury and posttraumatic stress disorder: A systematic review of the evidence. *Journal of Head Trauma Rehabilitation* 26(2):103-115.

Carter-Visscher, R., M. A. Polusny, M. Murdoch, P. Thuras, C. R. Erbes, and S. M. Kehle. 2010. Predeployment gender differences in stressors and mental health among US National Guard troops poised for Operation Iraqi Freedom deployment. *Journal of Traumatic Stress* 23(1):78-85.

Carty, J., M. L. O'Donnell, and M. Creamer. 2006. Delayed-onset PTSD: A prospective study of injury survivors. *Journal of Affective Disorders* 90(2-3):257-261.

CBO (Congressional Budget Office). 2012. *The Veterans Health Administration's Treatment of PTSD and Traumatic Brain Injury Among Recent Combat Veterans.* Washington, DC: Congressional Budget Office.

CDC (Centers for Disease Control and Prevention). 2011a. Suicidal thoughts and behaviors among adults aged ≥18 years—United States, 2008–2009. *Morbidity and Mortality Weekly Report* 60(s13):1-22.

———. 2011b. Vital signs: Overdoses of prescription opioid pain relievers—United States, 1999–2008. *Morbidity and Mortality Weekly Report* 60(43):1487-1492.

———. 2012. *National suicide statistics at a glance.* http://www.cdc.gov/ViolencePrevention/suicide/statistics/trends02.html (accessed April 13, 2012).

Cooper, D. B., J. E. Kennedy, M. A. Cullen, E. Critchfield, R. R. Amador, and A. O. Bowles. 2011. Association between combat stress and post-concussive symptom reporting in OEF/OIF service members with mild traumatic brain injuries. *Brain Injury* 25(1):1-7.

Corkin, S., T. J. Rosen, E. V. Sullivan, and R. A. Clegg. 1989. Penetrating head injury in young adulthood exacerbates cognitive decline in later years. *Journal of Neuroscience* 9(11):3876-3883.

Corsellis, J. A., C. J. Bruton, and D. Freeman-Browne. 1973. The aftermath of boxing. *Psychological Medicine* 3(3):270-303.

Cosgrove, D. J., Z. Gordon, J. E. Bernie, S. Hami, D. Montoya, M. B. Stein, and M. Monga. 2002. Sexual dysfunction in combat veterans with post-traumatic stress disorder. *Urology* 60(5):881-884.

Crowell, T. A., K. M. Kieffer, C. A. Siders, and R. D. Vanderploeg. 2002. Neuropsychological findings in combat-related posttraumatic stress disorder. *Clinical Neuropsychologist* 16(3):310-321.

Cucciare, M. A., S. Ghaus, K. R. Weingardt, and S. M. Frayne. 2011. Sexual assault and substance use in male veterans receiving a brief alcohol intervention. *Journal of Studies on Alcohol and Drugs* 72(5):693-700.

Dagan, Y., P. Lavie, and A. Bleich. 1991. Elevated awakening thresholds in sleep stage 3-4 in war-related post-traumatic stress disorder. *Biological Psychiatry* 30(6):618-622.

DCoE (Defense Centers For Excellence for Psychological Health and Traumatic Brain Injury). 2011. *Department of Defense Suicide Event Report: Calendar Year 2010 Annual Report.* Washington, DC: National Center for Telehealth and Technology, Defense Centers for Excellence for Psychological Health and Traumatic Brain Injury.

Dedert, E. A., K. T. Green, P. S. Calhoun, R. Yoash-Gantz, K. H. Taber, M. M. Mumford, L. A. Tupler, R. A. Morey, C. E. Marx, R. D. Weiner, and J. C. Beckham. 2009. Association of trauma exposure with psychiatric morbidity in military veterans who have served since September 11, 2001. *Journal of Psychiatric Research* 43(9):830-836.

Department of the Army. 2012. *Army 2020: Generating Health and Discipline in the Force.* Washington, DC: Department of Defense.

Dikmen, S., J. Machamer, N. Temkin, and A. McLean. 1990. Neuropsychological recovery in patients with moderate to severe head injury: 2 year follow-up. *Journal of Clinical and Experimental Neuropsychology* 12(4):507-519.

Dikmen, S., J. Machamer, and N. Temkin. 1993. Psychosocial outcome in patients with moderate to severe head injury: 2-year follow-up. *Brain Injury* 7(2):113-124.

Dikmen, S. S., N. R. Temkin, J. E. Machamer, A. L. Holubkov, R. T. Fraser, and H. R. Winn. 1994. Employment following traumatic head injuries. *Archives of Neurology* 51(2):177-186.

Dikmen, S. S., J. E. Machamer, H. Winn, and N. R. Temkin. 1995. Neuropsychological outcome at 1-year post head injury. *Neuropsychology* 9(1):80-90.

Dikmen, S. S., J. D. Corrigan, H. S. Levin, J. MacHamer, W. Stiers, and M. G. Weisskopf. 2009. Cognitive outcome following traumatic brain injury. *Journal of Head Trauma Rehabilitation* 24(6):430-438.

Dikmen, S., J. Machamer, J. R. Fann, and N. R. Temkin. 2010. Rates of symptom reporting following traumatic brain injury. *Journal of the International Neuropsychological Society* 16(3):401-411.

Dobie, D. J., D. R. Kivlahan, C. Maynard, K. R. Bush, T. M. Davis, and K. A. Bradley. 2004. Posttraumatic stress disorder in female veterans: Association with self-reported health problems and functional impairment. *Archives of Internal Medicine* 164(4):394-400.

Doctor, J. N., J. Castro, N. R. Temkin, R. T. Fraser, J. E. Machamer, and S. S. Dikmen. 2005. Workers' risk of unemployment after traumatic brain injury: A normed comparison. *Journal of the International Neuropsychological Society* 11(6):747-752.

DOD (Department of Defense). 2009a. *DOD/VA Code Proposal Final.* http://www.cdc.gov/nchs/data/icd9/Sep08TBI.pdf (accessed October 29, 2012).

———. 2009b. *Status of Drug Use in Department of Defense Personnel: Fiscal Year 2008 Drug Testing Statistical Report.* Falls Church, VA: Office of the Assistant Secretary of Defense for Health Affairs.

Dow, B. M., J. R. Kelsoe, Jr., and J. C. Gillin. 1996. Sleep and dreams in Vietnam PTSD and depression. *Biological Psychiatry* 39(1):42-50.

Drew, R. H., D. I. Templer, B. A. Schuyler, T. G. Newell, and W. G. Cannon. 1986. Neuropsychological deficits in active licensed professional boxers. *Journal of Clinical Psychology* 42(3):520-525.

Dutra, L., K. Grubbs, C. Greene, L. L. Trego, T. L. McCartin, K. Kloezeman, and L. Morland. 2011. Women at war: Implications for mental health. *Journal of Trauma and Dissociation* 12(1):25-37.

DVBIC (Defense and Veterans Brain Injury Center). 2012. *DOD Numbers for Traumatic Brain Injury Worldwide — Totals*. Silver Spring, MD: Department of Defense.

Edens, E. L., W. Kasprow, J. Tsai, and R. A. Rosenheck. 2011. Association of substance use and VA service-connected disability benefits with risk of homelessness among veterans. *American Journal on Addictions* 20(5):412-419.

Eisen, S. V., M. R. Schultz, D. Vogt, M. E. Glickman, A. R. Elwy, M. L. Drainoni, P. E. Osei-Bonsu, and J. Martin. 2012. Mental and physical health status and alcohol and drug use following return from deployment to Iraq or Afghanistan. *American Journal of Public Health* 102(S1):S66-S73.

Elbogen, E. B., H. Wagner, S. R. Fuller, P. S. Calhoun, P. M. Kinneer, and J. C. Beckham. 2010. Correlates of anger and hostility in Iraq and Afghanistan war veterans. *American Journal of Psychiatry* 167(9):1051-1058.

Elder, G. A., and A. Cristian. 2009. Blast-related mild traumatic brain injury: Mechanisms of injury and impact on clinical care. *Mount Sinai Journal of Medicine* 76(2):111-118.

Engdahl, B. E., R. E. Eberly, T. D. Hurwitz, M. W. Mahowald, and J. Blake. 2000. Sleep in a community sample of elderly war veterans with and without posttraumatic stress disorder. *Biological Psychiatry* 47(6):520-525.

Engel, C. C., Jr., X. Liu, B. D. McCarthy, R. F. Miller, and R. Ursano. 2000. Relationship of physical symptoms to posttraumatic stress disorder among veterans seeking care for gulf war-related health concerns. *Psychosomatic Medicine* 62(6):739-745.

Erbes, C. R., M. E. Kaler, T. Schult, M. A. Polusny, and P. A. Arbisi. 2011. Mental health diagnosis and occupational functioning in National Guard/reserve veterans returning from Iraq. *Journal of Rehabilitation Research and Development* 48(10):1159-1170.

Fann, J. R., A. Leonetti, K. Jaffe, W. J. Katon, P. Cummings, and R. S. Thompson. 2002. Psychiatric illness and subsequent traumatic brain injury: A case control study. *Journal of Neurology, Neurosurgery, and Psychiatry* 72(5):615-620.

Fann, J. R., B. Burington, A. Leonetti, K. Jaffe, W. J. Katon, and R. S. Thompson. 2004. Psychiatric illness following traumatic brain injury in an adult health maintenance organization population. *Archives of General Psychiatry* 61(1):53-61.

Fear, N. T., M. Jones, D. Murphy, L. Hull, A. C. Iversen, B. Coker, L. Machell, J. Sundin, C. Woodhead, N. Jones, N. Greenberg, S. Landau, C. Dandeker, R. J. Rona, M. Hotopf, and S. Wessely. 2010. What are the consequences of deployment to Iraq and Afghanistan on the mental health of the UK Armed Forces? A cohort study. *Lancet* 375(9728):1783-1797.

Federman, E. B., R. M. Bray, and L. A. Kroutil. 2000. Relationships between substance use and recent deployments among women and men in the military. *Military Psychology* 12(3):205-220.

Ferrier-Auerbach, A. G., S. M. Kehle, C. R. Erbes, P. A. Arbisi, P. Thuras, and M. A. Polusny. 2009. Predictors of alcohol use prior to deployment in National Guard soldiers. *Addictive Behaviors* 34(8):625-631.

Flynn, P. M., and B. S. Brown. 2008. Co-occurring disorders in substance abuse treatment: Issues and prospects. *Journal of Substance Abuse and Treatment* 34(1):36-47.

Fontana, A., and R. Rosenheck. 2008. Treatment-seeking veterans of Iraq and Afghanistan: Comparison with veterans of previous wars. *Journal of Nervous and Mental Disease* 196(7):513-521.

Frayne, S. M., M. R. Seaver, S. Loveland, C. L. Christiansen, A. Spiro, 3rd, V. A. Parker, and K. M. Skinner. 2004. Burden of medical illness in women with depression and posttraumatic stress disorder. *Archives of Internal Medicine* 164(12):1306-1312.

Frayne, S. M., V. Y. Chiu, S. Iqbal, E. A. Berg, K. J. Laungani, R. C. Cronkite, J. Pavao, and R. Kimerling. 2011. Medical care needs of returning veterans with PTSD: Their other burden. *Journal of General Internal Medicine* 26(1):33-39.

Friedman, M. 2003. *Post Traumatic Stress Disorder*. Kansas City, MO: Compact Clinicals.

Fritch, A. M., M. Mishkind, M. A. Reger, and G. A. Gahm. 2010. The impact of childhood abuse and combat-related trauma on postdeployment adjustment. *Journal of Traumatic Stress* 23(2):248-254.

Gahm, G. A., B. A. Lucenko, P. Retzlaff, and S. Fukuda. 2007. Relative impact of adverse events and screened symptoms of posttraumatic stress disorder and depression among active duty soldiers seeking mental health care. *Journal of Clinical Psychology* 63(3):199-211.

Gale, C. R., I. J. Deary, S. H. Boyle, J. Barefoot, L. H. Mortensen, and G. D. Batty. 2008. Cognitive ability in early adulthood and risk of 5 specific psychiatric disorders in middle age: The Vietnam Experience Study. *Archives of General Psychiatry* 65(12):1410-1418.

Galovski, T. E., J. Mott, Y. N. Young-Xu, and P. A. Resick. 2011. Gender differences in the clinical presentation of PTSD and its concomitants in survivors of interpersonal assault. *Journal of Interpersonal Violence* 26(4):789-806.

Gaylord, K. M., D. B. Cooper, J. M. Mercado, J. E. Kennedy, L. H. Yoder, and J. B. Holcomb. 2008. Incidence of posttraumatic stress disorder and mild traumatic brain injury in burned service members: Preliminary report. *Journal of Trauma: Injury, Infection, and Critical Care* 64(2):s200-s206.

Gellis, L. A., P. R. Gehrman, S. Mavandadi, and D. W. Oslin. 2010a. Predictors of sleep disturbances in Operation Iraqi Freedom/Operation Enduring Freedom veterans reporting a trauma. *Military Medicine* 175(8):567-573.

Gellis, L. A., S. Mavandadi, and D. W. Oslin. 2010b. Functional quality of life in full versus partial posttraumatic stress disorder among veterans returning from Iraq and Afghanistan. *Primary Care Companion to the Journal of Clinical Psychiatry* 12(3).

Gerber, D. J., and J. C. Schraa. 1995. Mild traumatic brain injury: Searching for the syndrome. *Journal of Head Trauma Rehabilitation* 10(4):28-40.

Gibbons, S. W., E. J. Hickling, S. D. Barnett, P. L. Herbig-Wall, and D. D. Watts. 2012. Gender differences in response to deployment among military healthcare providers in Afghanistan and Iraq. *Journal of Women's Health* 21(5):496-504.

Gilbertson, M. W., T. V. Gurvits, N. B. Lasko, S. P. Orr, and R. K. Pitman. 2001. Multivariate assessment of explicit memory function in combat veterans with posttraumatic stress disorder. *Journal of Traumatic Stress* 14(2):413-432.

Gilbertson, M. W., M. E. Shenton, A. Ciszewski, K. Kasai, N. B. Lasko, S. P. Orr, and R. K. Pitman. 2002. Smaller hippocampal volume predicts pathologic vulnerability to psychological trauma. *Nature Neuroscience* 5(11):1242-1247.

Glenn, D. M., J. C. Beckham, M. E. Feldman, A. C. Kirby, M. A. Hertzberg, and S. D. Moore. 2002. Violence and hostility among families of Vietnam veterans with combat-related posttraumatic stress disorder. *Violence and Victims* 17(4):473-489.

Goldstein, L. E., A. M. Fisher, C. A. Tagge, X. L. Zhang, L. Velisek, J. A. Sullivan, C. Upreti, J. M. Kracht, M. Ericsson, M. W. Wojnarowicz, C. J. Goletiani, G. M. Maglakelidze, N. Casey, J. A. Moncaster, O. Minaeva, R. D. Moir, C. J. Nowinski, R. A. Stern, R. C. Cantu, J. Geiling, J. K. Blusztajn, B. L. Wolozin, T. Ikezu, T. D. Stein, A. E. Budson, N. W. Kowall, D. Chargin, A. Sharon, S. Saman, G. F. Hall, W. C. Moss, R. O. Cleveland, R. E. Tanzi, P. K. Stanton, and A. C. McKee. 2012. Chronic traumatic encephalopathy in blast-exposed military veterans and a blast neurotrauma mouse model. *Science Translational Medicine* 4(134):1-16.

Grafman, J., A. M. Salazar, H. Weingartner, and D. Amin. 1986. Face memory and discrimination: An analysis of the persistent effects of penetrating brain wounds. *International Journal of Neuroscience* 29(1-2):125-139.

Grafman, J., B. S. Jonas, A. Martin, A. M. Salazar, H. Weingartner, C. Ludlow, M. A. Smutok, and S. C. Vance. 1988. Intellectual function following penetrating head injury in Vietnam veterans. *Brain* 111(Pt 1):169-184.

Grafman, J., B. Jonas, and A. Salazar. 1990. Wisconsin card sorting test performance based on location and size of neuroanatomical lesion in Vietnam veterans with penetrating head injury. *Perceptual and Motor Skills* 71(3 Pt 2):1120-1122.

Graham, D. P., and A. L. Cardon. 2008. An update on substance use and treatment following traumatic brain injury. *Annals of the New York Academy of Sciences* 1141:148-162.

Gray, M. J., E. E. Bolton, and B. T. Litz. 2004. A longitudinal analysis of PTSD symptom course: Delayed-onset PTSD in Somalia peacekeepers. *Journal of Consulting and Clinical Psychology* 72(5):909-913.

Green, B. L., M. C. Grace, J. D. Lindy, and G. C. Gleser. 1990. War stressors and symptom persistence in posttraumatic stress disorder. *Journal of Anxiety Disorders* 4(1):31-39.

Grieger, T. A., S. J. Cozza, R. J. Ursano, C. W. Hoge, P. E. Martinez, C. C. Engel, and H. J. Wain. 2006. Posttraumatic stress disorder and depression in battle-injured soldiers. *American Journal of Psychiatry* 163(10):1777-1783.

Groswasser, Z., G. Reider, II, K. Schwab, A. K. Ommaya, A. Pridgen, H. R. Brown, R. Cole, and A. M. Salazar. 2002. Quantitative imaging in late TBI. Part II: Cognition and work after closed and penetrating head injury: A report of the Vietnam Head Injury study. *Brain Injury* 16(8):681-690.

Grubaugh, A. L., J. Monnier, K. M. Magruder, R. G. Knapp, and B. C. Frueh. 2006. Female veterans seeking medical care at Veterans Affairs primary care clinics: Psychiatric and medical illness burden and service use. *Women and Health* 43(3):41-62.

Guerra, V. S., and P. S. Calhoun. 2011. Examining the relation between posttraumatic stress disorder and suicidal ideation in an OEF/OIF veteran sample. *Journal of Anxiety Disorders* 25(1):12-18.

Gurvits, T. V., L. J. Metzger, N. B. Lasko, P. A. Cannistraro, A. S. Tarhan, M. W. Gilbertson, S. P. Orr, A. M. Charbonneau, M. M. B. S. Wedig, and R. K. M. D. Pitman. 2006. Subtle neurologic compromise as a vulnerability factor for combat-related posttraumatic stress disorder: Results of a twin study. *Archives of General Psychiatry* 63(5):571-576.

Hankin, C. S., K. M. Skinner, L. M. Sullivan, D. R. Miller, S. Frayne, and T. J. Tripp. 1999. Prevalence of depressive and alcohol abuse symptoms among women VA outpatients who report experiencing sexual assault while in the military. *Journal of Traumatic Stress* 12(4):601-612.

Haskell, S. G., C. A. Brandt, E. E. Krebs, M. Skanderson, R. D. Kerns, and J. L. Goulet. 2009. Pain among veterans of Operations Enduring Freedom and Iraqi Freedom: Do women and men differ? *Pain Medicine* 10(7):1167-1173.

Haskell, S. G., K. S. Gordon, K. Mattocks, M. Duggal, J. Erdos, A. Justice, and C. A. Brandt. 2010. Gender differences in rates of depression, PTSD, pain, obesity, and military sexual trauma among Connecticut war veterans of Iraq and Afghanistan. *Journal of Women's Health* 19(2):267-271.

Hassija, C. M., M. Jakupcak, S. Maguen, and J. C. Shipherd. 2012. The influence of combat and interpersonal trauma on PTSD, depression, and alcohol misuse in US Gulf War and OEF/OIF women veterans. *Journal of Traumatic Stress* 25(2):216-219.

Hawkins, E. J., G. T. Lapham, D. R. Kivlahan, and K. A. Bradley. 2010. Recognition and management of alcohol misuse in OEF/OIF and other veterans in the VA: A cross-sectional study. *Drug and Alcohol Dependence* 109(1-3):147-153.

Heitger, M. H., R. D. Jones, C. M. Frampton, M. W. Ardagh, and T. J. Anderson. 2007. Recovery in the first year after mild head injury: Divergence of symptom status and self-perceived quality of life. *Journal of Rehabilitation Medicine* 39(8):612-621.

Heltemes, K. J., A. L. Dougherty, A. J. MacGregor, and M. R. Galarneau. 2011. Alcohol abuse disorders among US service members with mild traumatic brain injury. *Military Medicine* 176:147-150.

Highfill-McRoy, R. M., G. E. Larson, S. Booth-Kewley, and C. F. Garland. 2010. Psychiatric diagnoses and punishment for misconduct: The effects of PTSD in combat-deployed marines. *BMC Psychiatry* 10:88.

Hill, J. J., 3rd, B. H. Mobo, Jr., and M. R. Cullen. 2009. Separating deployment-related traumatic brain injury and posttraumatic stress disorder in veterans: Preliminary findings from the Veterans Affairs traumatic brain injury screening program. *American Journal of Physical Medicine and Rehabilitation* 88(8):605-614.

Himmelfarb, N., D. Yaeger, and J. Mintz. 2006. Posttraumatic stress disorder in female veterans with military and civilian sexual trauma. *Journal of Traumatic Stress* 19(6):837-846.

Hirsch, K. A. 2009. Sexual dysfunction in male Operation Enduring Freedom/Operation Iraqi Freedom patients with severe post-traumatic stress disorder. *Military Medicine* 174(5):520-522.

Hoge, C. W., C. A. Castro, S. C. Messer, D. McGurk, D. I. Cotting, and R. L. Koffman. 2004a. Combat duty in Iraq and Afghanistan, mental health problems, and barriers to care. *New England Journal of Medicine* 351(1):13-22.

Hoge, C. W., K. Wright, P. Bliese, A. Adler, and J. Thomas. 2004b. *Prevalence and Screening of Mental Health Problems Among US Combat Soldiers Pre- and Post- Deployment.* Silver Spring, MD: Walter Reed Army Institute of Research.

Hoge, C. W., J. L. Auchterlonie, and C. S. Milliken. 2006. Mental health problems, use of mental health services, and attrition from military service after returning from deployment to Iraq or Afghanistan. *Journal of the American Medical Association* 295(9):1023-1032.

Hoge, C. W., A. Terhakopian, C. A. Castro, S. C. Messer, and C. C. Engel. 2007. Association of posttraumatic stress disorder with somatic symptoms, health care visits, and absenteeism among Iraq war veterans. *American Journal of Psychiatry* 164(1):150-153.

Hoge, C. W., D. McGurk, J. Thomas, A. L. Cox, C. C. Engel, and C. A. Castro. 2008. Mild traumatic brain injury in US soldiers returning from Iraq. *New England Journal of Medicine* 358(5):453-463.

Holbrook, T. L., D. B. Hoyt, M. B. Stein, and W. J. Sieber. 2002. Gender differences in long-term posttraumatic stress disorder outcomes after major trauma: Women are at higher risk of adverse outcomes than men. *Journal of Trauma—Injury, Infection and Critical Care* 53(5):882-888.

Holsinger, T., D. C. Steffens, C. Phillips, M. J. Helms, R. J. Havlik, J. C. S. Breitner, J. M. Guralnik, and B. L. Plassman. 2002. Head injury in early adulthood and the lifetime risk of depression. *Archives of General Psychiatry* 59(1):17-22.

Horner, M. D., P. L. Ferguson, A. W. Selassie, L. A. Labbate, K. Kniele, and J. D. Corrigan. 2005. Patterns of alcohol use 1 year after traumatic brain injury: A population-based, epidemiological study. *Journal of the International Neuropsychological Society* 11(3):322-330.

Hyman, J., R. Ireland, L. Frost, and L. Cottrell. 2012. Suicide incidence and risk factors in an active duty US military population. *American Journal of Public Health* 102(1 Suppl):S138-S146.

Hyun, J. K., J. Pavao, and R. Kimerling. 2009. Military sexual trauma. *PTSD Research Quarterly* 20(2):1-8.

Ilgen, M. A., K. R. Conner, M. Valenstein, K. Austin, and F. C. Blow. 2010. Violent and nonviolent suicide in veterans with substance-use disorders. *Journal of Studies on Alcohol and Drugs* 71(4):473-479.

Inman, D. J., S. M. Silver, and K. Doghramji. 1990. Sleep disturbance in post-traumatic stress disorder: A comparison with non-PTSD insomnia. *Journal of Traumatic Stress* 3(3):429-437.

IOM (Institute of Medicine). 2006. *Posttraumatic Stress Disorder: Diagnosis and Assessment.* Washington, DC: The National Academies Press.

———. 2008a. *Gulf War and Health, Volume 6: Physiologic, Psychologic, and Psychosocial Effects of Deployment-related Stress.* Washington, DC: The National Academies Press.

———. 2008b. *Treatment of Posttraumatic Stress Disorder: An Assessment of the Evidence.* Washington, DC: The National Academies Press.

———. 2009. *Gulf War and Health, Volume 7: Long-Term Consequences of Traumatic Brain Injury.* Washington, DC: The National Academies Press.

———. 2010. *Returning Home from Iraq and Afghanistan: Preliminary Assessment of Readjustment Needs of Veterans, Service Members, and their Families.* Washington, DC: The National Academies Press.

Irwin, C., S. A. Falsetti, R. B. Lydiard, J. C. Ballenger, C. D. Brock, and W. Brener. 1996. Comorbidity of posttraumatic stress disorder and irritable bowel syndrome. *Journal of Clinical Psychiatry* 57(12):576-578.

Iverson, K. M., A. M. Hendricks, R. Kimerling, M. Krengel, M. Meterko, K. L. Stolzmann, E. Baker, T. K. Pogoda, J. J. Vasterling, and H. L. Lew. 2011. Psychiatric diagnoses and neurobehavioral symptom severity among OEF/OIF VA patients with deployment-related traumatic brain injury: A gender comparison. *Women's Health Issues* 21(4 Suppl):S210-S217.

Jacobson, I. G., M. A. Ryan, T. J. Hooper, T. C. Smith, P. J. Amoroso, E. J. Boyko, G. D. Gackstetter, T. S. Wells, and N. S. Bell. 2008. Alcohol use and alcohol-related problems before and after military combat deployment. *Journal of the American Medical Association* 300(6):663-675.

Jakupcak, M., D. Conybeare, L. Phelps, S. Hunt, H. A. Holmes, B. Felker, M. Klevens, and M. E. McFall. 2007. Anger, hostility, and aggression among Iraq and Afghanistan war veterans reporting PTSD and subthreshold PTSD. *Journal of Traumatic Stress* 20(6):945-954.

Jakupcak, M., J. Cook, Z. Imel, A. Fontana, R. Rosenheck, and M. McFall. 2009. Posttraumatic stress disorder as a risk factor for suicidal ideation in Iraq and Afghanistan war veterans. *Journal of Traumatic Stress* 22(4):303-306.

Jakupcak, M., M. T. Tull, M. J. McDermott, D. Kaysen, S. Hunt, and T. Simpson. 2010a. PTSD symptom clusters in relationship to alcohol misuse among Iraq and Afghanistan war veterans seeking post-deployment VA health care. *Addictive Behaviors* 35(9):840-843.

Jakupcak, M., S. Vannoy, Z. Imel, J. W. Cook, A. Fontana, R. Rosenheck, and M. McFall. 2010b. Does PTSD moderate the relationship between social support and suicide risk in Iraq and Afghanistan war veterans seeking mental health treatment? *Depression and Anxiety* 27(11):1001-1005.

Jakupcak, M., K. D. Hoerster, A. Varra, S. Vannoy, B. Felker, and S. Hunt. 2011. Hopelessness and suicidal ideation in Iraq and Afghanistan war veterans reporting subthreshold and threshold posttraumatic stress disorder. *Journal of Nervous and Mental Disease* 199(4):272-275.

Jones, E., A. Thomas, and S. Ironside. 2007. Shell shock: An outcome study of a first world war "PIE" unit. *Psychological Medicine* 37(2):215-223.

Jordan, B. K., C. R. Marmar, J. A. Fairbank, W. E. Schlenger, R. A. Kulka, R. L. Hough, and D. S. Weiss. 1992. Problems in families of male Vietnam veterans with posttraumatic stress disorder. *Journal of Consulting and Clinical Psychology* 60(6):916-926.

Jorge, R. E., R. G. Robinson, D. Moser, A. Tateno, B. Crespo-Facorro, and S. Arndt. 2004. Major depression following traumatic brain injury. *Archives of General Psychiatry* 61(1):42-50.

Jorge, R. E., S. E. Starkstein, S. Arndt, D. Moser, B. Crespo-Facorro, and R. G. Robinson. 2005. Alcohol misuse and mood disorders following traumatic brain injury. *Archives of General Psychiatry* 62(7):742-749.

Kang, H. K., and T. A. Bullman. 2009. Is there an epidemic of suicides among current and former US military personnel? *Annals of Epidemiology* 19(10):757-760.

Kaplan, M. S., B. H. McFarland, N. Huguet, and M. Valenstein. 2012. Suicide risk and precipitating circumstances among young, middle-aged, and older male veterans. *American Journal of Public Health* 102(S1):S131-S137.

Kehle, S. M., A. G. Ferrier-Auerbach, L. A. Meis, P. A. Arbisi, C. R. Erbes, and M. A. Polusny. 2011a. Predictors of postdeployment alcohol use disorders in National Guard soldiers deployed to Operation Iraqi Freedom. *Psychology of Addictive Behaviors* 26(1):42-50.

Kehle, S. M., M. K. Reddy, A. G. Ferrier-Auerbach, C. R. Erbes, P. A. Arbisi, and M. A. Polusny. 2011b. Psychiatric diagnoses, comorbidity, and functioning in National Guard troops deployed to Iraq. *Journal of Psychiatric Research* 45(1):126-132.

Kennedy, J. E., M. S. Jaffee, G. A. Leskin, J. W. Stokes, F. O. Leal, and P. J. Fitzpatrick. 2007. Posttraumatic stress disorder and posttraumatic stress disorder-like symptoms and mild traumatic brain injury. *Journal of Rehabilitation Research and Development* 44(7):895-920.

Kennedy, J. E., F. O. Leal, J. D. Lewis, M. A. Cullen, and R. R. Amador. 2010. Posttraumatic stress symptoms in OIF/OEF service members with blast-related and non-blast-related mild TBI. *NeuroRehabilitation* 26(3):223-231.

Kimerling, R., K. Gima, M. W. Smith, A. Street, and S. Frayne. 2007. The Veterans Health Administration and military sexual trauma. *American Journal of Public Health* 97(12):2160-2166.

Kimerling, R., A. E. Street, J. Pavao, M. W. Smith, R. C. Cronkite, T. H. Holmes, and S. M. Frayne. 2010. Military-related sexual trauma among veterans health administration patients returning from Afghanistan and Iraq. *American Journal of Public Health* 100(8):1409-1412.

Kinder, L. S., K. A. Bradley, W. J. Katon, E. Ludman, M. B. McDonell, and C. L. Bryson. 2008. Depression, posttraumatic stress disorder, and mortality. *Psychosomatic Medicine* 70(1):20-26.

Kline, A., M. Falca-Dodson, B. Sussner, D. S. Ciccone, H. Chandler, L. Callahan, and M. Losonczy. 2010. Effects of repeated deployment to Iraq and Afghanistan on the health of New Jersey Army National Guard troops: Implications for military readiness. *American Journal of Public Health* 100(2):276-283.

Kline, A., D. S. Ciccone, M. Falca-Dodson, C. M. Black, and M. Losonczy. 2011. Suicidal ideation among National Guard troops deployed to Iraq: The association with postdeployment readjustment problems. *Journal of Nervous and Mental Disease* 199(12):914-920.

Koenen, K. C., T. E. Moffitt, R. Poulton, J. Martin, and A. Caspi. 2007. Early childhood factors associated with the development of post-traumatic stress disorder: Results from a longitudinal birth cohort. *Psychological Medicine* 37(2):181-192.

Koenigs, M., and J. Grafman. 2009. Posttraumatic stress disorder: The role of medial prefrontal cortex and amygdala. *Neuroscientist* 15(5):540-548.

Kolkow, T. T., J. L. Spira, J. S. Morse, and T. A. Grieger. 2007. Post-traumatic stress disorder and depression in health care providers returning from deployment to Iraq and Afghanistan. *Military Medicine* 172(5):451-455.

Koso, M., and S. Hansen. 2006. Executive function and memory in posttraumatic stress disorder: A study of Bosnian war veterans. *European Psychiatry* 21(3):167-173.

Kremen, W. S., K. C. Koenen, C. Boake, S. Purcell, S. A. Eisen, C. E. Franz, M. T. Tsuang, and M. J. Lyons. 2007. Pretrauma cognitive ability and risk for posttraumatic stress disorder: A twin study. *Archives of General Psychiatry* 64(3):361-368.

Kulka, R. A., W. E. Schlenger, J. A. Fairbank, R. L. Hough, B. K. Jordan, C. R. Marmar, D. S. Weiss, and D. A. Grady. 1990. *Trauma and the Vietnam War Generation: Report of Findings from the National Vietnam Veterans Readjustment Study*. New York: Routledge.

Lande, R. G., B. A. Marin, A. S. Chang, and G. R. Lande. 2008. Survey of alcohol use in the US Army. *Journal of Addictive Diseases* 27(3):115-121.

Lane, M. E., L. L. Hourani, R. M. Bray, and J. Williams. 2012. Prevalence of perceived stress and mental health indicators among reserve-component and active-duty military personnel. *American Journal of Public Health* 102(6):1213-1220.

Langhinrichsen-Rohling, J., J. D. Snarr, A. M. Slep, R. E. Heyman, and H. M. Foran. 2011. Risk for suicidal ideation in the US Air Force: An ecological perspective. *Journal of Consulting and Clinical Psychology* 79(5):600-612.

Lannsjo, M., J. L. af Geijerstam, U. Johansson, J. Bring, and J. Borg. 2009. Prevalence and structure of symptoms at 3 months after mild traumatic brain injury in a national cohort. *Brain Injury* 23(3):213-219.

Lapierre, C. B., A. F. Schwegler, and B. J. LaBauve. 2007. Posttraumatic stress and depression symptoms in soldiers returning from combat operations in Iraq and Afghanistan. *Journal of Traumatic Stress* 20(6):933-943.

Larson, G. E., P. S. Hammer, T. L. Conway, E. A. Schmied, M. R. Galarneau, P. Konoske, J. A. Webb-Murphy, K. J. Schmitz, N. Edwards, and D. C. Johnson. 2011. Predeployment and in-theater diagnoses of American military personnel serving in Iraq. *Psychiatric Services* 62(1):15-21.

Lemaire, C. M., and D. P. Graham. 2011. Factors associated with suicidal ideation in OEF/OIF veterans. *Journal of Affective Disorders* 130(1-2):231-238.

Letz, R. 1990. The Neurobehavioral Evaluation System (NES): An international effort. In *Advances in Neurobehavioral Toxicology: Applications in Environmental and Occupational Health*, edited by B. L. Johnson, W. K. Anger, A. Durao and C. Xintaras. Chelsea, MI: Lewis Publishers.

Levin, H. S., H. E. Gary, Jr., H. M. Eisenberg, R. M. Ruff, J. T. Barth, J. Kreutzer, W. M. High, Jr., S. Portman, M. A. Foulkes, J. A. Jane, A. Marmarou, and L. F. Marshall. 1990. Neurobehavioral outcome 1 year after severe head injury: Experience of the traumatic coma data bank. *Journal of Neurosurgery* 73:699-709.

Lewis, V., M. Creamer, and S. Failla. 2009. Is poor sleep in veterans a function of post-traumatic stress disorder? *Military Medicine* 174(9):948-951.

Lipari, R. N., P. J. Cook, L. M. Rock, and K. Matos. 2008. *2006 Gender Relations Survey of Active Duty Members.* Arlington, VA: Defense Manpower Data Center.

Logan, J., N. A. Skopp, D. Karch, M. A. Reger, and G. A. Gahm. 2012. Characteristics of suicides among US Army active duty personnel in 17 US states from 2005 to 2007. *American Journal of Public Health* 102(S1):S40-S44.

Luethcke, C. A., C. J. Bryan, C. E. Morrow, and W. C. Isler. 2011. Comparison of concussive symptoms, cognitive performance, and psychological symptoms between acute blast-versus nonblast-induced mild traumatic brain injury. *Journal of the International Neuropsychological Society* 17(1):36-45.

Luxton, D. D., N. A. Skopp, and S. Maguen. 2010. Gender differences in depression and PTSD symptoms following combat exposure. *Depression and Anxiety* 27(11):1027-1033.

Macey, T. A., B. J. Morasco, J. P. Duckart, and S. K. Dobscha. 2011. Patterns and correlates of prescription opioid use in OEF/OIF veterans with chronic noncancer pain. *Pain Medicine* 12(10):1502-1509.

MacGregor, A. J., R. A. Shaffer, A. L. Dougherty, M. R. Galarneau, R. Raman, D. G. Baker, S. P. Lindsay, B. A. Golomb, and K. S. Corson. 2009. Psychological correlates of battle and nonbattle injury among Operation Iraqi Freedom veterans. *Military Medicine* 174(3):224-231.

MacGregor, A. J., P. P. Han, A. L. Dougherty, and M. R. Galarneau. 2012. Effect of dwell time on the mental health of US military personnel with multiple combat tours. *American Journal of Public Health* 102(1 Suppl):S55-S59.

Magruder, K. M., B. C. Frueh, R. G. Knapp, M. R. Johnson, J. A. Vaughan Iii, T. C. Carson, D. A. Powell, and R. Hebert. 2004. PTSD symptoms, demographic characteristics, and functional status among veterans treated in VA primary care clinics. *Journal of Traumatic Stress* 17(4):293-301.

Magruder, K. M., B. C. Frueh, R. G. Knapp, L. Davis, M. B. Hamner, R. H. Martin, P. B. Gold, and G. W. Arana. 2005. Prevalence of posttraumatic stress disorder in Veterans Affairs primary care clinics. *General Hospital Psychiatry* 27(3):169-179.

Maguen, S., L. Ren, J. O. Bosch, C. R. Marmar, and K. H. Seal. 2010. Gender differences in mental health diagnoses among Iraq and Afghanistan veterans enrolled in Veterans Affairs health care. *American Journal of Public Health* 100(12):2450-2456.

Maguen, S., D. D. Luxton, N. A. Skopp, G. A. Gahm, M. A. Reger, T. J. Metzler, and C. R. Marmar. 2011a. Killing in combat, mental health symptoms, and suicidal ideation in Iraq war veterans. *Journal of Anxiety Disorders* 25(4):563-567.

Maguen, S., D. D. Luxton, N. A. Skopp, and E. Madden. 2011b. Gender differences in traumatic experiences and mental health in active duty soldiers redeployed from Iraq and Afghanistan. *Journal of Psychiatric Research* 46(3):311-316

Maguen, S., D. S. Vogt, L. A. King, D. W. King, B. T. Litz, S. J. Knight, and C. R. Marmar. 2011c. The impact of killing on mental health symptoms in Gulf War veterans. *Psychological Trauma: Theory, Research, Practice, and Policy* 3(1):21-26.

Maguen, S., B. Cohen, L. Ren, J. Bosch, R. Kimerling, and K. Seal. 2012. Gender differences in military sexual trauma and mental health diagnoses among Iraq and Afghanistan veterans with posttraumatic stress disorder. *Womens Health Issues* 22(1):e61-e66.

Martin, S. L., D. A. Gibbs, R. E. Johnson, K. Sullivan, M. Clinton-Sherrod, J. L. Walters, and E. D. Rentz. 2010. Substance use by soldiers who abuse their spouses. *Violence Against Women* 16(11):1295-1310.

Martland, H. S. 1928. Punch drunk. *Journal of the American Medical Association* 91:1103-1107.

Marx, B. P., K. Brailey, S. P. Proctor, and E. al. 2009. Association of time since deployment, combat intensity, and posttraumatic stress symptoms with neuropsychological outcomes following Iraq war deployment. *Archives of General Psychiatry* 66(9):996-1004.

Mason, J., S. Southwick, R. Yehuda, S. Wang, S. Riney, D. Bremner, D. Johnson, H. Lubin, D. Blake, G. Zhou, et al. 1994. Elevation of serum free triiodothyronine, total triiodothyronine, thyroxine-binding globulin, and total thyroxine levels in combat-related posttraumatic stress disorder. *Archives of General Psychiatry* 51(8):629-641.

Mattiko, M. J., K. L. Olmsted, J. M. Brown, and R. M. Bray. 2011. Alcohol use and negative consequences among active duty military personnel. *Addictive Behaviors* 36(6):608-614.

McAllister, T. W. 2011. Neurobiological consequences of traumatic brain injury. *Dialogues in Clinical Neuroscience* 13(3):287-300.

McAllister, T. W., and M. B. Stein. 2010. Effects of psychological and biomechanical trauma on brain and behavior. *Annals of the New York Academy of Sciences* 1208:46-57.

McCarthy, J. F., M. Valenstein, H. M. Kim, M. Ilgen, K. Zivin, and F. C. Blow. 2009. Suicide mortality among patients receiving care in the Veterans Health Administration health system. *American Journal of Epidemiology* 169(8):1033-1038.

McCarthy, J. F., F. C. Blow, R. V. Ignacio, M. A. Ilgen, K. L. Austin, and M. Valenstein. 2012. Suicide among patients in the Veterans Affairs health system: Rural–urban differences in rates, risks, and methods. *American Journal of Public Health* 102(S1):S111-S117.

McCrea, M., G. L. Iverson, T. W. McAllister, T. A. Hammeke, M. R. Powell, W. B. Barr, and J. P. Kelly. 2009. An integrated review of recovery after mild traumatic brain injury (mTBI): Implications for clinical management. *Clinical Neuropsychologist* 23(8):1368-1390.

McDevitt-Murphy, M. E., J. L. Williams, K. L. Bracken, J. A. Fields, C. J. Monahan, and J. G. Murphy. 2010. PTSD symptoms, hazardous drinking, and health functioning among US OEF and OIF veterans presenting to primary care. *Journal of Traumatic Stress* 23(1):108-111.

McKee, A. C., R. C. Cantu, C. J. Nowinski, E. T. Hedley-Whyte, B. E. Gavett, A. E. Budson, V. E. Santini, H. S. Lee, C. A. Kubilus, and R. A. Stern. 2009. Chronic traumatic encephalopathy in athletes: Progressive tauopathy after repetitive head injury. *Journal of Neuropathology and Experimental Neurology* 68(7):709-735.

McKee, A. C., B. E. Gavett, R. A. Stern, C. J. Nowinski, R. C. Cantu, N. W. Kowall, D. P. Perl, E. T. Hedley-Whyte, B. Price, C. Sullivan, P. Morin, H. S. Lee, C. A. Kubilus, D. H. Daneshvar, M. Wulff, and A. E. Budson. 2010. TDP-43 proteinopathy and motor neuron disease in chronic traumatic encephalopathy. *Journal of Neuropathology and Experimental Neurology* 69(9):918-929.

McLay, R. N., W. P. Klam, and S. L. Volkert. 2010. Insomnia is the most commonly reported symptom and predicts other symptoms of post-traumatic stress disorder in US service members returning from military deployments. *Military Medicine* 175(10):759-762.

Mellman, T. A., R. Kulick-Bell, L. E. Ashlock, and B. Nolan. 1995. Sleep events among veterans with combat-related posttraumatic stress disorder. *American Journal of Psychiatry* 152(1):110-115.

Mellman, T. A., B. Nolan, J. Hebding, R. Kulick-Bell, and R. Dominguez. 1997. A polysomnographic comparison of veterans with combat-related PTSD, depressed men, and non-ill controls. *Sleep* 20(1):46-51.

MHAT-II. 2005. *Mental Health Advisory Team (MHAT-II): Operation lraqi Freedom (01F-11)* Washington, DC: Office of the Surgeon General, United States Army Medical Command, Office of the Surgeon Multinational Force-Iraq.

MHAT-III. 2006. *Mental Health Advisory Team (MHAT III): Operation Iraqi Freedom 04-06.* Washington, DC: Office of The Surgeon General, United States Army Medical Command, Office of the Surgeon Multinational Force-Iraq.

MHAT-IV. 2006. *Mental Health Advisory Team (MHAT IV): Operation Iraqi Freedom 05-07 Final Report.* Washington, DC: Office of the Surgeon General, United States Army Medical Command, Office of the Surgeon Multinational Force-Iraq.

MHAT-V. 2008. *Mental Health Advisory Team (MHAT-V) Operation Iraqi Freedom 06-08: Iraq; Operation Enduring Freedom 8: Afghanistan.* Washington, DC: Office of the Surgeon General, United States Army Medical Command, Office of the Surgeon Multinational Force-Iraq.

MHAT-VI. 2009. *Operation Iraqi Freedom 07-09. Mental Health Advisory Team (MHAT-VI).* Washington, DC: Office of The Surgeon General, US Army Medical Command, Office of the Surgeon Multinational Force-Iraq.

MHAT-VII. 2011. *Joint Mental Health Advisory Team 7 (J-MHAT 7) Operation Enduring Freedom 2010.* Washington, DC: Office of the Surgeon General, United States Army Medical Command, Office of the Command Surgeon HQ, USCENTCOM, Office of the Command Surgeon U.S. Forces Afghanistan.

Mickeviciene, D., H. Schrader, K. Nestvold, D. Surkiene, R. Kunickas, L. J. Stovner, and T. Sand. 2002. A controlled historical cohort study on the post-concussion syndrome. *European Journal of Neurology* 9(6):581-587.

Mickeviciene, D., H. Schrader, D. Obelieniene, D. Surkiene, R. Kunickas, L. J. Stovner, and T. Sand. 2004. A controlled prospective inception cohort study on the post-concussion syndrome outside the medicolegal context. *European Journal of Neurology* 11(6):411-419.

Milliken, C. S., J. L. Auchterlonie, and C. W. Hoge. 2007. Longitudinal assessment of mental health problems among active and reserve component soldiers returning from the Iraq war. *Journal of the American Medical Association* 298(18):2141-2148.

Monson, C. M., C. T. Taft, and S. J. Fredman. 2009. Military-related PTSD and intimate relationships: From description to theory-driven research and intervention development. *Clinical Psychology Review* 29(8):707-714.

Murdoch, M., J. B. Pryor, M. A. Polusny, and G. D. Gackstetter. 2007. Functioning and psychiatric symptoms among military men and women exposed to sexual stressors. *Military Medicine* 172(7):718-725.

Nash, D. L., J. Wilkinson, B. Paradis, S. Kelley, A. Naseem, and K. M. Grant. 2011. Trauma and substance use disorders in rural and urban veterans. *Journal of Rural Health* 27(2):151-158.

Nazarian, D., R. Kimerling, and S. M. Frayne. 2012. Posttraumatic stress disorder, substance use disorders, and medical comorbidity among returning US veterans. *Journal of Traumatic Stress* 25(2):220-225.

Neylan, T. C., C. R. Marmar, T. J. Metzler, D. S. Weiss, D. F. Zatzick, K. L. Delucchi, R. M. Wu, and F. B. Schoenfeld. 1998. Sleep disturbances in the Vietnam generation: Findings from a nationally representative sample of male Vietnam veterans. *American Journal of Psychiatry* 155(7):929-933.

North, C. S., S. J. Nixon, S. Shariat, S. Mallonee, J. C. McMillen, E. L. Spitznagel, and E. M. Smith. 1999. Psychiatric disorders among survivors of the Oklahoma City bombing. *Journal of the American Medical Association* 282(8):755-762.

Nunnink, S. E., G. Goldwaser, N. Afari, C. M. Nievergelt, and D. G. Baker. 2010. The role of emotional numbing in sexual functioning among veterans of the Iraq and Afghanistan wars. *Military Medicine* 175(6):424-428.

Oddy, M., M. Humphrey, and D. Uttley. 1978. Subjective impairment and social recovery after closed head injury. *Journal of Neurology, Neurosurgery, and Psychiatry* 41(7):611-616.

Office of National Drug Control Policy. 2010. Study shows increased misuse of prescription drugs in military. *ONDCP Update* 1(2):1-4.

Office of the Army Surgeon General. 2010. *Pain Management Task Force: Final Report.* Washington, DC: Department of Defense.

Omalu, B. I., S. T. DeKosky, R. L. Minster, M. I. Kamboh, R. L. Hamilton, and C. H. Wecht. 2005. Chronic traumatic encephalopathy in a National Football League player. *Neurosurgery* 57(1):128-134.

Omalu, B. I., S. T. DeKosky, R. L. Hamilton, R. L. Minster, M. I. Kamboh, A. M. Shakir, and C. H. Wecht. 2006. Chronic traumatic encephalopathy in a National Football League player: Part II. *Neurosurgery* 59(5):1086-1092.

Omalu, B. I., J. Bailes, J. L. Hammers, and R. P. Fitzsimmons. 2010. Chronic traumatic encephalopathy, suicides and parasuicides in professional american athletes: The role of the forensic pathologist. *American Journal of Forensic Medicine and Pathology* 31(2):130-132.

Omalu, B., J. Bailes, R. L. Hamilton, M. I. Kamboh, J. Hammers, M. Case, and R. Fitzsimmons. 2011a. Emerging histomorphologic phenotypes of chronic traumatic encephalopathy in American athletes. *Neurosurgery* 69(1):173-183.

Omalu, B., J. L. Hammers, J. Bailes, R. L. Hamilton, M. I. Kamboh, G. Webster, and R. P. Fitzsimmons. 2011b. Chronic traumatic encephalopathy in an Iraqi war veteran with posttraumatic stress disorder who committed suicide. *Neurosurgical Focus* 31(5):E3.

Op den Velde, W., J. E. Hovens, P. G. Aarts, E. Frey-Wouters, P. R. Falger, H. Van Duijn, and J. H. De Groen. 1996. Prevalence and course of posttraumatic stress disorder in dutch veterans of the civilian resistance during World War II: An overview. *Psychological Reports* 78(2):519-529.

Otis, J. D., K. Gregor, C. Hardway, J. Morrison, E. Scioli, and K. Sanderson. 2010. An examination of the co-morbidity between chronic pain and posttraumatic stress disorder on US veterans. *Psychological Services* 7(3):126-135.

O'Toole, B. I., R. P. Marshall, R. J. Schureck, and M. Dobson. 1998. Posttraumatic stress disorder and comorbidity in Australian Vietnam veterans: Risk factors, chronicity and combat. *Australian and New Zealand Journal of Psychiatry* 32(1):32-42.

Ouimette, P. C., J. Wolfe, and K. R. Chrestman. 1996. Characteristics of posttraumatic stress disorder-alcohol abuse comorbidity in women. *Journal of Substance Abuse* 8(3):335-346.

Ouimette, P., R. Cronkite, B. R. Henson, A. Prins, K. Gima, and R. H. Moos. 2004. Posttraumatic stress disorder and health status among female and male medical patients. *Journal of Traumatic Stress* 17(1):1-9

Palatini, P., and S. Julius. 1997. Heart rate and the cardiovascular risk. *Journal of Hypertension* 15(1):3-17.

Peterson, A. L., V. Wong, M. F. Haynes, A. C. Bush, and J. E. Schillerstrom. 2010. Documented combat-related mental health problems in military noncombatants. *Journal of Traumatic Stress* 23(6):674-681.

Phillips, C. J., C. A. Leardmann, G. R. Gumbs, and B. Smith. 2010. Risk factors for posttraumatic stress disorder among deployed US male Marines. *BMC Psychiatry* 10:52.

Picchioni, D., O. A. Cabrera, D. McGurk, J. L. Thomas, C. A. Castro, T. J. Balkin, P. D. Bliese, and C. W. Hoge. 2010. Sleep symptoms as a partial mediator between combat stressors and other mental health symptoms in Iraq war veterans. *Military Psychology* 22(3):340-355.

Pietrzak, R. H., M. B. Goldstein, J. C. Malley, D. C. Johnson, and S. M. Southwick. 2009a. Subsyndromal posttraumatic stress disorder is associated with health and psychosocial difficulties in veterans of Operations Enduring Freedom and Iraqi Freedom. *Depression and Anxiety* 26(8):739-744.

Pietrzak, R. H., D. C. Johnson, M. B. Goldstein, J. C. Malley, A. J. Rivers, C. A. Morgan, and S. M. Southwick. 2009b. Psychosocial buffers of traumatic stress, depressive symptoms, and psychosocial difficulties in veterans of Operations Enduring Freedom and Iraqi Freedom: The role of resilience, unit support, and postdeployment social support. *Journal of Affective Disorders* 120(1-3).

Pietrzak, R. H., D. C. Johnson, M. B. Goldstein, J. C. Malley, and S. M. Southwick. 2009c. Psychological resilience and postdeployment social support protect against traumatic stress and depressive symptoms in soldiers returning from Operations Enduring Freedom and Iraqi Freedom. *Depression and Anxiety* 26(8):745-751.

Pietrzak, R. H., M. B. Goldstein, J. C. Malley, A. J. Rivers, D. C. Johnson, and S. M. Southwick. 2010. Risk and protective factors associated with suicidal ideation in veterans of Operations Enduring Freedom and Iraqi Freedom. *Journal of Affective Disorders* 123(1-3):102-107.

Pietrzak, R. H., A. R. Russo, Q. Ling, and S. M. Southwick. 2011a. Suicidal ideation in treatment-seeking veterans of Operations Enduring Freedom and Iraqi Freedom: The role of coping strategies, resilience, and social support. *Journal of Psychiatric Research* 45(6):720-726.

Pietrzak, R. H., J. M. Whealin, R. L. Stotzer, M. B. Goldstein, and S. M. Southwick. 2011b. An examination of the relation between combat experiences and combat-related posttraumatic stress disorder in a sample of connecticut OEF-OIF veterans. *Journal of Psychiatric Research* 45(12):1579-1584.

Pietrzak, R. H., R. B. Goldstein, S. M. Southwick, and B. F. Grant. 2012. Psychiatric comorbidity of full and partial posttraumatic stress disorder among older adults in the United States: Results from wave 2 of the National Epidemiologic Survey on alcohol and related conditions. *American Journal of Geriatric Psychiatry* 20(5):380-390.

Pittman, J. O., A. A. Goldsmith, J. A. Lemmer, M. T. Kilmer, and D. G. Baker. 2012. Post-traumatic stress disorder, depression, and health-related quality of life in OEF/OIF veterans. *Quality of Life Research: An International Journal of Quality of Life Aspects of Treatment, Care and Rehabilitation* 21(1):99-103.

Polusny, M. A., S. M. Kehle, N. W. Nelson, C. R. Erbes, P. A. Arbisi, and P. Thuras. 2011. Longitudinal effects of mild traumatic brain injury and posttraumatic stress disorder comorbidity on postdeployment outcomes in National Guard soldiers deployed to Iraq. *Archives of General Psychiatry* 68(1):79-89.

Port, C. L., B. Engdahl, and P. Frazier. 2001. A longitudinal and retrospective study of PTSD among older prisoners of war. *American Journal of Psychiatry* 158(9):1474-1479.

Porter, M. D. 2003. A 9-year controlled prospective neuropsychologic assessment of amateur boxing. *Clinical Journal of Sport Medicine* 13(6):339-352.

Porter, M. D., and P. A. Fricker. 1996. Controlled prospective neuropsychological assessment of active experienced amateur boxers. *Clinical Journal of Sport Medicine* 6(2):90-96.

Possemato, K., M. Wade, J. Andersen, and P. Ouimette. 2010. The impact of PTSD, depression, and substance use disorders on disease burden and health care utilization among OEF/OIF veterans. *Psychological Trauma: Theory, Research, Practice, and Policy* 2(3):218-223.

Ramchand, R., T. L. Schell, B. R. Karney, K. C. Osilla, R. M. Burns, and L. B. Caldarone. 2010. Disparate prevalence estimates of PTSD among service members who served in Iraq and Afghanistan: Possible explanations. *Journal of Traumatic Stress* 23(1):59-68.

Ramchand, R., J. Acosta, R. M. Burns, L. H. Jaycox, and C. G. Pernin. 2011. *The War Within: Preventing Suicide in the US Military.* Santa Monica, CA: RAND Corporation.

Ratcliff, J. J., A. I. Greenspan, F. C. Goldstein, A. Y. Stringer, T. Bushnik, F. M. Hammond, T. A. Novack, J. Whyte, and D. W. Wright. 2007. Gender and traumatic brain injury: Do the sexes fare differently? *Brain Injury* 21(10):1023-1030.

Rauch, S. A., T. Favorite, N. Giardino, C. Porcari, E. Defever, and I. Liberzon. 2010. Relationship between anxiety, depression, and health satisfaction among veterans with PTSD. *Journal of Affective Disorders* 121(1-2):165-168.

Raymont, V., A. Greathouse, K. Reding, R. Lipsky, A. Salazar, and J. Grafman. 2008. Demographic, structural and genetic predictors of late cognitive decline after penetrating head injury. *Brain* 131(Pt 2):543-558.

Reeves, D. L., K. Winter, S. LaCour, K. Raynsford, G. Kay, and T. Elsmore. 1992. *Automated Neuropsychological Assessment Metrics Documentation: Vol. I. Test Administration Guide*. Silver Spring, MD: Office of Military Performance Assessment Technology.

Reger, M. A., G. A. Gahm, R. D. Swanson, and S. J. Duma. 2009. Association between number of deployments to Iraq and mental health screening outcomes in US Army soldiers. *Journal of Clinical Psychiatry* 70(9):1266-1275.

Richardson, L. K., B. C. Frueh, and R. Acierno. 2010. Prevalence estimates of combat-related post-traumatic stress disorder: Critical review. *Australian and New Zealand Journal of Psychiatry* 44(1):4-19.

Riviere, L. A., A. Kendall-Robbins, D. McGurk, C. A. Castro, and C. W. Hoge. 2011. Coming home may hurt: Risk factors for mental ill health in US reservists after deployment in Iraq. *British Journal of Psychiatry* 198:136-142.

Roebuck-Spencer, T. M., A. S. Vincent, D. A. Twillie, B. W. Logan, C. M. Lopez, C. K. Friedl, S. J. Grate, R. E. Schlegel, and K. Gilliland. 2012. Cognitive change associated with self-reported mild traumatic brain injury sustained during the OEF/OIF conflicts. *Clinical Neuropsychologist* 26(3):473-489.

Rosen, G. M., R. L. Spitzer, and P. R. McHugh. 2008. Problems with the post-traumatic stress disorder diagnosis and its future in *DSM-V*. *British Journal of Psychiatry* 192(1):3-4.

Rosenheck, R., and A. Fontana. 1994. A model of homelessness among male veterans of the Vietnam war generation. *American Journal of Psychiatry* 151(3):421-427.

Rundell, J. R. 2006. Demographics of and diagnoses in Operation Enduring Freedom and Operation Iraqi Freedom personnel who were psychiatrically evacuated from the theater of operations. *General Hospital Psychiatry* 28(4):352-356.

Ruzich, M. J., J. C. Looi, and M. D. Robertson. 2005. Delayed onset of posttraumatic stress disorder among male combat veterans: A case series. *American Journal of Geriatric Psychiatry* 13(5):424-427.

Salazar, A. M., J. Grafman, S. Schlesselman, S. C. Vance, J. P. Mohr, M. Carpenter, P. Pevsner, C. Ludlow, and H. Weingartner. 1986. Penetrating war injuries of the basal forebrain: Neurology and cognition. *Neurology* 36(4):459-465.

SAMHSA (Substance Abuse and Mental Health Services Administration). 2011. *Results from the 2010 National Survey on Drug Use and Health: Summary of National Findings.* Rockville, MD: Substance Abuse and Mental Health Services Administration.

Samuelson, K. W., T. C. Neylan, T. J. Metzler, M. Lenoci, J. Rothlind, C. Henn-Haase, G. Choucroun, M. W. Weiner, and C. R. Marmar. 2006. Neuropsychological functioning in posttraumatic stress disorder and alcohol abuse. *Neuropsychology* 20(6):716-726.

Sandweiss, D., D. Slymen, C. LeardMann, B. Smith, M. White, E. Boyko, T. Hooper, G. Gackstetter, P. Amoroso, and T. Smith. 2011. Preinjury psychiatric status, injury severity, and postdeployment posttraumatic stress disorder. *Archives of General Psychiatry* 68(5):496-504.

Saulle, M., and B. D. Greenwald. 2012. Chronic traumatic encephalopathy: A review. *Rehabilitation Research and Practice* 1-9.

Savoca, E., and R. Rosenheck. 2000. The civilian labor market experiences of Vietnam-era veterans: The influence of psychiatric disorders. *Journal of Mental Health Policy and Economics* 3(4):199-207.

Schneiderman, A. I., E. R. Braver, and H. K. Kang. 2008. Underdstanding sequelae of injury mechanisms and mild traumatic brain injury incurred during the conflicts in Iraq and Afghanistan: Persistent postconcussive symptoms and posttraumatic stress disorder. *American Journal of Epidemiology* 167(12):1446-1452.

Schnurr, P. P., and C. A. Lunney. 2008. Exploration of gender differences in how quality of life relates to posttraumatic stress disorder in male and female veterans. *Journal of Rehabilitation Research and Development* 45(3):383-393.

Schnurr, P. P., A. Spiro, 3rd, and A. H. Paris. 2000. Physician-diagnosed medical disorders in relation to PTSD symptoms in older male military veterans. *Health Psychology* 19(1):91-97.

Schwab, K., J. Grafman, A. M. Salazar, and J. Kraft. 1993. Residual impairments and work status 15 years after penetrating head injury: Report from the Vietnam Head Injury study. *Neurology* 43(1):95-103.

Seal, K. H., D. Bertenthal, S. Maguen, K. Gima, A. Chu, and C. R. Marmar. 2008. Getting beyond "Don't Ask; Don't Tell": An evaluation of US Veterans Administration postdeployment mental health screening of veterans returning from Iraq and Afghanistan. *American Journal of Public Health* 98(4):714-720.

Seal, K. H., T. J. Metzler, K. S. Gima, D. Bertenthal, S. Maguen, and C. R. Marmar. 2009. Trends and risk factors for mental health diagnoses among Iraq and Afghanistan veterans using Department of Veterans Affairs health care, 2002-2008. *American Journal of Public Health* 99(9):1651-1658.

Seal, K. H., G. Cohen, A. Waldrop, B. E. Cohen, S. Maguen, and L. Ren. 2011. Substance use disorders in Iraq and Afghanistan veterans in VA healthcare, 2001-2010: Implications for screening, diagnosis and treatment. *Drug and Alcohol Dependence* 116(1-3):93-101.

Seal, K. H., Y. Shi, G. Cohen, B. E. Cohen, S. Maguen, E. E. Krebs, and T. C. Neylan. 2012. Association of mental health disorders with prescription opioids and high-risk opioid use in US veterans of Iraq and Afghanistan. *Journal of the American Medical Association* 307(9):940-947.

Shea, M. T., A. A. Vujanovic, A. K. Mansfield, E. Sevin, and F. Liu. 2010. Posttraumatic stress disorder symptoms and functional impairment among OEF and OIF National Guard and reserve veterans. *Journal of Traumatic Stress* 23(1):100-107.

Shen, Y., and J. Arkes. 2009. *Effects of OEF/OIF Deployment Intensity on PTSD Diagnoses Among Still Active Population: Analysis of Enlisted and Officer Populations 2001-2006.* Monterey, CA: Naval Postgraduate School.

Shen, Y.-C., J. Arkes, B. W. Kwan, L. Y. Tan, and T. V. Williams. 2010. Effects of Iraq/Afghanistan deployments on PTSD diagnoses for still active personnel in all four services. *Military Medicine* 175(10):763-769.

Shen, Y. C., J. Arkes, and T. V. Williams. 2012. Effects of Iraq/Afghanistan deployments on major depression and substance use disorder: Analysis of active duty personnel in the US military. *American Journal of Public Health* 102(1 Suppl):S80-S87.

Shipherd, J. C., J. Stafford, and L. R. Tanner. 2005. Predicting alcohol and drug abuse in Persian Gulf War veterans: What role do PTSD symptoms play? *Addictive Behaviors* 30(3):595-599.

Shipherd, J. C., S. L. Pineles, J. L. Gradus, and P. A. Resick. 2009. Sexual harassment in the marines, posttraumatic stress symptoms, and perceived health: Evidence for sex differences. *Journal of Traumatic Stress* 22(1):3-10.

Shively, S., A. I. Scher, D. P. Perl, and R. Diaz-Arrastia. 2012. Dementia resulting from traumatic brain injury: What is the pathology? *Archives of Neurology* 69(10):1245-1251.

Silver, J. M., T. W. McAllister, and S. C. Yudofsky. 2011. *Textbook of Traumatic Brain Injury*. 2nd ed. Arlington, VA: American Psychiatric Publishing, Inc.

Skopp, N. A., M. A. Reger, G. M. Reger, M. C. Mishkind, M. Raskind, and G. A. Gahm. 2011. The role of intimate relationships, appraisals of military service, and gender on the development of posttraumatic stress symptoms following Iraq deployment. *Journal of Traumatic Stress* 24(3):277-286.

Skopp, N. A., L. Troimovich, Col. J. Grimes, L. Oetjen-Gerdes, and G. A. Gahm. 2012. Relations between suicide and traumatic brain injury, psychiatric diagnoses, and relationship problems, active component, US Armed Forces, 2001-2009. *Medical Surveillance Monthly Report* 19(2):7-11.

Slewa-Younan, S., S. van den Berg, I. J. Baguley, M. Nott, and I. D. Cameron. 2008. Towards an understanding of sex differences in functional outcome following moderate to severe traumatic brain injury: A systematic review. *Journal of Neurology, Neurosurgery, and Psychiatry* 79(11):1197-1201.

Smith, M. W., P. P. Schnurr, and R. A. Rosenheck. 2005. Employment outcomes and PTSD symptom severity. *Mental Health Services Research* 7(2):89-101.

Smith, T. C., M. A. Ryan, D. L. Wingard, D. J. Slymen, J. F. Sallis, and D. Kritz-Silverstein. 2008. New onset and persistent symptoms of posttraumatic stress disorder self reported after deployment and combat exposures: Prospective population based US military cohort study. *British Medical Journal* 336(7640):366-371.

Snarr, J. D., R. E. Heyman, and A. M. Smith Slep. 2010. Recent suicidal ideation and suicide attempts in a large-scale survey of the US Air Force: Prevalences and demographic risk factors. *Suicide and Life-Threatening Behavior* 40(6):544-552.

Spera, C., R. K. Thomas, F. Barlas, R. Szoc, and M. H. Cambridge. 2011. Relationship of military deployment recency, frequency, duration, and combat exposure to alcohol use in the Air Force. *Journal of Studies on Alcohol and Drugs* 72(1):5-14.

Spiro, A., 3rd, C. S. Hankin, D. Mansell, and L. E. Kazis. 2006. Posttraumatic stress disorder and health status: The veterans health study. *Journal of Ambulatory Care Management* 29(1):71-86.

Stahre, M. A., R. D. Brewer, V. P. Fonseca, and T. S. Naimi. 2009. Binge drinking among US active-duty military personnel. *American Journal of Preventive Medicine* 36(3):208-217.

Stecker, T., J. Fortney, R. Owen, M. P. McGovern, and S. Williams. 2010. Co-occurring medical, psychiatric, and alcohol-related disorders among veterans returning from Iraq and Afghanistan. *Psychosomatics: Journal of Consultation Liaison Psychiatry* 51(6):503-507.

Stein, M. B., and T. W. McAllister. 2009. Exploring the convergence of posttraumatic stress disorder and mild traumatic brain injury. *The American Journal of Psychiatry* 166(7):768-776.

Stern, R. A., D. O. Riley, D. H. Daneshvar, C. J. Nowinski, R. C. Cantu, and A. C. McKee. 2011. Long-term consequences of repetitive brain trauma: Chronic traumatic encephalopathy. *PM&R: The Journal of Injury, Function, and Rehabilitation* 3(10 Suppl 2):S460-S467.

Street, A. E., J. Stafford, C. M. Mahan, and A. Hendricks. 2008. Sexual harassment and assault experienced by reservists during military service: Prevalence and health correlates. *Journal of Rehabilitation Research and Development* 45(3):409-419.

Street, A. E., D. Vogt, and L. Dutra. 2009. A new generation of women veterans: Stressors faced by women deployed to Iraq and Afghanistan. *Clinical Psychology Review* 29(8):685-694.

Stulemeijer, M., S. P. van der Werf, B. Jacobs, J. Biert, A. B. van Vugt, J. M. Brauer, and P. E. Vos. 2006. Impact of additional extracranial injuries on outcome after mild traumatic brain injury. *Journal of Neurotrauma* 23(10):1561-1569.

Summerall, E. L. 2012. *Traumatic Brain Injury and PTSD.* http://www.ptsd.va.gov/professional/pages/traumatic-brain-injury-ptsd.asp (accessed September 11, 2012).

Suris, A., and L. Lind. 2008. Military sexual trauma: A review of prevalence and associated health consequences in veterans. *Trauma, Violence, and Abuse* 9(4):250-269.

Suris, A., L. Lind, T. M. Kashner, P. D. Borman, and F. Petty. 2004. Sexual assault in women veterans: An examination of PTSD risk, health care utilization, and cost of care. *Psychosomatic Medicine* 66(5):749-756.

Suris, A., L. Lind, T. M. Kashner, and P. D. Borman. 2007. Mental health, quality of life, and health functioning in women veterans: Differential outcomes associated with military and civilian sexual assault. *Journal of Interpersonal Violence* 22(2):179-197.

Taft, C. T., R. P. Weatherill, H. E. Woodward, L. A. Pinto, L. E. Watkins, M. W. Miller, and R. Dekel. 2009. Intimate partner and general aggression perpetration among combat veterans presenting to a posttraumatic stress disorder clinic. *American Journal of Orthopsychiatry* 79(4):461-468.

Tanielian, T., and L. H. Jaycox. 2008. *Invisible Wounds of War: Psychological and Cognitive Injuries, Their Consequences, and Services to Assist Recovery*. Santa Monica, CA: RAND Corporation.

Teasdale, G., and B. Jennett. 1974. Assessment of coma and impaired consciousness. A practical scale. *Lancet* 2(7872):81-84.

Teasdale, T. W., and A. W. Engberg. 2001. Suicide after traumatic brain injury: A population study. *Journal of Neurology, Neurosurgery, and Psychiatry* 71(4):436-440.

Terrio, H., L. A. Brenner, B. J. Ivins, J. M. Cho, K. Helmick, K. Schwab, K. Scally, R. Bretthauer, and D. Warden. 2009. Traumatic brain injury screening: Preliminary findings in a US Army brigade combat team. *Journal of Head Trauma Rehabilitation* 24(1):14-23.

Teten, A. L., J. A. Schumacher, S. D. Bailey, and T. A. Kent. 2009. Male-to-female sexual aggression among Iraq, Afghanistan, and Vietnam veterans: Co-occurring substance abuse and intimate partner aggression. *Journal of Traumatic Stress*.

Teten, A. L., J. A. Schumacher, C. T. Taft, M. A. Stanley, T. A. Kent, S. D. Bailey, N. J. Dunn, and D. L. White. 2010. Intimate partner aggression perpetrated and sustained by male Afghanistan, Iraq, and Vietnam veterans with and without posttraumatic stress disorder. *Journal of Interpersonal Violence* 25(9):1612-1630.

Teuber, H. L., and S. Weinstein. 1954. Performance on a formboard-task after penetrating brain injury. *Journal of Psychology* 38:177-190.

Thomas, J. L., J. E. Wilk, L. A. Riviere, D. McGurk, C. A. Castro, and C. W. Hoge. 2010. Prevalence of mental health problems and functional impairment among active component and National Guard soldiers 3 and 12 months following combat in Iraq. *Archives of General Psychiatry* 67(6):614-623.

Tolin, D. F., and E. B. Foa. 2006. Sex differences in trauma and posttraumatic stress disorder: A quantitative review of 25 years of research. *Psychological Bulletin* 132(6):959-992.

Trief, P. M., P. Ouimette, M. Wade, P. Shanahan, and R. S. Weinstock. 2006. Post-traumatic stress disorder and diabetes: Co-morbidity and outcomes in a male veterans sample. *Journal of Behavioral Medicine* 29(5):411-418.

Trofimovich, L., N. A. Skopp, D. D. Luxton, and M. A. Reger. 2012. Health care experiences prior to suicide and self-inflicted injury, active component, US Armed Forces, 2001-2010. *Medical Surveillance Monthly Report* 19(2):2-6.

Uddo, M., J. J. Vasterling, K. Brailey, and P. B. Sutker. 1993. Memory and attention in combat-related post-traumatic stress disorder (PTSD). *Journal of Psychopathology and Behavioral Assessment* 15(1):43-52.

VA (Department of Veterans Affairs). 2012. *Analysis of VA Health Care Utilization Among Operation Enduring Freedom (OEF), Operation Iraqi Freedom (OIF), and Operation New Dawn (OND) Veterans: Cumulative from 1st QTR FY 2002 through 3rd QTR FY 2012 (October 1, 2001–June 30, 2012)*. Washington, DC: Department of Veterans Affairs.

VA and DOD. 2009. *VA/DOD Clinical Practice Guidelines for Management of Concussion/Mild Traumatic Brain Injury (mTBI)*. Washington, DC: Department of Veterans Affairs, Department of Defense.

Vanderploeg, R. D., G. Curtiss, C. A. Luis, and A. M. Salazar. 2007. Long-term morbidities following self-reported mild traumatic brain injury. *Journal of Clinical and Experimental Neuropsychology* 29(6):585-598.

Vassallo, J. L., Z. Proctor-Weber, B. K. Lebowitz, G. Curtiss, and R. D. Vanderploeg. 2007. Psychiatric risk factors for traumatic brain injury. *Brain Injury* 21(6):567-573.

Vasterling, J. J., and S. Dikmen. 2012. Mild traumatic brain injury and posttraumatic stress disorder: Clinical and conceptual complexities. *Journal of the International Neuropsychological Society* 18(3):390-393.

Vasterling, J. J., K. Brailey, J. I. Constans, and P. B. Sutker. 1998. Attention and memory dysfunction in posttraumatic stress disorder. *Neuropsychology* 12(1):125-133.

Vasterling, J. J., C. Rogers, and E. Kaplan. 2000. Qualitative block design analysis in posttraumatic stress disorder. *Assessment* 7(3):217-226.

Vasterling, J. J., L. M. Duke, K. Brailey, J. I. Constans, A. N. Allain, Jr., and P. B. Sutker. 2002. Attention, learning, and memory performances and intellectual resources in Vietnam veterans: PTSD and no disorder comparisons. *Neuropsychology* 16(1):5-14.

Vasterling, J. J., M. Verfaellie, and K. D. Sullivan. 2009. Mild traumatic brain injury and posttraumatic stress disorder in returning veterans: Perspectives from cognitive neuroscience. *Clinical Psychology Review* 29(8):674-684.

Vasterling, J. J., S. P. Proctor, M. J. Friedman, C. W. Hoge, T. Heeren, L. A. King, and D. W. King. 2010. PTSD symptom increases in Iraq-deployed soldiers: Comparison with nondeployed soldiers and associations with baseline symptoms, deployment experiences, and postdeployment stress. *Journal of Traumatic Stress* 23(1):41-51.

Vasterling, J. J., K. Brailey, S. P. Proctor, R. Kane, T. Heeren, and M. Franz. 2012. Neuropsychological outcomes of mild traumatic brain injury, post-traumatic stress disorder and depression in Iraq-deployed US Army soldiers. *British Journal of Psychiatry* 201(3):186-192.

Vogt, D., R. Vaughn, M. E. Glickman, M. Schultz, M. L. Drainoni, R. Elwy, and S. Eisen. 2011. Gender differences in combat-related stressors and their association with postdeployment mental health in a nationally representative sample of US OEF/OIF veterans. *Journal of Abnormal Psychology* 120(4):797-806.

Wagner, T. H., K. M. Harris, B. Federman, L. Dai, Y. Luna, and K. Humphreys. 2007. Prevalence of substance use disorders among veterans and comparable nonveterans from the national survey on drug use and health. *Psychological Services* 4(3):149-157.

Wang, S., and J. Mason. 1999. Elevations of serum T3 levels and their association with symptoms in World War II veterans with combat-related posttraumatic stress disorder: Replication of findings in Vietnam combat veterans. *Psychosomatic Medicine* 61(2):131-138.

Wang, S., J. Mason, S. Southwick, D. Johnson, H. Lubin, and D. Charney. 1995. Relationships between thyroid hormones and symptoms in combat-related posttraumatic stress disorder. *Psychosomatic Medicine* 57(4):398-402.

Wechsler, D. 2009. *Wechsler Memory Scale—Fourth Edition (WMS-IV)*. San Antonio, TX: Pearson.

Weinstein, S., and H. L. Teuber. 1957. Effects of penetrating brain injury on intelligence test scores. *Science* 125(3256):1036-1037.

Wells, T. S., C. A. LeardMann, S. O. Fortuna, B. Smith, T. C. Smith, M. A. K. Ryan, E. J. Boyko, D. Blazer, and T. Millennium Cohort Study. 2010. A prospective study of depression following combat deployment in support of the wars in Iraq and Afghanistan. *American Journal of Public Health* 100(1):90-99.

Widome, R., S. M. Kehle, K. F. Carlson, M. N. Laska, A. Gulden, and K. Lust. 2011. Post-traumatic stress disorder and health risk behaviors among Afghanistan and Iraq war veterans attending college. *American Journal of Health Behavior* 35(4):387-392.

Wilk, J. E., P. D. Bliese, P. Y. Kim, J. L. Thomas, D. McGurk, and C. W. Hoge. 2010a. Relationship of combat experiences to alcohol misuse among US soldiers returning from the Iraq war. *Drug and Alcohol Dependence* 108(1-2):115-121.

Wilk, J. E., J. L. Thomas, D. M. McGurk, L. A. Riviere, C. A. Castro, and C. W. Hoge. 2010b. Mild traumatic brain injury (concussion) during combat: Lack of association of blast mechanism with persistent postconcussive symptoms. *Journal of Head Trauma Rehabilitation* 25(1):9-14.

Wilk, J. E., R. K. Herrell, G. H. Wynn, L. A. Riviere, and C. W. Hoge. 2012. Mild traumatic brain injury (concussion), posttraumatic stress disorder, and depression in US soldiers involved in combat deployments: Association with postdeployment symptoms. *Psychosomatic Medicine* 74(3):249-257.

Wojcik, B. E., F. Z. Akhtar, and L. H. Hassell. 2009. Hospital admissions related to mental disorders in US Army soldiers in Iraq and Afghanistan. *Military Medicine* 174(10):1010-1018.

Wojcik, B. E., C. R. Stein, K. Bagg, R. J. Humphrey, and J. Orosco. 2010. Traumatic brain injury hospitalizations of US Army soldiers deployed to Afghanistan and Iraq. *American Journal of Preventive Medicine* 38(1 Suppl):S108-S116.

Woodhead, C., S. Wessely, N. Jones, N. T. Fear, and S. L. Hatch. 2012. Impact of exposure to combat during deployment to Iraq and Afghanistan on mental health by gender. *Psychological Medicine* 42(9):1985-1996.

Woodward, S. H., M. M. Murburg, and D. L. Bliwise. 2000. PTSD-related hyperarousal assessed during sleep. *Physiology and Behavior* 70(1-2):197-203.

Wright, K. M., T. W. Britt, P. D. Bliese, and A. B. Adler. 2011a. Insomnia severity, combat exposure and mental health outcomes. *Stress and Health: Journal of the International Society for the Investigation of Stress* 27(4):325-333.

Wright, K. M., T. W. Britt, P. D. Bliese, A. B. Adler, D. Picchioni, and D. Moore. 2011b. Insomnia as predictor versus outcome of PTSD and depression among Iraq combat veterans. *Journal of Clinical Psychology* 67(12):1240-1258.

Wu, P. C., C. Lang, N. K. Hasson, S. H. Linder, and D. J. Clark. 2010. Opioid use in young veterans. *Journal of Opioid Management* 6(2):133-139.

Yaffe, K., E. Vittinghoff, K. Lindquist, D. Barnes, K. E. Covinsky, T. Neylan, M. Kluse, and C. Marmar. 2010. Posttraumatic stress disorder and risk of dementia among US veterans. *Archives of General Psychiatry* 67(6):608-613.

Yarvis, J. S., P. S. Bordnick, C. A. Spivey, and D. Pedlar. 2005. Subthreshold PTSD: A comparison of alcohol, depression, and health problems in Canadian peacekeepers with different levels of traumatic stress. *Stress, Trauma, and Crisis* 8(2-3):195-213.

Yehuda, R., R. S. Keefe, P. D. Harvey, R. A. Levengood, D. K. Gerber, J. Geni, and L. J. Siever. 1995. Learning and memory in combat veterans with posttraumatic stress disorder. *American Journal of Psychiatry* 152(1):137-139.

Zalewski, C., W. Thompson, and I. I. Gottesman. 1994. Comparison of neuropsychological test performance in PTSD, generalized anxiety disorder, and control Vietnam veterans. *Assessment* 1(2):133-142.

Zatzick, D. F., C. R. Marmar, D. S. Weiss, W. S. Browner, T. J. Metzler, J. M. Golding, A. Stewart, W. E. Schlenger, and K. B. Wells. 1997a. Posttraumatic stress disorder and functioning and quality of life outcomes in a nationally representative sample of male Vietnam veterans. *American Journal of Psychiatry* 154(12):1690-1695.

Zatzick, D. F., D. S. Weiss, C. R. Marmar, T. J. Metzler, K. Wells, J. M. Golding, A. Stewart, W. E. Schlenger, and W. S. Browner. 1997b. Post-traumatic stress disorder and functioning and quality of life outcomes in female Vietnam veterans. *Military Medicine* 162(10):661-665.

Zatzick, D. F., F. P. Rivara, G. J. Jurkovich, C. W. Hoge, J. Wang, M. Y. Fan, J. Russo, S. G. Trusz, A. Nathens, and E. J. Mackenzie. 2010. Multisite investigation of traumatic brain injuries, posttraumatic stress disorder, and self-reported health and cognitive impairments. *Archives of General Psychiatry* 67(12):1291-1300.

Zinzow, H. M., A. L. Grubaugh, J. Monnier, S. Suffoletta-Maierle, and B. C. Frueh. 2007. Trauma among female veterans: A critical review. *Trauma Violence Abuse* 8(4):384-400.

Zivin, K., H. M. Kim, J. F. McCarthy, K. L. Austin, K. J. Hoggatt, H. Walters, and M. Valenstein. 2007. Suicide mortality among individuals receiving treatment for depression in the Veterans Affairs Health System: Associations with patient and treatment setting characteristics. *American Journal of Public Health* 97(12):2193-2198.

Zouris, J. M., A. L. Wade, and C. P. Magno. 2008. Injury and illness casualty distributions among US Army and Marine Corps personnel during Operation Iraqi Freedom. *Military Medicine* 173(3):247-252.

# 5

# SCREENING, ASSESSMENT, AND TREATMENT

In this chapter, the committee assesses the approaches used in the Department of Defense (DOD) and Department of Veterans Affairs (VA) to identify service members and veterans with neurologic or psychologic health conditions and treat them. The committee reviews health screening and assessment practices and treatment interventions for six conditions that can affect readjustment after military deployment: traumatic brain injury (TBI), posttraumatic stress disorder (PTSD), major depressive disorder (MDD), substance-use disorders (SUDs), suicidal ideation, and comorbid conditions. Their assessment relies on clinical and scientific evidence to examine the efficacy of approaches that DOD and VA use in the management of those conditions.

The committee reviewed the clinical practice guidelines (CPGs) developed jointly by VA and DOD[1] and compared them with clinical guidelines developed by leading scientific and professional organizations. CPGs are statements and recommendations for clinical care that are informed by a systematic review of evidence and an assessment of the benefits and harms of alternative care options (IOM, 2011a). The committee also reviewed the research and policy literature as a basis for discussing standard-of-care recommendations that are presented throughout this chapter.[2]

The committee acknowledges that the presence of clinical guidelines does not ensure that people receive optimal evidence-based care. Poor dissemination practices and other barriers affect the extent to which clinicians use CPGs (Stein et al., 2009). The committee examined the sparse data available to address the question of whether military members and veterans actually *receive* evidence-based interventions offered in the VA and DOD health systems. Our inquiries to VA and DOD did not yield much about results of using clinical performance measures, metrics that are designed for assessing and monitoring clinical processes or patient outcomes.

The committee became aware of a few sources of clinical performance measures relevant to VA's monitoring of mental-health care delivery and discusses this information in each section. For example, the VA Office of Quality and Performance contracts with an external agency to

---

[1]Under the auspices of the VA/DOD Evidence Based Practice-Guidelines Work Group, representatives of VA and DOD serve on committees for developing, updating, and implementing joint CPGs for a number of physical- and mental-health conditions. VA/DOD joint guidelines exist for TBI, PTSD, MDD, and SUD but not for suicidal ideation and comorbid conditions.

[2]The literature review concentrated on new studies since publication of the CPGs and on synthesized analyses of randomized controlled trials.

conduct monthly standardized medical-record reviews of outpatient care as part of the External Peer Review Program and uses the data to monitor according to national performance measures. In addition, much of the data on implementation and monitoring of evidenced-based practices included in this chapter comes from an independent evaluation of the quality of VA mental-health and substance-use care. VA commissioned the RAND Corporation and Altarum Institute to perform the evaluation, which they conducted between 2006 and 2010 (Watkins and Pincus, 2011). The study was authorized by the Government Performance and Results Act of 1993 and Title 38 of the US Code, which require independent evaluations of large government programs. In general, studies have shown that the health care that VA provides for a number of conditions, such as diabetes and heart disease, is on par with or better than care provided in non-VA settings (Jha et al., 2003; Trivedi et al., 2011). However, as discussed in this chapter, VA's performance in mental health is not as strong, given the variation found among service networks and the low rate of delivery of some evidence-based practices (Watkins et al., 2011).

DOD has an extensive centralized Military Health System–wide database for population health management called the Military Health System Population Health Portal.[3] However, clinical performance measures in the dataset do not address mental-health care. In 2010, the Defense Health Board recommended to the assistant secretary of defense for health affairs that "evidence-based metrics for *processes* of mental health care" should be developed and monitored to address questions of mental health care quality and adequacy of clinical capacity/resources (Defense Health Board, 2010). The Defense Health Board added that DOD should evaluate clinician competence in providing evidence-based treatment and patience adherence to treatment.

As VA and DOD continue to advance their efforts to evaluate mental-health care services, they face a number of challenges, such as the lack of validated clinical performance measures that assess the full array of psychologic health services and the lack of appropriate benchmarks that VA and DOD can use to compare their performance. Measurement of clinical performance is not as advanced in mental health as it is in other types of care (Pincus et al., 2011; Watkins et al., 2010). That potentially presents opportunities for VA and DOD to collaborate with each other and with others in the field to advance clinical performance measurement aimed at improving the quality of mental health care and care for brain injury.

## ORGANIZATION OF THE CHAPTER

The chapter is organized in six main sections: TBI, PTSD, MDD, SUDs, suicidal ideation, and comorbid conditions. By structuring the chapter according to each condition, the committee does not mean to suggest that it is always the case that a single diagnosis can account for all symptoms or that a single set of clinical guidelines and evidenced-based treatments will address all symptoms. Many patients, particularly in military settings, present with complex problems that do not fall neatly into single diagnostic categories. *Comorbid*, *co-occurring*, and *dual diagnosis* are terms used to indicate that more than one disorder is occurring in the same person, simultaneously or sequentially, and that associated interactions between the illnesses affect the course and prognosis of each. This chapter uses the terms *comorbid* and *co-occurring*.

---

[3]The Military Health System Population Health Portal contains administrative health care data on TRICARE Prime/Plus enrollees who receive care through military treatment facilities and contracted providers.

Each section presents screening, assessment, and treatment interventions. In this chapter, *screening* refers to a process for identifying people who may be at risk for a specific disease that uses tests (or screening instruments), examinations, or other procedures. Screening instruments are helpful for identifying people who might have a disease but are not very useful for assessing progression, prognosis, or treatment efficacy (IOM, 2006). A person who has positive screening results should be referred for assessment by a medical professional for diagnosis and treatment. *Assessment* refers to a process for defining the nature of a problem, determining a diagnosis, and developing recommendations for addressing the problem or diagnosis (SAMHSA, 2009).

Within the discussion of screening, assessment, and treatment, the chapter describes the VA and DOD clinical guidance and practices used in the management of the selected conditions. The chapter often refers to screening processes achieved in the US military during the deployment cycle—the predeployment health assessment, the Post-Deployment Health Assessment (PDHA), and the Post-Deployment Health Re-Assessment (PDHRA) (Terrio et al., 2011). Predeployment health assessments are administered at home stations or at mobilization processing stations before deployment. The PDHA is conducted 3–10 days after deployment, and the PDHRA 90–180 days after deployment. On return from deployment, service members are required to complete assessment forms that ask about their deployment history and that screen for a number of physical and psychologic conditions, including TBI, PTSD, MDD, SUDs, and suicidal ideation. Health care providers followup with all service members on completion of the forms to make referrals to appropriate health care or community-based services if further evaluation or treatment is needed.

For each health condition, there is a discussion of the evidence underlying the validity of the screening and assessment instruments used by VA and DOD health practitioners. A review of treatment interventions includes a comparison of the VA and DOD recommended practices with recommendations in other relevant CPGs. Finally, we present information available on the extent to which VA and DOD are implementing evidenced-based interventions for screening, assessment, and treatment.

## TRAUMATIC BRAIN INJURY

A TBI is the result of a blow or jolt to the head or a penetrating head injury that disrupts the function of the brain. In 2007, DOD formally defined TBI as a "traumatically induced structural injury or physiological disruption of brain function as a result of an external force" (DCoE, 2012e). Such an injury may range from "mild"—a brief change in mental status or consciousness—to "severe," an extended period of unconsciousness or amnesia after the injury. The terms *concussion* and *mild TBI* are used interchangeably. See Chapter 4 for a full definition of TBI and for details about its prevalence in the military and veteran populations.

Numerous symptoms are associated with mild TBI, including headaches, dizziness, fatigue, inability to concentrate, memory problems, irritability, balance problems, vision change, and sleep disturbance. Most people who sustain a mild TBI usually recover completely with minimal intervention. A TBI classified as moderate or severe can result in short-term or long-term problems with independent function (IOM, 2009). As discussed in Chapter 4, TBIs of all severities, including a small fraction of mild cases, are known to be associated with adverse long-term neurologic outcomes, such as seizures, cognitive dysfunction, and neurodegeneration. The military emphasizes early assessment for TBI on the battlefield in recognition that delayed diagnosis might be detrimental to a service member's health and combat readiness (DOD, 2010b; Helmick, 2011).

To assess the efficacy of current screening and treatment approaches for mild TBI, the committee examined a number of clinical guidelines and DOD and VA policy directives for TBI. This section's emphasis is on mild TBI, inasmuch as such cases are the most common and the most frequently underrecognized and undertreated.

## Department of Defense and Department of Veterans Affairs Guidance for Screening for Mild Traumatic Brain Injury

Detecting mild TBI close to the time of injury is best for preventing symptoms, optimizing care, and improving outcomes; however, mild TBI can be difficult to identify. The rigor of combat operations and lack of observable head trauma may delay assessment. In addition, identifying a head injury often relies on self-reported symptoms, but service members may be reluctant to report symptoms because they do not want to be separated from their unit and wish to avoid any stigma associated with psychologic or psychiatric services. Moreover, the frequent presence of comorbid conditions, such as PTSD, complicates recognition of mild TBI based on symptoms alone.

DOD and VA have system wide screening and assessment procedures in place at multiple points of care to identify mild TBI in service members. A positive screen indicates the need for further evaluation to diagnose a TBI. Diagnosis cannot be made on the basis of a positive screening test alone.

### Department of Defense

In DOD, service members may be screened for TBI in a theater of combat operations, in MTFs, and on return from theater (postdeployment). In addition to screening, DOD requires all service members to undergo a baseline neurocognitive assessment before deployment.

#### *Neurocognitive Testing*

Neurocognitive testing helps to determine the degree of cognitive impairment after head injury. In 2006, a DOD expert panel concluded that neurocognitive assessment is an important part of a TBI evaluation (DVBIC, 2006). In May 2008, DOD issued guidance requiring each service to implement baseline predeployment neurocognitive assessment for service members with the Automated Neuropsychological Assessment Metrics (ANAM) tool (Casscells, 2008a). Developed, tested, and implemented by DOD, the ANAM is a computer-based assessment of cognitive functions likely to be affected by a concussion, including attention, concentration, reaction time, memory, processing speed, and decision making (DVBIC, 2006). The ANAM is not used as a TBI screening tool itself but serves as a baseline with which a post-TBI evaluation can be compared. Service members take the predeployment neurocognitive assessment within 12 months of deployment. Injured service members can be given a second ANAM test in theater, which should be administered 24–72 hours after injury if possible, and the results are compared with the original test scores to look for changes in cognitive function (DCoE, 2011b).

DOD policy does not require that all service members receive a postdeployment neurocognitive assessment, such as one with the ANAM, but recommends that care providers in theater consider postinjury neurocognitive testing as a component of the comprehensive TBI evaluation and return-to-duty assessment (DCoE, 2011b; GAO, 2011).

*Screening in Theater and in Medical Facilities*

During deployment, service members are screened for possible TBI, whether on the basis of self-reported symptoms or an event that occurred. In 2006, the Defense and Veterans Brain Injury Center (DVBIC) recommended screening service members in military operational settings (DVBIC, 2006); in the following year, the Army required screening of service members who were exposed to a blast or other injury event and had associated loss of consciousness, amnesia, or alteration in mental status, however brief (DVBIC, 2007). In June 2010, DOD broadened the screening criteria: all service members exposed to a "mandatory event"—regardless of initial symptoms—are screened for TBI and required to rest for 24 hours (DOD, 2010b). Mandatory events are defined as being in a vehicle associated with a blast, collision, or rollover; being within 50 m of a blast; a direct blow to the head or witnessed loss of consciousness; or command-directed, especially in a case with multiple blast events. The 24-hour rest period is mandatory regardless of the results of TBI screening (DOD, 2010b).

DOD's TBI screening tool, the Military Acute Concussion Evaluation (MACE), is suitable for use in theater and in medical facilities. The DVBIC developed the MACE in conjunction with national experts in sports concussion. The MACE has history and evaluation components. The history component can confirm the diagnosis of mild TBI after it is established that trauma has occurred and that the service member experienced an alteration in consciousness. The evaluation component, designed to be used easily by medics and corpsmen in combat theater, consists of a symptom inventory and a brief assessment of neurocognitive deficits in four domains: orientation, immediate memory, concentration, and delayed recall (DVBIC, 2006, 2008a; French et al., 2008).

The MACE is also used to screen wounded service members who are evaluated in tactical medical units that provide Level III care (resuscitative care, stabilization, and hospitalization), such as the Air Force Theater Hospital in Balad, Iraq, or in definitive care (Level IV) regional medical facilities outside the area of operations, such as the Landstuhl Regional Medical Center in Germany (these two types of facilities have somewhat different procedures for following up a positive screen). Of stateside inpatient MTFs that provide comprehensive care (Level V), only Walter Reed National Military Medical Center was conducting TBI screening since 2007 (DOD, 2010b).

*Postdeployment Screening*

In 2008, DOD started routine screening of Operation Enduring Freedom (OEF) and Operation Iraqi Freedom (OIF) service members for TBI immediately on their return from the combat theater and again 3–6 months after return as part of the required PDHA and PDHRA process (briefly described at the beginning of this chapter). Routine screening was not implemented until 2008, so many service members have never been screened for mild TBI (Iverson et al., 2009).

The TBI screen used in the DOD health assessments is a modified version of the Brief Traumatic Brain Injury Screen (BTBIS) (Schwab et al., 2007), which was validated by further research and adapted for use in the PDHA and PDHRA (Terrio et al., 2011). Returning service members report responses to four screening questions about exposure to an injury event, the later loss of or alterations in consciousness, the presence of symptoms at the time of injury, and the presence of current symptoms (see questions in Box 5.1). A positive response regarding at least one problem in each of the four questions means that the screen is positive. A service member who has a positive screen is referred for a full TBI evaluation (Helmick, 2011).

**BOX 5.1**
**TBI Screening Questions in DOD's PDHA and PDHRA**

**9.a. During this deployment, did you experience any of the following events? (Mark all that apply.)**

1. Blast or explosion (IED, RPG, land mine, grenade, etc.)
2. Vehicular accident/crash (any vehicle, including aircraft)
3. Fragment wound or bullet wound above your shoulders
4. Fall
5. Other event (for example, a sports injury to your head). Describe:

**9.b. Did any of the following happen to you, or were you told happened to you, IMMEDIATELY after any of the event(s) you just noted in question 9.a.? (Mark all that apply.)**

1. Lost consciousness or got "knocked out"
2. Felt dazed, confused, or "saw stars"
3. Didn't remember the event
4. Had a concussion
5. Had a head injury

**9.c. Did any of the following problems begin or get worse after the event(s) you noted in Question 9.a.? (Mark all that apply.)**

1. Memory problems or lapses
2. Balance problems or dizziness
3. Ringing in the ears
4. Sensitivity to bright light
5. Irritability
6. Headaches
7. Sleep problems

**9.d. In the past week, have you had any of the symptoms you indicated in 9.c.? (Mark all that apply.)**

1. Memory problems or lapses
2. Balance problems or dizziness
3. Ringing in the ears
4. Sensitivity to bright light
5. Irritability
6. Headaches
7. Sleep problems

SOURCE: DOD, 2008.

## Department of Veterans Affairs

In April 2007, VA started screening all OEF and OIF veterans who were receiving medical care in the Veterans Health Administration (VHA) for TBI; those who screen positive are offered further evaluation and treatment by clinicians who have expertise in TBI (VA, 2010c; VA and VHA, 2007). VHA's screening tool, the Traumatic Brain Injury Screening Instrument (TBISI), has four questions based on the BTBIS, the tool designed for active-duty military personnel (Carlson et al., 2010); see questions in Box 5.2.

**BOX 5.2**
**TBI Screening Questions in VA's TBISI**

**Section 1: During any of your OEF and OIF deployment(s), did you experience any of the following events? (Check all that apply.)**

1. Blast or explosion
2. Vehicular accident/crash *(including aircraft)*
3. Fragment wound or bullet wound above shoulders
4. Fall

**Section 2: Did you have any of these symptoms IMMEDIATELY afterwards? (Check all that apply.)**

1. Losing consciousness/ "knocked out"
2. Being dazed, confused or "seeing stars"
3. Not remembering the event
4. Concussion
5. Head injury

**Section 3: Did any of the following problems begin or get worse afterwards? (Check all that apply.)**

1. Memory problems or lapses
2. Balance problems or dizziness
3. Sensitivity to bright light
4. Irritability
5. Headaches
6. Sleep problems

**Section 4: In the past week, have you had any of the symptoms from section 3? (Check all that apply.)**

1. Memory problems or lapses
2. Balance problems or dizziness
3. Sensitivity to bright light
4. Irritability
5. Headaches
6. Sleep problems

SOURCE: GAO, 2008.

The screening process for TBI (see Figure 5.1) is executed as part of the VHA automated clinical reminder system used by clinicians at its medical facilities (Carlson et al., 2010). An

OEF or OIF veteran who reports having received a TBI diagnosis at some point is offered a referral; a veteran who reports no prior TBI diagnosis during deployment is asked to answer the four screening questions. The screen is positive if the veteran says yes to any response item in each of the four questions (GAO, 2008). A veteran who had a positive screen is offered a followup evaluation with a specialty provider at a specified medical center. VA clinicians have to document any refusal of specialty care in the veteran's electronic medical record (VA, 2010c).

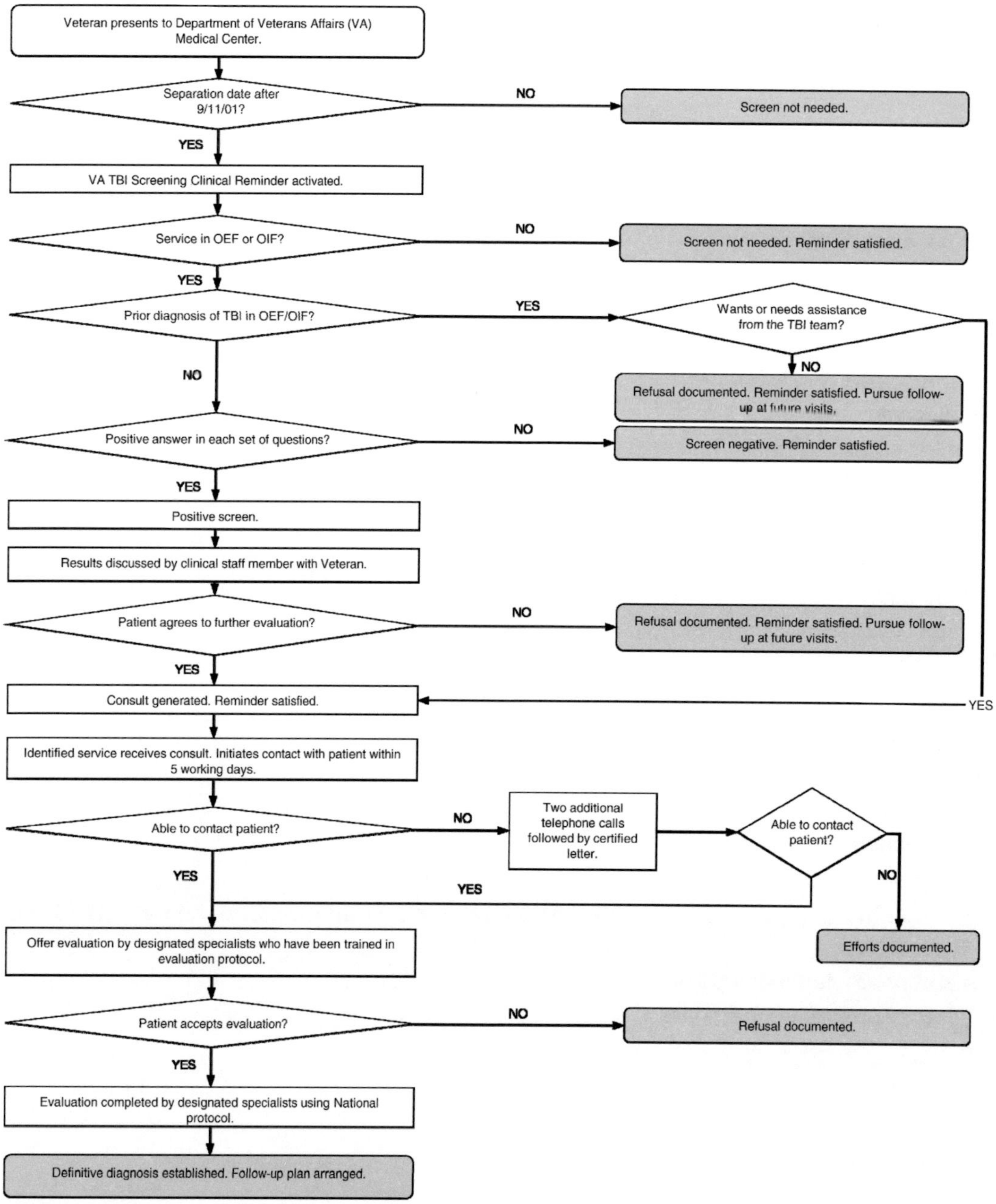


**FIGURE 5.1** Flow chart for VHA screening and evaluation of possible traumatic brain injury in OEF and OIF veterans.
SOURCE: VA, 2010c.

## Validity of Tools for Neurocognitive Assessment and Screening for Mild Traumatic Brain Injury

### Automated Neuropsychological Assessment Metrics

A 2010 comprehensive review of the DOD ANAM program, prepared by the Army's Office of the Surgeon General, states that the lack of clear scientific evidence supporting ANAM's effectiveness raises important questions about whether DOD is using the best available technology to assess cognitive function after head injury (Department of the Army, 2010a). Research data raise questions about the accuracy of the ANAM for detecting cognitive dysfunction—and recovery from this dysfunction—after mild TBI.

In one study, among 956 soldiers returning from Iraq or Afghanistan, a history of self-reported mild TBI or current postconcussive symptoms was not associated with poor ANAM performance (Ivins et al., 2009). In another study, 502 service members recently deployed to Iraq or Afghanistan who had self-reported TBI and predeployment and postdeployment ANAM testing were compared with 400 service members who had no history of TBI. The two groups performed similarly on predeployment testing. Of the entire group that reported TBI during deployment, 70% had no significant change in cognitive performance compared with their baseline ANAM test (Roebuck-Spencer et al., 2012). Research is under way to address questions about the ANAM (see Appendix D). This is an important subject of study because ANAM scores are being used to inform return-to-duty decisions.

### Military Acute Concussion Evaluation

Used both in theater and in medical facilities, the MACE is the most widely used TBI screen in DOD; however, there is some concern that it might fail to detect a large proportion of service members' concussions. Embedded in the MACE is the Standardized Assessment of Concussion (SAC), a brief cognitive screening tool developed to assess the acute effects of sports-related mild TBI. The SAC has demonstrated reliability, validity, sensitivity, and specificity in athletic cohorts (McCrea et al., 2003). The MACE, however, when administered more than 12 hours after injury in a military setting and compared with a clinical diagnosis of concussion, had a sensitivity of only 51% (specificity 64%) when a cutoff score of 27 was used. At the suggested cutoff score of 25, the sensitivity was even less at 20% (specificity 88%) (Coldren et al., 2010). Research is under way to determine the validity of this tool at earlier times and to attempt to improve its accuracy through comparison with predeployment scores (see Appendix D).

### Brief Traumatic Brain Injury Screen

Initial research with the BTBIS postdeployment TBI screen suggested that it was a reasonably accurate screening tool for TBI. In 2007, the BTBIS was administered to 596 soldiers returning from Iraq or Afghanistan and compared with two longer surveys—the Quarterly Survey and the Computerized TBI Questionnaire—that were used to elicit a history of TBI. The BTBIS had a sensitivity of 90% when compared with the Quarterly Survey and 88% when compared with the Computerized TBI Questionnaire. It had a specificity of 88% when compared with the Quarterly Survey and 97% when compared with the Computerized TBI Questionnaire (Schwab et al., 2007).

However, a 2011 study suggested that the false-negative rate of the DOD postdeployment TBI screen—which was adapted from the BTBIS—was high. Its four questions were compared with a brief structured clinical interview for mild TBI in 3,072 soldiers who were returning from a 15-month tour of duty in Iraq. The sensitivity and specificity of the DOD screening tool (positive response to all four items) were 60% and 96%, respectively. The sensitivity increased to 80%, with a slight decrease in specificity to 93%, when affirmative responses only to questions 1 and 2 were included. Thus, omission of the last two questions significantly reduced the false-negative rate from 40% to 20% (Terrio et al., 2011).

### Traumatic Brain Injury Screening Instrument

Research on the accuracy of the TBISI, the screening tool used by VA, is emerging (VA, 2012). The Government Accountability Office (GAO) emphasized the need for empirical evidence on the sensitivity and specificity of the VA TBI screening instrument in a 2008 report (GAO, 2008). A 2010 study revealed that the test–retest reliability of the VHA postdeployment TBI screen was low. In 44 OEF and OIF veterans referred for neuropsychologic evaluation after a positive TBI screen, agreement was low between answers to the original TBI screen and rescreening 6 months later for mechanism of injury and symptoms immediately after injury but high for current symptoms (Van Dyke et al., 2010). A recent psychometric study of the TBISI involving 500 OEF and OIF veterans concluded that the instrument appears to be reliable and valid. The results showed high internal consistency (0.77) and test–retest reliability (0.80), high sensitivity (0.94), and moderate specificity (0.59) (Donnelly et al., 2011).

## Implementation of Department of Defense and Department of Veterans Affairs Guidance for Screening for Mild Traumatic Brain Injury

This section presents information available to the committee on the extent to which DOD and VA are implementing and tracking screening procedures to identify possible TBI. The committee identified various sources of information but notes the lack of readily available centralized sources of data, particularly within DOD, on the numbers of people who are screened and have a positive screen.

### Department of Defense

#### *Neurocognitive Testing*

More than 1 million service members had received neurocognitive tests as of September 30, 2011 (DCoE, 2012a). The ANAM is not Web-enabled, and data are not stored in a centralized database; therefore, summary statistics comparing ANAM scores before and after injury are not available.

#### *Screening in Theater and in Medical Facilities*

Over 9,000 soldiers have been screened for mild TBI in theater since August 2010 (Department of the Army, 2012). An article in the popular press reported that from January to September 2011, nearly 1,400 service members had screened positive in Afghanistan and Iraq as part of the new mandatory evaluation requirements that broadened the screening criteria (Zoroya, 2011). DOD policy requires the documentation of all service members who were exposed to potential concussive events and the development of a medical quality-assurance program and metrics to track implementation of TBI screening procedures (DOD, 2010b). In response, US Central Command developed an automated reporting module called the Blast Exposure and Concussion Incident Report, but data have yet to be publicly released (USMedicine.com, 2012).

An article in *Military Medicine* raised concern about the quality of screening implementation, stating that "there is no standardized training or evaluation of administration competence on the MACE for medical providers in Iraq" (Coldren et al., 2010).

*Postdeployment Screening*

During FY 2009 and 2010, 2% of service members who were returning from tours of duty screened positive for TBI on the PDHA, and 4% on the PDHRA (DOD, 2012). In a study of 7,909 marines of the First Marine Expeditionary Force who were returning home during 2004–2006, 9% screened positive on the BTBIS. It appears that the investigators considered only responses on the first two questions of the screen. Of those who screened positive for TBI, 70.5% (500) were first identified with the screen (Drake et al., 2010).

### Department of Veterans Affairs

VA measures the rates of TBI screening of all veterans returning from Iraq and Afghanistan who present for medical care; the VA's Office of Quality and Performance (OQP) has set a target of screening 95% of all veterans (Sayer, 2009). From April 2007 to November 2012, over 644,000 veterans have been screened for TBI. This represents approximately 95% of those eligible for screening. Through July 2012, 127,901 (20%) of OEF/OIF/OND veterans have screened positive for TBI (Sayer, 2012).

## Department of Defense and Department of Veterans Affairs Guidance for Assessment and Diagnosis of Mild Traumatic Brain Injury

There is no biologic "gold standard" for diagnosing mild TBI. On the basis of a positive TBI screen test, further clinical evaluation is needed to make a diagnosis.

### Department of Defense

In DOD, the level of the medical care facility determines the nature of the assessment. In Level I and II facilities in theater, MACE screening results are used to determine the disposition of service members. Those who screen negative can return to active duty after 24 hours of rest. Those who screen positive receive concussion education or management of symptoms and can return to duty when they are asymptomatic at rest and then asymptomatic after exertion but no sooner than 24 hours after injury. Service members who receive a diagnosis of a second concussion in a 12-month period must rest for 7 days. Service members who suffer three or more concussions in a 12-month period cannot return to duty until a Recurrent Concussion Evaluation is completed by a neurologist or other qualified licensed provider who is knowledgeable about concussion. The evaluation includes the Neurobehavioral Symptom Inventory, the Acute Stress Disorder Questionnaire, a vestibular assessment, and neurobehavioral testing (no specific instrument is recommended). Neuroimaging (with computed tomography [CT] or magnetic resonance imaging) and a functional assessment are initiated at the discretion of the health care provider (DOD, 2010b).

In Level III and IV facilities, those who screen positive are referred to a TBI specialty center if they are still symptomatic; they are then evaluated by a trained nurse or physician (Dempsey et al., 2009). In Level V facilities, those who screen positive get education, PTSD or acute stress disorder (ASD) screening, neuroimaging, and basic cognitive testing (DOD, 2010b).

**Department of Veterans Affairs**

VA policy dictates that service members who screen positive be referred for a comprehensive TBI evaluation by a specialized team in VA's Polytrauma–TBI system of care (VA, 2010c). The Comprehensive TBI Evaluation includes the origin or etiology of the patient's injury, assessment for neurobehavioral symptoms (with the 22-question Neurobehavioral Symptom Inventory), a targeted physical examination, and a followup treatment plan. All TBI evaluations and diagnostic conclusions are documented with an electronic Comprehensive TBI Evaluation template (VA, 2010c).

**Comparison of Guidelines for Assessment and Diagnosis of Traumatic Brain Injury**

The strategy of using a brief TBI screen followed by a confirmatory evaluation in those who screen positive is particular to DOD and VA guidelines. Current civilian guidelines use self-reporting of injury mechanisms and symptoms as the sole means to trigger a diagnostic evaluation (CDC, 2003). The use of a separate screening process for those at risk is not addressed in civilian guidelines. Because neuroimaging studies are often used in the evaluation of civilian mild TBI—to exclude other diagnoses—guidelines for their use have been recommended (Holm et al., 2005; Jagoda et al., 2009; NICE, 2007).

The DOD in-theater TBI guidelines use the American College of Emergency Physicians (ACEP) recommendations for head CT scanning. Head CT scanning is recommended in head-trauma patients who suffer loss of consciousness or posttraumatic amnesia and have one or more of the following: headache, vomiting, age over 60 years, drug or alcohol intoxication, deficits in short-term memory, physical evidence of trauma above the clavicle, posttraumatic seizure, focal neurologic deficit, and coagulopathy. However, because most in-theater mild TBI involves blast and the ACEP guidelines were based on cohorts that were not injured by blasts, it is unclear how fully the ACEP guidelines identify clinically significant brain injury in military settings.

Civilian studies have suggested that comparison of preinjury baseline and postconcussion performance on neuropsychologic tests is the most sensitive and objective method for detecting the presence and resolution of cognitive postconcussion symptoms (Erlanger et al., 1999).

## Implementation of Department of Defense and Department of Veterans Affairs Guidance for Assessment and Diagnosis of Mild Traumatic Brain Injury

This section presents information available to the committee on the extent to which DOD and VA conduct followup and evaluation of service members and veterans who have positive TBI screens. The committee notes the lack of readily available, centralized sources of data within the DOD about the implementation of TBI assessment processes and the need for improved followup and evaluation of veterans who might have TBI.

### Department of Defense

The committee was unable to identify data on the number of service members that received comprehensive TBI evaluation because of a positive TBI screen or other clinical indication in either in-theater or postdeployment settings. In a recent report to Congress, DOD reported that systems for documenting and tracking potentially concussive events would allow DOD to obtain data to facilitate proper identification of and care for service members who are at risk for mild TBI (DOD, 2012).

### Department of Veterans Affairs

As of July 2012, 50,869 of the 127,901 OEF/OIF/OND veterans who screened positive received a confirmed diagnosis of TBI on the basis of a comprehensive TBI evaluation (7.9% of the total number who were screened) (Sayer, 2012).

VA implemented two performance measures to evaluate the degree to which veterans who have positive TBI screens are followed up and evaluated. One measure assesses whether veterans who have positive TBI screens are contacted within 14 working days to schedule a comprehensive evaluation for TBI; 84% of all cases is set as the target rate. The other measure assesses whether veterans have the comprehensive evaluation for TBI completed within 30 days of a positive screen; 75% of all cases is set as the target rate (Sayer, 2012).

Data suggest that VA needs to improve the rate of followup evaluations of those who screen positive for TBI. The rate of completion for comprehensive TBI evaluations varies considerably at the facility level. The rate of followup evaluation ranges from 48% to 99%, and the TBI diagnosis rate in those who screened positive ranges from 21% to 91% (Sayer, 2012). In an evaluation of a TBI screening program in one VA medical center, 52% of OEF and OIF veterans who had positive TBI screens had later appointments in a TBI polytrauma specialty clinic within 18 months of TBI screening (Sayer et al., 2011). Moreover, a 2008 GAO report found that some providers reported difficulties in implementing electronic requests for followup evaluations and did not always use a symptom checklist—to assess the presence and severity of symptoms associated with mild TBI—during followup evaluations (GAO, 2008).

## Department of Defense and Department of Veterans Affairs Guidance for Treatment for Mild Traumatic Brain Injury

The DVBIC published its recommendations for the Acute Management of Mild TBI in Military Operational Settings in 2006 (DVBIC, 2006) and updated them in 2008 (DVBIC, 2008b). The guidelines make recommendations in four aspects of care for mild TBI: symptom management, rest or return to duty, educational initiatives, and supportive therapies. The guidelines recognize that strong evidence supporting the use of pharmacologic treatment of patients for mild TBI is lacking; however, it provides some guidance on which medications to use for common mild-TBI complaints (such as headache). The overall treatment strategy relies on obtaining an initial symptom inventory first. Physical examination, later testing, and treatment options are then dictated by the particular symptoms endorsed by the service member. The guidelines recommend that treatment for mild TBI be managed with the guidance of an interdisciplinary team and that referrals for physical therapy, occupational therapy, speech and language therapy, pharmacy, audiology and vestibular care, and optometry be made when appropriate. They also recommend that coping strategies, stress management, and avoidance of excessive alcohol and drugs be communicated via patient education. Finally, they note that duty restrictions for service members who have TBI should be considered to protect them from risk of secondary injury or reexposure. For example, in the subacute phase (over 7 days), symptomatic patients should be considered for limited duty hours.

*VA/DOD Clinical Practice Guideline: Management of Concussion/Mild Traumatic Brain Injury* (VA and DOD, 2009b) was designed to provide guidance for treatment more than 7 days after mild TBI. The guidelines contain evidence-based recommendations for management at initial presentation, treatment for specific symptoms, and management of persistent symptoms. They also recommend patient education, screening for the presence of comorbid psychiatric problems (such as depression, PTSD, and SUD), and medications to treat for symptoms, such as headaches, depression and anxiety, and sleep disturbances.

The Defense Centers of Excellence for Psychological Health & Traumatic Brain Injury (DCoE) *Case Management of Concussion/Mild TBI* provides guidelines for managing postconcussive symptoms that last longer than about 4–6 weeks (DCoE, 2010). Case management for this subset of concussed service members entails identifying barriers to a service member's successful return to duty and assisting in developing a recovery care plan. That may involve education, facilitating medical appointments, and acting as liaison between the service member and VA.

## Comparison of Guidelines for Treatment for Mild Traumatic Brain Injury

In addition to the guidelines promulgated by VA and DOD, guidelines for treatment for civilian mild TBI have been published by the Ontario Neurotrauma Foundation (ONF) (Ontario Neurotrauma Foundation, 2011), the East Practice Management Work Group (Cushman et al., 2001), the Scandinavian Neurotrauma Committee (Ingebrigtsen et al., 2000), and the National Institute for Health and Clinical Excellence (NICE, 2007). Guidelines for the management of concussions in athletes have been published by the International Conference on Concussion in Sports (Aubry et al., 2002; McCrory et al., 2005, 2009), the American Academy of Neurology (AAN) (American Academy of Neurology, 1997), the Canadian Academy of Sports Medicine (Canadian Academy of Sport Medicine Concussion Committee, 2000), and McGill (Johnston et al., 2001). There is substantial overlap between those guidelines and the VA/DOD guidelines for treatment for mild TBI (see Table 5.1). All indicate that the vast majority of mild TBI cases will resolve within 7 days to 3 months (McCrea et al., 2003).

The greatest distinction among the guidelines is related to the timeframe after the injury (see Table 5.1). Some deal only with the acute phase (up to 1 week after injury), whereas others deal with the subacute phase (day 7 to 4–6 weeks after injury) or the chronic phase (more than 4–6 weeks after injury). There are some minor distinctions among the guidelines regarding treatment for headache. Headache is the most prominent symptom after mild TBI, occurring in 30%–90% of patients (Bazarian et al., 1999). All guidelines that address posttraumatic headache recommend pharmacotherapy, such as nonsteroidal anti-inflammatory drugs (NSAIDs) or amitriptyline, but some guidelines, such as those promulgated by the DCoE and the ONF, distinguish between tension headaches and migraine headaches; NSAIDs are recommended for tension headaches, whereas triptans, such as sumatriptan and rizatriptan, are recommended for migraine headaches. The ONF is the only one that recommends, in appropriate circumstances, prophylactic treatment for headaches with tricyclic antidepressants, venlafaxine, tizanidine, or other adjunctive therapies. In addition to or in lieu of pharmacologic treatments, nonpharmacologic treatment for headaches—such as sleep education, physical therapy, and relaxation—is also recommended by the DCoE and VA/DOD. The ONF cautions against overuse of headache medications because a patient may experience rebound symptoms that perpetuate headaches. All the guidelines caution against the use of narcotics to control headaches.

Memory loss, difficulty in concentrating, and difficulty in making decisions are cognitive deficits that are highly prevalent after mild TBI. Recommendations for cognition assessment and treatment are highly variable. The need for cognition assessment is articulated in all the guidelines, but there is no uniformity in which questionnaires or other measurement instruments should be used to assess the nature and degree of abnormalities. Treatment is also variable. The VA/DOD and DCOE guidelines are the only ones that provide for specific pharmacologic and nonpharmacologic interventions. The former are selective serotonin reuptake inhibitors and stimulants; the latter include reassurance, aerobic exercise, and sleep hygiene education. Finally, there is some variability regarding the specific psychiatric disorders and SUDs to assess for comorbidities (see Table 5.1).

## Subspecialty Recommendations

In the period after acute evaluation of and treatment for TBI, patients who remain symptomatic are referred for subspecialty care. Recommendations for treatment of military personnel for mild TBI have been published for various aspects of management, such as the role of neuropsychology (McCrea et al., 2009), rehabilitation psychology (McCrea et al., 2009), speech and language pathology (Cherney et al., 2010), audiology (Cherney et al., 2010), treatment for persistent cognitive dysfunction (Cozzarelli, 2010), cognitive rehabilitation (Helmick, 2010), physical therapy (Weightman et al., 2010), and occupational therapy (Radomski et al., 2009). Among civilians after mild TBI, the effectiveness of psychologic treatments (Snell et al., 2009), cognitive rehabilitation (Cappa et al., 2003; NIH, 1999; Rohling et al., 2009), and drug treatment for neurobehavioral disorders (Neurobehavioral Guidelines Working Group, 2006) have all been systematically reviewed. The effectiveness of cognitive rehabilitation for TBI was examined by a DVBIC-sponsored randomized controlled trial (RCT) (Vanderploeg et al., 2008). In 2011, the Institute of Medicine (IOM) recommended continuing use of cognitive rehabilitation therapy for people who had TBI despite the need for additional research to address shortcomings in the supporting evidence (IOM, 2011b). Many of those recommendations were published after the VA/DOD guidelines were released and are not reflected in documentation reviewed by the present committee. Therefore, the committee is unable to ascertain whether VA and DOD implement the recommendations in their practice standards.

**TABLE 5.1** Comparison of Department of Veterans Affairs and Department of Defense Guidelines with Other Guidelines for Mild Traumatic Brain Injury

| Aspect of Care | VA/DOD | DVBIC[a] | DCOE[b] | ONF[c] | 3rd ICC Sports[d] | NICE[e] |
|---|---|---|---|---|---|---|
| Target population | Military, postdeployment | Military in theater | Military | Civilians, athletes | Athletes | Civilians with mild to severe TBI |
| Postinjury period covered | Over 7 days | Acute | Over 4–6 weeks | Acute, subacute, chronic | Acute | Acute |
| Overall treatment strategy | Comprehensive assessment, management | Testing, referral, treatment based on symptoms | Case management | Comprehensive assessment, management | Assessment, management | Assessment, management en route to and in emergency room |
| Rates level of evidence supporting the recommendations | ✓ | | | ✓ | | |
| Treatment of headache | ✓ Pharmacologic, nonpharmacologic | ✓ | ✓ Pharmacologic, nonpharmacologic | ✓ Including prophylactic pharmacotherapy | | |
| Treatment of memory impairment, other cognitive symptoms | ✓ SSRI,[f] stimulants, nonpharmacologic methods | | ✓ SSRI, stimulants, nonpharmacologic methods | ✓ | ✓ Cognitive rest | |
| Treatment of balance problems | ✓ | | ✓ | ✓ | | |
| Treatment of irritability | ✓ | | ✓ | ✓ | | |
| Treatment of sleep disturbance | ✓ | | ✓ | ✓ | | |
| Treatment of mood changes | ✓ | | ✓ | ✓ | | |

| Aspect of Care | VA/DOD | DVBIC[a] | DCOE[b] | ONF[c] | 3rd ICC Sports[d] | NICE[e] |
|---|---|---|---|---|---|---|
| Indications for neuroimaging | ✓ | ✓ Highly detailed | | ✓ | ✓ | ✓ |
| Cognitive testing? | ✓ Reliable, standardized | ✓ Military Acute Concussion Evaluation | ✓ | ✓ Rivermead Post-Concussion Symptom Questionnaire | ✓ Maddock's questions or Standard Assessment of Concussion | |
| Indications for referral to specialist | ✓ | ✓ | ✓ | ✓ | | ✓ |
| Education recommended | ✓ | ✓ | ✓ | ✓ | | ✓ |
| Screening recommended for other disorders? | ✓ Psychiatric, SUDs[g] | ✓ Depression, acute stress reaction | ✓ Depression, PTSD, SUDs | ✓ Depression, anxiety, PTSD, SUDs, somatoform disorder | ✓ Depression | |

[a]Defense and Veterans Brain Injury Center.
[b]Defense Centers of Excellence for Psychological Health & Traumatic Brain Injury.
[c]Ontario Neurotrauma Foundation.
[d]International Conference on Concussion in Sports.
[e]National Institute for Health and Clinical Experience.
[f]Selective serotonin reuptake inhibitors.

### Guidelines for Management of Severe Traumatic Brain Injury

A number of civilian guidelines exist for the management of civilians who have more severe TBI. They include guidelines by the New Zealand Guidelines Group (2006), the Scottish Intercollegiate Guidelines Network (2009), and the Brain Trauma Foundation (BTF) (Brain Trauma Foundation et al., 2007; Bullock et al., 2006; Knuth et al., 2005). The committee is uncertain about the extent to which DOD and VA are evaluating the guidelines for the evidence base to support their best-practices recommendations. For example, the BTF published a series of guidelines for several aspects of field management of combat-related moderate to severe TBI, including pain management, assessment of oxygenation and blood pressure, airway management, brain-directed pharmacologic interventions, use of the Glasgow Coma Scale, triage and transport, and fluid resuscitation (Knuth et al., 2005). The BTF also published guidelines for several aspects of the management of civilian moderate to severe TBI, including steroids, nutrition, deep-vein thrombosis prophylaxis, hyperventilation, sedation, antiseizure prophylaxis, blood pressure and oxygenation, brain-oxygen monitoring, hyperosmolar therapy, intracranial-pressure monitoring, infection prophylaxis, cerebral perfusion, and hypothermia (Brain Trauma Foundation et al., 2007). The BTF published guidelines related to the surgical management of epidural hematoma, subdural hematoma, traumatic parenchymal lesions, posterior fossa mass lesions, and depressed cranial fractures (Bullock et al., 2006). The AAN published guidelines on the use of antiepileptic drugs after severe TBI (Chang et al., 2003).

### Implementation of Department of Defense and Department of Veterans Affairs Guidance for Treatment for Traumatic Brain Injury

This section presents information available to the committee on the extent to which DOD and VA monitor and implement their treatment guidelines. The committee notes a lack of data in that regard.

#### Department of Defense

The committee is not aware of any metrics used by DOD to assess the extent to which the TBI guidelines are being implemented and treatments provided. DOD outlines a number of subjects in need of quality and performance metrics in its 2008 report to Congress, *Comprehensive Approach to Psychological Health and Traumatic Brain Injury.* Regarding surveillance, the report states that "there is a need to further develop a robust system that allows tracking and monitoring of both TBI and mental health conditions and treatment outcomes" (Casscells, 2008b). In a later report to Congress, DOD reported its work with the VA on standardizing TBI-related diagnosis codes to facilitate proper diagnosis and tracking of clinical outcomes (DOD, 2011a). In that report, DOD described plans for a clinical-outcomes project in which standardized outcome assessments (functional status and quality of life) are administered to mild-TBI patients at intake, on discharge, and at predetermined followup times. The objective is to relate patient outcome with specific clinical practices and programs to determine clinical best practices (DOD, 2011a).

**Department of Veterans Affairs**

To support the implementation of the 2009 VA/DOD CPG for managing concussion and mild TBI, various educational interventions—including noninteractive Web-based education—have been implemented (DCoE, 2011e). However, the committee in not aware of the existence of performance measures related to the guidelines (Sayer, 2009).

### Summary

There are aspects of VA's and DOD's screening, assessment, and treatment interventions for mild TBI for which questions of efficacy and effectiveness have not been conclusively answered. Scientific evidence supporting ANAM's effectiveness in the assessment of cognitive function after head injury is insufficient. Additional psychometric studies are needed on VHA's TBI screening tool that are based on military cohorts. Studies are also needed to address the extent to which DOD's use of civilian guideline recommendations for head CT scanning identify clinically significant brain injury in military settings. Of the guidelines reviewed, the VA/DOD and DCOE guidelines are the only ones that provide for specific pharmacologic and nonpharmacologic interventions. RCTs are needed determine the efficacy of those interventions, for which there is not yet a strong evidence base. There is a lack of readily available, centralized sources of data on the implementation of TBI assessment processes and treatment outcomes. The limited data available suggest that there is a need for improved followup and evaluation of service members and veterans who might have TBI.

## POSTTRAUMATIC STRESS DISORDER

Posttraumatic stress disorder (PTSD) can result from the direct, personal experience or witnessing of an event that poses a perceived threat of death or serious injury (APA, 2000). Symptoms that are characteristic of PTSD include reexperiencing of the traumatic event, often through intrusive thoughts, flashbacks, or nightmares; avoidance of stimuli associated with the trauma; numbing of emotions; and hyperarousal, often manifested by difficulty in sleeping and lack of concentration. For a diagnosis of PTSD, symptoms of acute stress must persist for at least a month and cause substantial impairment in important aspects of daily life (IOM, 2006). (Chapter 4 presents the diagnostic criteria for defining PTSD and data on its prevalence in the military and veteran populations.)

PTSD can be difficult to diagnose and treat. No objective measure can confirm a diagnosis of PTSD; diagnosis ultimately rests on a careful and comprehensive clinical evaluation performed by a qualified professional (a psychologist, social worker, psychiatrist, or psychiatric nurse practitioner) under conditions of privacy and confidentiality (IOM, 2012). Determining appropriate treatment can be complicated because PTSD presents with varied psychosocial morbidity and functional impairment and is often comorbid with other psychiatric disorders, particularly SUD, major depression, and mild TBI. In addition, fear of negative consequences for a military career and the perceived stigma associated with mental-health problems may discourage service members and veterans from seeking treatment (Hoge et al., 2004; Nash et al., 2009).

To assess the efficacy of current screening, assessment, and treatment approaches for PTSD in DOD and VA, the committee reviewed the 2010 *VA/DoD Clinical Practice Guideline for the Management of Post-Traumatic Stress* (VA and DOD, 2010). The guideline documents evidence-based procedures for assessment and diagnosis of and treatment for posttraumatic stress in adults who are treated in any DOD or VA clinical setting. The committee compared key aspects of the recommended practices in the VA–DOD guideline with state-of-the-art clinical guidelines (reviewed later in this chapter) and evidence in the literature on the management of PTSD.

A substantial contribution to the body of literature on PTSD that is reflected in the present report is the recently published IOM report *Treatment for Posttraumatic Stress Disorder in Military and Veteran Populations: Initial Assessment* (IOM, 2012). In response to a congressional mandate to assess PTSD programs and services in DOD and VA, the Committee on the Assessment of Ongoing Efforts in the Treatment of Posttraumatic Stress Disorder conducted a thorough synthesis of evidence related to many aspects of PTSD. Its report covers the history, diagnostic criteria, epidemiology, and neurobiology of PTSD. It summarizes the DOD and VA health care systems and examples of PTSD programs and services offered and their prevention of and screening approaches for PTSD, including the tools and instruments most commonly used by DOD and VA. The report evaluates the evidence supporting the many options for PTSD treatment, including treatment for PTSD comorbid conditions and novel interventions. Findings from that report are discussed in this chapter.

## Prevention of Posttraumatic Stress Disorder

DOD supports a number of programs that are aimed at preventing the development of PTSD by building resilience and helping service members to anticipate some of the traumatic events that they may experience in a combat zone. For example, Army prevention programs include Battlemind and, most recently, the Comprehensive Soldier Fitness program that will be used for all Army personnel before deployment (Brusher, 2011; Casey, 2011). All four services have a variety of programs to help service members who have symptoms of PTSD to avoid chronic PTSD. VA attempts to prevent chronic PTSD by working with veterans who have symptoms and has programs that help veterans with PTSD to regain functioning in civilian life and to prevent further PTSD-related disability (IOM, 2012).

After examining prevention of and prophylaxis for PTSD in active-duty and veteran populations, the IOM Committee on the Assessment of Ongoing Efforts in the Treatment of Posttraumatic Stress Disorder concluded that "while there are a variety of DoD and VA programs that target PTSD prevention, it is important to note that, at present, none of them has evidence for their effectiveness in preventing or reducing PTSD or stress in service members or their families" (IOM, 2012). This committee agrees with that conclusion and with the need that the report highlights for systematic evaluation of such programs, ideally before widespread implementation.

## Provision of Services for Posttraumatic Stress Disorder

DOD provides PTSD services to service members in numerous programs, and settings, including counseling centers, general inpatient and outpatient mental-health services, and specialized treatment programs. PTSD care for service members includes programs that are DOD-wide and programs that are specific to the Army, Air Force, Navy, Marine Corps, reserves, or National Guard. Treatment for PTSD in DOD is provided by a variety of health professionals in the theater of war and in other settings on and off base. Many service members who have a diagnosis of PTSD receive counseling, medication, or both in an outpatient setting through a mental-health department (IOM, 2012).

VA provides PTSD services in VHA hospitals, outpatient clinics, community-based outpatient clinics (CBOCs), and Vet Centers. In addition, VA pays for some care delivered through outside providers. PTSD treatment delivered in outpatient clinics and CBOCs is through either general mental-health clinics or, less commonly, specialized programs provided by PTSD clinical teams, substance-use PTSD teams, and women's stress-disorder treatment teams. Hospitalizations for PTSD include both traditional inpatient stays and specialized programs involving short residential stays; the latter involve counseling and treatment with social, vocational, and recreational therapies (CBO, 2012).

## Department of Defense and Department of Veterans Affairs Guidance for Screening for Posttraumatic Stress Disorder

Evidence suggests that identifying PTSD early and referring people to treatment can decrease symptoms and lessen the severity of functional impairment (VA and DOD, 2010). PTSD screening instruments help to identify people who have PTSD symptoms and inform decisions about who should receive a full diagnostic assessment by a health professional. A diagnosis of PTSD cannot be made on the basis of a positive screening test alone.

The VA/DOD guideline specifies that all new patients be screened for symptoms of PTSD and then rescreened annually or more frequently if it is clinically indicated by clinical suspicion, recent trauma exposure, or history of PTSD. Figure 5.2 shows the process for initial evaluation and triage of patients who might have PTSD in a primary care setting as presented in the VA/ DOD guideline.

The guideline endorses the use of validated instruments for screening for PTSD. It suggests the use of a number of possible screening instruments but does not offer specific guidance on which one to use, citing insufficient evidence to support a recommendation of one PTSD screening tool vs another. The Primary Care PTSD Screen (PC-PTSD) is the instrument most commonly used by DOD and VA. The PC-PTSD (Prins et al., 2004) is a validated four-question screening measure designed for use in primary care settings (see Box 5.3).

### Department of Veterans Affairs

In the VA system, all veterans coming to VA for the first time are screened for PTSD. The PC-PTSD screening tool is incorporated into the VHA Clinical Reminder tracking system used in its medical facilities. A clinician accessing a veteran's electronic VA medical record is prompted to complete the screening. The reminder furnishes the four PC-PTSD questions to screen for risk factors associated with PTSD. A veteran who screens positive—defined by VA as a positive response to three or more questions, which is different from the scoring used by DOD—is evaluated further by a primary care provider or is referred to a mental-health clinician.

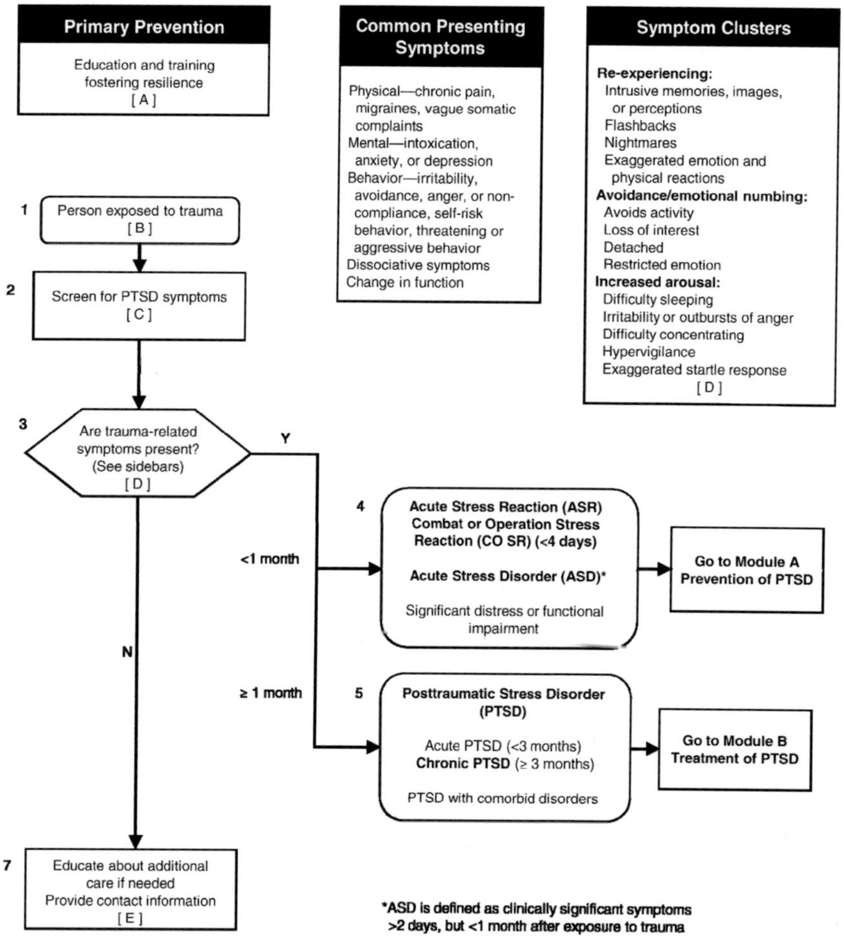


**FIGURE 5.2** Algorithm for initial evaluation of and triage for PTSD.
SOURCE: VA and DOD, 2010.

---

**BOX 5.3**
**The Primary Care PTSD Screen**

In your life, have you ever had any experience that was so frightening, horrible, or upsetting that, in the past month, you:

1. Have had nightmares about it or thought about it when you did not want to?
   YES / NO
2. Tried hard not to think about it or went out of your way to avoid situations that reminded you of it?
   YES / NO
3. Were constantly on guard, watchful, or easily startled?
   YES / NO
4. Felt numb or detached from others, activities, or your surroundings?
   YES / NO

SOURCE: Prins et al., 2004.

---

The veteran is also assessed for suicide risk (VA, 2007). Followup screening for PTSD is repeated every year for the first 5 years that the veteran is in VA care and every 5 years thereafter unless there is a clinical need more frequently (VA, 2010b). In addition, veterans seen in any of the roughly 300 VA Vet Centers are screened for PTSD.

The difference between PC-PTSD scoring thresholds used by DOD and VA hampers the ability to make valuable clinical and research comparisons between the two systems of care. The next section discusses research findings about PC-PTSD scoring methods.

### Validity of Tools for Screening for Posttraumatic Stress Disorder

A wide array of PTSD screening tools are available for identifying undiagnosed cases of PTSD (National Center for PTSD, 2004), but there is little evidence to support recommending one PTSD screening tool over another (VA and DOD, 2010). A systematic review of validated screening instruments for civilian PTSD found that instruments that have fewer items, simpler response scales, and simpler scoring methods perform as well as if not better than longer and more complex measures (Brewin, 2005). As mentioned previously, the VA and DOD use the four-item PC-PTSD screening tool.

Research with VA primary care patients has shown that the PC-PTSD is optimally efficient (yielding a sensitivity of 0.78 and a specificity of 0.87) when a cutoff score of 3 is used, meaning that patients answering yes to at least three questions should be considered for further evaluation for PTSD (Prins et al., 2004). Recent studies of the performance of the PC-PTSD in military populations also found that a cutoff of 3 has an acceptable level of sensitivity to identify people who have PTSD (the range is 0.76–0.83) and a high degree of specificity to identify people who do not have PTSD (the range is 0.82–0.92) (Bliese et al., 2008; Calhoun et al., 2010). However, given the measure's relative susceptibility to false positives (positive results in people who do not have PTSD), Calhoun et al. (2010) suggest that, within primary care, the PC-PTSD may be most advantageously used in the context of staged screening—using the PC-PTSD followed by another assessment tool. As mentioned above, DOD uses a staged approach in which a cutoff score of 2 on the PC-PTSD is followed by use of the PCL to assess symptom severity.

Research suggests that DOD postdeployment mental-health screening may fail to identify a sizable fraction of service members who need mental-health services because of service members' concerns about anonymity. In one study by (Warner et al., 2011b), a brigade of Army soldiers first completed the PDHA on returning from Iraq, and a subsample completed an anonymous survey that consisted of the same mental-health questions as were on the PDHA. Service members reported much higher rates regarding all mental-health concerns on the anonymous survey; of those who screened positive for PTSD or depression, 20.3% reported that they were uncomfortable about reporting their answers honestly on the PDHA (Warner et al., 2011a). Concerns related to stigma are a problem in the accurate assessment of PTSD and other psychopathologic conditions.

## Implementation of Department of Defense and Department of Veterans Affairs Guidance for Screening for Posttraumatic Stress Disorder

The section presents sparse information on the extent to which DOD and VA are implementing and tracking screening procedures to identify possible PTSD. The lack of VA data raises questions about how well it is implementing and assessing their screening practices to ensure the best possible result.

### Department of Defense

The Armed Forces Health Surveillance Center (AFHSC) reports PTSD screening rates on the basis of data from postdeployment health screenings (with the PDHA and the PDHRA). In the first quarter of 2010, about 10% of active and reserve service members who returned from OEF and OIF deployments screened positive on the PC-PTSD, which is included in the health assessments (DeFraites and Vythilingam, 2011). As mentioned above, research suggests that postdeployment health screenings may underestimate the number of service members who might have PTSD (Warner et al., 2011a).

Data from the RESPECT-Mil program show that from February 2007, when the program began, through the end of FY 2011, 76 clinics at 31 active RESPECT-Mil sites provided more than 1.6 million primary care visits by active-duty service members, of which 1.3 million visits—almost 80%—included screening for PTSD and depression. Although there is opportunity to improve screening, that rate shows that attention is being given to screening at the RESPECT-Mil sites. Of visits that included screening, nearly 13% (168,519) resulted in positive screens; 49% of positive screens resulted in primary care diagnoses of depression, possible PTSD, or both (DCoE, 2012b).

### Department of Veterans Affairs

In VA's Performance Management Program, VA uses several measures to see whether veterans are being screened for PTSD (AHRQ, 2012). The committee was unable to identify results of using those measures. Inquiries to VA about performance measures did not yield information about them.

One measure is the percentage of eligible patients who are screened for PTSD at required intervals. Another is the percentage of veterans who have positive PC-PTSD screens whose disposition is documented in the record. A disposition is defined as either a timeline for care; an arrangement for treatment, such as a mental-health appointment; or giving of instructions to a patient. A related measure looks at whether disposition is timely. *Timely* is defined as completion of the disposition by the next calendar day after a positive screen.

## Department of Defense and Department of Veterans Affairs Guidance for Assessment and Diagnosis of Posttraumatic Stress Disorder

Figure 5.3 shows the process presented in the VA/DOD guideline for managing the assessment and diagnosis of PTSD in patients who have a positive PTSD screen.

For patients who screen positive for PTSD, the VA/DOD guideline states that clinicians should perform a comprehensive clinical assessment to obtain relevant information to guide accurate diagnosis and appropriate clinical decision making. In a comprehensive clinical interview, a provider should focus on the traumatic event, danger to self or others, relevant history, physical and mental status examinations, relevant laboratory tests, psychosocial functioning, and possible comorbid conditions (such as SUDs and depression). The provider should assess the patient's symptoms against each of the 17 PTSD criteria in the *Diagnostic and Statistical Manual, Fourth Edition* (*DSM-IV*) and gather details about time of onset, frequency, course, severity, level of distress, and functional impairment. A functional assessment should evaluate the patient's current level of family, relationship, work or school, and social functioning and fitness for duty.

As part of the comprehensive assessment, there are several instruments to assist the clinician in making a PTSD diagnosis, documenting a traumatic event, and assessing symptom severity. Two main types of instruments are used in PTSD evaluations: structured (or semistructured) interview questions that a clinician asks and self-reporting questionnaires that a patient completes. Typically, both structured interviews and self-reporting questionnaires are used in clinical settings to measure PTSD symptoms (National Center for PTSD, 2012a).

The VA/DOD guideline recommends the use of structured interviews and specifically mentions the Clinician-Administered PTSD Scale (CAPS) to support a diagnosis of PTSD on the basis of symptoms related to each of the *DSM-IV* diagnostic criteria for PTSD. The CAPS (Blake et al., 1995) is a semistructured interview that should be administered by a trained health professional to determine whether a patient meets the *DSM-IV* diagnostic criteria for PTSD. It has the advantage of assessing the array of PTSD symptoms and their severity (frequency and intensity), but it cannot be used to determine the presence of comorbid psychiatric disorders. The CAPS contains 34 questions, 17 of which measure symptom frequency and 17 measure symptom intensity. A total symptom severity score (which ranges from 17 to 85) can be obtained by summing the scores on each of the 17 items. The CAPS generally takes about 40–60 minutes to administer (IOM, 2006).

The VA/DOD guideline also recommends the use of a validated self-administered checklist of symptoms and history of trauma exposure and specifically mentions the PTSD Checklist (PCL). The PCL (Blanchard et al., 1996; Weathers et al., 1991) assesses *DSM-IV* symptoms of PTSD and symptom severity. With the PCL, patients use a 1–5 scale to rate the frequency and intensity of their symptoms (IOM, 2006).

Acknowledging the high prevalence of psychiatric comorbidities in the PTSD population, the VA/DOD guideline states that screening for depression and other psychiatric disorders is warranted. The section "Comorbid Conditions" discusses the management of comorbid conditions.

**Department of Defense**

In DOD, as previously mentioned, a service member who has a positive result on the PC-PTSD should complete the PCL-C as part of the deployment health-assessment process and the RESPECT-Mil program before evaluation in a diagnostic interview. However, the deployment health assessments and the RESPECT-Mil program use different scoring thresholds for purposes of diagnosis and treatment. According to clinician training materials for the DOD deployment health assessment, a PCL score of less than 30 means no PTSD symptoms, scores of 30–39 correspond to mild PTSD symptoms, scores of 40–49 correspond to moderate PTSD symptoms, and a score of 50 or more means severe PTSD symptoms (Vythilingam et al., 2010).

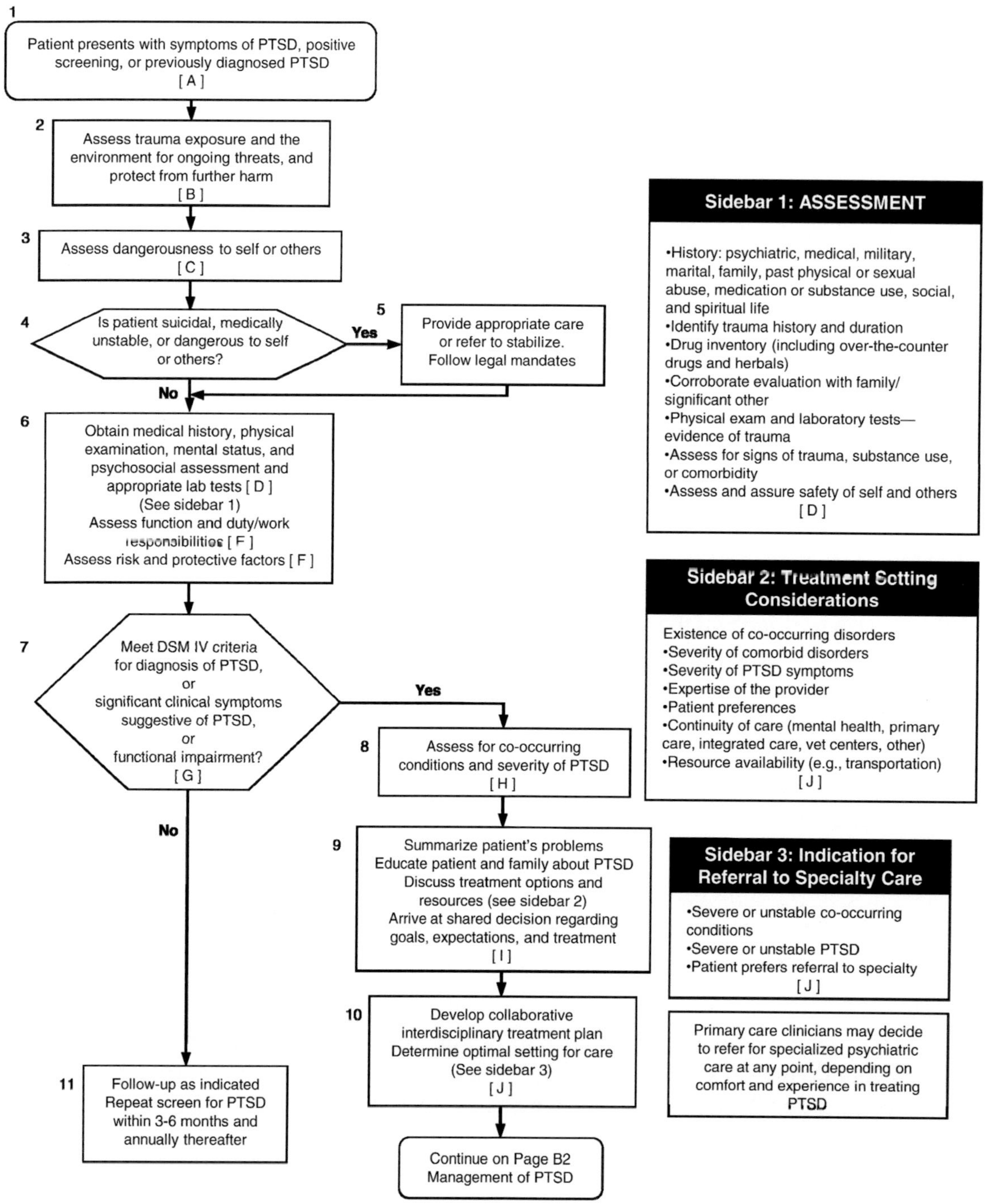


**FIGURE 5.3** Algorithm for the assessment and diagnosis of posttraumatic stress disorder.
SOURCE: VA and DOD, 2010.

According to the RESPECT-Mil clinician manual, a score of less than 13 means no PTSD, scores of 13–32 correspond to mild PTSD, and scores of 33 or greater correspond to moderate to severe PTSD. As a result of the different definitions for symptom severity, the treatment recommendations are inconsistent between the deployment health assessment and the RESPECT-Mil programs.

**Department of Veterans Affairs**

In the VA health system, a veteran who has a positive result on the PC-PTSD is evaluated further by the primary care provider or is referred to a mental-health clinician—such as a psychiatrist, psychologist, or trained clinician—for further evaluation. Patients referred for mental-health services must have an initial assessment within 24 hours and a first full evaluation appointment within 14 days. Established patients require followup appointments within 30 days (VA, 2010b). The PCL-C is the most widely used severity scale for veterans who have positive PC-PTSD screens, but its use is optional (VA, 2007). The VA National Center for PTSD indicates that a cut score should be based on prevalence and setting characteristics. For VA primary care settings, the suggested cut scores are 36–44; for VA specialty mental-health clinics, the suggested point range is 45–50 (National Center for PTSD, 2012b).

## Validity of Tools for Assessment of Posttraumatic Stress Disorder

The CAPS, the structured interview recommended in the VA/DOD guideline, is considered the gold standard in PTSD assessment (National Center for PTSD, 2012a). All the major CPGs for the management of PTSD recommend its use (Forbes et al., 2007; International Society for Traumatic Stress Studies, 2009; National Collaborating Centre for Mental Health, 2005; Ursano et al., 2004). Less frequently cited validated diagnostic instruments referred to in the guidelines include the Structured Clinical Interview for DSM-IV (Spitzer et al., 1992), the PTSD Symptom Scale–Interview Version (Foa et al., 1993), and the Structured Interview for PTSD (Davidson et al., 1997). See IOM's *Treatment for Posttraumatic Stress Disorder in Military and Veteran Populations: Initial Assessment* for a discussion of those and other instruments used in screening for and assessment of PTSD (IOM, 2012).

Among self-reported measures recommended by the VA/DOD guideline, the PCL is well validated and is most frequently cited in the major CPGs for the management of PTSD (Forbes et al., 2007; International Society for Traumatic Stress Studies, 2009; National Collaborating Centre for Mental Health, 2005; Ursano et al., 2004). There are three versions of the PCL: in the "specific" version (PCL-S), symptoms are rated in relation to a particular event; in the "military" version (PCL-M), symptoms are rated in relation to an event experienced during military service; and in the "civilian" version (PCL-C), ratings are based on any stressful life experiences. The PCL-C and PCL-S are appropriate for a wide array of patients, including military personnel and veterans. The PCL can be scored in several ways, including combining methods to ensure that a patient meets both the symptom pattern and the severity threshold (National Center for PTSD, 2012b).

A review that synthesized 72 research studies that evaluated the psychometric properties of one or more versions of the PCL found the PCL to be a well-validated measure. In general, it is psychometrically sound and shows good temporal stability, internal consistency, test–retest reliability, and convergent validity (Wilkins et al., 2011). However, the VA National Center for PTSD states that "there is no absolute method for determining the correct cut score on the PCL" (National Center for PTSD, 2012b). On the basis of the PCL's total symptom severity score (which ranges from 17 to 85), studies have shown considerable variability in the PCL's sensitivity and specificity depending on the cutoff score used. For example, studies' recommended cutoff scores to indicate a positive screen in veteran populations were 28, 31, 38, and 48 (McDonald and Calhoun, 2010). In their review of the diagnostic accuracy of the PCL,

McDonald and Calhoun (2010) concluded that the variability in the PCL's sensitivity and specificity suggests that interpretation of a score depends on the characteristics of a respondent's setting and the goal of assessment. Specifically, more studies of the PCL's diagnostic accuracy in Iraq and Afghanistan war veterans are needed. Wilkins et al. (2011) expounded on the PCL's strengths and limitations and emphasized that caution should be used if the PCL is expected to differentiate PTSD from similar disorders or to be used to assess treatment-related change in symptoms.

Although the PCL threshold recommended by VA is consistent with the thresholds reported in the literature, the committee is not aware of the evidence underlying the specific thresholds used in DOD's deployment health assessment and RESPECT-Mil programs.

### Implementation of Department of Defense and Department of Veterans Affairs Guidance for Assessment and Diagnosis of Posttraumatic Stress Disorder

This section presents the information on the extent to which DOD and VA conduct followup and evaluation of service members and veterans who have positive PTSD screens. The data suggest that DOD and VA need to improve their assessment practices to ensure the best possible patient care.

#### Department of Defense

The AFHSC reports depression referral rates according to data from the PDHA and the PDHRA. In the first quarter of 2010, the percentage of active-duty and reserves who had positive PTSD screens and who received referrals to mental-health primary or specialty care increased from about 20% to 40% over a 4-year period and achieved the 2010 target referral rate of 40% (DeFraites and Vythilingam, 2011). The committee is not aware how the targets are determined.

The committee did not find data from the RESPECT-Mil program on rates of followup and assessment of service members who were seen in primary care settings and who had positive PTSD screens.

#### Department of Veterans Affairs

VA reports that the numbers of referrals to diagnosis and to treatment cannot be determined, because such referrals are not coded consistently in the administrative medical record (IOM, 2012). Some data on the assessment process are available from a recent evaluation and from the Office of Inspector General (OIG).

In 2006, VA contracted with the Altarum Institute and RAND to conduct an independent evaluation of the quality of VA mental-health and substance-use care (Watkins and Pincus, 2011). The evaluation included PTSD-related measures calculated for a cohort of veterans who had PTSD that were identified for each fiscal year from FY 2004 through FY 2008. The PTSD cohort selection was based on *International Classification of Diseases, Ninth Revision* codes in the administrative records and reflected at least one inpatient episode or two outpatient visits (for any mental-health or non-mental-health diagnosis) in a fiscal year.

In FY 2007, of patients in the PTSD cohort who were defined as experiencing a new treatment episode (NTE),[4] fewer than 5.6% had documentation of assessment for PTSD symptoms with a standard instrument within 30 days. Standard instruments included the PCL and the CAPS. That low rate is noteworthy given that the VA/DOD guideline recommends that clinicians use a standard assessment tool to inform clinical assessment. In addition, the extent of improvement needed in VA's implementation of assessment practices is underscored in light of more recent VA policy that calls for providing patients referred for mental-health services with an initial assessment within 24 hours and a full evaluation within 14 days (VA, 2010b).

In response to concerns about belated mental-health assessments for veterans returning from Iraq and Afghanistan, Congress called for an investigation by the OIG. The OIG concluded that "VHA does not have a reliable and accurate method of determining whether they are providing patients timely access to mental health care services. VHA did not provide first-time patients with timely mental health evaluations and existing patients often waited more than 14 days past their desired date of care for their treatment appointment." The OIG made a series of recommendations for revision of existing measures and for evaluation of possible alternative measures, staffing analysis, and improvements in data collection (VA Office of Inspector General, 2012). The committee is concerned about the OIG's findings and underscores the importance of those recommendations for providing timely health care to our veterans.

## Department of Defense and Department of Veterans Affairs Guidance for Treatment for Posttraumatic Stress Disorder

In general, treatment for PTSD symptoms includes three broad intervention categories: psychotherapy (based on psychology techniques), pharmacotherapy (using prescription medication), and education (including coping mechanisms for the patient and family members).

First-line psychotherapy treatments recommended by the VA/DOD guideline are trauma-focused psychotherapy that includes components of exposure or cognitive restructuring or stress inoculation training (SIT). Specifically, the approach may include an exposure-based therapy, such as prolonged exposure (PE); a cognitive-based therapy, such as cognitive processing therapy (CPT); stress management therapy (such as SIT); or eye-movement desensitization and reprocessing (EMDR). In addition, the guideline identifies other approaches as having possible benefit in treating for PTSD, including relaxation techniques, imagery-reversal therapy, brief psychodymamic therapy, hypnosis, and group therapy. Dialectical behavioral therapy or family and couples therapy are not recommended as first-line treatment for PTSD. The guideline states that the treatment approach selected should reflect symptom severity, clinician expertise, and patient preference. In VA, CPT and PE must be available to all who need and want it (VA, 2008a). Data presented later in this section suggest that there are shortcomings in the implementation of that policy.

With respect to the use of technology for the delivery of treatment, the VA/DOD guideline does not recommend Internet-based interventions for treatment for PTSD; however, it supports the use of telephone delivery and videoconferencing, particularly to overcome geographic distance or other barriers to care. Although controlled trials of technology-based

---

[4]Defined by either the exacerbation of a condition that requires psychiatric inpatient care or the initiation of outpatient treatment after a break of 5 or more months without care.

delivery of PTSD treatments are under way, there are no definitive conclusions about its effectiveness (IOM, 2012).

Among the pharmacotherapy interventions, first-line agents recommended by the VA/DOD guideline are mainly the antidepressants SSRIs and serotonin norepinephrine reuptake inhibitors (SNRIs). If needed, the guideline suggests that the use of second-line agents, such as mirtazapine, nefazodone, tricyclic antidepressants (TCAs), and monoamine oxidase inhibitors (MAOIs) be considered. In addition, the guideline recommends the atypical antipsychotics risperidone or olanzapine as adjunctive treatment with antidepressants.

## Comparison of Guidelines for Treatment for Posttraumatic Stress Disorder

In addition to the recommendations by the VA/DOD guideline, major CPGs for treatment for PTSD have been published by the American Psychiatric Association (APA) (Ursano et al., 2004), the United Kingdom National Institute of Health and Clinical Excellence (NICE) (National Collaborating Centre for Mental Health, 2005), the Australian National Health and Medical Research Council (Forbes et al., 2007), and the International Society for Traumatic Stress Studies (ISTSS) (International Society for Traumatic Stress Studies, 2009). Table 5.2 compares treatment recommendations and their various systems for indicating their strength (IOM, 2012).

**TABLE 5.2** Guideline Recommendations for Treatment for Posttraumatic Stress Disorder

| Treatment Modality | VA/DOD | APA | NICE | NHMRC | ISTSS |
|---|---|---|---|---|---|
| *Psychotherapy* | | | | | |
| Exposure therapy | A | I | | | A |
| Prolonged exposure | A | I | | A | A |
| Virtual reality exposure | | | | | |
| Other exposure therapies | | | | | |
| Cognitive-based therapies | A | I | A | A | A |
| Trauma-focused cognitive | A | | | A | A |
| Behavioral therapy | I | | | | |
| Cognitive processing therapy | | | | | |
| Internet-based | I | | | | |
| Eye movement desensitization and reprocessing | A | II | A | A (with in vivo exposure) | A |
| Stress inoculation training | A | II | | | A |
| Group therapy | C | III | | | |
| Hypnosis | C | | | | |
| Imagery rehearsal therapies | C | II | | | |
| Psychodynamic psychotherapy | C | II | | C (stress management) | D |
| Patient education | C | | | | |

| Treatment Modality | VA/DOD | APA | NICE | NHMRC | ISTSS |
|---|---|---|---|---|---|
| Relaxation | C | | | | |
| Dialectic behavioral therapy | I | | | | |
| Acceptance and commitment therapy | I | | | | |
| Family therapy | I | | | | |
| *Pharmacotherapy* | | | | | |
| Antidepressants | | | | | |
| SSRI | A | I | B | B | A |
| SNRI | A | I | | | A |
| Tricyclic and MOAIs | B | II | B | B | A |
| Mirtazapine | B | III | B | B | A |
| Nefazodone | D | | | | A |
| Anticonvulsants | D | III | | | Not efficacious |
| Antipsychotics | | | | | |
| Conventional | I | | | | |
| Atypical | B (as adjunct) | III | | | A (as adjunct) |
| | I (as monotherapy) | | | | C (quetiapine) |
| Benzodiazepines and GABAergic drugs | D (benzodiazepine) | III | | | Not efficacious |
| Antiadrenergic drugs | | III | | | |
| Prazosin | B (for sleep); C (for global PTSD) | | | | |
| Guanfacine | D | | | | |
| Clonidine | I | | | | Not efficacious |
| Other drugs | | | | | |
| Buspirone | I | | | | |
| Nonbenzodiazepine hypnotics | I | | | | |
| Bupropion | I | Not endorsed | | C | |
| Trazodone | I | | | C | |
| Gabapentin | I | | | Not efficacious | |
| Lamotrigine | I | | | | |
| Propranolol | I | II | | Not efficacious | |
| D-Cycloserine | | | | | |
| *Complementary and alternative medicines* | I | | | | |

NOTE: VA/DOD: A = good evidence that the intervention improved outcomes; B = a fair amount of evidence supported the use of the intervention; C = the working group did not make a recommendation for or against the routine use of the intervention as the risk-benefit ratio was too close to make a general recommendation; D = presence of evidence that either the intervention was harmful or the risks outweighed the benefits offered by it; I = evidence was lacking, of insufficient quality, or conflicting; therefore a recommendation could not be made for or against providing the treatment routinely. APA: I = intervention recommended with substantial clinical confidence; II = intervention recommended with moderate clinical confidence; III = intervention recommended on the basis of individual circumstances. NICE: A = intervention was supported by a consistent body of evidence, including at least one RCT; B = treatment was supported by well-conducted clinical trials but no RCTs had tested the intervention; C = treatment was supported by expert committee reports or opinion but good clinical studies were absent; GPP (good practice point) = treatment was considered good practice by the guideline development group. NHMRC: 5-point scale (A, B, C, D, GPP) with A indicating that a treatment had the strongest evidence supporting its use and D indicating that a particular treatment had very weak evidence supporting its use. GPP = treatments deemed to be effective based on expert consensus opinion despite lacking empirical evidence. ISTSS: A = evidence for a particular treatment was based on RCTs; B = evidence was based on well-designed studies without randomization or placebo comparison; C = evidence was based on naturalistic clinical studies and clinical observations; D = evidence was based on long-standing and widespread clinical practice that had yet to be tested empirically; E = evidence was based on long-standing practice by a selected group of clinicians that had not been tested empirically; F = a new treatment that had not been tested empirically.

SOURCE: IOM, 2012.

### Psychosocial Treatments

In its review of the guideline recommendations for psychosocial treatments for PTSD (see Table 5.2), the earlier IOM committee drew the following conclusions:

> There are many similarities among the recommendations of the reviewed guidelines. . . . All the guidelines strongly support the use of trauma-focused psychotherapy treatment for PTSD in adults and children with an emphasis on trauma-focused CBT, such as PE and CT. All but one of the guidelines recommended against the use of psychologic debriefing soon after exposure to trauma (IOM, 2012).

That committee noted that eye-movement desensitization and reprocessing (EMDR) is one example of the variation in the guidelines assessment of a specific therapy. EMDR was given the highest rating in all but one of the guidelines. The APA guideline gave it a second-tier rating. What contributed to that difference among the guidelines was how the absence of support for the use of eye movements in EMDR was addressed.

After reviewing the psychosocial treatments whose efficacy had been examined in RCTs or open trials, IOM (2012) found that the vast majority of treatments that have been examined via RCTs are in the general group of psychosocial therapies called cognitive behavioral therapy (CBT). They include exposure therapies such as prolonged exposure (PE), stress inoculation training or anxiety-management programs, cognitive therapies such as cognitive processing therapy (CPT), and EMDR. RCTs have shown that cognitive therapy alone results in PTSD symptom reduction and improved mood and functioning (IOM, 2012).

In addition, the earlier committee considered the evidence base for numerous other psychosocial therapies, including psychodynamic psychotherapy, brief eclectic psychotherapy, hypnosis, relaxation, stress inoculation training, interpersonal therapy, skills training in affect and interpersonal regulation, and group therapy. That committee found that, with the exception of CBT-based group therapy, the efficacy of the other psychosocial therapies is supported by only a few RCTs. Small RCTs and open trials of acceptance and commitment therapy have been conducted and warrants further review. Until the results from the four ongoing RCTs are available, there is insufficient evidence for the efficacy of virtual reality exposure programs that integrate computer graphics and head-mounted visual displays as a tool to deliver PE to reduce PTSD symptoms (IOM, 2012). See IOM (2012) for a full discussion of the evidence supporting the use of various psychosocial therapies for PTSD.

### Pharmacologic Treatments

As shown in Table 5.2, PTSD treatment guidelines, including the 2010 VA/DOD guideline, all recommend the use of antidepressants, specifically, an SSRI or an SNRI, in treatment for chronic PTSD. The US guidelines—VA/DOD, ISTSS, and APA—all recommend the use of SSRIs or the SNRI antidepressant venlafaxine as a first-line therapy with status equal to that of psychotherapy. The UK and Australian guidelines recommend pharmacotherapy only as a second choice unless a patient declines psychotherapy or manifests particular clinical features (IOM, 2012).

The recently published IOM report (IOM, 2012) also cited reviews and meta-analyses that found good evidence that pharmacotherapy reduces symptoms in chronic PTSD, including combat-related PTSD (see Ipser and Stein, 2012; Stein et al., 2006; Stewart and Wrobel, 2009). See IOM 2012 for a full discussion of the evidence supporting the use of various pharmacologic treatments for PTSD.

### Emerging Therapies

Guideline recommendations do not show strong evidence supporting the use of various innovative or alternative treatments for PTSD, such as couple and family therapy and complementary and alternative medicine (CAM), which includes yoga, contemplative treatments, and acupuncture. IOM (2012) concluded that these treatments do not have a substantial evidence base; evidence of the effectiveness of these therapies for PTSD is based on small RCTs, case studies, or anecdotal reports.

## Implementation of Department of Defense and Department of Veterans Affairs Guidance for Treatment for Posttraumatic Stress Disorder

This section presents information available to the present committee on the extent to which DOD and VA provide treatment for service members and veterans who have PTSD. There is a striking lack of data to inform conclusions about the extent to which PTSD treatments are offered, delivered, and completed and about whether they are leading to improved patient outcomes.

### Department of Defense

The AFHSC reports PTSD referral rates on the basis of data from the postdeployment health screenings (PDHA and PDHRA). In the first quarter of 2010, 65% of active-duty and reserve personnel who had a positive PTSD screen and who received a referral to mental-health primary or specialty care were engaged in treatment, that is, had a mental-health–related clinic encounter during the 180 days after their return. That reached the 2010 target referral rate of 65%

(DeFraites and Vythilingam, 2011). The committee does not know how the targets are determined.

**Department of Veterans Affairs**

VA reports that there is no mechanism for tracking the delivery of evidence-based therapies in the VA centralized databases. The VHA is developing progress-note templates for CPT, PE, and other evidence-based treatments that will allow documentation of care in the computerized record in a manner that will facilitate the collection of centralized aggregate data (IOM, 2012). The committee obtained the data discussed below, which suggest that many veterans are not getting necessary treatment and that most of those who are do not complete the full course.

VA reported to the Congressional Budget Office (CBO) that 40% of OEF and OIF veterans initiating CPT or PE therapy complete a full course of therapy, which is typically at least nine treatment sessions ideally administered weekly (Seal et al., 2010). The CBO report states that veterans who completed PE therapy attended an average of 11 sessions, whereas those who did not complete therapy attended an average of five sessions; results were similar for patients undergoing CPT. A recently published study found that of 49,425 veterans with newly diagnosed PTSD in VA, fewer than 10% completed the recommended treatment in the first year of diagnosis (Seal et al., 2010).

As mentioned previously, VA contracted with Altarum Institute and RAND to conduct an independent evaluation of the quality of VA mental-health and substance-use care (Watkins and Pincus, 2011). The evaluation included PTSD-related measures calculated for a cohort of veterans who had PTSD. In FY 2007, 27.9% of veterans in the PTSD cohort in a new treatment episode had documentation of an adequate trial (at least 60 days) of SSRIs or a documented reason for discontinuing. Only 19.9% in the PTSD cohort who received psychotherapy had documentation of receiving at least one visit for CBT (including behavioral therapy and cognitive therapy) in the study period. Some 16.3% of veterans in the PTD cohort received VA's Specialized Intensive PTSD Programs (SIPP) within 60 days of a new treatment episode, and 25.3% received SIPP during the study period. Veterans over 65 years old and veterans who resided in rural areas had the lowest use of SIPP, and there was considerable variation among the Veterans Integrated Service Networks.

To improve implementation of treatment regimens, VA is undertaking a national effort to disseminate evidence-based psychotherapies for PTSD and other mental-health conditions throughout the VA health care system. Since 2007, VA has been working to disseminate CPT and PE therapy for PTSD. Competence-based training of VA mental-health care providers in the delivery of those therapies is a component of the initiative. It involves experientially based workshop training followed by weekly consultation for 6 months with an expert in the treatment (Karlin et al., 2010). As of May 31, 2010, VA had provided training to over 2,700 VA mental-health staff in the delivery of CPT or PE, and some staff have been trained in the delivery of both (Karlin, 2010). Additional efforts to promote communication and sharing of best practices throughout VA include the PTSD national mentoring program and the appointment of evidenced-based coordinators at each medical center. The committee is impressed by the training of clinicians in evidence-based therapies (PE and CPT) and commends VA on its psychotherapy dissemination efforts. What remains a question to the committee is how much the treatments are actually offered, delivered, and completed and whether they are leading to improved patient outcomes.

### Summary

The VA/DOD clinical guidelines for PTSD are in line with the available evidence base and state-of-the-art clinical guidelines put forth by other professional organizations (such as APA and NICE). The VA/DOD guidelines suggest standards for the screening for and assessment of PTSD that are generally reasonable and evidence based. They also make treatment recommendations that are in line with the evidence base and other state-of-the-art guidelines. VA has undertaken a large, impressive effort to disseminate the evidence-based therapies PE and CPT for PTSD. It is to be commended for that effort and for its success in training large numbers of clinicians. The committee has concerns, however, about the timeliness of assessments and treatment delivery for veterans who need them. On the basis of the relatively modest data that we could access, wait times are too long, and appropriate assessment and treatment delivery are delayed beyond what is acceptable. The committee also has concerns about how well the dissemination effort has "penetrated" into practice. To judge by the data that we reviewed, most veterans who have PTSD do *not* receive evidence-based psychotherapy (many receive SSRIs but not necessarily in adequate dosage or for an adequate duration), and most of those who receive it do not complete an adequate course of treatment.

## MAJOR DEPRESSIVE DISORDER

Diagnosis of major depressive disorder (MDD) is based on the presence of depressed mood or a marked reduction in or loss of interest or pleasure in all or nearly all activities for most of the day and the presence of at least four additional symptoms, such as substantial change in weight, change in sleeping patterns, fatigue, feelings of worthlessness, and suicidal ideation (APA, 2000). To warrant the diagnosis, symptoms must persist for at least 2 weeks and involve substantial impairment in functioning. Chapter 4 presents the diagnostic criteria of MDD and gives details about the prevalence of MDD in the military and veteran populations.

To assess the efficacy of current screening, assessment, and treatment approaches to MDD in DOD and VA, the committee reviewed the *VA/DOD Clinical Practice Guideline for Management of Major Depressive Disorder (MDD), May 2009* (VA and DOD, 2009a). The guideline is intended to assess, diagnose, and treat for MDD in the military and veteran populations and is intended to be used in the primary care setting. Here, the committee assesses key aspects of the recommended practices in the VA/DOD guideline in light of evidence in the literature and other clinical guidelines for the management of MDD.

### Department of Defense and Department of Veterans Affairs Guidance for Screening for Major Depressive Disorder

Among service members and veterans, systematic screening for depression is especially vital considering its prevalence, its associated risk of suicide, and the perceived stigma that deters the receipt of mental-health care. The VA/DOD guideline for MDD recommends annual screening in the primary-care setting. Figure 5.4 shows the process presented in the VA/DOD guideline for the initial assessment (including screening) and diagnosis of MDD in primary care.

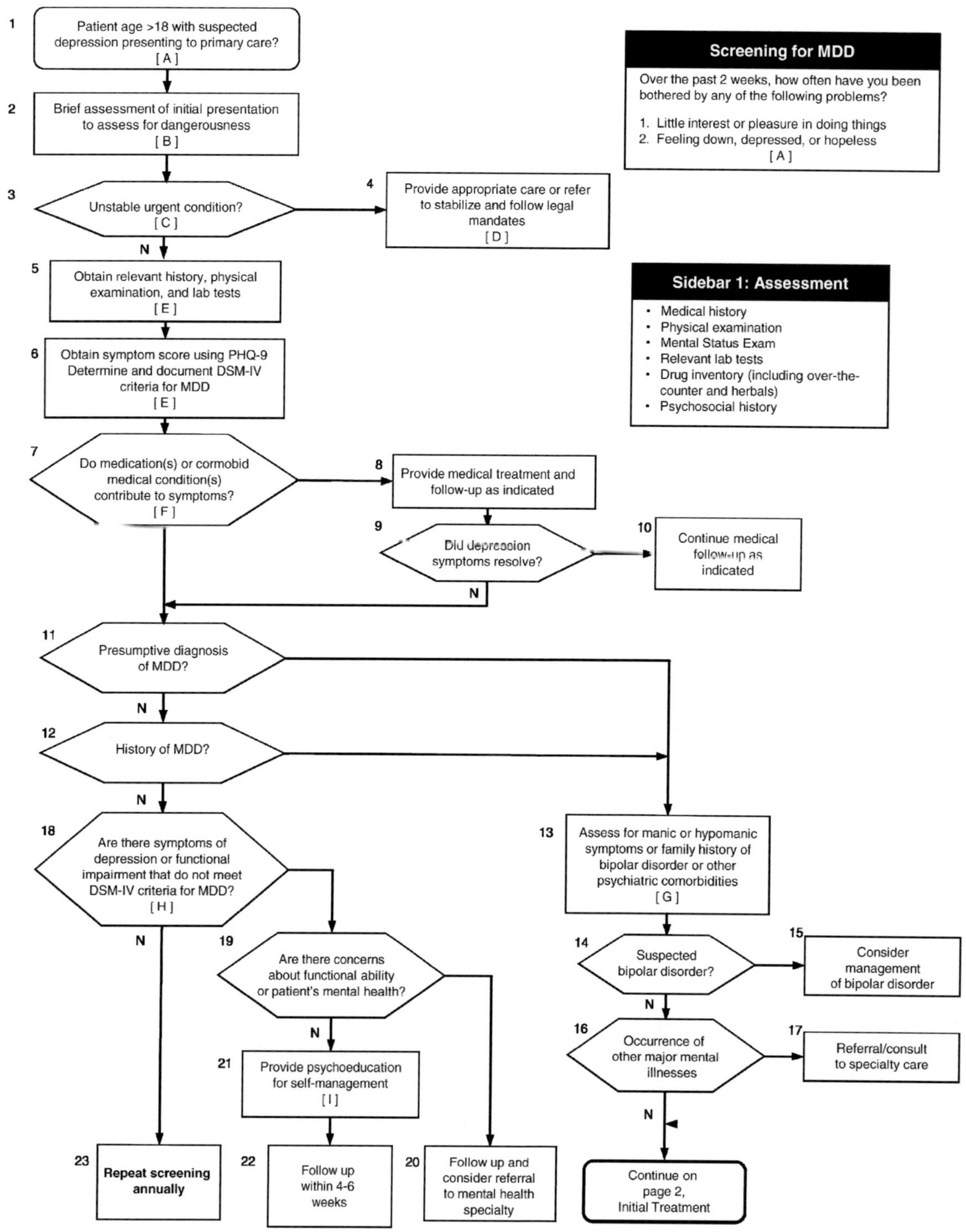


**FIGURE 5.4** Algorithm for initial assessment and diagnosis of MDD in primary care.
SOURCE: VA and DOD, 2009a.

To screen for MDD, the guideline recommends the use of a standardized screening tool, the Patient Health Questionnaire (PHQ-2), which is a validated two-item screen (see Box 5.4). A PHQ-2 score ranges from 0 to 6. Patients who screen positive on the PHQ-2 should be given a more detailed quantitative questionnaire and a full clinical interview that includes evaluation for suicide risk.

**BOX 5.4**
**Patient Health Questionnaire-2 (PHQ-2)**

Over the past 2 weeks, how often have you been bothered by any of the following problems?

Little interest or pleasure in doing things.
0 = Not at all
1 = Several days
2 = More than half the days
3 = Nearly every day

Feeling down, depressed, or hopeless.
0 = Not at all
1 = Several days
2 = More than half the days
3 = Nearly every day

SOURCE: Kroenke et al., 2003.

### Department of Defense

In DOD, depression screening occurs routinely as a component of periodic health assessments, the PDHA and PDHRA, which are briefly described in the introduction to this chapter. It also occurs routinely in primary care settings. The US Army Medical Command implemented the RESPECT-Mil, which provides primary care–based screening, assessment, treatment, and referral of active-duty personnel who have PTSD or depression. DOD is implementing a triservice expansion of the program (DCoE, 2012b). Service members who present in RESPECT-Mil clinics are screened for depression and for PTSD at every primary care provider visit. To screen for depression, both the deployment health assessment and RESPECT-Mil use the PHQ-2 questions. The screen is considered positive if a service member indicates that either one or both symptoms are present either "more than half the days" or "nearly every day." Service members who screen positive are evaluated further with the nine-item PHQ-9 (Department of the Army, 2010b; Vythilingam et al., 2010).

### Department of Veterans Affairs

In the VA health system, all veterans who come to VA for the first time are screened for depression. The PHQ-2 screening tool is incorporated into the VHA clinical-reminder tracking system. A clinician who accesses a veteran's electronic VA medical record is prompted to complete the screening. The reminder presents the two PHQ-2 questions; a cutoff score of 3 is used to define a positive screen. Veterans who screen positive are assessed for suicide risk and then, if it is warranted, evaluated by either a primary care provider or a mental-health specialist. The PHQ-2 should be completed annually by all patients who are seen in a primary care setting (VA, 2010b). VA has several care-management models that integrate mental-health and primary care and in which depression screening and treatment take place. Such programs include Translating Initiatives for Depression into Effective Solutions (TIDES), the Behavioral Health Laboratory, the Post-Deployment Integrated Care Initiative, and Patient-Care Alignment Teams. In addition, veterans seen in any of the roughly 300 Vet Centers are screened for depression.

### Validity of Tools for Screening for Major Depressive Disorder

Evidence supports the practice of screening for depression in primary care (US PSTF, 2009; Yano et al., 2012), as recommended by the VA/DOD MDD guideline. In reviewing evidence on the accuracy of screening instruments to identify depressed adults, the US Preventive Services Task Force (USPSTF) found little evidence to support recommending one screening tool over another. It concluded that asking the two questions on the PHQ-2 may be as effective as using more complex instruments (USPSTF, 2009). A recent systematic review found that the PHQ-2 has good sensitivity (83%) and specificity (92%) for detecting depressive disorders with a cutoff score of 3 (Kroenke et al., 2010). A separate study, an RCT of screening for depression in primary care, suggests that using a threshold score of 2 is superior to detecting cases on the basis of a score of 3 or more (Arroll et al., 2010). Using a score of 2 or more, the PHQ-2 screen had a sensitivity of 86% and a specificity of 78%. Using a score of 3 or more, the study reported a sensitivity of 61% and a specificity of 92%. VA currently uses a cutoff score of 3 on the PHQ-2 as the basis of a positive MDD screen.

### Implementation of Department of Defense and Department of Veterans Affairs Guidance for Screening for Major Depressive Disorder

This section presents information available to the committee on the extent to which DOD and VA are implementing and tracking screening procedures to identify MDD. The sparse data suggest that there is room for improvement in DOD and VA screening practices for MDD.

#### Department of Defense

The AFHSC reports depression-screening rates by using data from the PDHA and the PDHRA. In the first quarter 2010, about 10% of active and reserve service members who had returned from OEF and OIF deployments screened positive on the PHQ-2 (DeFraites and Vythilingam, 2011).

Data from the RESPECT-Mil program show that from February 2007 through the end of FY 2011, 76 clinics at 31 active RESPECT-Mil sites provided more than 1.6 million primary care visits to active-duty service members, of which 1.3 million visits included screening for PTSD and depression. That represents an overall 80% screening rate for active-duty primary care visits to participating clinics since the program began. Of visits with screening, nearly 13% (168,519) resulted in positive screens; and 49% of positive screens resulted in a primary care diagnosis of depression, possible PTSD, or both (DCoE, 2012b).

#### Department of Veterans Affairs

Under VA's Performance Management Program, VA uses several measures to see whether veterans are being screened for depression (AHRQ, 2012). The committee was unable to identify results of using those measures, and inquiries to VA about performance measures did not yield information about them.

One measure is the percentage of eligible patients who are screened annually for depression with the PHQ-2 or PHQ-9. Another is the percentage of veterans who have a positive screen during their annual depression screening and have a disposition documented in the record. A disposition is defined as a timeline for care; an arrangement for treatment, such as a mental-health appointment; or the giving of instructions to the patient. A separate measure looks at whether documentation of the disposition is timely, which is defined as completion of the disposition by the next calendar day after a positive screen.

A study that used 2002 data on a national sample of VA medical outpatients found that overall about 85% of eligible veterans (18,245) were screened for depression in the study year. However, patients who were more likely to screen positive (veterans who were younger, were unmarried, or had more medical comorbidity) were less likely to be screened (Desai et al., 2006).

## Department of Defense and Department of Veterans Affairs Guidance for Assessment and Diagnosis of Major Depressive Disorder

For patients who screen positive for depression, the VA/DOD guideline states that the primary care provider should perform a clinical interview that focuses on relevant history, physical and mental-status examinations, relevant laboratory tests, drug inventory, and comorbid conditions. Providers should also evaluate the patient with a standardized assessment tool, the PHQ-9, and should assess for symptoms, symptom severity, and effects on daily functioning. See Figure 5.4 above for the process presented in the VA/DOD guideline for managing the assessment and diagnosis of MDD in primary care.

The PHQ-9 is a validated self-administered or interviewer-administered instrument that assesses the nine *DSM, Fourth Edition, Text Revision (DSM-IV-TR)* criterion symptoms and effects on functioning. It also assesses severity and treatment response. See questions in Box 5.5.

**BOX 5.5**
**PHQ-9 Questions***

**Over the last 2 weeks, how often have you been bothered by**

1. Little interest or pleasure in doing things
2. Feeling down, depressed, or hopeless
3. Trouble falling or staying asleep, or sleeping too much
4. Feeling tired or having little energy
5. Poor appetite or overeating
6. Feeling bad about yourself—or that you are a failure or have let yourself or your family down
7. Trouble concentrating on things, such as reading the newspaper or watching television
8. Moving or speaking so slowly that other people could have noticed. Or the opposite—being so fidgety or restless that you have been moving around a lot more than usual
9. Thoughts that you would be better off dead, or hurting yourself in some way

The first nine questions have a possible answer of:

- Not at all
- Several days
- More than half the days

- Nearly every day

---

**10. How difficult have these problems made it for you to do your work, take care of things at home, or get along with other people?**

Question 10 has a possible answer of:

- Not difficult at all
- Somewhat difficult
- Very difficult
- Extremely difficult



Each of the first nine items on the PHQ is scored 0–3, providing a 0–27 severity score. A total score of 10–14 is classified as meaning mild MDD, a score of 15–19 means moderate MDD, and a score of 20 or higher means severe MDD. A diagnosis is further modified as having complications if it co-occurs with PTSD, SUD, psychosis, suicide risk, mania, significant social stressors, or war-related conditions; and it is considered chronic if symptoms persist for more than 2 years despite treatment (VA and DOD, 2009a).

### Department of Defense

In deployment health assessments, DOD uses a variation of the PHQ-9, the PHQ-8, which omits the suicide-screening item because suicide screening and assessment do not occur until the diagnostic interview. Clinicians are to administer the PHQ-8 to service members who have positive PHQ-2 screens. They are to provide depression education or support counseling and *consider* referral to mental-health care for service members who have mild or moderate symptoms (a PHQ-8 score of 10–18) and *make* a referral for service members who have severe symptoms (a PHQ-8 score of 19 or higher) (Vythilingam et al., 2010). In the RESPECT-Mil program, service members who have positive PHQ-2 screens will complete the PHQ-9 (Department of the Army, 2010b). Treatment recommendations are to provide an antidepressant or psychotherapy for scores of 10–19 and an antidepressant and psychotherapy for scores of 20 or higher (Oxman et al., 2008).

### Department of Veterans Affairs

VA uses the PHQ-9—it is integrated into the clinical reminder—but not exclusively, inasmuch as the choice of instrument is determined by the care provider. However, the clinical reminder will prompt clinicians to perform the PHQ-9 test if a PHQ-2 test is positive (a score of 3 or higher). Any patient who has a PHQ-9 score over 10 or a response to question 9 of the PHQ-9 other than "not at all" must have an assessment for suicide risk and disposition by a provider within a day of the positive screen (VA, 2007).

## Validity of Tools for Assessment and Diagnosis of Major Depressive Disorder

The PHQ-9 has been found to be a reliable and valid measure of depressive disorders and depression severity (Kroenke et al., 2001). One systematic review of the psychometric literature on the PHQ-9 reported a sensitivity of 88% and a specificity of 88% when a cutoff score of 10 was used (Wittkampf et al., 2007). Because of the risk of overdiagnosis with that level of specificity, researchers concluded using a cutoff score of 10 is acceptable in patient populations that have a relatively high prevalence of MDD (Wittkampf et al., 2007).

## Implementation of Department of Defense and Department of Veterans Affairs Guidance for Assessment and Diagnosis of Major Depressive Disorder

This section presents information available to the committee on the extent to which DOD and VA conduct followup and evaluation of service members and veterans who have positive MDD screens. The information raises questions about how well DOD and VA are implementing and tracking their assessment practices to ensure the best possible patient care.

### Department of Defense

The AFHSC reports depression referral rates by using data from the PDHA and PDHRA. In the first quarter of 2010, the proportion of active-duty and reserve personnel referred to mental-health primary or specialty care, substance-abuse care, chaplains, or Military OneSource for further evaluation or treatment had increased from about 25% to 60% over a 4-year period, surpassing the 2010 target referral rate of 40% (DeFraites and Vythilingam, 2011).

The committee did not find data from the RESPECT-Mil program on rates of followup and assessment of service members who were seen in primary care settings and who had positive MDD screens.

### Department of Veterans Affairs

Under VA's Performance Management Program, VA collects two performance measures related to depression and suicide risk assessment (AHRQ, 2012). The committee was unable to identify results of using those measures, and inquiries to VA about performance measures did not yield information about them.

One measure is the percentage of patients who screen positive on a depression screen (PHQ-2 or PHQ-9) and have a suicide-risk evaluation completed within 24 hours. The other measure is the percentage of patients who screen positive on the depression screen (PHQ-2 or PHQ-9) and on the PTSD screen (PC-PTSD) and have a suicide-risk evaluation completed within 24 hours.

A study that used 2002 data from a national sample of VA medical outpatients found that veterans who had depressive symptoms were not being assessed as recommended. The results showed that overall 84.9% of eligible patients (18,245) were screened for depression in the study year. Although 8.8% screened positive, only about half (54.0%) the patients who screened positive received recommended followup evaluation for diagnostic confirmation and only 1.1% of those who screened positive received a new depression diagnosis (Desai et al., 2006).

## Department of Defense and Department of Veterans Affairs Guidance for Treatment for Major Depressive Disorder

For initial treatment for mild or moderate MDD, the VA/ DOD guideline advocates the use of monotherapy—either psychotherapy or pharmacotherapy with a single antidepressant.

Combination treatment with pharmacotherapy and psychotherapy should be used for moderate to severe MDD or for patients who have a poor response to monotherapy. The guideline advises that patients who receive a diagnosis of mild or moderate MDD may be treated in primary care. Patients who have severe MDD or any complicated MDD and comorbidities should be referred to specialty care for treatment. Figure 5.5 is the algorithm from the VA/DOD guideline for treatment for MDD in primary care.

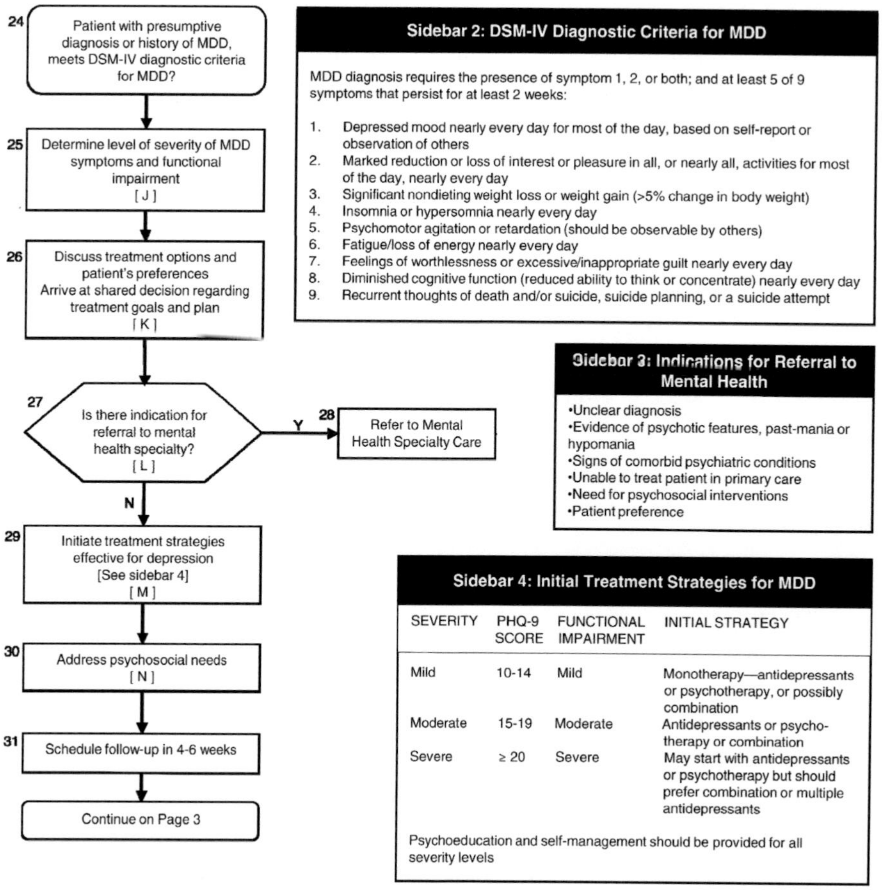


**FIGURE 5.5** Algorithm for treatment of MDD in primary care.
SOURCE: VA and DOD, 2009a.

The recommended first-line medications include SSRIs, such as sertraline and paroxetine, and SNRIs, such as bupropion and mirtazapine. The guideline notes that all the SSRIs, excluding fluvoxamine, may be used as first-line agents in the treatment of adults for MDD. Patients who do not remit or are intolerant to one SSRI may be switched to another SSRI or to another class of antidepressant, such as TCAs or MAOIs. Augmentation may be considered for those who show only partial response to an SSRI.

The recommended first-line psychotherapies include CBT, interpersonal psychotherapy (IPT), problem-solving therapy (PST), and behavior therapy, including behavioral activation (BA). Second-line interventions include short-term psychodynamic psychotherapy, couple-focused and marital-focused therapies, client-centered counseling, and acceptance and mindfulness therapies, such as acceptance and commitment therapy (ACT). The guideline also cites computer-based CBT as an alternative to traditional individual or group psychotherapy. Guided self-help is listed as an option for mild to moderate depression.

The guideline recommends individual CBT, 16–20 sessions long, as a monotherapy for patients who have moderate depression. CBT in combination with pharmacotherapy is a recommended option for patients who do not respond to monotherapy and for patients who have severe, recurrent MDD (defined as three or more episodes).

Individual IPT is recommended for adults who have uncomplicated mild to moderate MDD. The recommended treatment is 16–20 sessions delivered by mental-health professionals who are trained in this modality. PST can be used for uncomplicated mild to moderate MDD, particularly in the primary care setting, and can be delivered by primary care physicians or nurses. Six sessions, delivered over the course of 3 months, is a recommended option for patients who have uncomplicated mild to moderate MDD.

Electroconvulsive therapy (ECT) should be considered for patients who have severe MDD and cannot tolerate or have not responded to several trials of antidepressant treatment unless a patient has substantial comorbid medical conditions that would increase the risks associated with ECT.

The guideline recommends against the use of vagus nerve stimulation (VNS) as an intervention for treatment-resistant depression because when it was published, in 2009, VNS had not been demonstrated to be safe and effective. The controversy over the use of VNS is discussed later.

Among the possible complementary and alternative treatments, the guideline recommends the use of exercise as an adjunct to other empirically supported treatments for depression, particularly antidepressant medication. It recommends the consideration of light therapy for some patients who have MDD, particularly if they have seasonal affective disorder. The guideline suggests that St. John's wort may be used by patients who have mild MDD and who have a strong preference for herbal treatments. The guideline does not recommend acupuncture as a treatment for MDD on the basis of insufficient evidence to determine its efficacy.

After initiation of treatment, the patient should be periodically assessed to determine treatment effects. The PHQ-9 should be used to monitor treatment response 4–6 weeks after initiation of treatment, after each change in treatment, and periodically until full remission is achieved. In patients who reach full remission, assessment of symptoms should be continued periodically to monitor for relapse or recurrence.

A VHA 2008 directive states that all veterans who have depression (or anxiety disorders) must have access to CBT, ACT, or IPT. Medical centers and large community-based outpatient clinics (CBOCs) must provide adequate staff capacity to deliver evidence-based psychotherapy when it is clinically indicated. Large and middle-sized CBOCs may provide the services through telemental health when necessary (VA, 2008a). In addition to the required evidence-based treatments, VA offers a variety of treatments that fit into the CAM category and have almost no evidence base, such as spirituality group, relaxation group, relaxation yoga group, group ear acupuncture, socialization group, Tai-Chi group, and yoga nidra group. Many of those approaches have been used for relaxation in other settings.

## Comparison of Guidelines for Treatment for Major Depressive Disorder

In this section, the VA/DOD guideline is compared with evidence-based CPGs for the management of MDD developed by APA (2010) and NICE (2009). Table 5.3 compares treatment recommendations in the guidelines and uses their rating systems to indicate the strength of the evidence supporting them.

**TABLE 5.3** Summary of Guideline Recommendations for Treatment for Depression

| Treatment Modality | VA/DOD | APA | NICE |
|---|---|---|---|
| *Psychotherapy* | | | |
| Cognitive behavioral therapy (CBT) | A | I | ✓ |
| Interpersonal psychotherapy (IPT) | A | I | ✓ |
| Problem-solving therapy (PST) | A | I | ✓ |
| Behavioral therapy/behavioral activation | A | | ✓ |
| Computer-based cognitive behavioral therapy | B | | ✓First-line |
| Couple/marital-focused therapies | C | II | ✓ |
| Guided self-help (GSH) | B | | ✓ First-line |
| Client-centered counseling | C | | ✓ when other treatments are declined |
| Acceptance and Mindfulness | | | |
| Dialectical behavioral therapy | C | | |
| Mindfulness-based cognitive therapy | A | | ✓ |
| Acceptance and commitment therapy | No rating | | |
| Psychodynamic psychotherapy | C | II | ✓ when other treatments are declined |
| Group therapy | B (CBT) | III | ✓ CBT First-line |
| *Pharmacotherapy* | | | |
| Antidepressants | | | |
| SSRI | First-line (excluding Fluvoxamine) | I | ✓ |
| SNRI | First-line | I | |
| Bupropion | First-line | I | |
| Mirtazapine | First-line | I | |
| Tricyclic (TCA) | | I | |
| MAOIs | B If poor response w/other; no strength rating | I | |
| *Somatic Treatment* | | | |
| Electroconvulsive therapy | A | A | ✓ |

| Treatment Modality | VA/DOD | APA | NICE |
|---|---|---|---|
| Vagus nerve stimulation | D | III | |
| Transcranial magnetic stimulation | | II | |
| *Complementary and Alternative Treatments* | | | |
| Exercise | A (as adjunct) | | ✓ First-line |
| Light therapy | B (seasonal only) | III | |
| St. John's wort | B | III | X |
| Acupuncture | I | | |
| S-adenosyl methione (SAM-e) | | III | |

NOTE: VA/DOD: A = good evidence that the intervention improved outcomes; B = a fair amount of evidence supported the use of the intervention; C = the working group did not make a recommendation for or against the routine use of the intervention as the risk-benefit ratio was too close to make a general recommendation; D = presence of evidence that either the intervention was harmful or the risks outweighed the benefits offered by it; I = evidence was lacking, of insufficient quality, or conflicting; therefore a recommendation could not be made for or against providing the treatment routinely. APA: I = intervention recommended with substantial clinical confidence; II = intervention recommended with moderate clinical confidence; III = intervention recommended on the basis of individual circumstances. NICE: No rating system was used. For purposes of this report, √ denotes that use of the treatment was recommended; X indicates that the recommendation advises against the use of the treatment.

**Treatment Strategy**

Overall, the VA/DOD, APA, and NICE guidelines are consistent in recommending monotherapy as the initial treatment of choice for mild or moderate MDD. The VA/DOD guideline advocates the use of either pharmacotherapy alone or psychotherapy alone for mild or moderate MDD, whereas the APA and NICE guidelines suggest that psychotherapy alone may be the preferred initial treatment for mild and moderate MDD to be followed by the use of medication if symptoms persist. Research shows that the efficacy of psychotherapy for mild to moderate MDD is about the same as that of pharmacotherapy (Cuijpers et al., 2011; Thase, 2011).

Controversy surrounds the utility of antidepressants for treatment for mild depression. Because of small effect sizes, several reviews and meta-analyses have raised questions about the interpretation of results of RCTs. Examples of published reviews and meta-analyses relevant to the debate include (Hegerl et al., 2012; Pigott et al., 2010; Stewart et al., 2012; Thase, 2011; Vohringer and Ghaemi, 2011).

For moderate and severe MDD, all the guidelines recommend the use of pharmacotherapy alone or in combination with psychotherapy. RCTs in the Sequenced Treatment Alternatives to Relieve Depression (STAR*D) Study, funded by the National Institute of Mental Health, have shown that people whose depression is resistant to initial antidepressant treatment can achieve remission when treated with a secondary strategy. Patients benefited from either augmenting or switching medications or from augmenting with or switching to cognitive therapy; however, remission may take longer to achieve with the use of cognitive therapy (Warden et al., 2007). The meta-analysis by Cuijpers et al. (2011) concluded that combined treatment is more effective than psychotherapy alone and pharmacotherapy alone even for chronic depression. However, a more recent systematic review of the evidence could not provide clear evidence supporting the augmentation of pharmacotherapy with psychotherapy in treatment for chronic depression (von Wolff et al., 2012).

### Psychotherapies

On the basis of extensive research support, all the guidelines recommend CBT and IPT as first-line psychotherapy treatments. They also recommend PST and BA. Cuijpers et al. (2011) found only small differences between types of efficacious psychotherapies, including CBT, IPT, PST, nondirective supportive therapy, and BA. Compared with the other guidelines, the NICE guideline places a higher priority on a group-based format vs an individual format for delivering psychotherapy. The APA guideline does not strongly support the use of a group format for CBT or IPT, because a meta-analyses of their relative effectiveness did not include patients who had rigorously defined MDD. The NICE guideline also makes a stronger recommendation for the use of guided self-help materials and computer-based applications. A recent systematic literature review of computer-based psychologic treatments for depression and a meta-analysis of 19 RCTs support the efficacy and effectiveness of computer-based psychologic treatments for depression in diverse settings and in different populations (Richards and Richardson, 2012).

For patients who have moderate depression, the VA/DOD guideline recommends 16–20 sessions of individual CBT for MDD as a monotherapy, whereas the NICE guideline recommends six to eight sessions (face to face or via telephone), taking place over 9–12 weeks. A synthesis of findings of systematic reviews and trials encompassing 1,716 patients who had MDD or depressive symptoms found that brief CBT and PST (up to eight sessions) are efficacious for acute-phase treatment for depression in primary care (Nieuwsma et al., 2011). That does not appear to be the case for patients who have depressive relapse. A recent systematic review concluded that there is inadequate evidence to determine the effectiveness of brief (low-intensity) interventions (such as mindfulness-based cognitive therapy) for the prevention of relapse or recurrence of depression (Rodgers et al., 2012).

Regarding couple-focused therapy, the VA/DOD guideline notes that there is a smaller body of evidence than for other interventions and therefore recommends its use only for mild to moderate depression in patients who are experiencing marital distress. The findings from a Cochrane Collaboration support that recommendation. The authors concluded that the available evidence suggests that there is no reason to consider marital therapy as more or less effective than individual therapy even when it is associated with marital distress (Barbato and D'Avanzo, 2006).

Although there is a promising empirical base for ACT, a recent review of 18 RCTs found that ACT was not superior to control conditions for distress problems (anxiety and depression) (Powers et al., 2009). Additional research with larger samples and more rigorous designs is needed before more definitive claims can be made about the effectiveness of ACT (Montgomery et al., 2011). Given the lack of evidence supporting ACT as a first-line treatment for MDD, it is worth noting that a VA directive stipulates that veterans who have depression must have access to ACT as one of the treatments (VA, 2008a). ACT is on a priority list of psychotherapies for depression that is part of VA's initiative to disseminate evidence-based psychotherapies. VA has already provided training in ACT to hundreds of its clinicians.

### Pharmacologic Therapies

Each of the three guidelines recommends SSRIs as first-line pharmacotherapy. The APA and VA/DOD guidelines also recommend the SNRIs, bupropion, and mirtazapine as first-line medications. Second-generation antidepressants, such as SSRIs and SNRIs, are more commonly prescribed over first-generation antidepressants, such as TCAs and MAOIs, because they have lower toxicity (Qaseem et al., 2008). Research shows no clinically meaningful differences in efficacy between the various classes of antidepressant medications. Therefore, prescribing decisions should depend largely on side-effect profile, patient preference and previous experience with treatments, propensity to cause discontinuation symptoms, and safety in overdose (APA, 2010; NICE, 2009). The NICE guideline advocates the use of SSRIs "because SSRIs are equally effective as other antidepressants and have a favourable risk–benefit ratio."

**Somatic Treatments**

Each of the guidelines advises the use of ECT for severe MDD. In contrast with the VA/DOD guideline, the APA guideline considers VNS an option for treatment-resistant cases. In 2005, the Federal Drug Administration (FDA) approved the use of VNS in patients who had not responded to at least four trials of antidepressant medication or ECT. However, the role of VNS is the subject of debate (APA, 2010). In 2007, the Centers for Medicare and Medicaid Services decided not to provide coverage for VNS therapy and stated that the only well-designed trial had not demonstrated benefit and the observational studies had biases that made conclusions difficult (Phurrough et al., 2007). A recent systematic review and meta-analysis concluded that insufficient data are available to determine the efficacy of VNS (Martin and Martin-Sanchez, 2012).

Transcranial magnetic stimulation (TMS) is considered a recommended treatment only by APA, which noted that results of RCT had been variable. The treatment had received FDA approval in 2008 for people who had MDD and had not responded to antidepressants. A recent meta-analysis of TMS found that it appeared to be effective although at 4 weeks of followup there had been no further improvement beyond that at the end of treatment (Allan et al., 2011).

**Complementary and Alternative Treatments**

There are few data on complementary and alternative treatments for MDD. NICE is the only guideline that recommends exercise as a stand-alone first-line treatment; the VA/DOD and APA guidelines consider exercise a helpful adjunct to the treatment plan for MDD. A recent Cochrane Collaboration review combined data from 30 trials and found that exercise seemed to improve the symptoms of depression; however, a much smaller effect on depression was found when the analysis included only methodologically robust trials (Rimer et al., 2012).

The three guidelines differ in their recommendations for light therapy, but each acknowledges that although a number of studies have addressed efficacy they have notable methodologic limitations. On the basis of eight trials, the VA/DOD guideline recommends light therapy only for seasonal MDD. NICE does not recommend light therapy, arguing that studies are difficult to interpret because of equivocal results and methodologic differences. APA gives light therapy its lowest rating for strength of evidence, stating that it appeared effective for seasonal affective disorder and nonseasonal MDD generally in short-term, placebo-controlled trials. A Cochrane Collaboration review of the evidence on light therapy concluded that its benefit is modest, although promising, for nonseasonal depression, but that the results need to be interpreted with caution because of the limited data (for example, many studies were short term or lacked systematic reporting of adverse effects) and the heterogeneity of studies (Tuunainen et al., 2004).

The NICE guideline advises against any use of St John's wort for depression because of the stated uncertainty about appropriate doses, variation in potencies of preparations, and potential interactions with other drugs; however, the VA/DOD and APA guidelines suggest that use of St. John's wort may be considered for those who prefer alternative therapies. There is greater consensus about its use in mild to moderate MDD and less for use in more severe MDD (Freeman et al., 2010).

The APA Task Force on Complementary and Alternative Medicine reviewed the available data from RCTs on commonly used CAM treatments for MDD (acupuncture, omega-3 fatty acids, *S*-adenosyl methione (SAM-e), light therapy, exercise, mindfulness psychotherapies, folate, and St. John's wort). The task force's consensus was that although the treatments appear promising, more rigorous and larger studies are needed to determine whether any of them should be formally indicated for MDD (Freeman et al., 2010).

Overall, in light of the results of the guideline comparison and recent research studies, the committee concluded that the VA/DOD guideline recommends state-of-the-art treatment approaches. The one exception, as discussed above, is VA's emphasis on the use of ACT despite its lack of efficacy in treating for MDD.

## Implementation of Department of Defense and Department of Veterans Affairs Guidance for Treatment for Major Depressive Disorder

This section presents information available to the committee on the extent to which DOD and VA provide treatment for service members and veterans who have received a diagnosis of MDD. There is a striking lack of data to inform questions about the extent to which depression treatments are offered, delivered, and completed and whether they are leading to improved patient outcomes.

### Department of Defense

The AFHSC reports rates of depression treatment by using data from the PDHA and the PDHRA. In the first quarter of 2010, 67% of active-duty and reserve personnel who received a referral had a health-related clinical encounter within 180 days of return; this slightly exceeded the 2010 target referral rate of 65% (DeFraites and Vythilingam, 2011).

The DOD's Military Health System Population Health Portal, a centralized database for population health management, includes measures for assessing antidepressant medication and followup care for mental-health hospitalizations, but the committee was unable to identify results of the use of the measures. The specifications for depression-related measures are based on the Antidepressant Medication Management (AMM) measure in the Healthcare Effectiveness Data and Information Set (HEDIS) that the National Committee for Quality Assurance (NCQA) reports annually regarding the commercial, Medicare, and Medicaid markets. One measure focuses on compliance with medication regimens for treating MDD. Two rates are reported for the measure: the percentage of patients who have diagnoses of a new episode of major depression and who were treated with antidepressant medication and remained on the treatment for at least 12 weeks ("effective acute phase treatment") and the percentage who remained on medication for at least 6 months ("effective continuation phase treatment"). The other measure assesses followup therapy to patients after they have been hospitalized for mental illness. Two rates are reported for the measure: the percentage of patients who were hospitalized for selected mental-health disorders and who received followup within 7 days of discharge and the percentage who received followup within 30 days of discharge (MHSPHP, 2012).

**Department of Veterans Affairs**

VA reports that there is no mechanism for tracking the delivery of evidence-based therapies in the VA centralized databases. VHA is developing progress-note templates for evidence-based treatments that will allow documentation of care in the computerized record in a manner that will facilitate the collection of centralized aggregate data (IOM, 2012). The committee obtained the data discussed below, which suggest that many veterans are not getting necessary treatment and that most of those who are getting it are not completing the full course.

In 2006, VA contracted with Altarum Institute and RAND to conduct an independent evaluation of the quality of VA mental-health and substance-use care (Watkins and Pincus, 2011). The evaluation included several depression-related measures calculated for a cohort of veterans who had MDD and were identified for each fiscal year from FY 2004 through FY 2008. The MDD cohort selection was based on *International Classification of Diseases, Ninth Revision* codes in the administrative records and reflected at least one inpatient episode or two outpatient visits (for any mental-health or non-mental-health diagnosis) of a given patient in a given fiscal year.

In FY 2007, of patients in the MDD cohort and defined as experiencing a new treatment episode, 49% received a 12-week supply of antidepressants within 12 weeks, and 31% received a 180-day supply within 180 days. In addition, 60% of veterans in the MDD cohort who had at least one filled prescription for an antidepressant received a 12-week supply within 12 weeks. (That measure is one of the rates in the NCQA HEDIS AMM measure, which is also reported by DOD, as mentioned above.) Those results suggest that adequate followup care is needed to improve patients' adherence to treatment.

Indicators used to measure followup assessment examined whether there was documentation that a patient responded to treatment, including side effects and adherence. About one-fourth of veterans in the MDD cohort who were receiving psychotherapy had documentation of an assessment of response to psychotherapy, and 55% of those who received at least one prescription for psychiatric medications had documentation of assessment of response. Those findings reflect a need for improvement in continuing patient care and assessment once treatment is provided.

Treatment rates also appeared to be low. For the indicator used to assess use of evidenced-based treatments for MDD as documented in administrative and medical-record data, 31% of those in the MDD cohort who received psychotherapy had documentation of at least one visit for CBT (including behavioral therapy and cognitive therapy). The researchers noted that it is possible that some veterans were receiving evidence-based treatments other than those measured. For example, they were unable to assess whether veterans received IPT, an evidence-based psychotherapy often used instead of CBT.

To improve implementation of treatment regimens, VA is undertaking a national effort to disseminate throughout its health care system evidence-based psychotherapies for depression and other mental-health conditions. Since 2007, VA has been working to disseminate CBT and ACT. It began working to disseminate IPT in 2011. Competence-based training of VA mental-health care providers in the delivery of those therapies is a component of the strategic plan. Such training involves experientially based workshop training followed by weekly consultation for 6 months with an expert in the treatment (Karlin et al., 2010). As of March 31, 2010, VA has provided training for 330 VA mental-health staff in the delivery of CBT or ACT, and some staff have been trained in the delivery of both (Karlin, 2010).

Overall, the committee commends VA on its effort to improve the implementation of CBT for depression, but it questions the inclusion of ACT in the psychotherapy dissemination effort. As discussed above, there is a lack of evidence supporting ACT as a first-line treatment for MDD. The committee is confounded by VA's directive stipulating access to ACT as one of the treatments for depression (VA, 2008a) and its decision to include ACT in the national training and rollout of evidence-based psychotherapies.

### Summary

Overall, our review suggests that the screening for, diagnostic assessment of, and treatment for depression through DOD and VA is consistent with current standards and guidelines for care. The measures that are used have adequate psychometric properties and are among those advocated by experts in the field. With the exception of ACT, the VA/DOD guidelines for the assessment and treatment of depression are by and large consistent with other practice guidelines—those developed by APA and NICE—in the field. What remains questionable to the committee is how much the treatments are actually offered, delivered, and completed and whether they are leading to improved patient outcomes.

## SUBSTANCE-USE DISORDERS

The term *substance-use disorders* encompasses different substances—such as alcohol, opioids, cocaine, cannabis, prescription medications, and nicotine—and various disorders that are associated with their use, including abuse, dependence, intoxication, withdrawal, and resulting psychiatric problems. Substance *abuse* and *dependence* constitute formal diagnostic categories that are described in Chapter 4. Substance *misuse* is often used to characterize use that is thought to be clinically significant insofar as it is associated with specific adverse consequences, it but does not meet the diagnostic criteria (Kleber et al., 2006).

As prevalence data in Chapter 4 show, a substantial number of service members and veterans of OEF and OIF have had diagnoses of SUDs, and the numbers have been increasing since the conflicts began. Because SUDs have harmful effects on physical, psychologic, and social well-being, it is important to identify and evaluate people who are at risk for SUDs and to treat those who have a diagnosis of substance abuse or dependence. The goals of treatment include abstinence or reduction in substance use, relapse prevention, and improvement in psychologic and social functioning. The specific type of intervention or treatment will depend on the type of substances used, the intensity of use, and the patient's individual needs. SUDs commonly occur with other mental-health conditions (such as PTSD and depression) and with chronic medical illnesses (such as diabetes) that also require treatment. For many, a SUD is a chronic disorder that requires multiple interventions and continuing monitoring.

To assess the efficacy of current screening, assessment, and treatment approaches to SUDs in DOD and VA, the committee reviewed the *VA/DOD Clinical Practice Guideline for the Management of Substance Use Disorders (SUD), August 2009* (VA and DOD, 2009c). The

VA/DOD guideline applies to adult patients who have substance-use conditions that are treated in a VA/DOD clinical setting, including patients who have both substance-use and other health conditions and patients who have any level of severity ranging from hazardous and problematic use to SUDs. The guideline is relevant to all health care professionals who provide or direct treatment services to patients who have substance-use conditions in any VA/DOD health care setting, including specialty SUD care. The committee focused on the management of patients who have dependence on alcohol or opioids and to a smaller extent patients who have dependence on cocaine and cannabis. The committee did not address nicotine dependence in its assessment, because nicotine, although strongly linked with important medical consequences, rarely causes the behavioral or social harm seen with alcohol or illicit-drug dependence (Kleber et al., 2006).

Recently, the IOM Committee on Prevention, Diagnosis, Treatment, and Management of Substance Use Disorders in the U.S. Armed Forces completed a comprehensive assessment of the current policies and programs in place in the different branches of the military that pertain to the prevention of, screening for, diagnosis of, and treatment for SUDs in active-duty service members, members of the National Guard and reserves, and military dependents. The 2010 National Defense Authorization Act in Sec. 596 authorized the *Comprehensive Plan on Prevention, Diagnosis, and Treatment of Substance Use Disorders and Disposition of Substance Abuse Offenders in the Armed Forces*, which mandated an internal program review by DOD (DOD, 2011b) and an external review by an independent organization, such as IOM. See IOM's *Substance Use Disorders in the U.S. Armed Forces* (IOM, 2013) for all the committee's major findings and recommendations for improvements in SUD prevention, diagnosis, and treatment for active-duty service members, military dependents, and members of the reserves.

## Provision of Substance-Use Disorder Services

### Department of Defense

DOD substance-use screening, assessment, and treatment services for all beneficiaries are provided through the direct military health care system and TRICARE-authorized providers in the private sector. Current policy permits substance-use treatment in TRICARE-authorized hospitals, clinics, and certified freestanding treatment facilities. TRICARE does not cover substance-abuse care delivered in an individual provider's office and has in place yearly and lifetime limits on some forms of care that may affect the delivery of appropriate care. DOD reported to Congress that TRICARE is actively pursuing modification of the policies to expand coverage of substance-abuse treatment in primary care (DOD, 2011b).

DOD policy does not address the standardized collection of clinical and administrative data and outcome measures that would be useful for monitoring the provision of SUD prevention, diagnosis, and treatment services. Nor does it address the degree to which clinical practice recommendations related to SUD assessment and treatment are implemented (DOD, 2011b).

### Department of Veterans Affairs

VA provides SUD services in SUD-specific settings that include inpatient programs, residential rehabilitation treatment programs, outpatient programs that provide intensive treatment (at least 3 hours per day 3 days per week) or low-intensity or medication-assisted treatment services. VA also provides SUD-related care in non-SUD settings, such as primary care clinics, mental-health clinics, and specialized programs for treating PTSD (GAO, 2010).

### Prevention of Substance-Use Disorders

In IOM's *Substance Use Disorders in the U.S. Armed Forces*, the committee stated that "effective prevention has the potential to minimize the need for diagnosis, treatment, and management of SUDs and reduce the enormous social and economic costs of alcohol and drug dependence." That report cites the 2011 National Drug Control Strategy, which identifies the military personnel, veterans, and their families as important populations for receiving substance-abuse prevention services (IOM, 2013).

DOD SUD-prevention services range from individual screening and counseling services to large multimedia campaigns. Strategies include implementing policies and programs that regulate alcohol availability and pricing, deglamorize alcohol use, and promote personal responsibility and good health. Despite the military's efforts to address problems with substance use, there has been little formal evaluation of the effectiveness of programs, and program implementation is not widespread or sufficiently targeted to high-risk populations, such as service members who have PTSD (Ames and Cunradi, 2004; DOD, 2011b; Seal et al., 2011).

### Department of Defense and Department of Veterans Affairs Guidance for Screening for Substance-Use Disorders

The VA/DOD SUD guideline recommends universal screening for alcohol use; however, it does not recommend universal screening for other drug use, because there is a lack of evidence of the efficacy of screening for substances other than alcohol and tobacco (Polen et al., 2008). Neither the military nor VA conducts universal screening for the misuse of nonalcoholic substances. However, DOD policy requires drug testing (urine analysis) for a variety of illegal and legal drugs under various circumstances—in new military entrants, for probable cause, for medical reasons, and so on (DOD, 1994). In February 2012, DOD announced an expansion of its drug-testing program to include widely abused prescription medications that contain hydrocodone and benzodiazepines. Service members who have approved prescriptions for those medications will not be subject to disciplinary action for using them within the dosage and time prescribed. VA policy guidance states that health care providers should use targeted case-finding methods to identify substance use in patients and evaluate signs and symptoms of substance use in patients who have other relevant conditions, such as other mental-health disorders, hepatitis C, and HIV (VA, 2008a).

The VA/DOD SUD guideline calls for annual screening of patients in general care and mental-health care settings to identify unhealthy alcohol use. The guideline's reference to unhealthy alcohol use encompasses drinking behavior that includes severe alcohol dependence as defined by *DSM-IV* (see Chapter 4) and drinking above limits established by the National Institute on Alcohol Abuse and Alcoholism (NIAAA) (NIAAA, 2008). NIAAA recommends maximum alcohol limits of no more than 14 drinks in a week and no more than four drinks in a day for men and no more than seven drinks in a week and no more than three drinks in a day for women.[5] Drinking above the recommended limits is called risky or hazardous drinking. Figure 5.6 shows the process for screening for and initial assessment of substance use as presented in the VA/DOD guideline.

The VA/DOD guideline recommends annual screening for unhealthy alcohol use with one of two brief, standardized screening instruments: the AUDIT Consumption Questions (AUDIT-C) (Babor et al., 2001) and the version of the Single-Item Alcohol Screening Questionnaire (SASQ) recommended by NIAAA (2008).[6] The AUDIT-C comprises the first three questions on the 10-item Alcohol Use Disorders Identification Test (AUDIT), which was developed by the World Health Organization (WHO) for use in primary care settings to identify persons whose alcohol consumption has become hazardous or harmful. The three-item AUDIT-C asks about quantity and frequency of drinking and is scored on a scale of 0 to 12. The screen is considered positive for unhealthy alcohol use if the total score for a patient's responses is 4 or higher for men or 3 or higher for women. However, when the points are all from Question 1 (that is, the scores for Questions 2 and 3 are zero), a patient is considered to be drinking below recommended limits (see Box 5.6).

The version of the SASQ recommended by NIAAA comprises a single item that asks about heavy drinking in the preceding year. A positive screen is any report of having five or more drinks for men or four or more for women on an occasion in the preceding year (see Box 5.7).

For patients who screen positive or who have clinical conditions that contraindicate alcohol use, the VA/DOD guideline recommends assessing current alcohol consumption relative to NIAAA's recommended limits. If they are exceeded, brief alcohol counseling by a clinician or counselor (often termed brief intervention) is recommended. Brief interventions can be a single session or multiple sessions involving motivational interviewing techniques focused on drinking-related consequences and benefits of reducing alcohol use.

The guideline recommends referral to specialty SUD care for addiction treatment for a patient who has an AUDIT-C score of 8 or higher or who meets one of the following criteria: needs additional evaluation, does not respond to brief intervention, has a *DSM* diagnosis of alcohol or other substance dependence, or has received previous treatment for SUDs. In addition, any DOD active-duty member involved in an incident in which substance use is suspected to be a contributing factor is required to be referred to specialty SUD care for evaluation.

---

[5]NIAAA recommendations are based on definitions of a standard drink as 12 oz of beer, 5 oz of wine, and 1.5 oz of hard liquor (80-proof spirits).

[6]The AUDIT-C and SASQ are first-line screening instruments recommended by the VA/DOD guideline, but the guideline also identifies other commonly used screening tests (for example, the CAGE questionnaire augmented with the 10-item AUDIT instrument).

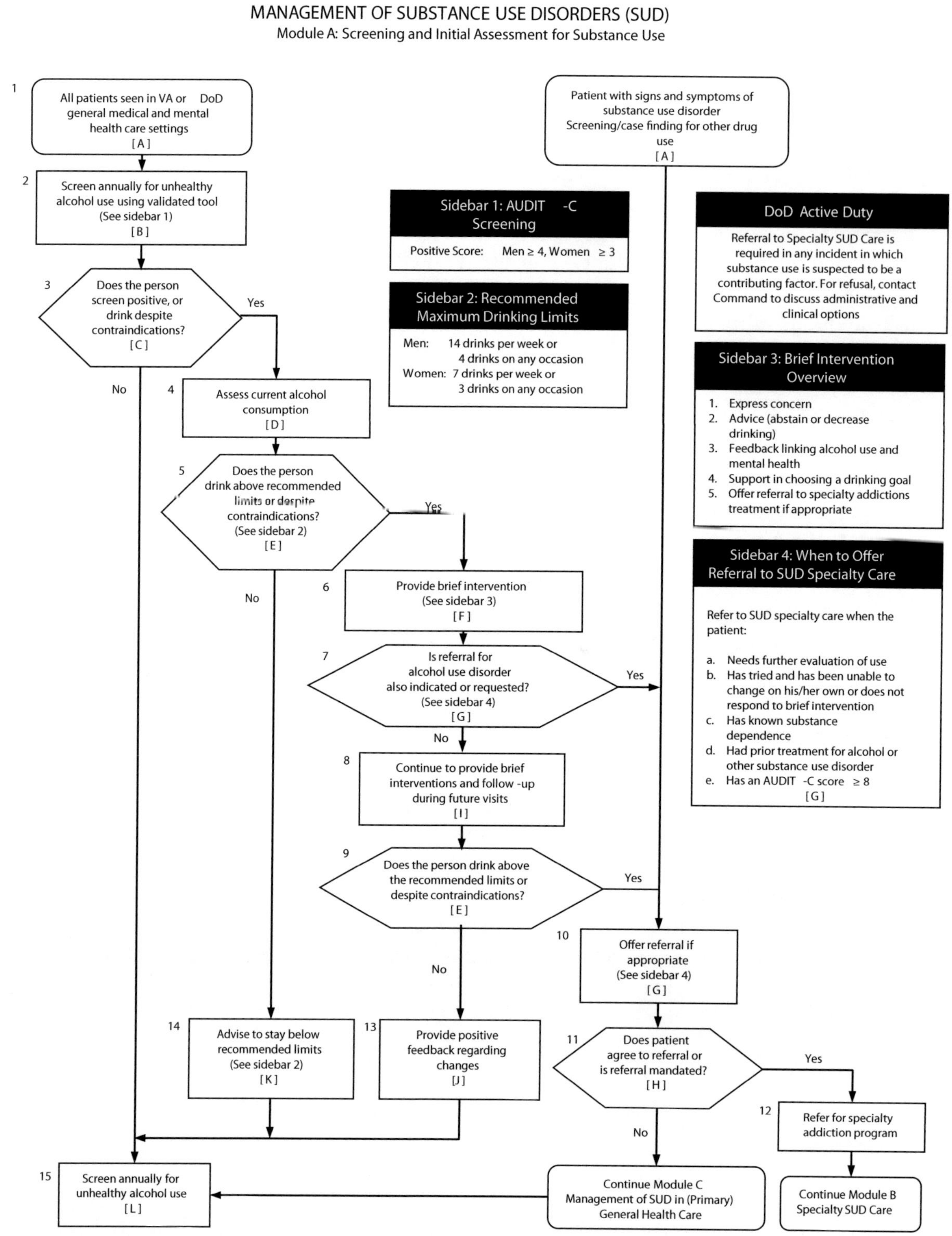


**FIGURE 5.6** Algorithm for screening for and initial assessment of substance use.
SOURCE: VA and DOD, 2009c.

**BOX 5.6**
**AUDIT Consumption Questions (AUDIT-C)**

**How often did you have a drink containing alcohol in the past year?**
0 = Never
1 = Monthly or less
2 = Two to four times per month
3 = Two to three times per week
4 = Four or more times per week

**On days in the past year when you drank alcohol how many drinks did you typically drink?**
0 = 0-2 drinks
1 = 3 or 4 drinks
2 = 5 to 6 drinks
3 = 7 to 9 drinks
4 = 10 or more drinks

**How often did you have six or more drinks on one occasion in the past year?**
0 = Never
1 = Less than monthly
2 = Monthly
3 = Weekly
4 = Daily or almost daily

SOURCE: Babor et al., 2001.

**BOX 5.7**
**Single-Item Alcohol Screening Questionnaire (SASQ)**

**Do you sometimes drink beer, wine or other alcoholic beverages?**
Yes or No
**If Yes,**
**How many times in the past year have you had…**
5 or more drinks in a day *(men)*
4 or more drinks in a day *(women)*

SOURCE: HHS, 2005.

## Department of Defense

In DOD, routine alcohol screening with the AUDIT-C occurs during DOD's periodic health assessments, the PDHA and the PDHRA, which are briefly described in the introduction to this chapter. In addition, urinalysis testing is random and applied to all personnel.

Commanders may order a drug test if there is suspicion of drug use. In May 2012, DOD also implemented new practices for its urinalysis drug testing programs to screen for some of the most commonly abused prescription medications (for example, hydrocodone and benzodiazepines). It is too early to tell whether these new measures will affect the prevalence of prescription drug abuse in the military (IOM, 2013). Screening may occur at medical appointments, but DOD does not mandate a common set of screening tools and processes in primary care settings.

### Department of Veterans Affairs

VA implemented routine screening for alcohol misuse in 2004 and since 2006 has required that the AUDIT-C be used for screening in either an outpatient or an inpatient setting. VA policy stipulates that all veterans coming to VA for the first time must be screened for alcohol misuse and again annually for patients in primary care, appropriate medical specialty care settings, and mental-health care services (VA, 2008a). In 2008, the VHA clinical-reminder tracking system used at its medical facilities incorporated the AUDIT-C questions; the system prompts clinicians to conduct appropriate followup (for example, brief intervention or referral to specialty care) on the basis of patient responses.

## Validity of Tools for Screening for Substance-Use Disorders

In 2004, the USPSTF found good evidence that screening in primary care settings can accurately identify patients whose levels or patterns of alcohol consumption place them at risk for increased morbidity and mortality. The USPSTF also found good evidence that brief behavioral-counseling interventions produce small to moderate reductions in alcohol consumption (HHS, 2004). Similarly, results of a 2007 Cochrane Collaboration meta-analysis of 22 RCTs (which enrolled 7,619 participants) showed that male but not female participants who received brief intervention had lower alcohol consumption than the control group after followup of a year or longer (Kaner et al., 2007).

### Screening, Brief Intervention, and Referral to Treatment Model

Clinical guidance for the management of SUDs developed by VA/DOD, APA (Connery and Kleber, 2007; Kleber et al., 2006), NIAAA (2008), and NICE (2011) are consistent in recommending the SBIRT model, a comprehensive mental-health approach for the prevention of and intervention in risky alcohol use. The model includes screening for at-risk drinking, providing a brief intervention, and providing referral to specialty substance-use treatment for those who have alcohol dependence (IOM, 2012a; SAMHSA, 2011).

Evidence supporting the efficacy of the SBIRT model is not yet as plentiful or compelling for drug misuse as it is for alcohol misuse. It is also important to note that the effectiveness of SBIRT programs can depend on their fidelity, application, and comprehensiveness (SAMHSA, 2011), and significant staff training and continuing monitoring are needed to sustain their effective implementation.

### Alcohol Use Disorders Identification Test-Consumption Questions

Extensive research shows that the AUDIT-C is an effective screening instrument for alcohol misuse in men and women and that the optimal screening threshold (maximizing sensitivity and specificity) for alcohol misuse is a cut score of 4 in men and a cut score of 3 in women (Bradley et al., 2003, 2007; Dawson et al., 2005).

### Single-Item Alcohol Screening Questionnaire

Findings from a cross-sectional study showed that the single screening question recommended NIAAA accurately identifies unhealthy alcohol use in a sample of primary care patients. The sensitivity and specificity (81.8% and 79.3%, respectively) of the single-question screen was comparable to that reported for longer instruments in other studies, including the AUDIT, which is among the best validated options for alcohol screening in primary care settings (Smith et al., 2009).

## Implementation of Department of Defense and Department of Veterans Affairs Guidance for Screening for Substance-Use Disorders

Below is information available to the committee on the extent to which DOD and VA are implementing and tracking screening procedures to identify possible SUD. The sparse information shows lapses in the DOD and VA's identification of and followup with patients with substance use problems. It raises concerns about how well the DOD and VA are implementing and monitoring their SUD screening practices.

### Department of Defense

DOD's internal review of SUD programs and policies (DOD, 2011b) found that with the exception of the deployment cycle, evidence-based screening tools are not consistently used among the military services. Non-active-duty service-member beneficiaries who screen positive for SUDs in primary care are probably referred to the TRICARE network, and this decreases the likelihood of patient followup for care. Furthermore, DOD stated that staff shortages may prevent adequate screening and identification of at-risk substance-use behavior, particularly during high-demand periods, such as when many service members are returning from deployment (DOD, 2011b). In IOM's *Substance Use Disorders in the U.S. Armed Forces*, the committee found that current DOD policy and screening practices to detect the use of drugs and alcohol are relatively inefficient and identify only a portion of drug users at risk for developing SUDs (IOM, 2013). That committee strongly emphasized the need for systematic and routine substance use screenings in DOD health care settings and improvements in the monitoring of prescriptions.

### Department of Veteran Affairs

Under VA's Performance Management Program, VA uses several performance measures to see whether veterans are being screened for SUD (AHRQ, 2012). The committee was unable to identify results of using those measures, and inquiries to VA about performance measures did not yield information about them.

One measure assesses the percentage of eligible patients who are seen in outpatient or inpatient settings and screened annually for alcohol misuse with the three-item AUDIT-C. Another measure assesses the percentage of veterans who are screened for alcohol misuse with AUDIT-C and meet or exceed a threshold score of 5 and who have timely brief alcohol counseling. The VA/DOD guideline indicates that although AUDIT-C scores greater than 4 points in men and greater than 3 points in women mean a positive screen, an AUDIT-C score of 5 or more is appropriate for performance measurement in a setting where brief alcohol counseling is required for everyone who screens positive for alcohol misuse.

In response to a recent GAO review of VA's provision of SUD services, VA reported that in FY 2009 about 96% of a sample of veterans seen in VA medical centers throughout the nation received the recommended screening for alcohol misuse (GAO, 2010). Although SUD screening rates in VA are high, research suggests that relatively few of those who screen positive receive guideline-recommended brief intervention, referral to treatment, or followup. In a national sample of 1,508 OEF and OIF veterans who were screened in an outpatient setting, 40% screened positive for potentially hazardous drinking. Of the veterans who had potentially hazardous drinking behavior, 31% reported being counseled to cut back on or abstain from drinking. The likelihood of risk-reduction counseling increased with the severity of alcohol misuse (higher AUDIT-C scores). Those findings are based on data collected in 2005 from the Survey of Healthcare Experiences (SHEP); the response rate was 21%, and nonresponders were more likely to be male and to have served in active-duty units vs those in the reserves or National Guard (Calhoun et al., 2008).

In another study that compared a national sample of OEF and OIF veterans with a sample of non-OEF and non-OIF veterans, researchers examined rates of documented brief interventions and rates of referrals to treatment. The study sample included outpatients who were screened for alcohol misuse in 2006–2007. About half of all the veterans who screened positive for alcohol misuse had brief interventions or referrals for treatment documented in the medical record. The difference in rates between OEF and OIF veterans (50.9%) and the other veterans (52.3%) was not statistically significant. Researchers noted one possible study limitation: the study sample reflects a period that preceded VA's implementation of a performance measure that requires documentation of brief intervention for patients who screen positive for alcohol misuse and the implementation of the electronic clinical reminder that facilitates appropriate screening and followup (Hawkins et al., 2010). In fact, a recent study found that implementation of the clinical reminder for brief interventions is associated with increases in the prevalence of documented brief alcohol interventions in VA. The percentage of patients with alcohol misuse who had documentation of brief intervention increased from 5.5% prior to the implementation of the clinical reminder to 29% after implementation (Lapham et al., 2012).

Findings from Bradley et al. (2011) suggest that many veterans, particularly black veterans, are being missed by clinical screening. Using a national sample of 6,861 patients in VA outpatient care in 2007–2008, the study compared AUDIT-C results that were documented during routine outpatient care (referred to as the "clinical screen") with AUDIT-C results collected by a mailed survey. Alcohol-screening results were considered discordant if patients screened positive on the clinical screen or on the mailed survey screen but not both. About twice as many patients screened positive for alcohol misuse on the mailed survey screen as on the clinical screen: 11.1% (765) and 5.7% (6,096), respectively. About 60% (468) screened positive on the mail survey and negative on the clinical screen. Only 1.5% (93) of patients screened negative on the mail survey and positive on the clinical screen. The researchers found that discordance was significantly higher in black patients than in white patients; however, they noted the difference might be due to a greater tendency among black patients to attempt to answer questions in a manner viewed favorably by the researchers or to variation in the administration of the AUDIT-C.

**Department of Defense and Department of Veterans Affairs Guidance for Assessment and Diagnosis of Substance-Use Disorders**

After screening for SUD, a clinical interview may be needed for further assessment of a substance-use problem against diagnostic criteria and for determination of the type and intensity of treatment needed. Figure 5.7 shows the process presented in the VA/DOD guideline for assessing, diagnosing, and treating for SUDs in a primary care setting.

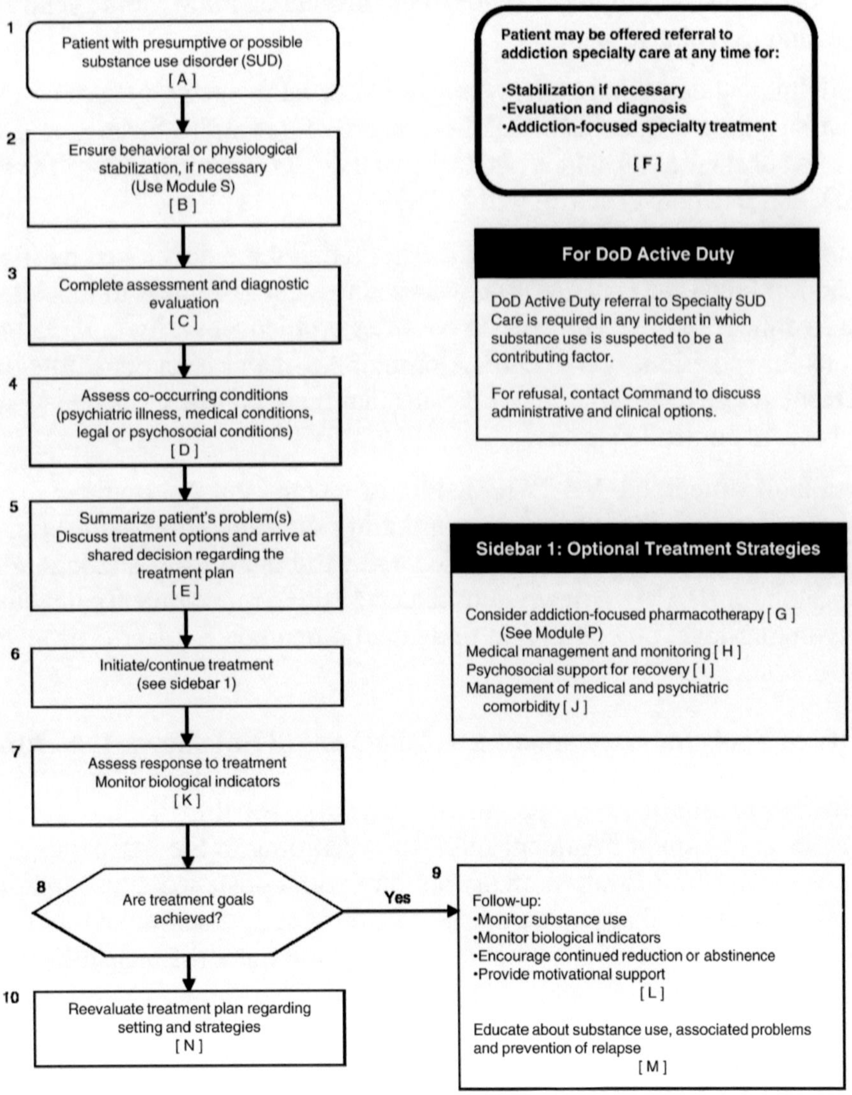


**FIGURE 5.7** Algorithm for SUD care in primary care.
SOURCE: VA and DOD, 2009c.

The VA/DOD guideline instructs providers to conduct a comprehensive biopsychosocial assessment that covers physical, emotional, cognitive, behavioral, emotional, and environmental domains. The assessment should gather information about the patient's personal and family medical, psychologic, social, and alcohol-use and drug-use history. Providers should conduct appropriate laboratory tests (for example, for sexually transmitted diseases and liver function) and a mental-status examination. The guideline emphasizes that co-occurring disorders are common with SUDs and should be identified as part of the comprehensive assessment. A provider's documented summary of the assessment serves as the basis of the treatment plan.

The guideline does not exclusively endorse the use of any particular instrument as the basis of a comprehensive assessment; however, the Addiction Severity Index (ASI) (McLellan et al., 1980) is identified as an accepted tool. The ASI is a standardized, rater-administered interview that assesses seven functional domains considered important in an overall addiction evaluation: medical status, employment status, legal problems, family and social relations, drug use, alcohol use, and psychiatric status.

The guideline indicates that patients may be referred to specialty care on the basis of the following indications for treatment: an AUDIT-C score of 8 or more for men and women, hazardous use of a substance, substance abuse, substance dependence, risk of relapse, suspected or possible SUD, and mandated referral within DOD.

The guideline identifies care-placement criteria that were developed by the American Society of Addiction Medicine (ASAM) and are used to steer providers in the determination of the appropriate treatment setting. The criteria consider problem severity in making recommendations for specific levels of care. Although ASAM criteria constitute the most widely accepted placement system, the guideline indicates that there is little evidence to support its validity on the basis of controlled trials.

After initial treatment, the VA/DOD guideline recommends periodically reassessing a patient's response to treatment (for example, continuing substance use, medication side effects, and emerging symptoms) by using a standardized and valid instrument and laboratory tests. The Brief Addiction Monitor (BAM), a newly introduced 17-item questionnaire developed by VA that measures symptom-level outcomes and functional outcomes, is offered as an example of a monitoring instrument.

## Validity of Tools for Assessment and Diagnosis of Substance-Use Disorders

The outcomes of an effective assessment are a valid, reliable diagnosis and referral to the most appropriate level of care of treatment services. According to the Substance Abuse and Mental Health Services Administration, many public-sector substance-abuse treatment systems define assessment procedures that require use of a level-of-care assessment tool (often the ASAM criteria) and a comprehensive addiction severity and outcome measure, such as the ASI (Center for Substance Abuse Treatment, 2005).

### Addiction Severity Index

The ASI, developed in VA, is considered the most widely used clinical and research assessment instrument for people who have SUDs. It is a semistructured interview used to assess SUD severity and quantifies change over time in problems commonly associated with substance abuse. In clinical settings, it is useful for treatment planning and outcome evaluation in that it identifies problems in need of targeted intervention. The ASI should be administered, scored, and interpreted by a trained technician or clinician. Good reliability and validity have been demonstrated in a variety of settings (Alcohol and Drug Abuse Institute Library, 2012). Extensive use of the ASI and changes in the SUD field over the years has revealed its limitations. Research is going on to remedy gaps in content and psychometric deficiencies (Cacciola et al., 2011).

### Addiction Medicine Patient Placement Criteria, Second Edition-Revised

As mentioned, ASAM has uniform criteria for treatment planning and placement for clients who have addiction and co-occurring disorders. The current edition, ASAM PPC-2R (Mee-Lee et al., 2001), includes criteria for comorbid mental-health and substance-related disorders. The criteria are used to match intensity of service to severity of illness in a continuum of care and to prescribe a treatment level that can accomplish treatment objectives (American Society of Addiction Medicine, 2012).

The ASAM PPC-2R has not undergone much validity testing, but it is widely accepted by public and private treatment programs and has been used to guide addiction treatment placement in more than half the states. Other placement instruments are considered simpler to use than ASAM PPC-2R but are less sensitive to the needs of people who have SUDs and do not differentiate between mental and substance-related symptoms (Center for Substance Abuse Treatment, 2005).

### Brief Addiction Monitor

As a treatment monitoring instrument, the BAM, if fully implemented, could be used to evaluate outcomes and effectiveness of SUD treatments throughout the VA system (GAO, 2010). The first study to evaluate the BAM's psychometric properties revealed good validity (Cacciola et al., 2012), but further research is warranted.

## Implementation of Department of Defense and Department of Veterans Affairs Guidance for Assessment and Diagnosis of Substance-Use Disorders

This section presents information available to the committee on the extent to which DOD and VA conduct followup and evaluation of service members and veterans who have positive SUD screens. The information shows significant gaps in DOD and VA SUD assessment and referral to treatment. The significant number of service members and veterans who are at risk of SUD but are not receiving needed interventions is a serious concern.

### Department of Defense

DOD is missing opportunities to intervene with service members who have high levels of drug or alcohol consumption. Data shows that treatment providers may fail to identify at-risk substance users who need referral to specialty care. Additionally, many patients may be offered a referral, but choose not to accept it, or encounter barriers, such as concerns about confidentiality, that prevent visits to specialty care (Glass et al., 2010; Milliken et al., 2007). In FY 2010, there were over 24,000 referrals of soldiers to the Army Substance Abuse Program; of those referred, about 50% enrolled. Although 12% of soldiers reported alcohol problems on the PDHRA, only 2% have been referred for further evaluation or treatment (Department of the Army, 2012). Among soldiers returning from Iraq, Milliken et al. (2007) found that soldiers frequently reported alcohol problems but were rarely referred for alcohol treatment and were infrequently followed up. Of 56,350 active-duty soldiers, 6,669 (11.8%) endorsed alcohol misuse, 134 (0.2%) were referred, and only 29 were seen within 90 days (Milliken et al., 2007). Some of the possible reasons cited include the stigma associated with receiving any form of mental-health care and concerns related to present military policies; SUD treatment triggers involvement of a soldier's commander, and failure to comply with the treatment program can have adverse career ramifications (Burnett-Zeigler et al., 2011; Milliken et al., 2007).

In response to the concerns over confidentiality and possible stigma, the Army implemented a pilot program, Confidential Alcohol Treatment and Education Pilot (CATEP), which allows service members to refer themselves for alcohol-abuse treatment without notifying their chains of command. In its *Comprehensive Plan*, DOD reported that it will evaluate the findings from CATEP to determine the effect of waiving the policy requirement for command notification (unless a soldier's condition poses a threat to safety, security, or mission) (DOD, 2011b). Under current DOD policy for active-duty members, clinical providers convene with command to review the treatment plan and goals. Service members who fail to engage in recommended treatment are informed that such a decision could result in involuntary separation from military service.

### Department of Veteran Affairs

In VA, rates of referral to SUD treatment indicate a large number of veterans with alcohol misuse appear not to be receiving referrals. Hawkins et al. (2010) reported that half the veterans who screened positive for alcohol misuse had a documented brief intervention or referral to alcohol treatment. In GAO's assessment of VA's SUD services, providers reported that limitation in resources was a factor in decisions about referrals for treatment (GAO, 2010).

## Department of Defense and Department of Veterans Affairs Guidance for Treatment for Substance-Use Disorders

### Withdrawal Management

Detoxification and withdrawal management is often a necessary first step toward treatment of those who have SUDs. The VA/DOD guideline defines withdrawal management from a substance as "non-pharmacologic and/or pharmacologic medical care with a goal of safely transitioning a patient from active use to sustained treatment for the patient's substance use disorder."

Pharmacologically supervised withdrawal is warranted only for alcohol, sedative hypnotics, and opioids; it is not warranted for stimulant and cannabis disorders.

For inpatient treatment for alcohol withdrawal, the VA/DOD guideline recommends the use of benzodiazepines as first-line treatment with other agents (such as beta-blockers and clonidine) as adjuncts in some patients. For opioid withdrawal, the guideline recommends initial stabilization and then short or extended tapering with buprenorphine and naloxone or methadone in 4–7 days in an inpatient setting. Withdrawal management should be followed by appropriate pharmacologic maintenance or behavioral therapies.

### Addiction-Focused Treatment

In general, the VA/DOD guideline recommends the use of addiction-focused pharmacotherapy and psychosocial treatments after patients who were dependent on alcohol or opioids have undergone successful withdrawal.

Figure 5.8 shows the process presented in the VA/DOD guideline for treating patients who have a diagnosis of SUD with medications.

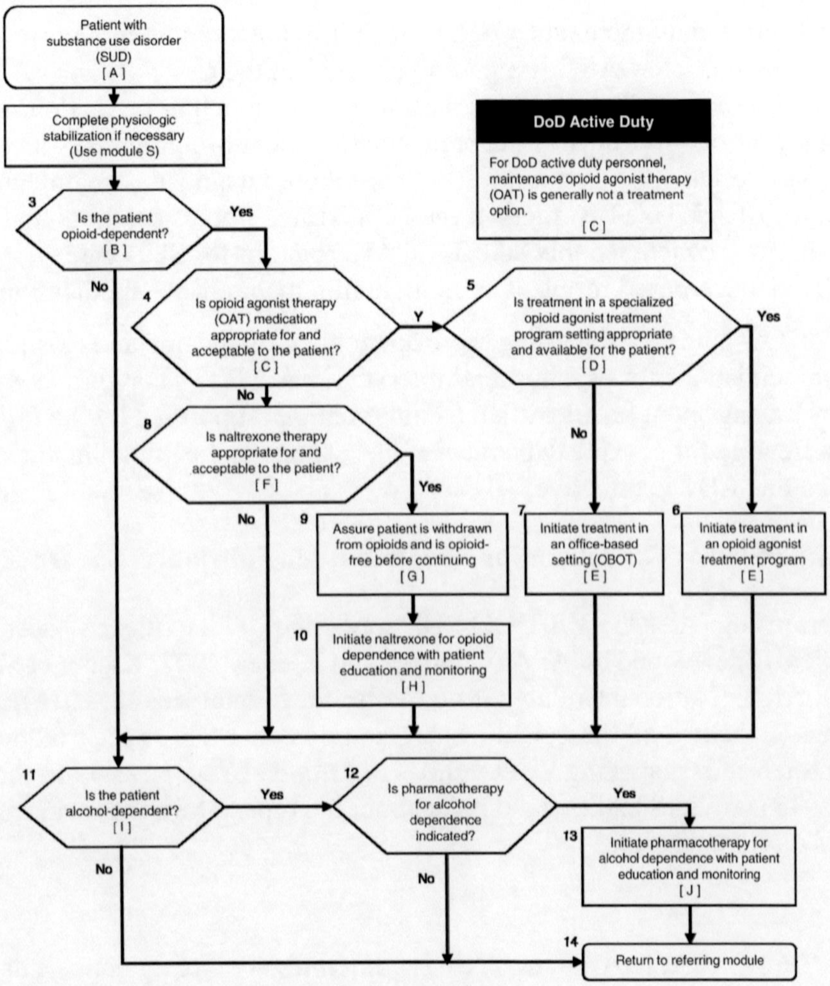


**FIGURE 5.8** Algorithm for addiction-focused pharmacotherapy.
SOURCE: VA and DOD, 2009c.

For patients with alcohol-use disorders (AUDs), the first-line pharmacotherapies recommended by the VA/DOD guideline are oral naltrexone and/or acamprosate[7]; both are FDA approved for this indication. The guideline discusses psychosocial interventions that research has shown to be effective: behavioral couples counseling, cognitive behavioral coping skills training, community reinforcement, motivational enhancement, and 12-step facilitation.

For patients who are dependent on opioids, the VA/DOD guideline recommends as first-line treatment methadone or the sublingual combination product of buprenorphine and naloxone. Those drugs are used in opioid-agonist treatment (OAT), which consists of administering one of the opioid-agonist medications in combination with a variety of medical, counseling, and rehabilitative services. OAT can be delivered through a VHA-licensed OAT clinic or through office-based treatment; however, buprenorphine is the only medication approved for office-based OAT. As adjunct interventions in pharmacotherapy, the guideline identifies cognitive behavioral therapy (CBT) and contingency management as effective psychosocial therapies for opioid dependence.

[7]The guideline recommends injectable naltrexone when medication adherence is an important concern.

For DOD active-duty members, OAT is generally not a treatment option. DOD has reported to Congress that TRICARE is pursuing changes in the *Code of Federal Regulations* that would permit the use of opioid agonists and partial agonists (such as methadone and buprenorphine) for opioid-dependence maintenance treatment of non-active-duty beneficiaries (DOD, 2011b). The recent IOM Committee on Prevention, Diagnosis, Treatment, and Management of Substance Use Disorders in the U.S. Armed Forces supports that change in policy. That committee concluded that "the TRICARE benefit for SUD care should provide coverage for all evidence-based forms of care, including maintenance medications" (IOM, 2013).

The VA/DOD guidance regarding the management of cocaine and marijuana use is limited to recommendations for psychosocial interventions. CBT, behavioral couples therapy, and contingency management are identified as interventions supported by the most evidence of effectiveness in treating for cocaine dependence. For cannabis, the guideline indicates that there is some evidence that CBT is effective.

## Comparison of Guidelines for Treatment for Substance-Use Disorders

This section compares the VA/DOD SUD guidelines with evidence-based CPGs for the management of SUD developed by APA (Connery and Kleber, 2007; Kleber et al., 2006), NIAAA (2008), NICE (National Collaborating Centre for Mental Health, 2011), and WHO (2009). As discussed below, all the guidelines are mainly consistent in their recommendations for specific treatments for managing SUD. IOM's *Substance Use Disorders in the U.S. Armed Forces* (IOM, 2013) provides additional details about the types of SUD pharmacotherapies and psychotherapies discussed below.

### Alcohol

The VA/DOD, APA, NIAAA, and NICE guidelines are largely consistent in their recommendations for specific treatments for managing alcohol dependence. Standard clinical practice for treatment for alcohol dependence supports the use of complementary approaches—medications, professional counseling, and mutual help groups—to address the neurobiologic, psychologic, and social aspects of alcohol dependence. Table 5.4 compares treatment recommendations of these guidelines and their various systems for indicating their strength.

**TABLE 5.4** Summary of Guideline Recommendations for Treating for Alcohol-Use Disorders

| Treatment Modality | VA/DOD | APA | NIAAA | NICE |
|---|---|---|---|---|
| Management of withdrawal | | | | |
| Thiamine | | I | ✓ | ✓ |
| Benzodiazepines | A | I | ✓ | ✓ |
| Anticonvulsants, beta adrenergic blockers or antipsychotics agents | C (adjunct therapy) | II (adjunct therapy) | ✓ (adjunct therapy) | |
| Psychotherapy | | | | |
| Motivational Interventions | First line | I | ✓ | ✓ |
| Twelve Step Facilitation (TSF)/Mutual-help groups (e.g., Alcoholics Anonymous) | First line | I | ✓ | ✓ |
| Cognitive behavioral therapy (CBT) | First line | I | ✓ | ✓ |
| Couple/marital-focused therapies | First line | I | ✓ | ✓ |

| Treatment Modality | VA/DOD | APA | NIAAA | NICE |
|---|---|---|---|---|
| Community reinforcement approach | First line | I | ✓ | ✓ |
| Group therapy | | II | | |
| Pharmacotherapy | | | | |
| Naltrexone | A | I | ✓ | First line |
| Acamprosate | A | I | ✓ | First line |
| Disulfiram | B | II | ✓ | Second line |
| Topiramate | | | ✓ | |

NOTE: VA/DOD: A = good evidence that the intervention improved outcomes; B = a fair amount of evidence supported the use of the intervention; C = the working group did not make a recommendation for or against the routine use of the intervention as the risk-benefit ratio was too close to make a general recommendation; D = presence of evidence that either the intervention was harmful or the risks outweighed the benefits offered by it; I = evidence was lacking, of insufficient quality, or conflicting; therefore, a recommendation could not be made for or against providing the treatment routinely. APA: I = intervention recommended with substantial clinical confidence; II = intervention recommended with moderate clinical confidence; III = intervention recommended on the basis of individual circumstances. NIAAA and NICE: No rating system was used. For purposes of this report, √ denotes that use of the treatment was recommended.

*Pharmacotherapy*

The VA/DOD, APA, NIAAA, and NICE guidelines are consistent in recommending the use of benzodiazepines for the management of alcohol withdrawal before the initiation of treatment for alcohol dependence. The VA/DOD guideline is the only one that does not mention the administration of thiamine. All guidelines except NICE also suggest the use of anticonvulsants, beta adrenergic blockers, or antipsychotics as adjuncts to benzodiazepines in treatment for alcohol-withdrawal syndrome.

All the guidelines state that after successful withdrawal by people who have moderate or severe alcohol dependence, medications for alcohol dependence used in conjunction with brief support or more extensive psychosocial therapy can be effective in primary care and specialty care medical settings.

FDA has approved three medications for the treatment of alcohol dependence: disulfiram, acamprosate, and naltrexone (in daily oral and monthly injectable formulations). Those medications for alcohol-dependent patients have well-established efficacy. They have been shown to help patients to reduce drinking, avoid relapse to heavy drinking, and achieve and maintain abstinence (NIAAA, 2008).

Each guideline recommends naltrexone and acamprosate as first-line pharmacologic treatments for alcohol dependence. Disulfiram is considered to be an effective adjunct to a comprehensive treatment program for patients who are motivated to abstain. NIAAA is the only guideline that suggests the use of topiramate, an anticonvulsant, to treat for alcohol dependence; it notes that FDA has not approved the drug for this purpose. The NICE guideline indicates that the evidence does not show an advantage of topiramate over other pharmacologic interventions for alcohol dependence. Several reviews of the evidence have concluded that topiramate is more efficacious than placebo in reducing drinking and improving other self-reported drinking outcomes. However, results of controlled trials reveal topiramate-induced adverse side effects, and this suggests that more research is needed to determine optimal dosing strategies to minimize side effects while maximizing therapeutic benefit (Arbaizar et al., 2010; Johnson and Ait-Daoud, 2010; Shinn and Greenfield, 2010).

The guidelines are in agreement that there is no evidence that combining any of the medications to treat alcohol dependence improves outcomes over the use of any one medication alone, according to the Combining Medications and Behavioral Interventions (COMBINE) clinical trial sponsored by NIAAA (Anton et al., 2006).

*Psychotherapy*

All the guidelines are in agreement that pharmacotherapy for alcohol dependence is most effective when combined with behavioral counseling that is focused on encouraging abstinence, adherence to the medication, and participation in community support groups. The guidelines indicate that there is evidence of the effectiveness of a number of psychosocial interventions for treatment for AUD, including CBT, couples therapy, community reinforcement, and couple or marital-focused therapies. There is no clear evidence that any one of those approaches is the treatment of choice or can be accurately matched to specific patient characteristics (VA and DOD, 2009c).

All the guidelines recommend that clinicians use motivational techniques during therapeutic encounters with patients and encourage patient participation in 12-step programs, such as Alcoholics Anonymous, which research has found to be associated with improved addiction outcomes compared with baseline (VA and DOD, 2009c). Twelve-step facilitation (TSF) refers to formal psychotherapy administered by a professional that is intended to foster a patient's active participation in Alcoholics Anonymous or other 12-step mutual-help programs. The NICE guideline states that the evidence is not strong enough to support motivational techniques or TSF as stand-alone alcohol-treatment interventions.

Only the NICE guideline offers specific guidance for the delivery of psychologic interventions, for example, that CBT and behavioral couples therapy should usually consist of one 60-minute session per week for 12 weeks and community reinforcement of eight 50-minute sessions over 12 weeks.

**Opioids**

The VA/DOD, APA, and WHO guidelines are mainly consistent in their recommendations for specific treatments for opioid dependence. Standard treatment is the use of OAT combined with psychosocial interventions. Table 5.5 compares treatment recommendations of these guidelines and their various systems for indicating their strength.

*Pharmacotherapy*

For medically supervised opioid withdrawal, the VA/DOD, APA, and WHO guidelines recommend the substitution of the opioid with methadone, buprenorphine, or buprenorphine combined with naloxone and then gradual tapering. The APA and WHO guidelines also support the use of clonidine to reduce the severity of opioid-withdrawal symptoms. The APA guideline states that the use of clonidine combined with naltrexone has been demonstrated to be a safe and effective approach for rapid detoxification.

**TABLE 5.5** Summary of Guideline Recommendations for Treating for Opioid Dependence

| Treatment Modality | VA/DOD | APA | WHO |
|---|---|---|---|
| Management of withdrawal | | | |
| Buprenorphine or Buprenorphine/naloxone | B | I | ✓ |
| Methadone | B | I | ✓ |
| Clonidine or clonidine/naltrexone | | II | ✓ |
| Psychotherapy | | | |
| Cognitive behavioral therapy (CBT) | adjunct | II (adjunct) | ✓ (adjunct) |
| Contingency management | adjunct | II (adjunct) | ✓ (adjunct) |
| Psychodynamic therapy | | III (adjunct) | |
| Self-help groups | | III (adjunct) | |
| Family therapy | | III (adjunct) | |
| Pharmacotherapy | | | |
| Methadone | A (first-line) | I | First line |
| Buprenorphine | A (first-line buprenorphine/ naloxone combo) | I | Second line |
| Naltrexone | C | I | ✓ |

NOTE: VA/DOD: A = good evidence that the intervention improved outcomes; B = a fair amount of evidence supported the use of the intervention; C = the working group did not make a recommendation for or against the routine use of the intervention as the risk-benefit ratio was too close to make a general recommendation; D = presence of evidence that either the intervention was harmful or the risks outweighed the benefits offered by it; I = evidence was lacking, of insufficient quality, or conflicting; therefore, a recommendation could not be made for or against providing the treatment routinely. APA: I = intervention recommended with substantial clinical confidence; II = intervention recommended with moderate clinical confidence; III = intervention recommended on the basis of individual circumstances. WHO: No rating system was used. For purposes of this report, √ denotes that use of the treatment was recommended.

The VA/DOD, APA, and WHO guidelines recommend maintenance treatment with methadone or buprenorphine as the primary treatment for opioid dependence. Maintenance treatment with naltrexone is considered an alternative strategy for preventing relapse although all the guidelines indicate that naltrexone's value is often limited by the lack of patient adherence and low treatment retention.

*Psychotherapy*

All three guidelines consider psychosocial treatment—primarily CBT and contingency management—effective as a component of a comprehensive treatment plan for patients who have opioid dependence. A recent review by the Cochrane Collaboration found that there was not enough evidence to conclude that psychosocial treatments alone are adequate to treat people for opioid abuse and dependence (Mayet et al., 2005).

**Cannabis**

There is no evidence that supports the use of any specific pharmacotherapy for marijuana withdrawal or dependence. Although further study of psychosocial therapies for treatment for marijuana dependence is necessary, studies suggest that adding contingency management to behavioral interventions is efficacious in reducing marijuana use (Budney et al., 2000).

**Stimulants**

No pharmacologic treatment for people who are dependent on stimulants, such as cocaine and amphetamines, is approved by FDA. Research to determine the most efficacious psychosocial interventions for reducing use of stimulants is still evolving. The Cochrane Collaboration reviewed 27 RCTs of the efficacy of psychosocial treatments for dependence on cocaine, amphetamine, and other stimulants. Comparisons of interventions favored treatment with some form of contingency management to reduce the use of stimulants (Knapp et al., 2007).

## Implementation of Department of Defense and Department of Veterans Affairs Guidance for Treatment for Substance-Use Disorders

This section presents information available to the committee on the extent to which DOD and VA provide treatment for service members and veterans who have diagnoses of SUD. There is a striking lack of data to inform questions about the extent to which SUD treatments are offered, delivered, and completed and about whether they are leading to improved patient outcomes. The available data show that many service members and veterans in need of SUD treatment are not receiving it.

**Department of Defense**

As discussed previously, referral rates for treatment of service member are very low (Department of the Army, 2012; Milliken et al., 2007); consequently, few service members are receiving treatment. A 2009 survey of 585 Michigan Army National Guard service members returning from Iraq and Afghanistan found that 36% met the criteria for alcohol misuse according to the AUDIT (10-item screen). Of the 36%, 31% reported receiving any mental-health services in the preceding year, but only 2.5% reported receiving specific substance-abuse treatment. The researchers pointed to other research that suggested the stigma attached to receiving mental-health treatment is a reason for the low rates of treatment (Burnett-Zeigler et al., 2011).

On the basis of TRICARE data on pharmacological SUD treatments for active-duty service members diagnosed with SUD, the earlier IOM committee declared, "It is apparent that the use of these medications is not an integral part of SUD treatment for most individuals despite the evidence for their effectiveness" (IOM, 2012). That committee found

> when one compares the number of ADSMs diagnosed with alcohol use disorders (6,175) with the number who received either naltrexone (1,034, some of which would have been prescribed for alcohol dependence, but some for opioid dependence), antabuse (605), and camparal (619), it is clear that many individuals with alcohol use disorders did not receive medication therapy. Among those diagnosed with drug use disorders (2,900), only 400 were prescribed buprenorphine.

**Department of Veteran Affairs**

VA reports that there is no mechanism for tracking the delivery of evidence-based therapies in the VA centralized databases. VHA is developing progress-note templates for evidence-based treatments that will allow documentation of care in the computerized record in a manner that will facilitate the collection of centralized aggregate data (IOM, 2012). The committee obtained the data discussed below, which suggest that many veterans are not getting necessary treatment and that most of those who are getting it are not completing the full course.

In 2006, VA contracted with Altarum Institute and the RAND Corporation to conduct an independent evaluation of the quality of VA mental-health and substance-use care (Watkins and Pincus, 2011). One aspect of the study assessed the availability of evidenced-based practices related to SUDs by using VA facility survey data collected in May 2007 and October 2009. The Altarum–RAND team administered surveys to 139 parent-facility service areas (PFSAs).[8] Although there was substantial growth in the availability of OAT (with either buprenorphine or methadone) among PFSAs, from 45% to 81%, the researchers concluded that OAT may warrant more widespread implementation inasmuch as it is available in fewer than 90% of the PFSAs. The availability of intensive outpatient treatment for SUD dropped slightly from 95% of the PFSAs in 2007 to 91% in 2009. Psychosocial interventions for SUD had a high rate of availability and remained stable from 2007 to 2009, in 98% and 99% of PFSAs, respectively.

The Altarum–RAND team collected data on three performance measures that address use of evidence-based practices for treatment for SUD as documented in VA medical records and administrative data. The SUD-related measures were calculated for a cohort of veterans who had SUD and were identified for each fiscal year from FY 2004 through FY 2008.[9] For FY 2007, the study team observed low rates of relapse-prevention therapy, maintenance pharmacotherapy, and contingency management in veterans in the SUD cohort. Specifically, about one-fifth of patients in the SUD cohort (21.5%) received psychotherapy with documentation of relapse-prevention therapy, one-fourth (24.8%) in the SUD cohort that had opiate dependence had documentation that maintenance pharmacotherapy was offered or contraindicated within 30 days of a new treatment episode, and only 1.0% had documentation that they had received contingency management.

Regarding rates of pharmacotherapy for opioid dependence, another recent study by Oliva et al. found similar rates for FY 2008 (27.3% of those with an opioid-use disorder) and substantial facility-level variability in the proportion of patients who were treated with OAT, ranging from 0% to 66%. Slightly over 40% of facilities treated under 5% of their patients with OAT (Oliva et al., 2012). It should be noted that both this study and the Altarum–RAND evaluation were conducted before the VHA national mandate of access to buprenorphine OAT established by the VHA handbook *Uniform Mental Health Services in VA Medical Centers and Clinics* (VA, 2008a).

---

[8]The study team defined a PFSA as VA service area that is anchored, in most cases, by a VA medical center and supporting community-based outpatient clinics. PFSAs have nonoverlapping geographic areas of responsibility.
[9]The SUD-cohort selection was based on *International Classification of Diseases, Ninth Revision* codes in the administrative records and reflected at least one inpatient episode or two outpatient visits (for any mental-health or non-mental-health diagnosis) in a given fiscal year.

The Altarum–RAND evaluation found that in FY 2007 about 15% of veterans in the SUD cohort who were in a new treatment episode[10] initiated treatment within the first 2 weeks of the episode, and about 14% became engaged with treatment (defined as two or more outpatient visits) within a month of the new treatment episode. One-fourth received followup care within 90 days of the new treatment episode. On those measures, the data showed statistically significant variation by sex: women had higher rates of treatment initiation, treatment engagement, and treatment followup. There was also statistically significant variation in all three indicators by OEF or OIF status.

Another measure related to treatment engagement, collected in VA's Performance Management Program, is the percentage of patients who maintain treatment involvement for at least 90 days after beginning a new treatment episode. In FY 2009 about 52% of veterans who entered VA specialty SUD treatment programs stayed in them for at least 90 days (GAO, 2010). However, a recent study raised a question about the utility of this measure: an analysis of patient-level data found that it was not associated with improvements in clinical outcomes (Harris et al., 2009).

Regarding types of treatment interventions provided to veterans who are alcohol-dependent, the Altarum–RAND evaluation found that 71.3% had documentation of a brief intervention, current specialty care, or a completed referral to specialty mental-health care during FY 2007 and that 16.4% had documentation in the medical record that pharmacotherapy (naltrexone, disulfiram, or acamprosate) was offered or contraindicated within 30 days of a new treatment episode.

Other studies corroborate the underuse of medications for AUD in VA. Harris et al. (2010) examined pharmacy-record data to determine the rate at which patients fill prescriptions for naltrexone, disulfiram, or acamprosate. Of the roughly one-fourth of a million VHA patients who have AUDs, 3% filled at least one prescription for those medications in FY 2007. The rate was 3.4% in FY 2009 (Harris et al., 2012).

Possible reasons for the underuse of pharmacotherapies for alcohol and opioid dependence in the VA may include providers' lack of awareness of or training in pharmacotherapy and reluctance to use them (GAO, 2010).

The present committee notes that to improve implementation of treatment regimens, VA has made extensive efforts to train clinicians in specialty substance-use care to deliver evidence-based therapies, such as CBT and contingency management (Karlin et al., 2010); however, there have been relatively few efforts to evaluate outcomes or to document the quality of implementation of treatment.

**Summary**

Overall, the VA/DOD guidelines for the management of SUD reflect evidence-based approaches to screening and assessment of and treatment for SUD. Taken together, the research studies and policy assessments of the effectiveness of practices in the military and VA show that more needs to done to improve dissemination of the practices, to understand the barriers to improvements in care for SUDs, and to determine which practices produce the best clinical

---

[10]Defined by either the exacerbation of a condition that requires psychiatric inpatient care or the initiation of outpatient treatment after a break of 5 or more months without care.

outcomes. VA has recently undertaken a number of national efforts to improve its SUD services that, according to VA officials, may address multiple challenges that VA faces in providing SUD services. VA's efforts include increasing access to SUD services, promoting evidence-based treatments for SUDs, and assessing SUD services and monitoring treatment effectiveness.

## SUICIDAL IDEATION

Suicide is a leading cause of deaths of US service members (Trofimovich et al., 2012). Research has shown that unrecognized or untreated mental-health disorders are a major risk factor for suicide in the general population. At least 90% of people who die by suicide have a mental illness at the time of their death. The most common is MDD, followed by SUD, but almost all the psychiatric disorders are associated with increased suicide rates (Moscicki, 2001). Data from the DOD Suicide Event Report, the standardized suicide-surveillance effort throughout the services, illustrate the relationship between psychiatric problems and suicide attempts and suicide in military members. Of the 863 service members who attempted suicide in 2010, 63.7% had a history of at least one documented psychiatric disorder, and 37.3% had at least two co-occurring diagnoses. Nearly 40% of service members who attempted suicide had a diagnosis of a mood disorder, most frequently MDD (17.7%), and 26.07% had a diagnosis of anxiety disorder, most frequently PTSD (8.1%); 23.4% had a known history of substance abuse; fewer than 10% had documentation of personality disorders; and fewer than 5% had sustained a TBI (2.43%) or had a diagnosis of psychotic disorder (1.27%). The rates of psychiatric disorders are slightly lower in the 281 military members who died by suicide in 2010. Slightly over 40% had a history of at least one documented behavioral-health disorder, and one-fourth had at least two co-occurring diagnoses (DCoE, 2011d). Although those rates are informative, the rates of undetected psychiatric disorders in service members who either attempted suicide or died by suicide are unclear. Chapter 4 further defines the scope of the problem of suicide in military and veteran populations by presenting rates of suicide and suicide attempts; it also provides details about risk factors for suicide and suicidal ideation.

In this section, to assess the efficacy of current screening, assessment, and treatment approaches for suicidal ideation, the committee examines a number of major clinical guidelines, policy directives, and research studies related to the management of suicidal ideation in DOD and VA populations. As noted previously, VA and DOD have collaborated in the development of CPGs for several health conditions, including TBI, PTSD, MDD, and SUDs. Those CPGs address the assessment of suicidality as only one component of the management of the diagnostic condition without a focus on the management of suicidality as the core issue. There is no joint VA/DOD evidence-based CPG specifically for assessing and treating patients who have suicidal thoughts and behaviors, but such a guideline is under development. VA and DOD have chartered a working group to draft a joint VA/DOD CPG that will provide clinicians with evidence-based guidance on the assessment and management of a person who has suicidal ideation (Woodson, 2011).

In DOD, the *Air Force Guide for Managing Suicidal Behavior* (*MSB*) is a recognized example of DOD clinical guidance (Air Force Medical Operations Agency, undated; DOD, 2010a). Noting the variability in clinical practices for the management of suicidal behaviors among the services, the DOD Task Force on the Prevention of Suicide by Members of the

Armed Forces recommended the development of clinical practice standards to promote systemwide use of evidence-based practices (DOD, 2010a).

## Suicide-Related Terminology

The use of standardized suicide-related terminology for the purposes of clinical care, surveillance, and research is a fundamental issue in the literature on suicide and suicidal ideation. A 2002 IOM report on reducing suicide in the nation emphasized the need for universally accepted definitions for suicide and suicidal behaviors to facilitate efforts in the field (IOM, 2002). Echoing the need for standardization, a 2008 VA-chartered Blue Ribbon Work Group on Suicide Prevention in the Veteran Population recommended that VHA collaborate with other federal agencies to create uniform definitions (Blue Ribbon Work Group on Suicide Prevention in the Veteran Population, 2008). In response, VA collaborated with the Centers for Disease Control and Prevention (CDC) to develop the Self-Directed Violence Classification System (SDVCS). Both VA and DOD have adopted the classification system as the basis of data collection and reporting and eventually for the purpose of risk assessment and case management (Brenner et al., 2011; DCoE, 2011a).

The SDVCS defines two types of self-directed violence—thoughts and behaviors—and defines various characteristics associated with each, including whether the thoughts and behaviors are suicide related. The nomenclature uses the term *suicidal ideation* to describe thoughts of engaging in suicide-related behavior. The thoughts may or may not involve suicidal intent, which is defined as the presence of "past or present evidence (implicit or explicit) that an individual wishes to die, means to kill him/herself, and understands the probable consequences of his/her actions or potential actions." Suicidal behavior encompasses the "acts or preparation toward self-directed violence," "behavior that is self-directed and deliberately results in injury or the potential for injury to oneself," and "evidence, whether implicit or explicit, of suicidal intent." Suicide is death caused by self-directed injurious behavior with any intent to die as a result of the behavior (Brenner et al., 2011).

## Suicide Prevention

The DOD and VA have many programs, policies, and interventions in place to prevent and manage suicidal ideation in service members and veterans. Bagley et al. (2010) systematically reviewed the state of evidence on suicide prevention for military and veteran populations. The researchers identified seven studies of military personnel containing interventions that may reduce the risk of suicide. Their review found that multifaceted interventions for active duty military personnel are supported by consistent evidence, although of very mixed quality. There were insufficient studies of US veterans to reach conclusions. The Blue Ribbon Work Group produced an overview of key components of VA's suicide-prevention strategy (Blue Ribbon Work Group on Suicide Prevention in the Veteran Population, 2008).

RAND conducted an assessment of DOD suicide-prevention programs offered by each military service (Ramchand et al., 2011). Its report covers an array of suicide interventions that address primary prevention (targeting the entire population), secondary prevention (targeting selected groups on the basis of common risk factors), indicated prevention (targeting people who have detectable symptoms), and dimensions of self-care and environmental safety (limiting lethal means) and postvention (interventions for survivors and bereaved after a suicide loss).

Ramchand et al. (2011) indicate there is evidence that restricting access to lethal means is an effective way to prevent suicide and conclude that suicide-prevention programs should limit gun availability to persons deemed to be at high risk of suicide.

**Restricting Access to Lethal Means**

As discussed in Freeman et al. (2003), research shows unequivocal evidence of an association between firearm possession and increased risk of suicide. Guns are the primary method of suicide by service members and veterans; these groups are known to have high rates of gun ownership (Claassen and Knox, 2011). A recent population-based study of veterans found that they were twice as likely as nonveterans to die by suicide and 58% more likely than nonveterans to use firearms rather than other suicide methods to end their lives (Kaplan et al., 2007). According to the DOD Suicide Event Report program for calendar year 2010, of the 281 military members in all services who died by suicide, 175 (62%) used firearms to kill themselves. Of those who used firearms, 136 (78%) used non-military-issue firearms, and a much smaller number, 39, used military-issue firearms. That underscores the importance of assessing and addressing access to non-military-issue firearms, as well as military-issue firearms, by people who are at risk for suicide (DCoE, 2011d).

International experts who reviewed the literature on suicide-prevention interventions have concluded that restriction of access to lethal means is one of the few suicide-prevention policies that has proven effectiveness. A systematic review on suicide prevention by Mann et al. (2005) concluded that among methods used to reduce suicide (physician education, restricting lethal means, public education, screening programs, and mass-media education), restricting access to lethal methods and education of physicians in MDD recognition and treatment were found to prevent suicide.

As discussed later, DOD gun-safety protocols for military-issued weapons exist, but the guidance on lethal-means counseling and restricting gun access is vague. Current DOD policy does not have provisions for restricting access to privately owned firearms for those believed to be at risk for suicide. In fact, the FY 2011 National Defense Authorization Act (PL 111-383, Section 1062) prohibits the secretary of defense from issuing any regulation or policy on legally owned personal firearms or ammunition kept by troops or civilian employees off base and from collecting any information on their guns or ammunition.[11] More recently, however, DOD military leaders have been quoted in the popular press as stating that they are considering policy that "will allow separation of privately owned firearms from those believed to be at risk of suicide" (Jordan, 2012).

## Department of Defense and Department of Veterans Affairs Guidance for Screening for Suicidal Ideation

In the absence of a joint VA/DOD CPG for the management of suicidal behavior, screening and assessment of suicidal ideation in VA and DOD is guided by a variety of policies and programs.

---

[11] PL 111-383: 111th Congress, Jan 7, 2011.

### Department of Defense

DOD uses a set of questions that specifically ask about suicidal thoughts and risk factors to screen for suicide risk (shown in Table 5.6). The questions are administered as part of DOD's periodic health assessments, the PDHA and the PDHRA, which are briefly described in the introduction to this chapter. All service members meet in person with a provider, who conducts a full clinical interview that includes specific questions pertaining to suicide assessment.

**TABLE 5.6** Periodic Health-Assessment Suicide-Screening Questions

| Periodic Health Assessment Questions Asked by Mental-Health Professionals or Certified Health Care Providers During Person-to-Person Interviews | Responses |
|---|---|
| Over the past month, have you been bothered by thoughts that you would be better off dead or of hurting yourself in some way? | Yes, no |
| If "yes," ask "How often have you been bothered by these thoughts?" | Very few days<br>More than half the time<br>Nearly every day |
| Have you ever had thoughts of actually hurting yourself?<br>If "yes," ask the following four questions: | Yes, no |
| Have you thought about how you might actually hurt yourself? | No, yes<br>If yes, how? |
| How likely do you think it is that you will act on these thoughts about hurting yourself or ending your life over the next month? | Not at all likely<br>Somewhat likely<br>Very likely |
| Is there anything that would prevent or keep you from harming yourself? | No, yes<br>If yes, what? |
| Have you ever attempted to harm yourself in the past? | No, yes<br>If yes, when? |
| Assess other risk factors for suicide, including interpersonal conflicts, social isolation, current alcohol or substance abuse, hopelessness, severe agitation or anxiety, diagnosis of depression or other psychiatric disorder, recent loss, financial stress, legal disciplinary problems, serious physical illness | Yes, no |

SOURCE: Adapted from Vythilingam et al., 2010.

According to DOD training materials for administering the periodic health assessments (Vythilingam et al., 2010), respondents to these questions are designated as being at high risk for suicide if they have an active desire to commit suicide in addition to having no self-control, having no external supports, or having comorbid alcohol abuse, PTSD, or MDD; high-risk patients are given an emergency mental-health referral and provided with safe transportation to a mental-health clinic or emergency room. Respondents are designated as being at intermediate risk of suicide if they have current suicidal thoughts but no active plan for committing suicide (the suicidal thoughts may or may not be accompanied by other risk factors); intermediate-risk patients are referred to a mental-health specialist for an assessment within 48 hours or monitored by primary care clinicians at each visit, depending on the clinicians' judgment. Health records of service members who are determined to be a danger to themselves or to others are flagged with a "behavioral health alert" (Woodson, 2011).

The Air Force *MSB* guide recommends that clinical staff use a one-item screening question for patients seen in a mental-health setting. The question is adapted from the National Depression Screening Project (Greenfield et al., 2000). "Over the past two weeks, how often have you had thoughts about wanting to commit suicide"? People who respond "sometimes," "frequently," or "always" undergo further assessment. A negative screen is the endorsement of "never" or "rarely" (Air Force Medical Operations Agency).

**Department of Veterans Affairs**

VA screens for suicide risk in primary care if patients screen positive for PTSD or MDD, in which case screening for suicide risk is mandatory. The suicide risk assessment includes having a patient respond to the questions in Box 5.8, which are included in two clinical tools for providers—*Suicide Risk Assessment Guide: Reference Manual* (VA, undated-a) and *Suicide Risk Assessment Pocket Card* (VA, undated-b)—and are incorporated into the VA clinical-reminder system in the electronic patient record.

**BOX 5.8**
**VA Suicide-Assessment Questions**

Are you feeling hopeless about the present/future? If yes, ask:
Have you had thoughts about taking your life? If yes, ask:
When did you have these thoughts, and do you have a plan to take your life?
Have you ever had a suicide attempt?

SOURCE: VA, undated-a.

Any reference to suicidal ideation, intent, or plans mandates a referral to specialty mental-health care for a mental-health assessment. When there is a referral or request for mental-health services, veterans must receive an initial evaluation within 24 hours (Kemp, 2011).

## Evidence Related to Screening for Suicide Risk

There is no widely accepted and scientifically validated tool for screening for suicide risk, partly because of the complex set of biologic, psychologic, and social factors associated with suicide. On the basis of insufficient evidence on the accuracy of screening tools in identifying suicide risk in the primary care setting, the USPSTF found no evidence that screening for suicide risk reduces suicide attempts or mortality. The USPSTF found that commonly used screening instruments—the Scale for Suicidal Ideation, the Scale for Suicidal Ideation–Worst, and the Suicidal Ideation Questionnaire—have not been validated for assessing suicide risk in primary care settings and that there has been little testing of the Symptom-Driven Diagnostic System for Primary Care (USPSTF, 2004).

In its assessment of DOD screening practices, the 2010 Task Force on the Prevention of Suicide by Members of the Armed Forces concluded that "current screening efforts are not effective in identifying Service Members at risk for suicide and tend to perpetuate negative feelings about mental health care, which leads to further stigma." In addition, the task force found that "current screening efforts are not effective in identifying Service Members who have significant moral and ethical problems resulting from their combat experience, resulting in a sense of guilt and loss of self-worth that places them at risk for suicide." The task force recommendations included ensuring service member receive routine mental-fitness assessment and wellness education and encouraging service members to obtain referrals to appropriate caregivers for concerns beyond a chaplain's scope of expertise and experience (DOD, 2010a).

In examining VA's suicide-prevention programs, the Blue Ribbon Work Group found that suicide-screening processes being implemented in VA primary care clinics go beyond the current evidence and may have unintended effects. The Work Group cited a lack of sufficient evidence to support mandatory suicide screening in non-mental-health settings. The Work Group recommended that VA revise and reevaluate the current policies regarding mandatory suicide screening assessments, stating that "this screening process, as designed, affects a large number of veterans, is time consuming, potentially stigmatizing, likely to be variable in implementation, and not evidence-based, and may result in unnecessary referrals to specialty mental health services" (Blue Ribbon Work Group on Suicide Prevention in the Veteran Population, 2008). In 2010, VA reported to Congress that a work group had reviewed VA practices and the evidence base on screening for and evaluation of suicide risk and recommended continuation of VA's existing policy (VA, 2010b).

## Implementation of Department of Defense and Department of Veterans Affairs Guidance for Screening for Suicidal Ideation

This section presents information available to the committee on the extent to which DOD and VA are implementing and tracking screening procedures to identify people who are at risk for suicide. The information raises questions about how well DOD and VA are implementing, tracking, and assessing their screening practices to ensure the best possible result.

### Department of Defense

The US Army Medical Command's RESPECT-Mil program provides primary care–based screening, assessment, treatment, and referral of active-duty personnel who have PTSD or MDD. Since 2007, 1.3 million visits have involved screening for PTSD and MDD. Of those, more than 13,600 (1%) involved suicidality and received mental-health intervention (DCoE, 2012c). Identification of suicide risk appears to be improving: over half the 13,600 visits involving suicidality were reported in 2011.

### Department of Veteran Affairs

Under its Performance Management Program, VA uses three performance measures related to screening and suicide-risk assessment (AHRQ, 2012). The committee was unable to identify results of using those measures, and inquiries to VA about performance measures did not yield information about them.

One measure is the percentage of patients who screen positive on a screen for MDD (PHQ-2 or PHQ-9 or endorsement of question 9 on the PHQ-9) and have a suicide-risk evaluation completed within 24 hours. Another is the percentage of eligible patients who screen positive on the PTSD screen (PC-PTSD) and who have a suicide-risk evaluation completed within 24 hours. A third measure combines the populations of the first two to assess the percentage of patients who screen positive for MDD (on the PHQ-2 or PHQ-9) or positive for PTSD (on the PC-PTSD) and who have a suicide-risk evaluation completed within 24 hours.

## Department of Defense and Department of Veterans Affairs Guidance for Assessment and Diagnosis of Suicidal Ideation

Available guidance in VA and DOD (such as the VA/DOD CPGs for PTSD, MDD, and SUDs and the Air Force *MSB* guide) emphasizes the importance of a formal assessment to determine suicide risk. Generally, the guidelines recommend the identification of risk factors and the use of a direct line of questioning to elicit details about suicidal thoughts and intent (for example, the VA/DOD MDD guideline recommends a group of questions modified from Hirschfeld and Russell, 1997). The Air Force *MSB* guide, refers to 31 suicide-assessment instruments on the basis of a comprehensive review by Brown (2000). Of those, the *MSB* guide recommends the Suicide Status Form-II, Suicide Tracking Form-I, and the Beck Scale for Suicide Ideation (Air Force Medical Operations Agency). Recently, the DOD/VA Suicide Prevention Tools Working Group compiled a descriptive summary of suicide assessment and prevention tools. The working group identified 26 clinical and 14 nonclinical suicide-prevention tools; of these, 25 were classified as aiming to assess suicidal ideation. The group's report did not make any recommendations about the tools reviewed (DCoE, 2011f).

In the VA, the *VA Suicide Risk Assessment Guide: Reference Manual* (VA, undated-a) provides guidance to clinicians to support determinations of high-risk people. Suicide-prevention coordinators in each VA medical facility play a key role in, among other things, assessing and monitoring high-risk people, providing direct clinical care for veterans who are at increased risk for suicide, and tracking and reporting suicidal behavior. In 2008, a VHA directive established the use of "flags" in the electronic medical records of patients who are assessed as having a high risk of suicidal behavior (VA, 2008b).

### Validity of Tools for Assessment of Suicide Risk

The purpose of a comprehensive suicide-risk assessment is, in addition to estimating the risk of suicidal behavior, to guide clinical action. In general, the greater the number of risk factors and the fewer the protective factors, the higher the risk of suicide and suicidal behavior. Many approaches to suicide-risk assessment emphasize the importance of systematically eliciting patient information in a number of key domains. For example, the APA *Practice Guideline for the Assessment and Treatment of Patients with Suicidal Behaviors* identifies five domains of a suicide assessment: the patient's current presentation (such as suicidal thoughts, plans, behaviors, and intent), previous psychiatric illness and treatment, history of self-harming behavior and family history of suicide or mental illness, psychosocial situation (for example, relationships, employment, finances, and domestic or sexual abuse), and individual strengths and vulnerabilities, such as coping skills and personality traits. Once risk factors are identified, the clinician should focus interventions on factors that can be modified, for example, treating psychiatric symptoms, increasing social support, and removing access to lethal means (APA, 2003).

Suicide-specific assessment instruments can assist providers in clinical assessment of suicidal ideation and behavior. However, assessment instruments are not a substitute for clinical judgment; no single test or panel of tests accurately identifies the emergence of a suicide crisis (Fowler, 2012). An array of suicide-assessment instruments are available (IOM, 2002). Recently, the VA's Evidence-based Synthesis Program completed a systematic review to determine what assessment tools are effective in assessing risk of suicidal self-directed violence in veteran and military populations. The researchers found that evaluation of the effectiveness of risk-assessment tools is lacking. They noted there is a dearth of evidence from prospective studies that examined associations between suicide-prevention assessment tools and suicidal self-directed violence outcomes (Haney et al., 2012).

As described by Brown (2000), numerous suicide-assessment instruments have demonstrated adequate internal reliability and concurrent validity, but the predictive validity of most suicide measures has not been established. The Scale for Suicide Ideation and the Beck Hopelessness Scale are among the few instruments that have been found to yield scores that represent important risk factors for suicide (Brown, 2000). Factors that contribute to the difficulty of determining the predictive validity of suicide-assessment measures include the low base rate of suicidal behavior and the high false-positive rates associated with the use of such relatively distal variables as psychiatric diagnosis, demographics, and self-reported psychologic states (Fowler, 2012). Brown (2000) concluded that further research that uses large samples and a prospective design is needed to investigate the predictive validity of standardized measures of suicide attempts and suicide.

To address the need for measures that are predictive of suicide, researchers at Columbia University compared the psychometric properties of the Columbia-Suicide Severity Rating Scale (C-SSRS) with those of other measures. Posner et al. (2011) found that the C-SSRS, which assesses both behavior and ideation, could reliably predict a suicide attempt in those who had previously attempted suicide. The researchers concluded that the tool can help to determine who is most at risk for suicide by pinpointing the threshold at which a person's suicidal thinking is severe enough to warrant professional intervention.

As an example of research on the predictive validity of a suicide-assessment tool that addresses specific populations, Breshears et al. (2010) sought to validate objective personality measures for use with those who have a history of TBI; the goal was to understand suicide risk better. The researchers investigated the Personality Assessment Inventory (PAI) Suicide Potential Index and Suicide Ideation scale as predictors of suicidal behavior in military personnel. They analyzed medical records of 154 veterans who had TBI and documented instances of suicidal behavior in the 2 years after PAI administration. The results suggest that the PAI may assist in assessing suicide risk in those who have TBI, particularly when population-based cutoffs are considered (on a score range of 0 to 20, a score of 15 or higher yields a sensitivity of 90.9% and a specificity of 95.1%). However, the relatively small number of suicides (11) raises questions as to the generalizability of the findings and some statistical issues (Breshears et al., 2010).

In addition to the need for diagnostic tests that can predict suicide risk accurately, there is an issue regarding the capabilities of those who conduct the risk assessments. On the basis of RAND's research on the DOD suicide-prevention program (Ramchand et al., 2011), the DOD Task Force on the Prevention of Suicide by Members of the Armed Forces reported that military health care providers (including mental-health care providers) and chaplains are insufficiently trained to deliver evidence-based assessment, management, and treatment to service members who exhibit suicide-related behaviors. The task force recommended that all military health care providers and chaplains receive training and continuing education in evidence-informed suicide-risk assessment, management, and treatment planning (DOD, 2010a).

## Implementation of Department of Defense and Department of Veterans Affairs Guidance for Assessment and Diagnosis of Suicidal Ideation

There appear to be very few data on the extent to which DOD and VA conduct suicide-risk assessments of service members and veterans who might be at risk for suicide.

### Department of Defense

The committee is unaware of any metrics in DOD for tracking the number of service members that have received suicide-risk assessment in the Military Health System.

### Department of Veteran Affairs

VA contracted with Altarum Institute and RAND to conduct an independent evaluation of the quality of VA mental-health care and substance-use care (Watkins and Pincus, 2011). The evaluation included one performance indicator related to suicide assessment in VA. On the basis of medical-record data from FY 2007, the Altarum–RAND team found 81% of study veterans had documentation of an assessment for suicidal ideation. Women were 9 percentage points more likely than men to have a documented assessment for suicidal ideation; OEF and OIF veterans were significantly more likely than non-OEF and non-OIF veterans to have a documented assessment for suicidal ideation or to have their symptoms reassessed. The research team surveyed all VA facilities nationwide in 2007 and again in 2009 to assess the availability of basic and specialized services. The unit of analysis was a parent-facility service area (PFSAs).[12] In 2009, all PFSAs reported having policies for flagging and 99% policies for tracking veterans who express suicidal thoughts. Results of the May 2007 survey indicated that 44% of the PFSAs reported having policies for flagging and 29% policies for tracking veterans who express suicidal thoughts (Watkins and Pincus, 2011).

## Department of Defense and Department of Veterans Affairs Guidance for Treatment for Suicidal Ideation

The Air Force *MSB* guide recommends that treatment plans specifically target suicidal symptoms and risk factors (Air Force Medical Operations Agency, undated). The guideline notes that treatment plans that target only a psychiatric diagnosis are insufficiently specific and may fail to address the multidimensional nature of suicide risk fully. Yet, with the exception of the Air Force *MSB* guide, the primary focus of the current DOD and VA treatment guidelines is on the therapeutic approaches that target the individual specific disorders that are the subjects of the guideline (MDD, PTSD, SUD, and TBI). Less emphasis is placed on the treatment of patients who may also have suicidal symptoms, although the VA/DOD guideline for MDD includes an appendix that has specific guidance for managing suicidality. The forthcoming VA/DOD guideline on assessing and managing suicidal behaviors may provide more detailed guidance. In this section, we highlight the few recommendations for treating suicidal thoughts and behaviors in the various existing VA/DOD guidelines for MDD (VA and DOD, 2009a), PTSD (VA and DoD, 2010), and SUD (VA and DoD, 2009c).

---

[12]The study team defined a PFSA as VA service area that is anchored, in most cases, by a VA medical center and supporting community-based outpatient clinics. PFSAs have nonoverlapping geographic areas of responsibility.

The VA/DOD MDD guideline discusses the use of behavioral therapy and pharmacotherapy under specific circumstances in the treatment of patients who have a diagnosis of MDD and are exhibiting suicidal behaviors. In patients who have a history of suicide attempts, CBT is recommended for reducing the risk of further suicide attempts. The guideline notes that one RCT found that a 10-session CBT led to 50% fewer suicide attempts than enhanced usual care (tracking and referral) without reducing rates of suicidal ideation (Brown et al., 2005). When antidepressant pharmacotherapy is used to treat MDD, clinicians are encouraged to inform patients that a slight increase in suicidal ideation may occur in the early phase of treatment. Clinicians are warned to use tricyclic antidepressants cautiously in patients who are at high risk for suicide and only when consultation with an appropriate specialist guides the therapy. Electroconvulsive therapy (ECT) should be considered in patients who have severe MDD and severe suicidality.

The VA/DOD guideline for PTSD provides some guidance in the use of two psychotherapies in patients who are at risk for suicide. The guideline alerts clinicians to use caution when considering exposure-based therapies (ETs) for patients who are at substantial risk for suicide. ET has not been studied in patients who have health problems that preclude exposure to intense physiologic arousal and some patients may experience an increased level of distress when confronting trauma memories. Although there is insufficient evidence to recommend for or against dialectical behavior therapy (DBT) as first-line treatment for PTSD, the guideline indicates that DBT can be considered for patients who have borderline personality disorder typified by parasuicidal behaviors (attempted self-injury in which the aim is not death). The guideline cites studies that identify DBT as a promising treatment for suicide but acknowledges the need for further research.

The VA/DOD guidelines for MDD, PTSD, and SUD address the sequencing of treatment for suicidal ideation in the context of comorbidity with these conditions. The guidelines indicate that if severe suicidality is identified during the clinical assessment, the clinician should first concentrate on management of suicide risk before initiating treatment for any other condition. In addition, The VA/DOD MDD guideline and the Air Force *MBS* guide recommend that clinicians adopt a systematic approach for making clinical decisions about potentially suicidal patients that involves identifying risk factors, classifying the level of suicide risk, and using that information to determine the course of action.

Although it is not specifically endorsed in DOD or VA clinical guidelines, the Collaborative Assessment and Management of Suicidality (CAMS) is an approach that some Air Force clinics and other military settings are using to monitor and manage suicidal behavior. CAMS is a therapeutic framework that targets suicide as the primary focus of assessment and problem-focused intervention. The Suicide Status Form (SSF) is used to guide assessment, treatment, and continuing suicide risk until suicidality resolves (Jobes, 2012). Six published correlational studies and one RCT support the use of CAMS and the SSF; additional RCTs and CAMS-related projects are under way (Jobes, 2012). In a US Air Force Study (n = 55), use of CAMS was related to more rapid resolution of suicidal thinking and decreases in emergency-department and primary care visits (Jobes et al., 2005).

In 2008, VA implemented a safety planning protocol for use with patients who are at high risk for suicide. A safety plan is a predetermined priority list of coping strategies, sources of support, and help-seeking behaviors that patients can refer to during vulnerable periods. As a therapeutic technique, a safety plan plays a role in the continuing mental-health treatment in outpatient settings (Stanley and Brown, 2008). As used in VHA, the safety plan involves the following steps: recognition of signs of increasing risk, use of coping strategies to manage episodes of suicidal ideation, use of social contacts that can distract from suicidal ideation and provide support, contact with family members or friends who can assist in resolving an episode of high-risk suicidal ideation, contact with professionals and agencies, and reduction in access to lethal means (Claassen and Knox, 2011). Protocol requires that the plan be included in the patient's medical record and that a copy be given to the patient.

## Evidence Related to Treatment for Suicidal Ideation

Research shows that 90% of people who committed suicide had psychiatric and mood disorders and that more than 80% had not received treatment at the time of death (Mann et al., 2005). Thus, a primary component of suicide prevention is prompt evidence-based treatment for psychiatric illness. Therapeutic approaches for addressing suicidality should target specific psychiatric disorders (such as MDD and PTSD), associated symptoms (such as anxiety), and the predominant psychodynamic or psychosocial stressors (APA, 2003).

Prescribed medications should be those necessary to treat for underlying disorders (IOM, 2002). There is evidence that lithium treatment for bipolar disorder significantly reduces suicide rates (APA, 2003; IOM, 2002). In a meta-analysis of 33 studies of the efficacy of lithium, Baldessarini et al. (2001) found that lithium reduces the incidence of completed suicide by 13-fold. Other studies of antipsychotic medications have found that clozapine is associated with significant decreases in suicide attempts by people who have schizophrenia or schizoaffective disorder (APA, 2003; IOM, 2002).

Meta-analyses of RCTs have not found independent benefit regarding suicide or suicide attempts in studies of the use of antidepressants for mood and other psychiatric disorders. Few studies prospectively used suicidal behavior as an outcome measure (Mann et al., 2005).

Although numerous studies have documented the efficacy of psychotherapy, especially CBT, in treating for mental disorders that increase suicide risk, such as MDD and PTSD, far fewer studies have documented the direct effects of therapy on suicidal behavior (IOM, 2002). Some studies have shown promising results for CBT as an intervention to reduce suicide (see a systematic review by Tarrier et al., 2008), but the use of small samples limits the ability to reach conclusions about efficacy from these studies (Hawton et al., 2000; Tarrier et al., 2008).

## Implementation of Department of Defense and Department of Veterans Affairs Gun-Safety Protocols

Gun-safety protocols for military-issued weapons are part of the standard of care for suicidal patients in VA and DOD clinical settings, but there is evidence that implementation may be inconsistent.

### Department of Defense

In the military, the standard practice for service members who are at risk for suicide consists of "lethal-means counseling," removing service members from weapon-carrying duties, and putting the service members' weapons in the base armory for safekeeping. But there are no clear guidelines, decision tree, or risk stratification to guide a clinician. A key recommendation by the 2010 DOD Task Force on the Prevention of Suicide by Members of the Armed Forces (DOD, 2010a) is to

> establish clear DoD, Joint and Service guidance for removal and subsequent re-issue of military weapon and ammunition for Service Members recognized to be at risk for suicide. The guidance should emphasize a collaborative, team approach to the decision-making process and specify documentation requirements.

**Department of Veterans Affairs**

In the VA system, the Office of Inspector General evaluated the extent to which VA mental-health care providers consistently developed suicide-prevention safety plans (SPSPs) for patients assessed as being at high risk for suicide. Inspectors evaluated SPSP practices in 45 facilities during January 1–September 30, 2010. Of the 469 medical records reviewed, 412 (88%) had documented SPSPs; of the 469,389 (83%) fully addressed the six essential components of the safety plan. Reducing the potential for use of lethal means is one of the components (VA Office of Inspector General, 2011).

## Summary

Suicide remains a paramount problem in the military despite substantial efforts. Although there are no VA/DOD joint evidence-based CPGs for screening for, assessing, or treating for suicidal thoughts and behaviors, a work group has been formed to draft such joint guidelines. The Air Force *MSB* guide is a recognized example in DOD, and the 2003 APA "Practice Guidelines for the Assessment and Treatment of Patients with Suicidal Behaviors" represents the prevailing national standard.

A substantial array of programs and resources has been developed by VA/DOD in an effort to enhance suicide prevention. However, there remains a lack of standardization or coordination. In fairness, the overall evidence base on screening and assessment approaches is sparse, in part because of challenges related to predicting and reducing the number of events that occur in a small proportion of the population. Consequently, there has been widespread controversy about the optimal approach. DOD screens as part of the PDHA, whereas VA assesses suicide risk in people who screen positive for PTSD or MDD.

Both DOD and VA recognize the importance of formal assessment of suicide risk. There are evidence-based approaches, such as those outlined by APA. Although DOD and VA have compiled resources, a standardized approach remains to be established and implemented. Likewise, there is a recognized need to improve the training of VA and DOD health care providers and chaplains in assessing suicide risk.

Interventions for suicidal ideation have focused principally on treatment for underlying psychiatric conditions. However, in accord with the prevailing evidence base, approaches should also focus on monitoring and managing suicidal behavior, as exemplified by CAMS (used by the US Air Force) and a safety plan (used by VA). The most compelling evidence-based approach to suicide prevention emphasizes the importance and potential favorable effects of restricting access to lethal means. In the case of service members and veterans, firearms constitute the leading lethal means of suicide. Standard practices have been developed that entail "lethal-means counseling" by DOD and "suicide-prevention safety plans" in VA, but a more robust and effective standardized complement of policies, procedures, and practices needs to be established and reliably implemented throughout DOD and VA.

## COMORBID CONDITIONS

The terminology used to describe the presence of more than one distinct health condition in a person is variable. Some common terms are *comorbidity, dual diagnosis, co-occurring disorders,* and *multimorbidity*; however, there is no consensus regarding the definitions of these terms (Center for Substance Abuse Treatment, 2006; de Groot et al., 2003; Valderas et al., 2009). That is important because the lack of consensus about how to define and measure the concept of multiple health conditions complicates attempts to study their effects on an array of outcomes—for example, death, functional status, and health care quality—and to develop clinical guidance on their management. Moreover, comorbidity is associated with worse health outcomes, more complex clinical management, and increased health care costs (Valderas et al., 2009).

According to Valderas et al. (2009), there are several characteristics associated with definitions of comorbidity. Some definitions are based on health conditions linked to classification systems, such as *ICD* and *DSM;* others are not. Definitions either identify one central disease, referred to as the index condition, which is relative to secondary conditions, or take an approach in which no particular condition is privileged over any other, as implied by the term *multimorbidity*. One dimension of comorbidity is the chronology of multiple health conditions. Conditions may be present simultaneously or during a period but not simultaneously; and they can appear in a particular sequence regardless of the period. Morbidity burden and patient complexity are other concepts associated with comorbidity (Valderas et al., 2009).

Among military and veteran personnel, rates of comorbid diagnosis are high; the most common overlapping disorders are PTSD, SUD, MDD, and postconcussive symptoms attributed to mild TBI. (See Chapter 4 for a full discussion of each condition and its associated comorbidities, including prevalence.)

DOD data show many service members are receiving diagnoses of more than one mental-health condition, and the trend is increasing slightly. In 2007, throughout the armed forces (excluding reserves and National Guard), 35,226 persons received 46,482 mental-health diagnoses,[13] for an average of 1.32 diagnoses per person. The average number of diagnoses increased to 1.38 in 2008, 1.42 in 2009, and 1.43 in 2010 (AFHSC, 2010).

In the veteran population, the rates of comorbidity are substantial. Carlson et al. (2010) examined rates of clinician-diagnosed psychiatric disorders in a sample of 13,201 OIF and OEF veterans who had been screened for TBI and found that over 80% of veterans who screened positive had psychiatric diagnoses. In an evaluation of VA mental-health programs, the Altarum–RAND evaluation team examined data for a FY 2008 cohort of 906,394 veterans who had at least one mental-health diagnosis.[14] Among those veterans, 53% had a mental-health diagnosis

---

[13] *Mental health diagnosis* is defined as a diagnostic code for PTSD, MDD, bipolar disorder, alcohol dependence, or substance dependence and at least one inpatient encounter or two outpatient encounters on separate days for the recorded diagnostic code; cases were counted by using the earliest medical encounter for a given person.

[14] The cohort consisted of veterans whose VHA use records contained at least one of 38 study-relevant *ICD-9-CM* diagnosis codes for the five study conditions (MDD, PTSD, SUD, schizophrenia, and bipolar disorder) and at least one inpatient episode or two outpatient visits annually for any diagnosis.

other than their cohort-qualifying diagnosis, 50% had at least one physical-health comorbidity, and 23% had co-occurring SUD. From an economic standpoint, RAND found that treating mental-health problems that co-occur with SUD substantially increases the cost of treatment per veteran. On the average in the FY 2008 study cohort, the per-veteran cost of treating a mental-health condition with co-occurring SUD was $20,903, compared with $11,342 for PTSD only, $14,202 for depression only, and $12,600 for SUD only (Watkins and Pincus, 2011).

Clinical management of the complex array of symptoms that is typical of patients who have comorbid conditions is challenging (Lew et al., 2008). Comorbidities require clinical attention at the point of diagnosis and throughout the process of treatment. Comorbid medical and psychiatric conditions are important to recognize because they can modify clinical determinations of prognosis, patient or provider treatment priorities, selection of interventions, and the setting where care will be provided. Current evidence-based practices to identify and treat people for conditions also may be less accurate or effective when conditions co-occur (Carlson et al., 2009).

As described in other sections of this chapter, substantial evidence-based clinical guidance exists for the management of individual health conditions that are prevalent among service members and veterans. However, there are no empirically validated therapies for comorbid PTSD, MDD, and postconcussive disorders, which may be confounded by substance use (Lew et al., 2008). No evidence was found to support particular sequencing of treatments in implementing practice recommendations of individual guidelines.

In the absence of a strong evidence base related to comorbid conditions, clinical judgment based on systematic symptom monitoring and the patient relationship is needed in deciding which specific treatments to implement, for which patients, and under which treatment conditions (National Center for PTSD, 2010a; Otis et al., 2011). As discussed below, experts agree that, given the lack of evidence on efficacious treatments for comorbid conditions, best practices involve treating for symptoms regardless of etiology by using current CPGs (Brenner et al., 2009; National Center for PTSD, 2010a, 2010b; Otis et al., 2011).

## Department of Defense and Department of Veterans Affairs Guidance for Comorbid Conditions

The various VA/DOD clinical guidelines reviewed by the committee acknowledge that few published trials can provide clinicians with guidance in treating for conditions that are complicated by comorbid illness. The guidance given is generally in the form of background information about commonly occurring comorbid conditions with some recommendations for patient management. Among the VA/DOD guidelines, the PTSD guideline provides the most extensive and detailed guidance for the management of comorbid conditions. In general, the recommendations in the guidelines are consistent and can be categorized into a few central themes, as summarized below.

### Assessment of the Presence of Comorbid Conditions

Each VA/DOD guideline states that in performing patient clinical assessments clinicians should determine whether comorbid medical or psychiatric conditions are present and are possible causes of the patient's symptoms. The VA/DOD MDD guideline identifies bipolar disorder, PTSD, SUD, suicidality and homicidality, and psychosis as conditions that commonly occur with MDD. The VA/DOD PTSD guideline recommends that providers assess PTSD patients for MDD and other psychiatric disorders, patterns of current and past use of substances, pain and sleep disturbances, physical and cognitive health symptoms, and high-risk behaviors. The TBI guideline indicates that patients with concussion or mild TBI should be screened for psychiatric symptoms and comorbid psychiatric disorders, including MDD, PTSD, and SUD. The SUD guideline emphasizes that SUD correlates highly with PTSD and other psychologic disorders, infectious diseases, and nicotine dependence.

In addition to medical and psychiatric comorbid conditions, the guidelines recommend that people be assessed for any important unmet psychosocial needs or situational stressors, such as financial difficulties, problematic family relationships, poor social support, or occupational problems.

**Priority Setting in Treatment for Symptoms**

Overall, the guidelines recommend that management of patients who have comorbidities focus on identifying and treating for the symptoms that are causing the most impairment regardless of cause or diagnosis. Of all the guidelines, the TBI guideline expresses this most directly:

> The expected outcome of intervention should be to improve the identified problem areas, rather than discover a disease etiology or "cure." The presence of comorbid psychiatric problems such as a major depressive episode, anxiety disorders (including post-traumatic stress disorder), or substance abuse—whether or not these are regarded as etiologically related to the mild TBI—should be treated aggressively using appropriate psychotherapeutic and pharmacologic interventions (VA, 2009).

**Treatment for Comorbid Disorders**

The VA/DOD guidelines indicate that presence of comorbid conditions should be considered in choosing treatments. Each guideline refers clinicians to specific VA/DOD guidelines for information about best practices in treatment for individual disorders (such as MDD, PTSD, SUD, and mild TBI).

The individual guidelines provide some minimal guidance about treating for comorbidities. For example, the VA/DOD guideline for MDD states that a patient who has a depressive disorder and a coexisting mental-health disorder that complicates treatment (such as a history of hypomania or a manic episode, PTSD, psychosis, or SUD) may require the use of multiple psychotropic medications and ancillary services, which may include the use of mood-stabilizing medications, antipsychotics, multiple antidepressants, benzodiazepines, case management, family support, peer support, group therapy, or mobile treatment units. The guideline also identifies the potential contraindications for ECT in patients who recently had an intracerebral hemorrhage, which may have occurred in TBI.

For the management of concurrent PTSD and SUD, the VA/DOD PTSD guideline indicates that there is insufficient evidence to recommend using or not using any specific psychosocial approach to addressing PTSD that is comorbid with SUD. The guideline (VA and DOD, 2010) states further that "no systematic findings indicate harm to patients provided integrated treatment for co-occurring SUD and PTSD and there is recognition that both conditions ought to be addressed." The guideline recommends addiction-focused pharmacotherapy in addition to any indicated pharmacotherapy for coexisting PTSD and the provision of specialty psychosocial treatment and adjunctive services.

The VA/DOD TBI guideline states that treatment for psychiatric or behavioral symptoms after concussion or mild TBI should be based on individual factors and on the nature and severity of symptoms and may include both psychotherapeutic and pharmacologic treatment. People who sustain a concussion or mild TBI and present with anxiety symptoms or irritability should be offered a several-week trial of pharmacologic agents. For the management of sleep dysfunction, the guideline recommends evaluating for potential comorbid psychiatric conditions, including MDD and anxiety, and, if they are present, considering the use of standard medications to improve sleep.

In connection with sequencing of various treatments, the PTSD guideline recommends treating for comorbid mental-health conditions concurrently with PTSD treatment, although a stated exception is severe substance dependence that requires medical detoxification before other forms of treatment. With respect to co-occurring TBI, the PTSD guideline (VA and DOD, 2010) states that "there is no evidence to support withholding PTSD treatments while addressing post-concussive symptoms" and that "physical or cognitive symptoms, such as headaches or memory problems, or other persistent post-concussive symptoms should be treated symptomatically whether or not concussion/mTBI is thought to be one of the causal factors."

**Referrals and Coordination of Care**

Each VA/DOD guideline encourages providers to consider the existence of comorbid conditions when deciding whether to treat patients in the primary care setting or to refer them for specialty mental-health care. For example, the PTSD guideline states that referral to specialty mental-health care is indicated if a patient who has PTSD has comorbid mental disorders that are severe or unstable. The examples given include patients whose MDD is accompanied by suicidality, patients who have substance dependence, and patients who have concurrent psychotic or bipolar disorder.

All the guidelines emphasize the importance of communication and coordination of care between primary care and mental-health care providers if a patient is referred to specialty care for treatment for comorbid conditions. The VA/DOD MDD guideline mentions that care management—"a clinical approach to coordinate the management of several chronic health conditions that may be integrated into primary care settings"—may be appropriate for those who have a variety of medical and psychiatric comorbid conditions that require integrated care.

The PTSD guideline states that integrated care, in which the physical-health and mental-health needs of patients are addressed in a single setting by a multidisciplinary provider team, has the potential to reduce the perceived stigma associated with help-seeking. As discussed later, the SUD guideline indicates that a growing body of research is demonstrating that integrated services produce better outcomes for people who have co-occurring disorders, particularly serious or complex conditions.

**Clinician Toolkits**

The Defense Centers of Excellence for Psychological Health & Traumatic Brain Injury developed a clinical tool, *Co-Occurring Conditions Toolkit: Mild Traumatic Brain Injury and*

*Psychological Health,* to guide primary care providers in assessing and managing patients when multiple diagnoses may be present. The toolkit synthesizes evidenced-based approaches from VA/DOD CPGs that address concussion, PTSD, MDD, chronic opioid therapy, and SUD. It is organized by symptom (such as sleep, mood, attention, and chronic pain) and identifies the probable etiology of symptoms (such as concussion, PTSD, MDD, chronic pain, headache, and SUD). Screening, assessment, and treatment steps are recommended. Information regarding potential side effects of particular drugs on co-occurring disorders is provided with specific drug information (doses, side effects, and safety warnings) (DCoE, 2011c).

## Implementation of Department of Defense and Department of Veterans Affairs Guidance for Comorbid Conditions

VA contracted with the Altarum Institute and RAND to conduct an independent evaluation of the quality of VA mental-health and substance-use care (Watkins and Pincus 2011). One of the research questions examined was whether veterans who have dual diagnoses (including co-occurring SUD and the mental-health diagnoses included in the evaluation) are receiving integrated care that manages both conditions. In this context, *integrated care* refers to mental-health and substance-abuse treatment delivered by a single clinical team or a clinician who is cross-trained in mental health and SUD. The performance indicator developed for the evaluation is the proportion of veterans who have co-occurring SUD with documentation of any visits that treated them for both SUD and the mental-health disorder on the same day within 3 months of a new treatment episode. For FY 2007, the study found that 47% of veterans in the co-occurring SUD cohort had a visit that treated them for the mental-health condition and a visit that treated them for SUD on the same day. The authors noted that VHA care for co-occurring SUD may be fairly well coordinated, if not integrated, inasmuch as it is likely that visits occurring on the same day reflect care that is more integrated than visits that are separated by months (Watkins and Pincus, 2011).

## Evidence Related to Treatment for Comorbid Conditions

There is little evidence on the best approaches for the assessment and treatment of patients who have comorbidities. The literature is insufficient to determine whether diagnostic or even screening instruments commonly used for assessing the symptoms of a particular condition perform accurately when a person has more than one condition. Nor does the literature support any one instrument over others. Examples of studies with those findings were related to instruments for detecting MDD in patients who also have mild TBI (Guillamondegui et al., 2011) and for screening for and diagnosing mild TBI in patients who have PTSD (Carlson et al., 2011).

As described below, findings from several studies demonstrate the lack of knowledge about whether evidence-based treatments for a single condition are effective when conditions co-occur or unique therapies are necessary for people who have multiple conditions.

### Traumatic Brain Injury and Posttraumatic Stress Disorder

In 2009, the VA Office of Mental Health Services (OMHS) and Office of Rehabilitation Services sponsored a consensus panel to make practice recommendations related to the diagnosis and management of PTSD, pain, and a history of mild TBI in veterans. The panel reviewed results of a systematic review of evidence on the epidemiology, assessment, and treatment of adults who had mild TBI and PTSD. The reported prevalence of comorbid TBI and PTSD varied widely among the studies reviewed. No published studies addressed the relative accuracy of diagnostic tests used for assessing mild TBI or PTSD when one condition co-occurs with the other. And no published studies evaluated treatments for the symptoms of mild TBI and PTSD together (Carlson et al., 2009). The consensus panel recommended the use of current VA/DOD CPGs for treating for PTSD, mild TBI, and pain in patients who meet diagnostic criteria for at least two of these disorders concurrently. The panel noted that there was no evidence to support modifying the current CPGs for treatment for comorbid PTSD, mild TBI, and pain (National Center for PTSD, 2010b).

**Posttraumatic Stress Disorder and Substance-Use Disorder**

In 2009, VA's OMHS convened a consensus panel to develop recommendations related to the clinical management of veterans who had comorbid SUD and PTSD. The panel's recommendations were informed by results in 52 articles on the assessment and treatment of veterans who had co-occurring SUD and PTSD (the report notes that an exhaustive review of the literature was not conducted). The panel found there are findings to support the provision of integrated treatment for SUD and PTSD, and no findings indicated harm to clients who received integrated treatment for co-occurring SUD and PTSD. The review of the research does not suggest the necessity of stabilizing SUD in patients fully before they receive any services for PTSD. And the data do not clearly identify one specific treatment as the "gold standard" (National Center for PTSD, 2010a). In the absence of guidelines that specifically address treatment for comorbid PTSD and SUD, the panel concluded that the use of current VA/DOD CPGs for PTSD and SUD is appropriate for treating patients who simultaneously meet the diagnostic criteria for these disorders. The panel's recommendations state that in general treatments of patients for both PTSD and SUD can be effectively delivered concurrently (National Center for PTSD, 2010a).

With respect to specific treatments, the panel urged VA SUD and PTSD specialists to use effective first-stage treatment strategies, such as use of motivational interviewing principles and Seeking Safety, a treatment model specifically for co-occurring SUD and PTSD (National Center for PTSD, 2010a). Seeking Safety is a strongly recommended treatment in the 2008 VHA Handbook for Uniform Mental Health Services in VA Medical Centers and Clinics (VA, 2008a).

There is little evidence that supports any particular treatments for co-occurring PTSD and SUD, but some treatments are available (see Foa et al., 2009; Gulliver and Steffen, 2010). Of the existing treatments, Seeking Safety is the most researched (Foa et al., 2009). Seeking Safety is a manualized treatment (having a set protocol of actions) for people who have comorbid PTSD and substance abuse or dependence. Its primary goal is to reduce both PTSD and SUD by focusing on safe coping skills that are addressed through cognitive, behavioral, interpersonal, and case-management approaches (Boden et al., 2012). The International Society for Traumatic Stress Studies guidelines classify the level of evidence for Seeking Safety as Level A, which is evidence that is based on randomized, well-controlled clinical trials for people who have PTSD. As reported by Desai et al. (2008) and Boden et al. (2012), various studies have shown that clients appeared to respond positively to the Seeking Safety intervention, and it outperformed treatment as usual. To test how Seeking Safety fares when incorporated into the VA SUD programs, Boden et al. (2012) conducted a randomized controlled effectiveness trial with 117 veterans who had diagnoses of SUD and co-occurring PTSD symptoms. They concluded that findings provided support for the feasibility and benefit of addressing PTSD and SUD simultaneously and early in SUD treatment as opposed to requiring separate or sequential treatments or a period of abstinence before PTSD-focused care. A review of the evidence by the National Center for PTSD was more tempered: the authors noted that RCT results, although promising, were equivocal and thus concluded that Seeking Safety should probably be combined with other treatments to ensure that all problematic behaviors decrease (Gulliver and Steffen, 2010).

### Depression and Substance-Use Disorder

Over the last 20 years, results of well-controlled trials have shown that antidepressants reduced depressive symptoms in patients who have MDD and alcohol dependence. In most of the trials, however, antidepressant medications had virtually no effect in reducing excessive drinking (Pettinati and Dundon, 2011). Findings of a recent controlled trial (Pettinati et al., 2010) indicate that integrating or combining medications showed promising results in treating for co-occurring MDD and alcohol dependence. More depressed alcohol-dependent patients who received the combination of sertraline (an antidepressant) and naltrexone (to treat alcohol dependence) achieved abstinence from alcohol, had delayed relapse to heavy drinking, reported fewer serious adverse events, and tended not to be depressed by the end of treatment (Pettinati and Dundon, 2011). The researchers noted that those findings require replication before changes in clinical practice can be recommended.

The Cochrane Collaboration recently published findings of a systematic review of RCTs of the efficacy of antidepressant medication in treat depressed people who were dependent on opioids (such as morphine and heroin, codeine, oxycodone, and hydrocodone). The authors concluded that it was not possible to draw confident conclusions about the efficacy and safety of antidepressants for treatment for MDD in people who are dependent on opioids, because of clinical and methodologic differences between studies (Pani Pier et al., 2010).

With respect to psychotherapy for co-occurring MDD and SUD, Hides et al. (2010) systematically reviewed the few clinical trials that have examined the efficacy of CBT. They concluded there is minimal evidence of the effectiveness of CBT either alone or in combination with antidepressant medication for treatment for co-occurring MDD and SUD.

### Integrated Treatments and Care Models

There are several approaches to treatment for comorbid conditions: integrated (simultaneous treatment for the comorbid disorders by the same provider or clinical team), parallel (simultaneous treatment for each disorder but in different settings), sequential (treatment for one disorder followed by treatment for another), and single (treatment for only one disorder) (Foa et al., 2009; Pettinati and Dundon, 2011). An emerging body of literature reports promising results associated with integrated treatments according to principles inspired by integrated dual diagnosis treatment for co-occurring SUD and severe mental illness (Drake et al., 1998). Seeking Safety, mentioned above, is one example. Although there has been little research on and experience with integrated treatment for comorbid MDD and SUD, Pettinati and Dundon (2011) cite research demonstrating that integrated approaches (such as CBT with standard pharmacotherapy) are superior to other approaches. Otis et al. (2011) identified studies of the effectiveness of various integrated treatment approaches for veterans for combinations of pain, mild TBI, and PTSD, including cognitive processing therapy (CPT) for PTSD and CBT for chronic pain management in veterans who have comorbid chronic pain and PTSD, a sleep intervention program for veterans who have blast-induced mild TBI and headache, and a CPT-based treatment program for veterans who have comorbid PTSD and mild TBI. The authors concluded that "the results of these studies support an integrated approach to treatment and tailoring of existing evidence-based treatments to meet the specific needs of veterans."

Integrated-care models are evolving in VA. For example, the Patient Aligned Care Teams deliver comprehensive care coordinated by primary-care providers and specialists, and SUD and PTSD specialists coordinate treatment planning and delivery of SUD services that best meet the needs of patients who have co-occurring PTSD and SUD. Nonetheless, VA faces challenges in delivering comprehensive and fully integrated care for patients who have a complex cluster of medical, psychiatric, and psychosocial conditions. Reports from VA's consensus panels mentioned above (one addressing comorbid TBI, pain, and PTSD and the other addressing comorbid SUD and PTSD) emphasized that a major challenge for clinicians was the development of an interdisciplinary treatment plan that coordinates and incorporates input from all necessary specialty services. Obstacles cited include the long time needed to consult with clinicians in other disciplines and the lack of motivation of consulting practitioners who often do not receive clinical workload "credit" for such activities (National Center for PTSD, 2010a, 2010b). Similarly, Lew et al. (2008) highlighted aspects of VA's polytrauma rehabilitation centers and PTSD programs that undermine integrated care delivery.

### Summary

The co-occurrence of mental-health problems or the combination of mental-health problems with neurologic disorders places additional demands on treatments designed for one of these conditions in isolation. The current literature emphasizes the need for research to develop an evidence base and identify best practices for patients who have comorbid conditions. In addition to determining which interventions are efficacious in treating for comorbid conditions, research studies should examine facets of clinical effectiveness, such as treatment adherence, engagement, and tolerability (Brenner et al., 2009; Carlson et al., 2011; Dobscha et al., 2009; Lew et al., 2008; National Center for PTSD, 2010b). The great burden associated with comorbid conditions underscores the need for coordinated care among providers for the delivery of patient-centered care for all conditions experienced by service members and veterans.

It is not known whether simple adaptations of evidence-based treatments will be sufficient to preserve their efficacy or whether a fundamentally different treatment approach will be required. An example of the latter evolved for people who had dual diagnoses of SUD and severe mental illness with the development of integrated dual diagnosis treatment (Drake et al., 2001). That approach introduced such ideas as holistic case conceptualization and individualized staging of treatment components to address the complexity of the clinical manifestation of co-occurring disorders. The complexity of co-occurring PTSD, TBI, MDD, and SUD may necessitate the development of new treatment concepts to treat veterans of OEF and OIF.

## CONCLUSIONS

Overall, the VA and DOD clinical guidelines for screening, assessment, and treatment are in line with the available evidence base and the state-of-the-art CPGs put forth by various professional organizations. Screening for, assessment of, and treatment for brain injuries and psychologic problems are not always implemented in a consistent manner or in line with the evidence base between and within DOD and VA. The available data suggest that patients who need evidence-based care may not be receiving it.

VA's performance-measurement initiatives are at the forefront of mental-health care evaluation. The VA performance measures that the committee reviewed, which mostly examine processes of care, appear to be based on sound evidence. Measures related to patient health outcomes are lacking. VA could do more to make information about the mental-health measures being collected and their results systematically available. DOD has an established mechanism for collecting performance data—the Military Health System Population Health Portal—but lacks an emphasis on mental health. There is an opportunity for VA and DOD to synchronize their efforts in this field.

## FUTURE RESEARCH DIRECTIONS

As the committee reviewed the literature and examined the array of federally funded research on screening, assessment, and treatment of OEF and OIF service members and veterans (Appendix D), it identified several subjects for future research. The committee notes that a number of studies that are under way will shed light on the potential effectiveness of a variety of interventions. However, there are gaps in the empirical base that warrant additional systematic research:

- Studies of the psychometric properties of screening and assessment instruments to determine appropriate screening and diagnostic thresholds specifically for VA and DOD populations, determine the validity and reliability of VHA's TBI screening tool, and determine the accuracy of the DOD head computed-tomography guidelines (adapted from American College of Emergency Physicians guidelines) for detecting clinically significant brain injury in theater.
- RCTs to determine the efficacy of interventions that do not yet have a strong evidence base, including telehealth mental-health care delivery, Internet-based clinician training and treatment interventions, complementary medicine approaches (such as yoga), staged and stepped care, and TBI treatments recommended by VHA guidelines.
- Comparative-effectiveness trials to determine the effectiveness of group vs individual treatments, duration of psychotherapies, dose and duration in the use of SSRIs, and combination treatments.
- Studies of the effectiveness and efficacy of treatment interventions in producing improved desired outcomes in veterans and service personnel.
- Studies to identify what modifications, if any, need to be made in the current evidence-based treatment recommendations for each condition for the management of comorbid conditions.
- Research to assess consumer (patient and family) preferences for educational materials that explain the different evidence-based treatments that are available; such studies should determine the most effective formats for facilitating informed decision making.

## RECOMMENDATIONS

Screening, assessment, and treatment approaches for brain injuries and psychologic health problems are not always implemented between and within DOD and VA in a consistent manner or aligned with the evidence base. DOD and VA use different thresholds for some of the same mental-health screening and assessment instruments, such as the Primary Care PTSD screen and the PTSD Checklist for PTSD and the Patient Health Questionnaire for depression. Parts of VA and DOD clinical guidance lack recommendations for a specific assessment instrument and leave the selection of instrument to the clinician, for example, for suicide-risk assessments and TBI neurocognitive assessments.

The committee identified topics on which VA and DOD policies are out of step with the evidence base. There is a lack of clear scientific evidence supporting the effectiveness of the neurocognitive assessment tool (Automated Neuropsychological Assessment Metrics) used by DOD to assess cognitive function after a head injury. With respect to suicide prevention, DOD policy prohibits restricting access to privately owned weapons for those who might be at risk for of suicide, but research shows that restricting access to lethal means prevents suicides. VA has included Acceptance and Commitment Therapy for depression in its national rollout of evidenced-based treatments, however, there is not sufficient evidence to support its use as a first-line intervention. Moreover, the limited data that are available suggest that patients in need of evidence-based care might not be receiving it. The committee has serious concerns about inadequate and untimely clinical followup and low rates of delivery of evidence-based treatments, particularly psychotherapies to treat PTSD and depression and approved pharmacotherapies for substance use disorder.

**The committee recommends that the Department of Defense and the Department of Veterans Affairs select instruments and their thresholds for mental-health screening and assessment in a standardized way on the basis of the best available evidence. The committee also recommends that the two departments ensure that treatment offerings are aligned with the evidence base, particularly before national rollouts, and that all patients consistently receive first-line treatments as indicated.**

Unwarranted variability in clinical practices and deviations from the evidence base presents threats to high-quality patient care. Such variability also hampers opportunities to make research comparisons that can inform and improve the effectiveness of screening, assessment, and treatment practices. The committee notes that the emphasis on promoting evidence-based practices should not discourage the use of new or experimental interventions where there is reason to believe that they might lead to better outcomes than standard interventions.

In many ways, DOD and VA clinicians are at the forefront of providing evidence-based care for service members and veterans who have brain injuries and psychologic-health problems. But there are opportunities to improve processes of training and evaluating clinicians. DOD does not have a standardized process for assessing clinicians' competence to administer the Military Acute Concussion Evaluation for TBI. VA is implementing a robust clinician-training program to disseminate evidence-based psychotherapies, but the program appears to lack periodic clinician assessments beyond the 6-month training period to ensure that continued treatment fidelity is maintained. Current approaches for training clinicians on the management of comorbid conditions (by disseminating clinician resources, for example) are not adequate.

**The committee recommends that the Department of Defense and the Department of Veterans Affairs incorporate continuing supervision and education into programs that train clinicians in the use of selected assessment instruments and evidence-based treatments. Once clinicians are trained, the two departments should systematically and periodically evaluate them to assess the degree to which therapeutic interventions are accurately implemented according to a manual, protocol, or model as supported by evidence. The committee also recommends that the two departments place greater focus on coordinated, interdisciplinary care to ensure optimal treatment for service members and veterans.**

The committee determined that there are few data on whether screening, assessment, and treatment interventions in DOD and VA are being implemented according to clinical guidelines and VA and DOD policy. Minimal data is readily available on the numbers of people who have been screened and the extent to which followup is appropriate and timely for those who screen positive. There is a dearth of data on which treatments patients receive and whether the treatments were appropriate, timely, and delivered at the recommended intensity level (for example, individual vs group format and frequency and duration of sessions).

**The committee recommends that the Department of Defense and the Department of Veterans Affairs conduct systematic assessments to determine whether screening and treatment interventions are being implemented according to clinical guidelines and department policy. Data systems should be developed to assess treatment outcomes, variations among treatment facilities, and barriers to the use of evidence-based treatment.**

## REFERENCES


AFHSC (Armed Forces Health Surveillance Center). 2010. Supplemental report: Selected mental health disorders among active component members, US Armed Forces, 2001-2010. *Medical Surveillance Monthly Report* 17(11):2-5.

AHRQ (Agency for Healthcare Research and Quality). 2012. *National Quality Measures Clearinghouse.* www.qualitymeasures.ahrq.gov/browse/by-organization.aspx?alpha=V (accessed June 18, 2012).

Air Force Medical Operations Agency. undated. *Air Force Guide for Managing Suicidal Behavior: Strategies, Resources and Tools.* Brooks, TX: Air Force Medical Operations Agency.

Alcohol and Drug Abuse Institute Library. 2012. *Screening and Assessment Instruments: Addiction Severity Index—Baseline and Follow-Up. 5th Ed.* bit.ly/ASI_inst (accessed July 2, 2012).

Allan, C. L., L. L. Herrmann, and K. P. Ebmeier. 2011. Transcranial magnetic stimulation in the management of mood disorders. *Neuropsychobiology* 64(3):163-169.

American Academy of Neurology. 1997. *Practice Parameter: The Management of Concussion in Sports.* St. Paul, MN: Quality Standards Subcommittee, American Academy of Neurology.

American Society of Addiction Medicine. 2012. *The ASAM Patient Placement Criteria.* http://www.asam.org/publications/patient-placement-criteria (accessed July 3, 2012).

Ames, G., and C. Cunradi. 2004. Alcohol use and preventing alcohol-related problems among young adults in the military. *Alcohol Research and Health* 28(4):252-257.

Anton, R. F., S. S. O'Malley, D. A. Ciraulo, R. A. Cisler, D. Couper, D. M. Donovan, D. R. Gastfriend, J. D. Hosking, B. A. Hosking, B. A. Johnson, J. S. LoCastro, R. Longabaugh, B. J. Mason, M. E. Mattson, W. R. Miller, H. M. Pettinati, C. L. Randall, R. Swift, R. D. Weiss, L. D. Williams, and A. Zweban. 2006. Combined pharmacotherapies and behavioral interventions for alcohol dependence: The combine study: A randomized controlled trial. *Journal of the American Medical Association* 295(17):2003-2017.

APA (American Psychiatric Association). 2000. *Diagnostic and Statistical Manual of Mental Disorders (DSM-IV-TR)*, 4th Ed. Washington, DC: American Psychiatric Association.

———. 2003. *Practice Guideline for the Assessment and Treatment of Patients with Suicidal Behaviors.* Washington, DC: American Psychological Association.

———. 2010. *Practice Guideline for the Treatment for Patients with Major Depressive Disorder,* 3rd Ed. Arlington, VA: Workgroup on Major Depressive Disorder, American Psychiatric Association.

Arbaizar, B., T. Diersen-Sotos, I. Gomez-Acebo, and J. Llorca. 2010. Topiramate in the treatment of alcohol dependence: A meta-analysis. *Actas Españolas de Psiquiatría* 38(1):8-12.

Arroll, B., F. Goodyear-Smith, S. Crengle, J. Gunn, N. Kerse, T. Fishman, K. Falloon, and S. Hatcher. 2010. Validation of PHQ-2 and PHQ-9 to screen for major depression in the primary care population. *Annals of Family Medicine* 8(4):348-353.

Aubry, M., R. Cantu, J. Dvorak, T. Graf-Baumann, K. Johnston, J. Kelly, M. Lovell, P. McCrory, W. Meeuwisse, and P. Schamasch. 2002. Summary and agreement statement of the First International Conference on Concussion in Sport, Vienna 2001: Recommendations for the improvement of safety and health of athletes who may suffer concussive injuries. *British Journal of Sports Medicine* 36(1):6-10.

Babor, T. F., J. C. Higgins-Biddle, J. B. Saunders, and M. G. Monteiro. 2001. *AUDIT: Alcohol Use Disorders Identification Test: Guidelines for Use in Primary Care*, 2nd Ed. Geneva: The World Health Organization.

Bagley, S. C., B. Munjas, and P. Shekelle. 2010. A systematic review of suicide prevention programs for military or veterans. *Suicide and Life-Threatening Behavior* 40(3):257-265.

Baldessarini, R. J., L. Tondo, and J. Hennen. 2001. Treating the suicidal patient with bipolar disorder. Reducing suicide risk with lithium. *Annals of the New York Academy of Sciences* 932:24-38; discussion 39-43.

Barbato, A., and B. D'Avanzo. 2006. Marital therapy for depression. *Cochrane Database of Systematic Reviews*(2):CD004188.

Bazarian, J. J., T. Wong, M. Harris, N. Leahey, S. Mookerjee, and M. Dombovy. 1999. Epidemiology and predictors of post-concussive syndrome after minor head injury in an emergency population. *Brain Injury* 13(3):173-189.

Blake, D. D., F. W. Weathers, L. M. Nagy, D. G. Kaloupek, F. D. Gusman, D. S. Charney, and T. M. Keane. 1995. The development of a clinician-administered PTSD scale. *Journal of Traumatic Stress* 8(1):75-90.

Blanchard, E. B., J. Jones-Alexander, T. C. Buckley, and C. A. Forneris. 1996. Psychometric properties of the PTSD checklist (PCL). *Behaviour Research and Therapy* 34(8):669-673.

Bliese, P. D., K. M. Wright, A. B. Adler, O. Cabrera, C. A. Castro, and C. W. Hoge. 2008. Validating the primary care posttraumatic stress disorder screen and the posttraumatic stress disorder checklist with soldiers returning from combat. *Journal of Consulting and Clinical Psychology* 76(2):272-281.

Blue Ribbon Work Group on Suicide Prevention in the Veteran Population. 2008. *Report to James B. Peake, MD, Secretary of Veterans Affairs, June 30, 2008.* http://www.mentalhealth.va.gov/suicide_prevention/Blue_Ribbon_Report-FINAL_June-30-08.pdf (accessed October 13, 2012).

Boden, M. T., R. Kimerling, J. Jacobs-Lentz, D. Bowman, C. Weaver, D. Carney, R. Walser, and J. A. Trafton. 2012. Seeking safety treatment for male veterans with a substance use disorder and post-traumatic stress disorder symptomatology. *Addiction* 107(3):578-586.

Bradley, K. A., K. R. Bush, A. J. Epler, D. J. Dobie, T. M. Davis, J. L. Sporleder, C. Maynard, M. L. Burman, and D. R. Kivlahan. 2003. Two brief alcohol-screening tests from the alcohol use disorders identification test (audit): Validation in a female veterans affairs patient population. *Archives of Internal Medicine* 163(7):821-829.

Bradley, K. A., A. F. DeBenedetti, R. J. Volk, E. C. Williams, D. Frank, and D. R. Kivlahan. 2007. Audit-C as a brief screen for alcohol misuse in primary care. *Alcoholism, Clinical and Experimental Research* 31(7):1208-1217.

Bradley, K. A., G. T. Lapham, E. J. Hawkins, C. E. Achtmeyer, E. C. Williams, R. M. Thomas, and D. R. Kivlahan. 2011. Quality concerns with routine alcohol screening in VA clinical settings. *Journal of General Internal Medicine* 26(3):299-306.

Brain Trauma Foundation, American Association of Neurological Surgeons, and Congress of Neurological Surgeons. 2007. Guidelines for the management of severe traumatic brain injury. *Journal of Neurotrauma* 24(1 Suppl):S1-106.

Brenner, L., R. Breshears, L. Betthauser, K. Bellon, E. Holman, J. Harwood, M. Silverman, J. Huggins, and H. Nagamoto. 2011. Implementation of a suicide nomenclature within two VA healthcare settings. *Journal of Clinical Psychology in Medical Settings* (2):116-128.

Brenner, L. A., R. D. Vanderploeg, and H. Terrio. 2009. Assessment and diagnosis of mild traumatic brain injury, posttraumatic stress disorder, and other polytrauma conditions: Burden of adversity hypothesis. *Rehabilitation Psychology* 54(3):239-246.

Breshears, R. E., L. A. Brenner, J. E. Harwood, and P. M. Gutierrez. 2010. Predicting suicidal behavior in veterans with traumatic brain injury: The utility of the personality assessment inventory. *Journal of Personality Assessment* 92(4):349-355.

Brewin, C. R. 2005. Systematic review of screening instruments for adults at risk of PTSD. *Journal of Traumatic Stress* 18(1):53-62.

Brown, G. K. 2000. *A Review of Suicide Assessment Measures for Intervention Research with Adults and Older Adults.* Philadelphia, PA: University of Pennsylvania.

Brown, G. K., T. Ten Have, G. R. Henriques, S. X. Xie, J. E. Hollander, and A. T. Beck. 2005. Cognitive therapy for the prevention of suicide attempts: A randomized controlled trial. *Journal of the American Medical Association* 294(5):563-570.

Brusher, E. A. 2011. Chapter 4: Combat and operational stress control. In *Textbooks of Military Medicine: Combat and Operational Behavioral Health*, edited by E. C. Ritchie. Fort Detrick, MD: Office of the Surgeon General, Borden Institute.

Budney, A. J., S. T. Higgins, K. J. Radonovich, and P. L. Novy. 2000. Adding voucher-based incentives to coping skills and motivational enhancement improves outcomes during treatment for marijuana dependence. *Journal of Consulting and Clinical Psychology* 68(6):1051-1061.

Bullock, M. R., R. Chesnut, J. Ghajar, D. Gordon, R. Hartl, D. W. Newell, F. Servadei, B. C. Walters, and J. E. Wilberger. 2006. Guidelines for the surgical management of traumatic brain injury. *Neurosurgery* 58(3):S2-vi.

Burnett-Zeigler, I., M. Ilgen, M. Valenstein, K. Zivin, L. Gorman, A. Blow, S. Duffy, and S. Chermack. 2011. Prevalence and correlates of alcohol misuse among returning Afghanistan and Iraq veterans. *Addictive Behaviors* 36(8):801-806.

Cacciola, J. S., A. I. Alterman, B. Habing, and A. T. McLellan. 2011. Recent status scores for version 6 of the addiction severity index (ASI-6). *Addiction* 106(9):1588-1602.

Cacciola, J. S., A. I. Alterman, D. Dephilippis, M. L. Drapkin, C. Valadez, Jr., N. C. Fala, D. Oslin, and J. R. McKay. 2012. Development and initial evaluation of the Brief Addiction Monitor (BAM). *Journal of Substance Abuse Treatment* (Epub).

Calhoun, P. S., J. R. Elter, E. R. Jones, H. Kudler, and K. Straits-Troster. 2008. Hazardous alcohol use and receipt of risk-reduction counseling among US veterans of the wars in Iraq and Afghanistan. *Journal of Clinical Psychiatry* 69(11):1686-1693.

Calhoun, P. S., S. D. McDonald, V. S. Guerra, A. M. Eggleston, J. C. Beckham, K. Straits-Troster, and VA Mid-Atlantic MIRECC OEF/OIF Registry Workgroup. 2010. Clinical utility of the primary care—PTSD screen among US veterans who served since September 11, 2001. *Psychiatry Research* 178(2):330-335.

Canadian Academy of Sport Medicine Concussion Committee. 2000. Guidelines for assessment and management of sport-related concussion. *Clinical Journal of Sport Medicine* 10(3):209-211.

Cappa, S. F., T. Benke, S. Clarke, B. Rossi, B. Stemmer, C. M. van Heugten, and European Federation of Neurological Societies. 2003. EFNS guidelines on cognitive rehabilitation: Report of an EFNS task force. *European Journal of Neurology* 10(1):11-23.

Carlson, K., N. Greer, S. Kehle, R. MacDonald, L. Meis, I. Rutks, and T. J. Wilt. 2009. *The Assessment and Treatment of Individuals with History of Traumatic Brain Injury and Post-Traumatic Stress Disorder: A Systematic Review of the Evidence.* Minneapolis, MN: Evidence based Synthesis Program (ESP) Center.

Carlson, K. F., D. Nelson, R. J. Orazem, S. Nugent, D. X. Cifu, and N. A. Sayer. 2010. Psychiatric diagnoses among Iraq and Afghanistan war veterans screened for deployment-related traumatic brain injury. *Journal of Traumatic Stress* 23(1):17-24.

Carlson, K. F., S. M. Kehle, L. A. Meis, N. Greer, R. MacDonald, I. Rutks, N. A. Sayer, S. K. Dobscha, and T. J. Wilt. 2011. Prevalence, assessment and treatment of mild traumatic brain injury and posttraumatic stress disorder: A systematic review of the evidence. *Journal of Head Trauma Rehabilitation* 26(2):103-115.

Casey, G. W., Jr. 2011. Comprehensive soldier fitness: A vision for psychological resilience in the US Army. *American Psychologist* 66(1):1-3.

Casscells, S. W. 2008a. *Baseline Pre-deployment Neurocognitive Functional Assessment—Interim Guidance.* Washington, DC: Department of Defense.

———. 2008b. *Report to Congress in Response to National Defesnse Authorization Act, Fiscal Year 2007: House Report 109-452. Comprehensive Approach to Psychological Health and TBI.* Washington, DC: Department of Defense.

CBO (Congressional Budget Office). 2012. *The Veterans Health Administration's Treatment of PTSD and Traumatic Brain Injury Among Recent Combat Veterans.* Washington, DC: Congressional Budget Office.

CDC (Centers for Disease Control and Prevention). 2003. *Report to Congress on Mild Traumatic Brain Injury in the United States: Steps to Prevent a Serious Public Health Problem.* Atlanta, GA: National Center for Injury Prevention and Control, CDC.

Center for Substance Abuse Treatment. 2005. *Substance Abuse Treatment for Persons with Co-Occurring Disorders: Treatment Improvement Protocol (TIP) Series 42.* Rockville, MD: Substance Abuse and Mental Health Services Administration.

———. 2006. *Definitions and Terms Relating to Co-Occurring Disorders.* Rockville, MD: Substance Abuse and Mental Health Services Administration, and Center for Mental Health Services.

Chang, B. S., D. H. Lowenstein, and Quality Standards Subcommittee of the American Academy of Neurology. 2003. Practice parameter: Antiepileptic drug prophylaxis in severe traumatic brain injury: Report of the quality standards subcommittee of the American Academy of Neurology. *Neurology* 60(1):10-16.

Cherney, L. R., P. Gardner, J. A. Logemann, L. A. Newman, T. O'Neil-Pirozzi, C. R. Roth, and N. P. Solomon. 2010. The role of speech-language pathology and audiology in the optimal management of the service member returning from Iraq or Afghanistan with a blast-related head injury: Position of the communication sciences and disorders clinical trials research group. *Journal of Head Trauma Rehabilitation* 25(3):219-224.

Claassen, C. A., and K. L. Knox. 2011. Chapter 5: Assessment and management of high-risk suicidal states in postdeployment Operation Enduring Freedom and Operation Iraqi Freedom military personnel. In *Caring for Veterans with Deployment-Related Stress Disorders: Iraq, Afghanistan and Beyond*, edited by J. I. Ruzek, P. P. Schnurr, J. J. Vasterling, and M. J. Friedman. Washington, DC: American Psychological Association. Pp. 109-127.

Coldren, R. L., M. P. Kelly, R. V. Parish, M. Dretsch, and M. L. Russell. 2010. Evaluation of the military acute concussion evaluation for use in combat operations more than 12 hours after injury. *Military Medicine* 175(7):477-481.

Connery, H. S., and H. D. Kleber. 2007. Guideline watch (April 2007): Practice guideline for the treatment of patients with substance use disorders, 2nd edition. *Focus* 5(2).

Cozzarelli, T. A. 2010. Evaluation and treatment of persistent cognitive dysfunction following mild traumatic brain injury. *Journal of Special Operations Medicine* 10(1):39-42.

Cuijpers, P., F. Clignet, B. van Meijel, A. van Straten, J. Li, and G. Andersson. 2011. Psychological treatment of depression in inpatients: A systematic review and meta-analysis. *Clinical Psychology Review* 31(3):353-360.

Cushman, J. G., N. Agarwal, T. C. Fabian, V. Garcia, K. K. Nagy, M. D. Pasquale, A. G. Salotto, and East Practice Management Guidelines Work Group. 2001. Practice management guidelines for the management of mild traumatic brain injury: The East Practice Management Guidelines Work Group. *Journal of Trauma—Injury, Infection, and Critical Care* 51(5):1016-1026.

Davidson, J. R., S. W. Book, J. T. Colket, L. A. Tupler, S. Roth, D. David, M. Hertzberg, T. Mellman, J. C. Beckham, R. D. Smith, R. M. Davison, R. Katz, and M. E. Feldman. 1997. Assessment of a new self-rating scale for post-traumatic stress disorder. *Psychological Medicine* 27(1):153-160.

Dawson, D. A., B. F. Grant, F. S. Stinson, and Y. Zhou. 2005. Effectiveness of the derived Alcohol Use Disorders Identification Test (AUDIT-C) in screening for alcohol use disorders and risk drinking in the US general population. *Alcoholism: Clinical and Experimental Research* 29(5):844-854.

DCoE (Defense Centers of Excellence for Psychological Health and Traumatic Brain Injury). 2010. *Case Management of Concussion/Mild TBI.* Silver Spring, MD: Department of Defense.

———. 2011a. *All the Way Home: Preventing Suicide Among Service Members and Veterans.* Boston, MA: DoD/VA Annual Suicide Prevention Conference, March 13-17, 2011.

———. 2011b. *Clinical Recommendation: Indications and Conditions for In-Theater Post-Injury Neurocognitive Assessment Tool (NCAT) Testing.* Silver Spring, MD: Department of Defense.

———. 2011c. *Co-Occurring Conditions Toolkit: Mild Traumatic Brain Injury and Psychological Health, Revised September 2011.* Silver Spring, MD: Department of Defense.

———. 2011d. *Department of Defense Suicide Event Report: Calendar Year 2010 Annual Report.* Washington, DC: National Center for Telehealth and Technology, Defense Centers of Excellence for Psychological Health and Traumatic Brain Injury.

———. 2011e. *Guidance for Training, Education on Clinical Practice Guidelines.* Arlington, VA: Defense Centers of Excellence for Psychological Health and Traumatic Brain Injury.

———. 2011f. *Screening and Assessment Tools for Suicide Prevention: Compilation by the DOD/VA Suicide Prevention Tools Working Group.* Arlington, VA and Silver Spring, MD: Defense Centers of Excellence for Psychological Health and Traumatic Brain Injury.

———. 2012a. *Defense and Veterans Brain Injury Center.* Silver Spring, MD: Defense Centers of Excellence for Psychological Health and Traumatic Brain Injury.

———. 2012b. *Fact Sheet Summer 2012.* Silver Spring, MD: Defense Centers of Excellence for Psychological Health and Traumatic Brain Injury.

———. 2012c. *Overview of DCOE and DOD Suicide Prevention Efforts.* Silver Spring, MD: Defense Centers of Excellence for Psychological Health and Traumatic Brain Injury.

———. 2012d. *RESPECT-Mil: Re-Engineering Systems of Primary Care Treatment in the Military.* Washington, DC: Defense Centers of Excellence for Psychological Health and Traumatic Brain Injury.

———. 2012e. *Traumatic Brain Injury.* Silver Spring, MD: Defense Centers of Excellence for Psychological Health and Traumatic Brain Injury.

de Groot, V., H. Beckerman, G. J. Lankhorst, and L. M. Bouter. 2003. How to measure comorbidity: A critical review of available methods. *Journal of Clinical Epidemiology* 56(3):221-229.

Defense Health Board. 2010. *Memorandum: Findings Pertaining to Evidence-Based Metrics for Department of Defense Mental Health Pre-Clinical Program Effectiveness and Clinical Program Outcomes.* Falls Church, VA: Defense Health Board.

DeFraites, R., and M. Vythilingam. 2011. *DOD Deployment Mental Health Assessments: A Review and Update.* Falls Church, VA: Force Health Protection and Readiness.

Dempsey, K. E., W. C. Dorlac, K. Martin, R. Fang, C. Fox, B. Bennett, K. Williams, and S. Flaherty. 2009. Landstuhl Regional Medical Center: Traumatic brain injury screening program. *Journal of Trauma Nursing* 16(1):6-7, 10-12.

Department of the Army. 2010a. *The DOD Automated Neuropsychological Assessment Metric Program: A Critical Review of Supporting Documentation.* Falls Church, VA: Department of the Army Office of the Surgeon General.

———. 2010b. *Re-Engineering Systems of the Primary Care Treatment (of Depression and Post-Traumatic Stress Disorder) in the Military Documentation Form.* Fort Sam Houston, TX: United States Army Medical Command.

———. 2012. *Army 2020: Generating Health and Discipline in the Force.* Washington, DC: Department of Defense.

Desai, M., R. Rosenheck, and T. J. Craig. 2006. Case-finding for depression among medical outpatients in the veterans health administration. *Medical Care* 44(2):175-181.

Desai, R. A., I. Harpaz-Rotem, L. M. Najavits, and R. A. Rosenheck. 2008. Impact of the seeking safety program on clinical outcomes among homeless female veterans with psychiatric disorders. *Psychiatric Services* 59(9):996-1003.

Dobscha, S. K., M. E. Clark, B. J. Morasco, M. Freeman, R. Campbell, and M. Helfand. 2009. Systematic review of the literature on pain in patients with polytrauma including traumatic brain injury. *Pain Medicine* 10(7):1200-1217.

DOD (Department of Defense). 1994. *Directive 1010.1: Military Personnel Drug Abuse Testing Program.* Washington, DC: Department of Defense.

———. 2008. *DD Form 2796.* Washington, DC: Department of Defense.

———. 2010a. *The Challenge and the Promise: Strengthening the Force, Preventing Suicide and Saving Lives.* Washington, DC: Department of Defense Task Force on the Prevention of Suicide By Members of the Armed Forces.

———. 2010b. *Directive-Type Memorandum DTM 09-033: Policy Guidance for Management of Concussion/Mild Traumatic Brain Injury in the Deployed Setting*. Washington, DC: Department of Defense.

———. 2011a. *Report to Congress on Expenditures for Activities on Traumatic Brain Injury and Psychological Health, Including Posttraumatic Stress Disorder, for 2010.* Washington, DC: Department of Defense

———. 2011b. *Section 596 of the FY 2010 National Defense Authorization Act (NDAA) Comprehensive Plan on Prevention, Diagnosis, and Treatment of Substance Use Disorders (SUDS) and Disposition of Substance Use Offenders in the Armed Forces.* Washington, DC: Department of Defense.

———. 2012. *Report to Congress: Cognitive Rehabilitation Therapy for Traumatic Brain Injury for Fiscal Year 2011*. Washington, DC: Department of Defense.

Donnelly, K. T., J. P. Donnelly, M. Dunnam, G. C. Warner, C. J. Kittleson, J. E. Constance, C. B. Bradshaw, and M. Alt. 2011. Reliability, sensitivity, and specificity of the VA traumatic brain injury screening tool. *Journal of Head Trauma Rehabilitation* 26(6):439-453.

Drake, A. I., K. S. Meyer, L. M. Cessante, C. R. Cheung, M. A. Cullen, E. C. McDonald, and M. C. Holland. 2010. Routine TBI screening following combat deployments. *NeuroRehabilitation* 26(3):183-189.

Drake, R. E., C. Mercer-McFadden, K. T. Mueser, G. J. McHugo, and G. R. Bond. 1998. Review of integrated mental health and substance abuse treatment for patients with dual disorders. *Schizophrenia Bulletin* 24(4):589-608.

Drake, R. E., S. M. Essock, A. Shaner, K. B. Carey, K. Minkoff, L. Kola, D. Lynde, F. C. Osher, R. E. Clark, and L. Rickards. 2001. Implementing dual diagnosis services for clients with severe mental illness. *Psychiatric Services* 52(4):469-476.

DVBIC (Defense and Veterans Brain Injury Center). 2006. *Acute Management of Mild Traumatic Brain Injury in Military Operational Settings: Clinical Practice Guideline and Recommendations.* Washington, DC: Defense and Veterans Brain Injury Center.

———. 2007. *Joint Theater Trauma System Clinical Practice Guideline: Theater Screening and Management of Mild Traumatic Brain Injury (Concussion).* Silver Spring, MD: Department of Defense.

———. 2008a. *Consensus Conference on the Acute Management of Concussion/Mild Traumatic Brain Injury (mTBI) in the Deployed Setting*. Washington, DC: Defense and Veterans Brain Injury Center.

———. 2008b. *Updated Mild Traumatic Brain Injury (mTBI) Clinical Guidance.* Washington, DC: Defense and Veterans Brain Injury Center.

Erlanger, D. M., K. C. Kutner, J. T. Barth, and R. Barnes. 1999. Neuropsychology of sports-related head injury: Dementia pugilistica to post concussion syndrome. *Clinical Neuropsychologist* 13(2):193-209.

Foa, E., T. Keane, and M. Friedman. 2009. *Effective Treatments for PTSD, Practice Guidelines from the International Society for Traumatic Stress Studies, 2nd Ed.* New York: The Guilford Press.

Foa, E. B., D. S. Riggs, C. V. Dancu, and B. O. Rothbaum. 1993. Reliability and validity of a brief instrument for assessing post-traumatic stress disorder. *Journal of Traumatic Stress* 6(4):459-473.

Forbes, D., M. Creamer, A. Phelps, R. Bryant, A. McFarlane, G. J. Devilly, L. Matthews, B. Raphael, C. Doran, T. Merlin, and S. Newton. 2007. Australian guidelines for the treatment of adults with acute stress disorder and post-traumatic stress disorder. *Australian and New Zealand Journal of Psychiatry* 41(8):637-648.

Fowler, J. C. 2012. Suicide risk assessment in clinical practice: Pragmatic guidelines for imperfect assessments. *Psychotherapy* 49(1):81-90.

Freeman, M. P., M. Fava, J. Lake, M. H. Trivedi, K. L. Wisner, and D. Mischoulon. 2010. Complementary and alternative medicine in major depressive disorder: The American Psychiatric Association Task Force report. *Journal of Clinical Psychiatry* 71(6):669-681.

Freeman, T. W., V. Roca, and T. Kimbrell. 2003. A survey of gun collection and use among three groups of veteran patients admitted to veterans affairs hospital treatment programs. *Southern Medical Journal* 96(3):240-243.

French, L., M. McCrea, and M. Baggett. 2008. The Military Acute Concussion Evaluation (MACE). *Journal of Special Operations Medicine* 8(1):68-77.

GAO (Government Accountability Office). 2008. *VA Health Care: Mild Traumatic Brain Injury Screening and Evaluation Implemented for OEF/OIF Veterans, but Challenges Remain.* Washington, DC: GAO.

———. 2010. *VA Faces Challenges in Providing Substance Use Disorder Services and is Taking Steps to Improve These Services for Veterans*. Washington, DC: GAO.

———. 2011. *Department of Defense: Use of Neurocognitive Assessment Tools in Post-deployment Identification of Mild Traumatic Brain Injury.* Washington, DC: GAO.

Glass, J. E., B. E. Perron, M. A. Ilgen, S. T. Chermack, S. Ratliff, and K. Zivin. 2010. Prevalence and correlates of specialty substance use disorder treatment for Department of Veterans Affairs healthcare system patients with high alcohol consumption. *Drug and Alcohol Dependence* 112(1-2):150-155.

Greenfield, S. F., J. M. Reizes, L. R. Muenz, B. Kopans, R. C. Kozloff, and D. G. Jacobs. 2000. Treatment for depression following the 1996 National Depression Screening Day. *American Journal of Psychiatry* 157(11):1867-1869.

Guillamondegui, O. D., S. A. Montgomery, F. T. Phibbs, M. L. McPheeters, P. T. Alexander, R. N. Jerome, J. N. McKoy, J. J. Seroogy, J. J. Eicken, S. Krishnaswami, R. M. Salomon, and K. E. Hartmann. 2011. *Traumatic Brain Injury and Depression.* Rockville, MD: Agency for Healthcare Research and Quality.

Gulliver, S. B., and L. E. Steffen. 2010. *Towards Integrated Treatments for PTSD and Substance Use Disorders.* Washington, DC: National Center for PTSD.

Haney, E. M., M. E. O'Neil, S. Carson, A. Low, K. Peterson, L. M. Denneson, C. Oleksiewicz, and D. Kansagara. 2012. *Suicide Risk Factors and Risk Assessment Tools: A Systematic Review*. Portland, OR: Evidence-based Synthesis Program (ESP) Center.

Harris, A. H., K. Humphreys, T. Bowe, D. R. Kivlahan, and J. W. Finney. 2009. Measuring the quality of substance use disorder treatment: Evaluating the validity of the Department of Veterans Affairs continuity of care performance measure. *Journal of Substance Abuse and Treatment* 36(3):294-305.

Harris, A. H., D. R. Kivlahan, T. Bowe, and K. N. Humphreys. 2010. Pharmacotherapy of alcohol use disorders in the Veterans Health Administration. *Psychiatric Services* 61(4):392-398.

Harris, A. H., E. Oliva, T. Bowe, K. N. Humphreys, D. R. Kivlahan, and J. A. Trafton. 2012. Pharmacotherapy of alcohol use disorders by the Veterans Health Administration: Patterns of receipt and persistence. *Psychiatric Services* 63:679-685.

Hawkins, E. J., G. T. Lapham, D. R. Kivlahan, and K. A. Bradley. 2010. Recognition and management of alcohol misuse in OEF/OIF and other veterans in the VA: A cross-sectional study. *Drug and Alcohol Dependence* 109(1-3):147-153.

Hawton, K., E. Townsend, E. Arensman, D. Gunnell, P. Hazell, A. House, and K. van Heeringen. 2000. Psychosocial versus pharmacological treatments for deliberate self harm. *Cochrane Database of Systematic Reviews* (2):CD001764.

Hegerl, U., P. Schonknecht, and R. Mergl. 2012. Are antidepressants useful in the treatment of minor depression: A critical update of the current literature. *Current Opinion in Psychiatry* 25(1):1-6.

Helmick, K. 2010. Cognitive rehabilitation for military personnel with mild traumatic brain injury and chronic post-concussional disorder: Results of April 2009 consensus conference. *NeuroRehabilitation* 26(3):239-255.

Helmick, K. M. 2011. Continuum of care for traumatic brain injury in the Department of Defense. Paper read at 2011 Military Health System Conference, February 7, 2011, Washington, DC.

HHS (US Department of Health and Human Services). 2004. *United States Preventative Services Task Force: Screening and Behavioral Counseling Interventions in Primary Care to Reduce Alcohol Misuse: Recommendation Statement.* Rockville, MD: Agency for Healthcare Research and Quality, US Department of Health and Human Services.

———. 2005. *Helping Patients Who Drink Too Much. A Clinicians Guide.* Washington, DC: Department of Health and Human Services.

Hides, L., S. Samet, and D. I. Lubman. 2010. Cognitive Behaviour Therapy (CBT) for the treatment of co-occurring depression and substance use: Current evidence and directions for future research. *Drug and Alcohol Review* 29(5):508-517.

Hirschfeld, R. M., and J. M. Russell. 1997. Assessment and treatment of suicidal patients. *New England Journal of Medicine* 337(13):910-915.

Hoge, C. W., C. A. Castro, S. C. Messer, D. McGurk, D. I. Cotting, and R. L. Koffman. 2004. Combat duty in Iraq and Afghanistan, mental health problems, and barriers to care. *New England Journal of Medicine* 351(1):13-22.

Holm, L., J. D. Cassidy, L. J. Carroll, J. Borg, and WHO Collaborating Centre for Neurotrauma Task Force on Mild Traumatic Brain Injury. 2005. Summary of the WHO Collaborating Centre for Neurotrauma Task Force on Mild Traumatic Brain Injury. *Journal of Rehabilitation Medicine* 37(3):137-141.

Ingebrigtsen, T., B. Romner, and C. Kock-Jensen. 2000. Scandinavian guidelines for initial management of minimal, mild, and moderate head injuries. The Scandinavian Neurotrauma Committee. *Journal of Trauma-Injury Infection and Critical Care* 48(4):760-766.

International Society for Traumatic Stress Studies. 2009. *Effective Treatments for PTSD: Practice Guidelines from the International Society for Traumatic Stress Studies, 2nd Ed.* Edited by E. B. Foa, T. M. Keane, M. J. Friedman and J. A. Cohen. New York: Guilford Press.

IOM (Institute of Medicine). 2002. *Reducing Suicide: A National Imperative.* Washington, DC: The National Academies Press.

———. 2006. *Posttraumatic Stress Disorder: Diagnosis and Assessment.* Washington, DC: The National Academies Press.

———. 2009. *Gulf War and Health, Volume 7: Long-Term Consequences of Traumatic Brain Injury.* Washington, DC: The National Academies Press.

———. 2011a. *Clinical Guideline Practices We Can Trust.* Washington, DC: The National Academies Press.

———. 2011b. *Cognitive Rehabilitation Therapy for Traumatic Brain Injury: Evaluating the Evidence.* Washington, DC: The National Academies Press.

———. 2012. *Treatment for Posttraumatic Stress Disorder in Military and Veteran Populations: Initial Assessment.* Washington, DC: The National Academies Press.

———. 2013. *Substance Use Disorders in the US Armed Forces.* Washington, DC: The National Academies Press.

Ipser, J. C., and D. J. Stein. 2012. Evidence-based pharmacotherapy of post-traumatic stress disorder (PTSD). *International Journal of Neuropsychopharmacology* 15(6):825-840.

Iverson, G. L., J. A. Langlois, M. A. McCrea, and J. P. Kelly. 2009. Challenges associated with post-deployment screening for mild traumatic brain injury in military personnel. *Clinical Neuropsychologist* 23(8):1299-1314.

Ivins, B. J., R. Kane, and K. A. Schwab. 2009. Performance on the automated neuropsychological assessment metrics in a nonclinical sample of soldiers screened for mild TBI after returning from Iraq and Afghanistan: A descriptive analysis. *Journal of Head Trauma Rehabilitation* 24(1):24-31.

Jagoda, A. S., J. J. Bazarian, J. J. Bruns, Jr., S. V. Cantrill, A. D. Gean, P. K. Howard, J. Ghajar, S. Riggio, D. W. Wright, R. L. Wears, A. Bakshy, P. Burgess, M. M. Wald, and R. R. Whitson. 2009. Clinical policy: Neuroimaging and decisionmaking in adult mild traumatic brain injury in the acute setting. *Journal of Emergency Nursing* 35(2):e5-e40.

Jha, A. K., J. B. Perlin, K. W. Kizer, and R. A. Dudley. 2003. Effect of the transformation of the Veterans Affairs health care system on the quality of care. *New England Journal of Medicine* 348(22):2218-2227.

Jobes, D. A. 2012. The Collaborative Assessment and Management of Suicidality (CAMS): An evolving evidence-based clinical approach to suicidal risk. *Suicide and Life-Threatening Behavior* 42(6): 640-653.

Jobes, D. A., S. A. Wong, A. K. Conrad, J. F. Drozd, and T. Neal-Walden. 2005. The collaborative assessment and management of suicidality versus treatment as usual: A retrospective study with suicidal outpatients. *Suicide and Life-Threatening Behavior* 35(5):483-497.

Johnson, B. A., and N. Ait-Daoud. 2010. Topiramate in the new generation of drugs: Efficacy in the treatment of alcoholic patients. *Current Pharmaceutical Design* 16(19):2103-2112.

Johnston, K. M., M. Lassonde, and A. Ptito. 2001. A contemporary neurosurgical approach to sport-related head injury: The McGill Concussion Protocol. *Journal of the American College of Surgeons* 192(4):515-524.

Jordan, B. 2012. *DOD Could Renew Push to Restrict Personal Weapons*. http://www.military.com/daily-news/2012/06/21/DoD-could-renew-push-to-restrict-personal-weapons.html (accessed October 1, 2012).

Kaner, E. F., F. Beyer, H. O. Dickinson, E. Pienaar, F. Campbell, C. Schlesinger, N. Heather, J. Saunders, B. Burnand. 2007. Effectiveness of brief alcohol interventions in primary care populations. *Cochrane Database of Systematic Reviews* 2.

Kaplan, M. S., N. Huguet, B. H. McFarland, and J. T. Newsom. 2007. Suicide among male veterans: A prospective population-based study. *Journal of Epidemiology and Community Health* 61(7):619-624.

Karlin, B. E. 2010. Evidence based psychotherapy and psychogeriatrics update. Paper read at Presentation to the *13th Annual VA Psychology Leadership Conference of the Association of VA Psychologist Leaders*, May 14, 2010.

Karlin, B. E., J. I. Ruzek, K. M. Chard, A. Eftekhari, C. M. Monson, E. A. Hembree, P. A. Resick, and E. B. Foa. 2010. Dissemination of evidence-based psychological treatments for posttraumatic stress disorder in the veterans health administration. *Journal of Traumatic Stress* 23(6):663-673.

Kemp, J. E. 2011. *Witness Testimony: Understanding and Preventing Veteran Suicide, December 12, 2011.* Washington, DC: House Committee on Veterans Affairs.

Kleber, H. D., R. D. Weiss, R. F. Anton Jr., T. P. George, S. F. Greenfield, T. R. Kosten, C. P. O'Brien, B. J. Rounsaville, E. C. Strain, D. M. Ziedonis, G. Hennessy, and H. Smith Connery. 2006. *Practice Guideline for the Treatment of Patients with Substance Use Disorder.* Washington, DC: American Psychiatric Association.

Knapp, W. P., B. G. Soares, M. Farrel, and M. S. Lima. 2007. Psychosocial interventions for cocaine and psychostimulant amphetamines related disorders. *Cochrane Database of Systematic Reviews* 3:CD003023.

Knuth, T., P. B. Letarte, G. Ling, L. E. Moores, P. Rhee, D. Tauber, and A. Trask. 2005. *Guidelines for the Field Management of Combat Related Head Trauma.* New York: Brain Trauma Foundation.

Kroenke, K., R. L. Spitzer, and J. B. Williams. 2001. The PHQ-9: Validity of a brief depression severity measure. *Journal of General Internal Medicine* 16(9):606-613.

Kroenke K., R. L. Spitzer, and J. B. Williams. 2003. The Patient Health Questionnaire-2: Validity of a two-item depression screener. *Medical Care* 41(11):1284-1292.

Kroenke, K., R. L. Spitzer, J. B. Williams, and B. Lowe. 2010. The patient health questionnaire somatic, anxiety, and depressive symptom scales: A systematic review. *General Hospital Psychiatry* 32(4):345-359.

Lapham, G. T., C. E. Achtmeyer, E. C. Williams, E. J. Hawkins, D. R. Kivlahan, and K. A. Bradley. 2012. Increased documented brief alcohol interventions with a performance measure and electronic decision support. *Medical Care* 50(2):179-187.

Lew, H. L., R. D. Vanderploeg, D. F. Moore, K. Schwab, L. Friedman, J. A. Yesavage, T. M. Keane, D. L. Warden, and B. J. Sigford. 2008. Overlap of mild TBI and mental health conditions in returning OIF/OEF service members and veterans. *Journal of Rehabilitation Research and Development* 45(3):xi-xvi.

Mann, J. J., A. Apter, J. Bertolote, A. Beautrais, D. Currier, A. Haas, U. Hegerl, J. Lonnqvist, K. Malone, A. Marusic, L. Mehlum, G. Patton, M. Phillips, W. Rutz, Z. Rihmer, A. Schmidtke, D. Shaffer, M. Silverman, Y. Takahashi, A. Varnik, D. Wasserman, P. Yip, and H. Hendin. 2005. Suicide prevention strategies: A systematic review. *Journal of the American Medical Association* 294(16):2064-2074.

Martin, J. L., and E. Martin-Sanchez. 2012. Systematic review and meta-analysis of vagus nerve stimulation in the treatment of depression: Variable results based on study designs. *European Psychiatry* 27(3):147-155.

Mayet, S., M. Farrell, M. Ferri, L. Amato, and M. Davoli. 2005. Psychosocial treatment for opiate abuse and dependence. *Cochrane Database Systematic Reviews* (1):CD004330.

McCrea, M., K. M. Guskiewicz, S. W. Marshall, W. Barr, C. Randolph, R. C. Cantu, J. A. Onate, J. Yang, and J. P. Kelly. 2003. Acute effects and recovery time following concussion in collegiate football players: The NCAA Concussion Study. *Journal of the American Medical Association* 290(19):2556-2563.

McCrea, M., G. L. Iverson, T. W. McAllister, T. A. Hammeke, M. R. Powell, W. B. Barr, and J. P. Kelly. 2009. An integrated review of recovery after mild traumatic brain injury (mTBI): Implications for clinical management. *Clinical Neuropsychologist* 23(8):1368-1390.

McCrory, P., K. Johnston, W. Meeuwisse, M. Aubry, R. Cantu, J. Dvorak, T. Graf-Baumann, J. Kelly, M. Lovell, and P. Schamasch. 2005. Summary and agreement statement of the 2nd International Conference on Concussion in Sport, Prague 2004. *British Journal of Sports Medicine* 39(4):196-204.

McCrory, P., W. Meeuwisse, K. Johnston, J. Dvorak, M. Aubry, M. Molloy, and R. Cantu. 2009. Consensus statement on concussion in sport: The 3rd International Conference on Concussion in Sport held in Zurich, November 2008. *Journal of Athletic Training* 44(4):434-448.

McDonald, S. D., and P. S. Calhoun. 2010. The diagnostic accuracy of the PTSD checklist: A critical review. *Clinical Psychology Review* 30(8):976-987.

McLellan, A. T., L. Luborsky, G. E. Woody, and C. P. O'Brien. 1980. An improved diagnostic evaluation instrument for substance abuse patients. The addiction severity index. *Journal of Nervous and Mental Disease* 168(1):26-33.

Mee-Lee, D., G. D. Schulman, M. Fishman, D. R. Gastfriend, and J. H. Griffith. 2001. *ASAM Patient Placement Criteria for the Treatment of Substance-Related Disorders, Second Edition-Revised (ASAM-PPC-2R).* Chevy Chase, MD: American Society of Addiction Medicine Inc.

MHSPHP (Military Healthcare System Population Health Portal). 2012. *Methodology Document —Draft.* San Antonio, TX: Health Informatics Division.

Milliken, C. S., J. L. Auchterlonie, and C. W. Hoge. 2007. Longitudinal assessment of mental health problems among active and reserve component soldiers returning from the Iraq war. *Journal of the American Medical Association* 298(18):2141-2148.

Montgomery, K. L., J. S. Kim, and C. Franklin. 2011. Acceptance and commitment therapy for psychological and physiological illnesses: A systematic review for social workers. *Health and Social Work* 36(3):169-181.

Moscicki, E. K. 2001. Epidemiology of completed and attempted suicide: Toward a framework for prevention. *Clinical Neuroscience Research* 1:310-323.

Nash, W. P., C. Silva, and B. Litz. 2009. The historic origins of military and veteran mental health stigma and the stress injury model as a means to reduce it. *Psychiatric Annals* 39(8):789-794.

National Center for PTSD. 2004. *Iraq War Clinician Guide,* 2nd ed. White River Junction, VT: Department of Veterans Affairs.

———. 2010a. *Report of (VA) Consensus Conference: Practice Recommendations for Treatment of Veterans with Comorbid Substance Abuse and PTSD.* Washington, DC: Department of Veterans Affairs.

———. 2010b. *Report of (VA) Consensus Conference: Practice Recommendations for Treatment of Veterans with Comorbid TBI, Pain, and PTSD.* Washington, DC: Department of Veterans Affairs.

———. 2012a. *Assessment.* http://www.ptsd.va.gov/professional/pages/assessments/assessment.asp (accessed August 1, 2012).

———. 2012b. *Using the PTSD Checklist (PCL).* Washington, DC: US Department of Veterans Affairs.

National Collaborating Centre for Mental Health. 2005. *Post-traumatic Stress Disorder (PTSD): The Management of PTSD in Adults and Children in Primary and Secondary Care, Clinical Guideline 26.* London, UK: National Institute for Clinical Excellence.

———. 2011. *Alcohol-use Disorders: Diagnosis, Assessment and Management of Harmful Drinking and Alcohol Dependence.* Leicester, UK: The British Psychological Society.

Neurobehavioral Guidelines Working Group. 2006. Guidelines for the pharmacologic treatment of neurobehavioral sequelae of traumatic brain injury. *Journal of Neurotrauma* 23(10):1468-1501.

New Zealand Guidelines Group. 2006. *Evidence-Based Best Practice Guideline: Traumatic Brain Injury: Diagnosis, Acute Management and Rehabilitation.* Wellington, New Zealand: New Zealand Guidelines Group.

NIAAA (National Institute on Alcohol Abuse and Alcoholism). 2008. *Helping Patients Who Drink Too Much: A Clinician's Guide.* Washington, DC: National Institutes of Health.

NICE (National Institute for Health and Clinical Excellence). 2007. *Head Injury: Triage, Assessment, Investigation and Early Management of Head Injury in Infants, Children and Adults.* London, UK: National Institute for Health and Clinical Excellence.

———. 2009. *Depression: Treatment and Management of Depression in Adults Including Adults with Chronic Physical Health Problems.* London: National Institute for Health and Clinical Excellence.

Nieuwsma, J. A., R. B. Trivedi, J. McDuffie, I. Kronish, D. Benjamin, and J. W. J. Williams. 2011. *Brief Psychotherapy for Depression in Primary Care: A Systematic Review of the Evidence.* Washington, DC: Department of Veterans Affairs.

NIH (National Institutes of Health). 1999. Consensus development panel: Rehabilitation of persons with traumatic brain injury. *Journal of the American Medical Association* 282(10):974-983.

Oliva, E. M., A. H. Harris, J. A. Trafton, and A. J. Gordon. 2012. Receipt of opioid agonist treatment in the Veterans Health Administration: Facility and patient factors. *Drug and Alcohol Dependence* 122(3):241-246.

Ontario Neurotrauma Foundation. 2011. *Guidelines for Mild Traumatic Brain Injury and Persistent Symptoms.* Toronto, Canada: Ontario Neurotrauma Foundation.

Otis, J., R. McGlinchey, J. Vasterling, and R. Kerns. 2011. Complicating factors associated with mild traumatic brain injury: Impact on pain and posttraumatic stress disorder treatment. *Journal of Clinical Psychology.*

Oxman, T., A. J. Dietrich, J. John W. Williams, C. C. Engel, M. Friedman, P. Schnurr, S. Rosenberg, and S. L. Barry. 2008. *Three Component Model for Primary Care Management of Depression and PTSD (Military Version).* Bethesda, MD: Deployment Health Clinical Center.

Pani Pier, P., R. Vacca, E. Trogu, L. Amato, and M. Davoli. 2010. Pharmacological treatment for depression during opioid agonist treatment for opioid dependence. *Cochrane Database of Systematic Reviews* (9).

Pettinati, H. M., and W. D. Dundon. 2011. Comorbid depression and alcohol dependence: New approaches to dual therapy challenges and progress. *Psychiatric Times* 28(6).

Pettinati, H. M., D. W. Oslin, K. M. Kampman, W. D. Dundon, H. Xie, T. L. Gallis, C. A. Dackis, and C. P. O'Brien. 2010. A double-blind, placebo-controlled trial combining sertraline and naltrexone for treating co-occurring depression and alcohol dependence. *American Journal of Psychiatry* 167(6):668-675.

Phurrough, S., M. E. Salive, B. Lofton, and J. Schafer. 2007. *Decision Memo for Vagus Nerve Stimulation for Treatment of Resistant Depression (TRD) (CAG-00313R).* Washington, DC: Centers for Medicaid and Medicare Services.

Pigott, H. E., A. M. Leventhal, G. S. Alter, and J. J. Boren. 2010. Efficacy and effectiveness of antidepressants: Current status of research. *Psychotherapy and Psychosomatics* 79(5):267-279.

Pincus, H. A., B. Spaeth-Rublee, and K. E. Watkins. 2011. The case for measuring quality in mental health and substance abuse care. *Health Affairs* 30(4):730-736.

Polen, M. R., E. P. Whitlock, J. P. Wisdom, P. Nygren, and C. Bougatsos. 2008. *Screening in Primary Care Settings for Illicit Drug Use: Staged Systematic Review for the United States Preventive Services Task Force*. Rockville, MD: Agency for Healthcare Research and Quality.

Posner, K., G. K. Brown, B. Stanley, D. A. Brent, K. V. Yershova, M. A. Oquendo, G. W. Currier, G. A. Melvin, L. Greenhill, S. Shen, and J. J. Mann. 2011. The Columbia-Suicide Severity Rating Scale: Initial validity and internal consistency findings from three multisite studies with adolescents and adults. *American Journal of Psychiatry* 168(12):1266-1277.

Powers, M. B., M. B. Zum Vorde Sive Vording, and P. M. Emmelkamp. 2009. Acceptance and commitment therapy: A meta-analytic review. *Psychotherapy and Psychosomatics* 78(2):73-80.

Prins, A., P. Ouimette, R. Kimerling, R. P. Camerond, D. S. Hugelshofer, J. Shaw-Hegwer, A. Thrailkill, F. D. Gusman, and J. I. Sheikh. 2004. The Primary Care PTSD Screen (PC-PTSD): Development and operating characteristics. *Primary Care Psychiatry* 9(1):9-14.

Qaseem, A., V. Snow, T. D. Denberg, M. A. Forciea, and D. K. Owens. 2008. Using second-generation antidepressants to treat depressive disorders: A clinical practice guideline from the American College of Physicians. *Annals of Internal Medicine* 149(10):725-733.

Radomski, M. V., L. Davidson, D. Voydetich, and M. W. Erickson. 2009. Occupational therapy for service members with mild traumatic brain injury. *American Journal of Occupational Therapy* 63(5):646-655.

Ramchand, R., J. Acosta, R. M. Burns, L. H. Jaycox, and C. G. Pernin. 2011. *The War Within: Preventing Suicide in the US Military.* Santa Monica, CA: RAND Corporation.

Richards, D., and T. Richardson. 2012. Computer-based psychological treatments for depression: A systematic review and meta-analysis. *Clinical Psychology Review* 32(4):329-342.

Rimer, J., K. Dwan, D. A. Lawlor, C. A. Greig, M. McMurdo, W. Morley, and G. E. Mead. 2012. Exercise for depression. *Cochrane Database Systematic Reviews* 7.

Rodgers, M., M. Asaria, S. Walker, D. McMillan, M. Lucock, M. Harden, S. Palmer, and A. Eastwood. 2012. The clinical effectiveness and cost-effectiveness of low-intensity psychological interventions for the secondary prevention of relapse after depression: A systematic review. *Health Technology Assessment* 16(28):1-130.

Roebuck-Spencer, T. M., A. S. Vincent, D. A. Twillie, B. W. Logan, C. M. Lopez, C. K. Friedl, S. J. Grate, R. E. Schlegel, and K. Gilliland. 2012. Cognitive change associated with self-reported mild traumatic brain injury sustained during the OEF/OIF conflicts. *Clinical Neuropsychologist* 26(3):473-489.

Rohling, M. L., M. E. Faust, B. Beverly, and G. Demakis. 2009. Effectiveness of cognitive rehabilitation following acquired brain injury: A meta-analytic re-examination of Cicerone et al.'s (2000, 2005) systematic reviews. *Neuropsychology* 23(1):20-39.

SAMHSA (Substance Abuse and Mental Health Services Administration). 2009. Chapter 4: Screening and assessment. In *Substance Abuse Treatment: Addressing the Specific Needs of Women. Treatment Improvement Protocol (TIP) Series, NO. 51*. Rockville, MD: Substance Abuse and Mental Health Services Administration.

———. 2011. *Screening, Brief Intervention and Referral to Treatment (SBIRT) in Behavioral Healthcare*. Rockville, MD: Substance Abuse and Mental Health Services Administration.

Sayer, N. 2009. *Polytrauma/Blast-Related Injuries QUERI Center: Strategic Plan*. Washington, DC: Quality Enhancement Research Initiative (QUERI), Department of Veterans Affairs.

———. 2012. *Department of Veterans Affairs Quality Enhancement Research Initiative (QUERI) Polytrauma/Blast-Related Injuries QUERI Center Strategic Plan FY 2013 through FY 2015*. Washington, DC: Department of Veterans Affairs.

Sayer, N. A., D. Nelson, and S. Nugent. 2011. Evaluation of the Veterans Health Administration traumatic brain injury screening program in the upper Midwest. *Journal of Head Trauma Rehabilitation* 26(6):454-467.

Schwab, K. A., B. Ivins, G. Cramer, W. Johnson, M. Sluss-Tiller, K. Kiley, W. Lux, and D. Warden. 2007. Screening for traumatic brain injury in troops returning from deployment in Afghanistan and Iraq: Initial investigation of the usefulness of a short screening tool for traumatic brain injury. *Journal of Head Trauma Rehabilitation* 22(6):377-389.

Scottish Intercollegiate Guidelines Network. 2009. *Early management of patients with a head injury: A national clinical guideline*. Edinburgh, Scotland: NHS Quality Improvement Scotland.

Seal, K. H., S. Maguen, B. Cohen, K. S. Gima, T. J. Metzler, L. Ren, D. Bertenthal, and C. R. Marmar. 2010. VA mental health services utilization in Iraq and Afghanistan veterans in the first year of receiving new mental health diagnoses. *Journal of Traumatic Stress* 23(1):5-16.

Seal, K. H., G. Cohen, A. Waldrop, B. E. Cohen, S. Maguen, and L. Ren. 2011. Substance use disorders in Iraq and Afghanistan veterans in VA healthcare, 2001-2010: Implications for screening, diagnosis and treatment. *Drug and Alcohol Dependence* 116(1-3):93-101.

Shinn, A. K., and S. F. Greenfield. 2010. Topiramate in the treatment of substance-related disorders: A critical review of the literature. *Journal of Clinical Psychiatry* 71(5):634-648.

Smith, P. C., S. M. Schmidt, D. Allensworth-Davies, and R. Saitz. 2009. Primary care validation of a single-question alcohol screening test. *Journal of General Internal Medicine* 24(7):783-788.

Snell, D. L., L. J. Surgenor, E. J. Hay-Smith, and R. J. Siegert. 2009. A systematic review of psychological treatments for mild traumatic brain injury: An update on the evidence. *Journal of Clinical and Experimental Neuropsychology: Official Journal of the International Neuropsychological Society* 31(1):20-38.

Spitzer, R. L., J. B. Williams, M. Gibbon, and M. B. First. 1992. The structured clinical interview for DSM-III-R (SCID): History, rationale, and description. *Archives of General Psychiatry* 49(8):624-629.

Stanley, B., and G. K. Brown. 2008. *Safety Plan Treatment Manual to Reduce Suicide Risk: Veteran Version.* Washington, DC: Department of Veterans Affairs.

Stein, D. J., J. C. Ipser, and S. Seedat. 2006. Pharmacotherapy for post traumatic stress disorder (PTSD). *Cochrane Database of Systematic Reviews* 1.

Stein, D. J., J. C. Ipser, and N. McAnda. 2009. Pharmacotherapy of posttraumatic stress disorder: A review of meta-analyses and treatment guidelines. *CNS Spectrums* 14(1 Suppl 1):25-31.

Stewart, C. L., and T. A. Wrobel. 2009. Evaluation of the efficacy of pharmacotherapy and psychotherapy in treatment of combat-related post-traumatic stress disorder: A meta-analytic review of outcome studies. *Military Medicine* 174(5):460-469.

Stewart, J. A., D. A. Deliyannides, D. J. Hellerstein, P. J. McGrath, and J. W. Stewart. 2012. Can people with nonsevere major depression benefit from antidepressant medication? *Journal of Clinical Psychiatry* 73(4):518-525.

Tarrier, N., K. Taylor, and P. Gooding. 2008. Cognitive-behavioral interventions to reduce suicide behavior: A systematic review and meta-analysis. *Behavior Modification* 32(1):77-108.

Terrio, H. P., L. A. Nelson, L. M. Betthauser, J. E. Harwood, and L. A. Brenner. 2011. Postdeployment traumatic brain injury screening questions: Sensitivity, specificity, and predictive values in returning soldiers. *Rehabilitation Psychology* 56(1):26-31.

Thase, M. E. 2011. The small specific effects of antidepressants in clinical trials: What do they mean to psychiatrists? *Current Psychiatry Reports* 13(6):476-482.

Trivedi, A. N., S. Matula, I. Miake-Lye, P. A. Glassman, P. Shekelle, and S. Asch. 2011. Systematic review: Comparison of the quality of medical care in Veterans Affairs and non-Veterans Affairs settings. *Medical Care* 49(1):76-88.

Trofimovich, L., N. A. Skopp, D. D. Luxton, and M. A. Reger. 2012. Health care experiences prior to suicide and self-inflicted injury, active component, US Armed Forces, 2001-2010. *Medical Surveillance Monthly Report* 19(2):2-6.

Tuunainen, A., D. F. Kripke, and T. Endo. 2004. Light therapy for non-seasonal depression. *Cochrane Database Systematic Reviews* 2.

Ursano, R. J., C. Bell, S. Eth, M. Friedman, A. Norwood, B. Pfefferbaum, R. Pynoos, D. F. Zatzick, and D. M. Benedek. 2004. *Practice Guideline for the Treatment of Patients with Acute Stress Disorder and Posttraumatic Stress Disorder.* Arlington, VA: American Psychiatric Association.

USMedicine.com. 2012. *Technology Makes for Efficient Application of New mTBI Policy.* Lambertville, NJ: Marathon Medical Communications, Inc.

USPSTF (US Preventive Services Task Force). 2004. *Screening for Suicide Risk, Topic Page.* http://www.uspreventiveservicestaskforce.org/uspstf/uspssuic.htm (accessed October 22, 2012).

———. 2009. Screening for depression in adults: US Preventive Services Task Force recommendation statement. *Annals of Internal Medicine* 151(11):784-792.

VA (Department of Veterans Affairs). 2007. *Vista Clinical Reminders: User Manual* Washington, DC: Health Provider Systems Office of Information and Technology, Department of Veterans Affairs.

———. 2008a. *Uniform Mental Health Services in VA Medical Centers and Clinics.* Washington, DC: Department of Veterans Affairs.

———. 2008b. *VHA Directive 2008-036: Use of Patient Record Flags to Identify Patients at High Risk for Suicide.* Washington, DC: Department of Veterans Affairs.

———. 2010a. *Examining the Process of Suicide Prevention Outreach Efforts at the US Department of Veterans* Affairs, *Committee on Veterans' Affairs, Subcommittee on Oversight and Investigations.* Washington, DC: US Government Printing Office.

———. 2010b. *Programs for Veterans with Post-Traumatic Stress Disorder (PTSD).* Washington, DC: Department of Veterans Affairs, Veterans Health Administration.

———. 2010c. *VHA Directive 2010-012 Screening and Evaluation of Possible Traumatic Brain Injury in Operation Enduring Freedom (OEF) and Operation Iraqi Freedom (OIF) Veterans.* Department of Veterans Affairs.

———. 2012. *Quality Enhancement Research Initiative (QUERI): PT/BRI Queri TBI Screening and Evaluation Research Fact Sheet.* Washington, DC: Department of Veterans Affairs.

———. undated-a. *Suicide Risk Assessment Guide: Reference Manual.* www.mentalhealth.va.gov/docs/Suicide_Risk_Assessment_Guide.doc (accessed October 22, 2012).

———. undated-b. *Suicide Risk Assessment Pocket Card.* http://www.mentalhealth.va.gov/docs/Suicide-Risk-Assessment-Guide.pdf (accessed October 22, 2012).

VA and DOD. 2009a. *VA/DOD Clinical Practice Guideline for Management of Major Depressive Disorder (MDD).* Washington, DC: Department of Veterans Affairs and Department of Defense.

———. 2009b. *VA/DOD Clinical Practice Guidelines for Management of Concussion/Mild Traumatic Brain Injury (mTBI)* Washington, DC: Department of Veterans Affairs and Department of Defense.

———. 2009c. *VA/DOD Clinical Practice Guidelines for Management of Substance Use Disorders (SUD).* Washington, DC: Department of Veterans Affairs and Department of Defense.

———. 2010. *VA/DOD Clinical Practice Guideline for Management of Post-Traumatic Stress.* Washington, DC: Department of Veterans Affairs and Department of Defense.

VA and VHA (Veterans Health Administration). 2007. *VHA Directive 2007-013: Screening and Evaluation of Possible Traumatic Brain Injury in Operation Enduring Freedom (OEF) and Operation Iraqi Freedom (OIF) Veterans.* Washington, DC: Department of Veterans Affairs, Veterans Health Administration.

VA Office of Inspector General. 2011. *Combined Assessment Program Summary Report Re-evaluation of Suicide Prevention Safety Plan Practices in Veterans Health Administration Facilities.* Washington, DC: Department of Veterans Affairs.

———. 2012. *Veterans Health Administration: Review of Veterans' Access to Mental Health Care.* Washington, DC VA Office of Inspector General.

Valderas, J. M., B. Starfield, B. Sibbald, C. Salisbury, and M. Roland. 2009. Defining comorbidity: Implications for understanding health and health services. *Annals of Family Medicine* 7(4):357-363.

Van Dyke, S. A., B. N. Axelrod, and C. Schutte. 2010. Test-retest reliability of the traumatic brain injury screening instrument. *Military Medicine* 175:947-949.

Vanderploeg, R. D., K. Schwab, W. C. Walker, J. A. Fraser, B. J. Sigford, E. S. Date, S. G. Scott, G. Curtiss, A. M. Salazar, and D. L. Warden. 2008. Rehabilitation of traumatic brain injury in active duty military personnel and veterans: Defense and Veterans Brain Injury Center randomized controlled trial of two rehabilitation approaches. *Archives of Physical Medicine and Rehabilitation* 89(12):2227-2238.

Vohringer, P. A., and S. N. Ghaemi. 2011. Solving the antidepressant efficacy question: Effect sizes in major depressive disorder. *Clinical Therapeutics* 33(12):B49-B61.

von Wolff, A., L. P. Holzel, A. Westphal, M. Harter, and L. Kriston. 2012. Combination of pharmacotherapy and psychotherapy in the treatment of chronic depression: A systematic review and meta-analysis. *BMC Psychiatry* 12(1):61.

Vythilingam, M., J. Davison, C. Engel, and H. V. Ritschard. 2010. *Training to Administer DOD Deployment Mental Health Assessments.* Washington, DC: Department of Defense.

Warden, D., A. J. Rush, M. H. Trivedi, M. Fava, and S. R. Wisniewski. 2007. The STAR*D project results: A comprehensive review of findings. *Current Psychiatry Reports* 9(6):449-459.

Warner, C. H., G. N. Appenzeller, T. Grieger, S. Belenkiy, J. Breitbach, J. Parker, C. M. Warner, and C. Hoge. 2011a. Importance of anonymity to encourage honest reporting in mental health screening after combat deployment. *Archives of General Psychiatry* 68(10):1065-1071.

Warner, C. H., G. N. Appenzeller, J. R. Parker, C. M. Warner, and C. W. Hoge. 2011b. Effectiveness of mental health screening and coordination of in-theater care prior to deployment to Iraq: A cohort study. *American Journal of Psychiatry* 168(4):378-385.

Watkins, K. E., and H. A. Pincus. 2011. *Veterans Health Administration Mental Health Program Evaluation Capstone Report.* Santa Monica, CA: RAND Corporation.

Watkins, K. E., D. J. Keyser, B. Smith, T. E. Mannle, D. R. Kivlahan, S. M. Paddock, T. Mattox, M. Horvitz-Lennon, and H. A. Pincus. 2010. Transforming mental healthcare in the Veterans Health Administration: A model for measuring performance to improve access, quality, and outcomes. *Journal for Healthcare Quality* 32(6):33-42.

Watkins, K. E., H. A. Pincus, S. Paddock, B. Smith, A. Woodroffe, C. Farmer, M. E. Sorbero, M. Horvitz-Lennon, T. Mannle, Jr., K. A. Hepner, J. Solomon, and C. Call. 2011. Care for veterans with mental and substance use disorders: Good performance, but room to improve on many measures. *Health Affairs* 30(11):2194-2203.

Weathers, F., J. Huska, and T. M. Keane. 1991. *PTSD Checklist—Military Version (PCL-M).* http://www.metrowestneurofeedback.com/files/62410952_ptsd_checklist.pdf (accessed March 15, 2011).

Weightman, M. M., R. Bolgla, K. L. McCulloch, and M. D. Peterson. 2010. Physical therapy recommendations for service members with mild traumatic brain injury. *Journal of Head Trauma Rehabilitation* 25(3):206-218.

WHO (World Health Organization). 2009. *Guidelines for the Psychosocially Assisted Pharmacological Treatment of Opioid Dependence.* Geneva, Switzerland: WHO.

Wilkins, K. C., A. J. Lang, and S. B. Norman. 2011. Synthesis of the psychometric properties of the PTSD Checklist (PCL) military, civilian, and specific versions. *Depression and Anxiety* 28(7):596-606.

Wittkampf, K. A., L. Naeije, A. H. Schene, J. Huyser, and H. C. van Weert. 2007. Diagnostic accuracy of the mood module of the patient health questionnaire: A systematic review. *General Hospital Psychiatry* 29(5):388-395.

Woodson, J. 2011. *Military Suicide: An Update.* Washington, DC: House Armed Services Committee, Military Personnel Subcommittee.

Yano, E. M., E. F. Chaney, D. G. Campbell, R. Klap, B. F. Simon, L. M. Bonner, A. B. Lanto, and L. V. Rubenstein. 2012. Yield of practice-based depression screening in VA primary care settings. *Journal of General Internal Medicine* 27(3):331-338.

Zoroya, G. 2011. *More Troops' Mild Brain Trauma Diagnosed.* http://usatoday30.usatoday.com/news/military/story/2011-09-27/military-diagnoses-more-brain-injuries-trauma-battle-combat-policy/50575536/1 (accessed March 22, 2012).

# 6

# MILITARY FAMILIES

This chapter examines the effects of deployments to Operation Enduring Freedom (OEF) and Operation Iraqi Freedom (OIF) on the mental, emotional, and social well-being of military family members, including spouses, children, and caregivers. It also discusses issues related to the availability of programs and services for military families. Military family members are an important part of the readiness and well-being of the military force. The care and support of military families is considered a top national security policy priority in recognition of the integral role family members have in supporting service members and, therefore, the mission of the military. With that priority, various challenges arise. Throughout this chapter, the committee presents evidence that military family members have to deal with additional relationship problems, impairments in psychologic and physical well-being, responsibilities as caregivers of children or wounded service members, and overwhelming household duties. The committee's primary focus is on the impacts of deployment on military families, and not on the entire scope of experiences faced by military families. Given the exceptional demands that deployments to OEF and OIF have placed on military families and the impact that family concerns have on soldiers' well-being, there continues to be a need for military leaders to gain a better understanding of the needs of families and to use that understanding to implement more-effective coordinated programs and services for the good of military families and, thus, for the military as a whole.

## CHARACTERISTICS OF MILITARY FAMILIES

Military families are more diverse than most statistics or research might suggest. Many families do not meet the criteria used for official counts of military families and, therefore, are not included in the data (for example, common-law spouses). Because of that, this chapter reports information only about a subset of military families: those of service members in heterosexual marriages and parents with dependent children who live with them at least part of the time. The committee views the military's definition of family as narrow and out of step with the diversity in family arrangements in modern society. The committee found little or no information about parents or siblings of service members (who are sometimes relied upon for important caregiving responsibilities), unmarried partners, stepfamilies, children who are not legal dependents (for example, stepchildren or nonresidential children), gay families, service members acting as substitute parents, or other nontraditional family configurations. Most published studies focus on active-duty male military personnel married to civilian wives.

Because women constitute a relatively small number of service members, they are sometimes excluded from studies. As the number of women in the military continues to increase, it becomes even more important that they be included in research studies.

Despite the apparent popularity of marriage among military members, nonmarital intimate relationships are likely to become a more prominent feature of the relationships of service members in the future, as they are in the population as a whole, and methods of counting relationships may need to be amended as a result. The general population has been characterized in recent decades by rising tendencies for individuals to delay marriage and to cohabit before marriage (Copen et al., 2012). Delays in and alternatives to marriage might become more evident in the military, especially as policies change in the aftermath of discontinuing the "Don't Ask, Don't Tell" policy (McKean et al., 2011). Thus, marital status might become an increasingly inaccurate index of relationship patterns, and useful information about the health of intimate relationships of military members might be overlooked if tabulation methods are not adjusted.

## Defining Military Families

Multiple definitions of *family* are used in the Department of Defense (DOD), each tied to specific regulatory requirements. The most common definition uses eligibility for military identification cards, which are necessary for access to health care, military exchanges, and a variety of supportive services for families. Military identification cards are currently issued to spouses and unmarried children of service members—exceptions and additional categories are defined by children's ages, student status, or special needs and by whether the marriage ends in divorce or in death of the service member while on active duty. Spouses and unmarried children of reserve-component members are covered while the service member is on active duty for more than 30 consecutive days (DOD, 2012d). Stepchildren may or may not qualify for military identification cards, depending on such factors as age, student status, and the circumstances of the biologic parents.

Single service members are not irrelevant in a chapter focused on the implications of deployment for family life. Single service members might have completed or be in the process of establishing families; for example, they might have cohabiting partners or they might be in close relationships that are precursors to marriage. The population of single service members also includes previously married individuals who might be in the process of establishing a second family. All service members, especially those who do not have spouses or partners, might rely on parents, siblings, or other family members for substantial emotional or tangible support, especially if they encounter hardships, such as illness, wounds, or other major life challenges. However, little research has examined family issues as they relate to single service members.

## Demographic Characteristics of Military Families

This section describes the demographic characteristics of families of active-duty forces and selected reserve components. Because data presented here are derived from the DOD's annual demographic profiles of the military community (DOD, 2011b, 2012a) and represent all service members—not only those who have been deployed—they will not be identical to the data presented in Chapter 3, which include only service members who have been deployed.

**TABLE 6.1** Summary of Selected Demographic Characteristics for DOD Active-Duty and Selected Reserve Members

| Status | Percent of Active-Duty Members[a] | Percent of Selected Reserve and National Guard Members[b] |
|---|---|---|
| Percent married (enlisted, officers); (male, female) | 56.6 (54.0, 69.6); (58.5, 45.7) | 47.7 (43.7, 70.6); (50.1, 37.0) |
| Percent in dual-military marriages (sex of active-duty member: male, female) | 6.5[c] (3.9, 21.6) | 2.6[d] (1.3, 8.6) |
| Percent of married members in dual-military marriage (sex of active-duty member: male, female) | 11.5 (6.8, 47.3) | 5.5 (2.6, 23.3) |

[a]Includes 1,411,425 members of the four DOD active-duty branches (Army, Navy, Marine Corps, and Air Force). Limited data are included for the active-duty Coast Guard (Department of Homeland Security).
[b]Includes 855,867 members of the six reserve components (Army National Guard, Army Reserve, Navy Reserve, Marine Corps Reserve, Air National Guard, and Air Force Reserve) and the Coast Guard Reserve.
[c]Of these, 81.8% are enlisted members, and 18.2% are officers.
[d]Of these, 76.1% are enlisted members, and 23.9% are officers.
NOTE: Data are derived from a variety of sources, including the Active Duty Military Personnel Master File, the Active Duty Military Family File, the Reserve Components Common Personnel Data System, the Reserve Components Family File, and the Defense Enrollment and Eligibility Reporting System (DEERS).
SOURCE: DOD, 2012a.

## Marital Status of Active-Duty and Selected Reserve Members

### *Marriage Patterns*

Over two-thirds of active-duty and reserve officers are married, as are over half of enlisted active-duty service members and nearly half of those in the selected reserves (see Table 6.1). Reflecting the general makeup of the services, the great majority of both active-duty military (93.1%), and selected reserve (88.1%) spouses are female (DOD, 2011b). Male military members ages 18 to 41 are significantly more likely to have married at some point in their lives than are comparable civilians, particularly if they are black, Hispanic, or hold enlisted rank (Karney et al., 2012). On the basis of 1999 data from the Active Duty Survey of Military Personnel, Lundquist (2004) found that black service members in their early 20s were at least three times more likely to marry than their civilian counterparts and that the large marriage gap present between black and white civilians did not exist for those in the military.

Although less is known about the marital patterns of women serving in the military, they are less likely to be married than their male counterparts, a pattern not observed among civilians of similar age. Women in the military are also much more likely to be married to other service members: In 2011, female active-duty service members and women serving in the reserve component were more likely than their male counterparts to be married to a fellow service member. Nearly half of married women on active duty were married to another service member (DOD, 2012a).

In summary, military members are as likely or more likely to be married than their civilian counterparts, and this factor is particularly true for officers and members serving on active duty. Although the prevalence of marriage has been declining steadily in the civilian population, in the military it has been essentially level, having some fluctuations, over the past two decades.

*Divorce Patterns*

An estimated 4.1% of married enlisted members and 2.1% of married officers divorced between September 2010 and September 2011. This percentage is a substantial increase over 2000 rates, when an estimated 1.4% of married officers and 2.9% of married enlisted members had divorced during the previous year. This increase was especially steep for married enlisted soldiers (2.3% in 2000 compared with 4.0% in 2011, a 74% increase) and sailors (2.6% in 2000 compared with 4.6% in 2010, a 77% increase).

Among the selected reserve, an estimated 2.8% of married enlisted members and 1.9% of married officers divorced during the 1-year period before September 2010. This percentage shows modest increases above the 2000 rates, which were 2.4% for married enlisted members and 1.6% for married officers.

Data analyses by Karney et al. (2012), however, suggest that the apparent increase in divorce rates in military relative to civilian populations is not statistically significant and does not reflect a widening gap between civilians and military members, at least during the 4 years before and after the start of combat operations in Afghanistan in 2001. In fact, male military officers and enlisted members reported being currently divorced at either the same or lower rates than civilian men with comparable education, age, race or ethnicity, and employment status both before (1998–2001) and during the war (2002–2005) (Karney et al., 2012).

Marriages of women in the military are more likely to fail than those of men (Karney and Crown, 2007; Lundquist, 2006). Karney and Crown (2007) examined military personnel records to track the marital status of service members over a 10-year period (1996 to 2005) and found that rates of marital dissolution for female service members were more than double those of their male counterparts. Regarding marital dissolution and race, Lundquist (2006) found that black service members were 53% less likely to divorce than whites, unlike in the civilian population, in which blacks were 30% more likely to divorce than whites. When only one partner was in the military, white dual-military couples were 40% more likely to divorce than black couples.

In summary, although overall divorce rates in the general population have been falling during the past decade, divorce rates in the military have risen noticeably. Nonetheless, on the basis of comparisons of matched civilian and military men, Karney et al. (2012) concludes that men serving in the military are no more likely than their civilian counterparts to divorce and that this gap did not widen between 1996 and 2004. A subsequent section about deployment and married couples examines research on the impact that deployment has on marital dissolution.

**Family Responsibilities of Active-Duty and Selected Reserve Members**

Information on the family status of service members is presented in Table 6.2.

**TABLE 6.2** Family Status of DOD Active-Duty and Selected Reserve Members

| Status | Percent or Number of DOD Active-Duty Members | Percent or Number of Selected Reserve and National Guard Members |
|---|---|---|
| Percent with children (overall) | 44.2% | 43.3% |
| Percent married to civilian, with children | 36.1% | 32.5% |
| Percent dual-military with children | 2.8% | 1.5% |
| Percent single with children | 5.3% | 9.4% |
| Average number of children of members with children | 2.0 | 2.0 |
| Percent of children ages 0 to 5 | 42.6% | 28.8% |
| Percent married to civilian with no children | 14.0% | 12.7% |
| Percent dual-military with no children | 3.7% | 1.2% |
| Percent single with no children | 38.1% | 42.9% |
| Percent with family responsibilities[a] (enlisted, officers) | 59.0% (56.7%, 70.0%) | 56.4% (52.9%, 76.4%) |
| Average number of dependents of members with dependents | 2.4 | 2.4 |

[a]Members are classified as having family responsibilities if they have a dependent (spouse, children, other dependents) registered in the Defense Enrollment and Eligibility Reporting System (DEERS).
NOTE: Children category includes minor dependents age 20 or younger or age 22 and younger enrolled as full-time students.
SOURCE: DOD, 2012a.

Over half of active-duty and selected reserve members have family responsibilities—that is, are married or have children or have another dependent registered in the Defense Enrollment and Eligibility Reporting System (DEERS)—as do over two-thirds of active-duty officers. Among active-duty enlisted service members, Army-enlisted soldiers are more likely to have family responsibilities than enlisted members of other active-duty service branches (63.5% for Army enlisted, compared with 53.0% for Navy, 46.3% for Marines, and 55.7% for Air Force enlisted). Approximately half to two-thirds of enlisted members of the selected reserve across reserve components have family responsibilities, the exception being Marine reserve families, in which just over a quarter (27.1%) have responsibilities. The majority (67.1%) of active-duty single parents are male service members. However, female service members are much more likely than males to be single parents (12.1% vs 4.2%, respectively).

The large minority of minor dependent children of active-duty members are 5 years old or younger (42.6%), followed by 6 to 11 years (30.7%), 12 to 18 years (22.4%), and 19 to 22 years old (4.3%; includes full-time students). The children of selected reserve members tend to be older than those of active-duty members, 28.8% being ages 5 or younger, 29.7% being ages 6 to 11, 29.6% being ages 12 to 18, and 11.8% being ages 19 to 22.

A study examining marital transitions among service members found that almost one-third of service members (30%) had nonresidential children, a strikingly high percentage in a population where 64.8% of the members were younger than age 30 (Adler-Baeder et al., 2006). Almost all of the service members with nonresidential children had *only* nonresidential children, meaning that under military rules, they were defined as single, not as single parents. Among remarried respondents, 42.2% had children from a previous relationship.

In 2008, the *Military Family Life* project included two items related to marital transitions in a survey of a probability sample of 28,500 military spouses. The first item asked respondents, all of whom were married or separated, if they were currently living in a stepfamily; 20% indicated that they were. In addition, 35% of the participants indicated that they had a child from the service member's or spouse's prior relationship or were acting as parents for someone else's child, such as a grandchild, niece, or nephew. Thus, a substantial proportion of service members are living in stepfamilies or are acting as parents for the children of others.

A small proportion of active-duty (0.7%) and selected reserve (0.2%) members are responsible for one or more adult dependents, such as a parent, grandparent, sibling, disabled older child, or other adult claimed as a dependent in the DEERS system. In the large majority of cases, the dependents are females age 51 or older.

## DEPLOYMENT AND FAMILIES

### Rewards and Challenges of Military Service for Families

Understanding the effects of wartime deployments on military families requires some understanding of the baseline conditions of military life. The demands of military service may characterize other occupations, but rarely with the prevalence and frequency of demands that occur in military life (Castro et al., 2006). However, military service offers tangible and intangible benefits and supports that other occupations might lack.

#### Rewards of Military Service

Research about military families tends to focus more on negative than beneficial aspects, but the latter are nonetheless important. Rewards of military service can include personal growth from surmounting difficult challenges, increased appreciation of personal relationships, increased earnings from hazardous duty pay, and a sense of purpose from performing an important mission for the country (Newby et al., 2005a).

A review of studies of appraisals by veterans from a variety of combat and peacekeeping operations (Schok et al., 2008) found that most veterans reported positive aspects of their experiences, primarily in three domains: self-image, such as self-discipline, self-confidence, and coping; in social relationships, such as cooperating better and becoming more tolerant; and in personal growth and priorities in life, such as valuing life, recognizing the importance of family, and strengthening of faith. In a focus group, data gathered by Hosek et al. (2006) showed that service members reported similar themes, including satisfaction from using the skills they had acquired in training and fulfillment of a sense of duty.

Family members also reported increased closeness, patriotism, pride, civic responsibility, and personal growth (Werber et al., 2008). Being in the military can also provide a sense of community for military families and a social support system of other military families who understand the demands of military life. Although relocations can be stressful, military life provides families with the opportunity to see and live in different parts of the country or the world that would not otherwise be available to them.

**Challenges of Military Service**

Military service includes a number of stressors related to the structure of work (Adams et al., 2006; MacDermid Wadsworth and Southwell, 2011; van Steenbergen et al., 2008). Military work is demanding, often requiring long hours and physically tiring tasks (Huffman and Payne, 2006; Kavanagh, 2005), and even nondeployed units must work to prepare for future deployments and support currently deployed units. Service members may be assigned with little advance notice to a variety of duties that require repeated episodes of time away from their families (for example, temporary duty assignments, training, disaster relief, humanitarian aid, and combat), all of which may expose service members to danger (Kavanagh, 2005).

Service members and their families are required to relocate much more frequently than civilian families (every 2 to 3 years), with little opportunity to influence the choice of the next duty station (DOD, 1998; GAO, 2001). In 2010, 31% of military members (excluding unmarried service members living in barracks) moved, compared with 13% of civilians (US Census Bureau, 2011c). Rates of international relocations, which can be more challenging than domestic moves, are four times higher among military families than their civilian counterparts (Reinkober Drummet et al., 2003). Frequent obligatory moves are associated with frustration and decreased satisfaction with military life (GAO, 2001). Lack of support and isolation in the new community is particularly mentioned as a concern by spouses (Burrell et al., 2006). In addition to their emotional consequences, frequent relocations disrupt the ability of spouses to achieve educational or career goals (Burrell et al., 2006; Eby et al., 1997; Harrell et al., 2004). Relocations can require spouses to transfer certifications and change jobs or retrain. Military spouses are less likely than their civilian counterparts to work full-time, to average fewer work hours and fewer days in the year, and to earn less than spouses of civilians (Hosek et al., 2002; Lim and Schulker, 2010).

Beyond dealing with the occupational demands of the service members, military life also may impose codes of conduct for family members as well as service members, especially when living in military housing, using military support services, or when the service member occupies a leadership position (Segal, 1986). Military scrutiny and expectations for good conduct on and off duty may lead service members and their families to perceive a lack of privacy. Furthermore, the behavior of spouses and children can impact service members and their careers. For example, spouses' problematic behavior (e.g., traffic violations, financial problems, substance abuse) can come to official attention and result in pressure on service members to "control their family member" (Segal, 1986).

The high proportion of military women in dual-service marriages, when combined with the high rates of marital dissolution among military women, raises questions about the severity of the unique challenges faced by dual-military families in coordinating leaves between parents, arranging child care, and other challenges posed by dual commitments to military service (Bethea, 2007). As discussed by Huffman and Payne (2006), individuals in dual-military marriages have multiple roles—at the very least as spouse and as service member, and often as parent or active community member. In dual-military marriages, having multiple roles can have positive implications, but the difficulty of fulfilling obligations associated with each role can strain individuals, particularly for those with children. In addition, military-specific challenges, such as being in the presence of danger, working at a high pace, and frequent or long separations, are magnified in dual-military marriages.

## Impact of Deployments on Families

Deployments are not single events but complex configurations of predictable and unpredictable experiences. Deployments are diverse, varying along several dimensions. The most obvious dimension is *content*, such as exposure to trauma, physical demands, harsh living conditions, access to resources, and the ability to communicate with family. The dimensions of deployment *structure* include duration and frequency of individual deployments, which also leads to consideration of "dwell time" or the interval between repeated deployments. As deployments accumulate, cumulative duration becomes relevant. Although every deployment comprises a before, during, and after period, there are differences in the amount of advance notice service members receive and when, where, and for how long they must receive training before departing or after they return. Deployments have been categorized as both normative and catastrophic. The former is characterized by adequate time to prepare, by predictable duration and content, and by relatively mild emotional distress; the latter is characterized by little advance warning, uncertainty and danger, and prolonged emotional distress (McCubbin and Figley, 1983; Wiens and Boss, 2006). To the extent that every deployment comprises before, during, and after deployment periods, they have a predictable structure. The duration and content of these phases vary widely, however—raising caution about the confidence with which predictions can be made about the implications for families.

Several scholars have constructed stage models to describe the emotional experiences and coping challenges that are thought to characterize the deployment and reunion periods (Wiens and Boss, 2006); see also Mateczun and Holmes (1996), Peebles-Kleiger and Kleiger (1994), and Pincus et al. (2001) for more information about stage models. Although these stage models are appealing in their clarity and appear to be consistent with the findings of some empirical studies, no longitudinal studies have documented that these stages occur, occur in the proposed sequence, incorporate the proposed experiences or challenges, or display the proposed durations.

Although the number of published peer-reviewed studies of the impact of OEF and OIF deployments is rapidly increasing, large knowledge gaps remain. For example, many studies do not incorporate family factors or gather data from family members. The studies that do incorporate that information focus mostly on spouses and to a lesser extent on children. Little attention is given to the parents or the "significant others" of service members, a particularly concerning gap for single service members. Similar to studies of military families in general, most OEF and OIF studies focus on male military personnel married to civilian women and serving in the Army (Kelley et al., 2002). Many studies focus on negative consequences, especially posttraumatic stress disorder (PTSD), rather than other potential sequelae of deployment.

Almost no studies have been conducted that include prospective data from the predeployment period. A few have gathered data during deployment but rarely from service members and even more rarely from both service members and family members. Most research—even of the period during deployment—has been conducted following return from deployment, and most studies are cross-sectional rather than longitudinal (de Burgh et al., 2011). Two large longitudinal studies, currently in the data-collection phase, are likely to generate important data about the effects of military service and deployments on families in the coming years. The family component of the Millennium Cohort Study is recruiting 10,000 spouses of service members participating in a 20-year prospective study of four cohorts totaling 150,000 service members. Data gathered from these spouses will permit comparisons of families of combat-deployed, noncombat-deployed, and nondeployed service members (Crum-Cianflone et al., 2012). The RAND Corporation is conducting a prospective, longitudinal study of approximately 2,000 military families who are expected to experience a deployment. This study will follow the cohort for 3 years; data will be gathered across a number of domains every 4 months. The design includes measures that will be repeated before, during, and after the deployment phases. One of the primary goals is to understand both risk and protective factors across the deployment phases in an effort to define family readiness. Other key elements of this study include data collection from multiple respondents per family, including one child 11 to 17 years old. Measures include physical health, behavioral health, marital relationship, parenting, use of services, career intentions, and deployment experience (RAND Center for Military Health Policy, 2012).

**Theoretical Models**

Several theoretical approaches have been presented to account for families' experiences of deployment. Most of them take a systemic approach, recognizing that families have properties distinct from the characteristics of individual members. Systemic approaches also draw attention to patterns of information flow that can foster or impede adaptation to challenges within families.

The theoretical perspectives used to account for the impact of deployment on families focus on stress processes (see Karney and Crown, 2007; McCubbin, 1979; Patterson, 2002) or on patterns of family resilience (see Saltzman et al., 2011; Walsh, 2006; Wiens and Boss, 2006). Several approaches are based on the attachment theory, which posits that individuals develop internal working models for attachments to others during childhood that condition their responses not only to separations from primary attachment figures but also to interactions with future partners and children. Attachments vary in their characteristics and may be secure or insecure, the latter characterized by anxiety or avoidance. Deployment constitutes a significant challenge to attachment systems and, depending on the nature of attachment relationships among family members, can result in reactions ranging from adaptation that allows the family to function well during separation and incorporate the service member on his or her return and ranging to problematic arrangements that "close ranks" against the service member (Riggs and Riggs, 2011).

Finally, attention is being given to the conditions surrounding military families, including informal support from social networks of family, friends, colleagues, and others, as well as formal support from community agencies and programs. This perspective is prompted in part by greater recognition of the differences between the circumstances of active- and reserve-component families (Bowen and Martin, 2011; MacLean and Elder, 2007; Wiens and Boss, 2006).

**Characteristics of Deployments and Impact on Families**

Families appear to experience greater stress and anticipate more difficulties when deployments are longer (Booth et al., 2007; Orthner and Rose, 2002). In a systematic review of studies of deployment length, Buckman et al. (2011) concluded that longer deployments are associated with adverse effects on service members and their families, deployments having a possible threshold of 6 months, beyond which negative effects are more likely to occur.

Several studies suggest that cumulative duration of deployments might be more important than frequency of deployment or the duration of a single deployment for certain family-related outcomes (Chandra et al., 2011; Hurley, 2011). For example, Lara-Cinisomo et al. (2011) found that caregivers who experienced more months of deployment of military members during the past 3 years (but not a larger number of deployments) reported lower relationship satisfaction, more relationship hassles, and poorer emotional well-being. Mansfield et al. (2010) found that the number of cases of depression was larger among wives whose husbands had been deployed longer. Franklin (2011), however, found that reports of psychologic symptoms on the Air Force Community Assessment rose with both frequency and duration of deployment. For length of deployment, but not for frequency, the connection to relationship quality was mediated by psychologic symptoms. These findings probably underestimate the impact of the frequency of deployment because most studies exclude deployments lasting less than 30 days or deployments not in support of war operations. Thus, the number of service members' departures from and returns home are greatly underestimated, and the statistical effects associated with deployment frequency may be attenuated as a result.

There is considerable evidence that family-related concerns weigh heavily on service members during deployment. In each administration of the Army-led Mental Health Advisory Team (MHAT) surveys, concerns about being separated from family are among the foremost deployment concerns, as reported by about one-third of service members (MHAT-VII, 2011). Responses to the 2008 DOD Survey of Health-Related Behaviors indicated that service members who had been deployed recently were significantly more likely to report high family stress than were service members who had not been deployed; levels of these concerns did not change between 2002 and 2008 (Bray et al., 2010). In another study, British Forces service members surveyed during deployments to Iraq and Afghanistan reported poorer mental health when negative events occurred at home and when they perceived poor military support for their families. These findings were firm regardless of combat exposure but were somewhat weaker in the presence of strong military unit cohesion or military leadership (Mulligan et al., 2012). Skopp et al. (2011), in a large study that included pre- and postdeployment data from 2,583 Army soldiers, found that female soldiers with higher levels of combat exposure were significantly more likely to screen positive for PTSD if the strength of their intimate relationships had declined during deployment.

In their longitudinal study of more than 88,000 soldiers who served in Iraq, Milliken et al. (2007) found a fourfold increase in interpersonal problems from when they returned from deployment and a median of 6 months thereafter. The authors made special note of the cumulative burden of mental-health problems on family relationships and advocated greater mental-health resources for family members.

Baseline levels of perceived stress appear to have risen among Army spouses in recent years. The recent Army "Gold Book" indicated that more than half of all spouses reported experiencing stress in 2010 (56%, up from 46% in 2006) (Department of the Army, 2012). Supporting the notion of relatively high baseline rates of stressors, almost half of the spouses (44%) reported concern about finances, and two-thirds reported that they had less than $500 in savings accounts. More than half of the spouses were employed or were looking for work. Finally, 19% of spouses who responded indicated that they were in counseling, mostly for stress, family, and marital issues (Department of the Army, 2012).

Evidence assembled so far from both prior and current wars suggests that the likelihood of negative consequences for families rises with the amount of the service members' exposure to traumatic or life-altering experiences. Thus, military service by itself does not appear to significantly raise the probability of negative outcomes (MacLean and Elder, 2007), and the same appears to be largely true for uneventful deployments lacking exposures to trauma (although traumatic exposures can occur not only with combat but also with duties related to peacekeeping and natural disasters (Allen et al., 2010). In contrast, deployment to combat zones has been found to significantly predict a variety of negative outcomes, including marital conflict and intimate partner violence (IOM, 2008). When service members display negative psychologic symptoms, the likelihood of negative consequences for families rises substantially (de Burgh et al., 2011), and families who experience the injury or death of service members are almost certain to experience at least some negative consequences.

**Deployment and Married Couples**

The health of marriages is typically assessed in research by two key indicators: marital quality and marital dissolution, which refers to the end of the marital relationship, typically via divorce (Karney and Bradbury, 1995). Although marital quality is difficult to measure, to date, measurements have focused primarily on the levels of satisfaction expressed by each partner (Knapp and Lott, 2010). Ideally, stable marriages have not only avoided dissolution, but also avoided separation or consideration of divorce, although studies vary in which of those elements are included (Karney and Bradbury, 1995). Dissolution, although relatively straightforward to measure, is a limited indicator of marital health because divorce is only the outcome of a lengthy and uncertain process.

In this section, we review research related to the impact of deployments on marital quality and marital dissolution.

*Marital Quality Throughout the Deployment Cycle*

The IOM (2008) found strong evidence that service members returning from deployments to combat zones were more likely to have marital problems, including intimate partner violence, than people who were not deployed and that this pattern was particularly strong when veterans had been diagnosed with PTSD. Evidence based on studies of Vietnam veterans was judged insufficient to conclude the existence of a causal relationship between deployment and marital conflict or marital dissolution.

On the basis of the perspectives of service members themselves, marital quality in the military population appears to have declined in the past decade. Data gathered from service members during deployments to Iraq and Afghanistan, as part of the MHAT research program, revealed a steady downward trend in marital satisfaction each year between 2003 and 2009, from 79% agreeing or strongly agreeing that they were satisfied with their marriages in 2000 to 57% giving similar reports in 2009 (MHAT-VII, 2011). The declines were limited to enlisted members and were largest among junior enlisted males (pay grades E1 to E4). Service members' reports that they intended to seek a divorce also rose from 12.4% in 2003 to 21.9% in 2009, again being much more evident among junior enlisted members. The 2006 MHAT report (MHAT-IV, 2006) indicated that problems with infidelity rose from 4% to 15% between 2003 and 2006, and marital problems more than doubled—from 12% to 27%.

Several studies suggest that marital quality following deployment is in part a function of quality before deployment (Nelson Goff and Smith, 2005; Rosen et al., 1995). Nonetheless, reasons for declines in marital quality are complex, and research results so far are mixed, particularly with regard to which mediators and moderators are most consequential for which people under which conditions (de Burgh et al., 2011).

Researchers have articulated several concepts evident throughout the deployment cycle—ambiguity and uncertainty, relationship connection, and communication—that characterize the nature of the relationship between military service members and their spouses and that influence their experiences (Sahlstein et al., 2009; Wiens and Boss, 2006).

*Ambiguity* and *uncertainty* are dominant aspects in the lives of military couples. Before and following deployment, the service member may be physically present but psychologically absent at least to some extent, while during deployment he or she is physically absent but psychologically present (Sahlstein et al., 2009; Wiens and Boss, 2006). In a study of 50 Army wives with current or recent experience with deployment, Sahlstein et al. (2009) found that separations related to training before the deployment heightened concerns about relational uncertainties (for example, concerns for the future of the marriage), and wives often responded by either expressing support or distancing themselves communicatively from their husbands (for example, by being silent or starting arguments). In a longitudinal study of Army reservists by Faber et al. (2008), ambiguity led to worries about the safety of the service member, how to handle challenges at home, and how to react to one another following return.

Baptist et al. (2011) interviewed 30 soldiers and spouses (not married to each other) in Army couples who had experienced one deployment to OIF or OEF. They used both open-ended and quantitative measures of the perceived impact of deployment on their marriages. Because of ambiguity about how to reintegrate service members into household duties following deployment, spouses sometimes continued to manage tasks as they had during the deployment, suppressing their personal needs or preferences. The researchers labeled this a maladaptive process because it complicated reintegration. Both reservists and spouses in the Faber et al. (2008) study reported similar hesitancies.

Using a cross-sectional convenience sample of 220 service members living in 27 states who had returned from deployment in the past 6 months, Knobloch and Theiss (2011) examined relational uncertainty (lack of confidence in self, partner, or relationship) and interference from partners (perceptions that partners are making it harder to achieve goals by disrupting routines). Service members who were dissatisfied with their relationships were more likely to report symptoms of depression but only if they felt uncertain about their commitment to the relationship and perceived their partners as interfering with their plans and activities.

For military couples, preparing for deployment and deployment separation can affect feelings of *closeness* and *connection*, heightening feelings of relationship insecurity and feelings of a lack of connection to their partner that result in relationship distress. For example, in the Sahlstein et al. (2009) study, the primary tension that spouses experienced during deployment was between autonomy and connection, particularly as it related to parenting roles. Spouses needed to feel independent enough to assume primary responsibility for parenting but also needed to feel sufficiently connected to their partner for support.

Permeating almost all accounts of deployment-related experiences are themes related to *communication*. Before and during deployment, families reported dissatisfaction with the communication they receive from the military about the logistics of deployment and the welfare of the deployed service members (SteelFisher et al., 2008). During deployment, service members may lack access to communication facilities, and service members and spouses must make difficult decisions about what information to share and, given the wide array of communication modalities now available, how and when (Mulligan et al., 2012). Following return, service members and their partners must negotiate reintegration of the service member into the daily operations of the family and renew their intimate relationships (Baptist et al., 2011).

In the following sections, we describe a range of concerns and impacts as they relate to different stages of the deployment cycle.

*Marital Quality Predeployment*

Before deployment, families must make legal, logistical, and emotional preparations for separation and the possible injury or death of their service members (McCarroll et al., 2005). Although it is logical that families would find this period difficult, few prospective studies of family members have been published.

Studies of service members indicate that concerns about their families are an important element of their predeployment experience. Findings from a study of deployment during the first Gulf War (Kelley et al., 2001) suggested that Navy parents anticipating deployment suffered from separation anxiety, particularly mothers (whether married or single). Polusny et al. (2009) surveyed 522 service members in the Army National Guard about 1 month before deployment, comparing responses of soldiers who had or had not been previously deployed for OIF or OEF. Results showed that service members were on average in good mental health and that soldiers with or without prior deployments were similar in their levels of concern about the impact of the separation on their families. McCreary et al. (2003) surveyed 180 members of the Canadian military 48 hours before departure for a peacekeeping mission in Bosnia and found that self-reports of family concerns explained more than half the variability in measures of depression, hyper-alertness, anxiety, and somatic complaints.

Service members also worry about their partners' ability to cope. The 2003 Air Force Community Assessment survey of over 30,000 Air Force members serving on active duty asked members to rate their spouses' readiness to cope with deployment-related challenges. Approximately one-third of junior enlisted members and members married less than 3 years indicated that their spouses would have a serious or very serious problem coping with deployment. Protective factors included military-unit relationship quality, military leadership effectiveness, and tangible social support from community members (Spera, 2009).

Spouses themselves also reported elevated worries and psychologic symptoms prior to service members' deployments, although baseline levels of these issues in the military spouse population are not well documented. For example, members of a sample of 295 Army active-duty-component spouses recruited from Family Readiness Groups shortly before departure of a Brigade Combat Team for deployment (response rate 33%) reported scores on the Perceived Stress Scale that were substantially above the community norm. One-quarter of the spouses reported scores consistent with mild depressive symptoms, another half reported scores consistent with depression, and one in 10 reported symptoms of severe depression. Almost all spouses (90% or more) reported two stressors: "feeling lonely" and concerns about the "safety of the deployed spouse." Four additional stressors were reported by at least half the spouses:

"having problems communicating with my spouse," "raising a young child while my spouse is not present," "caring/raising/disciplining children with my spouse absent," and "balancing between work and family obligations/responsibilities." Levels of depression were not related to number of stressors or prior deployments or number of children at home (Warner et al., 2009).

*During Deployment*

Relationships are often a worry for military members during deployment. Since 2003, family separation has consistently been among the top concerns of service members stationed in Iraq and Afghanistan and has been more strongly related to mental health problems than to any other concern (MHAT-V, 2008). A study of Navy sailors assigned to carriers showed that concerns about the children, and especially the marriage and the spouse, were expressed by substantially more participants during deployment and following return than before deployment (McNulty, 2005).

Hurley (2011) observed in a study of 129 Army spouses that a substantial proportion developed heightened rejection sensitivity partway through deployment, fearful that their deployed partners had decided to leave the marriage. These fears were significantly and negatively related to relationship adjustment, even though participants could identify no precipitating reason for their fear; fears also appeared to increase with cumulative months of separation.

Hinojosa et al. (2012) delved into communication difficulties experienced by 20 reserve-component members of the Army and Marine Corps during deployment, exposing specific challenges related to expressions of emotion. According to the participants, each partner's worry about the other led them to withhold information because of fears about revealing their own vulnerability or exposing vulnerability in their partner. The diminished familiarity with one another's day-to-day lives created a sense of disconnectedness and additional difficulties between spouses.

Baptist et al. (2011) observed many of the same patterns, including the tension between spouses who not only engaged in high levels of contact to maintain strong emotional connections but also limited information to insulate one another from stressors at home or in the war zone. When spouses chose not to disclose stressors they had experienced, they foreclosed the possibility of receiving support from their partners. Similarly, Lara-Cinisomo et al. (2011) found that at-home caregivers who experienced difficulty expressing feelings to their deployed partners reported lower satisfaction and more hassles in their relationship. Earlier, Bowling and Sherman (2008) suggested that service members and their family members coped with the stresses of deployment by suppressing their emotional responses and that this suppression could impede processes of reconnecting with one another after return. During the current conflicts, the prospect of possible future deployments and separations might complicate the reestablishment of intimate relationships.

Mulligan et al. (2012) and others have observed that access to immediate communication with home during deployment can present challenges. Although it offers a practical and immediate way for service members to participate in family life, it also might involve service members in solving problems that could be resolved without their attention. The authors suggested that service members and spouses be taught strategies to determine how to make the best choices of methods, content, and timing of communication. Carter et al. (2011) examined the communication of 193 Army couples characterized on average by high levels of marital satisfaction during deployment, including both frequency and type of communication (interactive, such as instant messaging and telephone calls; and delayed, such as emails, letters, and care packages). Many of the couples exchanged emails, instant messages, and phone calls daily and typically exchanged letters and care packages once or twice per month. More than half also used video instant messaging once per month. Results showed that service members reported lower levels of PTSD symptoms following deployment when they had communicated more frequently with their spouses during deployment but only when marital satisfaction was high and only when delayed forms of communication, such as letters, emails, and care packages, were used.

In the MHAT studies, length of deployment was positively correlated with the percentage of deployed service members who indicated that they planned to obtain a divorce or to separate after their return; for example, the MHAT-V study estimated that about 6% of noncommissioned Army officers indicated plans to divorce at 1 month of deployment, compared with over 20% at 15 months of deployment (MHAT-V, 2008). Plans to divorce or separate also appeared to be inversely correlated with pay grade: The MHAT-V study reported that, in 2007, 17.0% of junior enlisted soldiers deployed for 9 months were considering getting a divorce, compared with 12.3% of noncommissioned officers and 3.6% of officers. Mulligan et al. (2012) studied 2,000 British service members during deployments to Iraq and Afghanistan. They found that both family problems (death or illness of a loved one, financial problems, or problems with children) and home and relationship breakdowns were negatively related to mental health by a large amount. Although high military-unit cohesion and effective military leadership fully mediated the relationship between relationship breakdown and mental health, family problems at home could not be completely compensated for by unit cohesion or military leadership. In addition, perceptions of poor military support for families at home were negatively related to mental health regardless of combat exposure, unit cohesion, or effective leadership.

Several studies have presented empirical data regarding the logistic, psychologic, and economic challenges experienced by marital partners during deployment. Logistic challenges include maintaining a household with only one adult present, such as management of maintenance, repair, and financial activity; providing all necessary care for children; maintaining employment; and arranging medical care or other services that are affected by military regulations (for example, reserve-component families may need to change medical providers when TRICARE coverage begins and ends) (SteelFisher et al., 2008). SteelFisher et al. (2008) conducted telephone interviews early in 2004 with 744 Army spouses associated with units that were deployed to the Persian Gulf during the first 4 years after the event on September 11, 2001 (9/11). Some of them had experienced an unexpected extension of their partners' deployment. Deployment-induced logistic problems included difficulty in communication (sent and received) with the deployed members (41.0%), problems with household and car maintenance (29.0%), and problems finding child care (16.2%). Chandra et al. (2010a) and Lara-Cinisomo et al. (2011) surveyed over 1,000 at-home caregivers of children ages 7 to 17 who applied to have their children attend "Operation Purple" camps and conducted qualitative interviews with 50 participants. Baseline data were gathered during the summer of 2008; followups were conducted 6 and 12 months later. More than half of the caregivers surveyed reported one or more of the following logistic challenges associated with deployment: taking on more responsibilities at home; helping children deal with life without the deployed parent; spending more time with children on homework; and talking to teachers about children's school performance. A substantial proportion of spouses (30–50%) relocated during deployment. Proximity to extended family members increased, but it meant leaving local military services and causing children to change schools and living arrangements (Flake et al., 2009).

Psychologic challenges experienced by both service members and their spouses include fears for the safety of the service member, feeling anxious and overwhelmed by deployment-related challenges and responsibilities, worry about children, and concerns about military leadership, as well as vulnerability to additional stressors that might arise. In SteelFisher et al. (2008), the most common adverse effects of deployment on well-being that were reported by spouses were psychologic: loneliness (78.2%), anxiety (51.6%), depression (42.6%), and fears about personal safety (23.6%). A notable minority of the sample reported adverse perceptions of the military, the most commonly cited problem being lack of accurate information surrounding the timing of deployment, given that an unexpected extension had occurred (48.4%). According to Wright et al. (2006), fear of injury or death constituted major factors in the psychologic health of spouses throughout the deployment cycle, but especially before and during deployment. Existing data suggested that these concerns and fears tended to center on military training and leadership, the possible injury or death of service members, and concerns about managing on their own if that occurred.

In Chandra et al. (2010a), approximately half of the at-home spouses reported feeling that people in the community did not understand what life was like for them, particularly if they were affiliated with the reserve component. In addition, difficulties associated with new household duties were associated with increased anxiety and feelings of being overwhelmed (Lara-Cinisomo et al., 2011). Chandra et al. (2010a) also found that emotional well-being declined over time among caregivers who were experiencing deployment, but well-being improved if deployment ended during the course of the study. Overall, there were several indications in Lara-Cinisomo et al. (2011) of the same sample that reserve-component families were more likely than active-component families to experience deployment-related difficulties. For example, caregivers in both National Guard and reserve families reported significantly greater household and relationship hassles, and caregivers in National Guard families reported poorer emotional well-being.

Allen et al. (2011) studied 300 couples with active-duty Army husbands and civilian wives who experienced a deployment within the previous year. Top concerns during the year for both husbands and wives were exposure to combat and the effects of the deployment on children. Husbands' other strongest concerns pertained to sexual frustration; wives' other strongest concerns pertained to loneliness and staying in touch, injury and fear of death, and reintegration and fears about potential changes in the service member. Infidelity was not a major concern reported by either husbands or wives.

Economic challenges associated with deployment can include loss of spousal employment or difficulty paying for child care or other household services usually provided by the deployed family member. Reserve-component members experience small income increases on average, although some lose income during deployment (Angrist and Johnson, 2000). In the SteelFisher et al. (2008) study, spouses of service members experiencing a deployment extension were more likely to report problems with work and to have scaled back or left work; they were also more likely to report problems in their marriages than spouses who did not experience an extension. Reported problems with overall health (21%) and perceived effects on jobs (18%) were more prevalent than financial problems (12%) or problems with their marriage (10%).

*Marital Quality on Return from Deployment*

Many of the same adjustments and role reallocations that must be completed as deployments begin must be completed again when service members return home (Bowling and Sherman, 2008; Pincus et al., 2001). Studies conducted after return from deployment emphasize the implications of psychologic symptoms of service members, but many other aspects of the reintegration experience may be consequential for adults and children.

Following World War II, Hill (1949) recognized that families' experiences following reintegration were partially a function of their experiences and behavior during deployment. Some families appeared to function exceptionally well during deployment, "closing ranks" as if the deployed service member was unneeded or irrelevant; other families had great difficulty continuing to perform even basic tasks in the absence of the service members. Families who seemed to function best were those that closed ranks only enough to fulfill important tasks but not so much that there was no place for the service member upon his return. Research conducted during the Vietnam era reinforced these observations, demonstrating that families who maintained the service members' psychologic presence during deployment seemed to adapt more effectively when difficulties occurred (McCubbin et al., 1975).

Although most studies fail to measure positive consequences of deployment, the Rosen et al. (1995) study of Army couples who experienced deployments associated with Operation Desert Storm in Iraq found that the five most common reunion events were positive: the soldier was pleased with the spouse's handling of finances or running of the household, the couple became closer, the spouse became more independent, and the soldier did more chores. All positive events were reported by at least one-third of the sample. The five least common reunion events reported by no more than 10% of the sample were the following: the spouse became more dependent, the soldier was critical of the spouse's handling of finances, the soldier resented the spouse's new friends, and the spouse resented the soldier's new friends.

Following deployment, the couples in Baptist et al. (2011) who had been able to maintain the ability to exchange mutual support with their partners also were more likely to report closeness in their marriages. Religious faith and belief in the importance of the military mission also were helpful. However, participants also reported suppressing, avoiding, or restraining sexual behavior with their spouses, all of which interfered with marital closeness (Baptist et al., 2011).

In a review of existing literature about reintegration following war-related separations, Vormbrock (1993) found that longer separations were related to more distress, detachment, and damage to the attachment relationship. Although both service members and spouses tended to engage in contact-seeking behavior, home-based spouses were more likely than service members to display detachment and anger. Rosen et al. (1995) gathered data from 776 Army wives 1 year after deployments to Operation Desert Storm to test Vormbrock's conclusions. Both Vormbrock and Rosen et al. found that separation distress was heightened by stressful events during the separation but lessened when adults had access to alternative attachment figures; however, revival of childhood attachments, such as those to parents, could undermine the marital relationship.

After deployment, Sahlstein et al. (2009) observed, "soldiers and spouses often found themselves struggling to know how, when, and what to communicate with one another." Families who were able to achieve a quick "return to normal" had maintained open lines of communication, working as a team throughout the deployment. In most couples, however, there were mismatches between the service member's willingness to share and the spouse's willingness to hear.

Baptist et al. (2011) also found that both husbands and wives reported withholding information from their spouses in efforts to protect them from distress. Wives reported continuing to perform household duties following husbands' return from deployment when they would have preferred greater involvement by husbands, and both husbands and wives reported restraining sexual desires. Although well intentioned, these decisions usually were made without consulting the partner about his or her preferences. Nelson Goff and Smith (2005) also observed that couples who were unable to reconnect following deployment were a function of both prior marital problems, such as infidelity, and difficulties in sharing information, exchanging comfort, and supporting each other.

Although reintegration processes are typically described as occurring over time, few studies have empirically documented the sequence, durations, or content of these processes, particularly as they relate to families. In several studies, members of families affiliated with the National Guard and reserves have reported greater difficulties or poorer outcomes associated with deployment (Chandra et al., 2010a; Lara-Cinisomo et al., 2011). Faber et al. (2008) observed that reservists experienced prolonged ambiguity about their family roles and greater adjustment difficulties when return to the civilian workforce did not go smoothly. Civilian spouses and children might need to change medical providers, and civilian communities might be poorly prepared to serve military families (Huebner et al., 2009).

*Summary of the Impact of Deployment on Marital Quality*

In summary, as a result of deployment, marital quality is affected by psychologic challenges, including worry and uncertainty, that appear more prevalent than logistic issues (for example, managing the household) or economic difficulties (for example, loss of spousal employment). Some stressors are specific to a particular phase of the deployment cycle (that is, predeployment, during deployment, and postdeployment), and may dissipate as families move through the deployment cycle (for example, worries about a service member's safety during deployment may lessen upon returning home). Others stressors are evident throughout (for example, communication issues) and may be a chronic symptom in a couple's relationship. Male service members and their wives share many of the same concerns, such as concerns about the well-being of children and the service member's safety, but also have separate ones. Dominant concerns among male service members include worries about the impact of separation on their families and worries about their spouses' ability to cope with deployment-related challenges, including loneliness and household responsibilities. (The concerns of female service members are probably similar; however, there is a lack of studies of female service members to confirm the similarity.) The most common stressors among female spouses include feelings of loneliness, fears about their spouses' death or injury, raising children alone, and problems communicating with their spouses. Spouses who are depressed and families that are members of the reserve component are more likely to experience deployment-related challenges. Families may also have positive experiences as a result of deployment, such as family bonding and increase competence in family functioning. Important to the understanding of the impact of deployment on marital quality is knowledge about what issues—individual or relational—may have been preexisting and not a symptom of deployment per se. Epidemiologic research that characterizes military spouses irrespective of their experiences with deployment is lacking. Other gaps in the research base are related to the normative course, duration, and sequence of stressors experienced by military families as a result of deployment.

**Marital Dissolution**

Many media outlets have reported "skyrocketing" divorce rates as a result of deployment-related stressors (Alvarez, 2007; Crary, 2005; Parsons, 2008), and such an expectation seems reasonable given lengthy and repeated family separations. The empirical evidence so far is mixed, possibly because insufficient time has elapsed for the consequences of deployment to have become fully evident.

As noted earlier, military divorce rates have risen in the past decade. This section examines several investigations that have been conducted to determine the role of deployments in these increases. Two explanations have been proposed to explain divorce rates in the military. According to the stress hypothesis, the stressors of military life erode the stability of marriages, suggesting a positive relationship between deployment and the likelihood of divorce. In contrast, the selection hypothesis suggests that the likelihood of divorce is tied to characteristics of the partners and their relationships (Karney and Crown, 2007) and thus would not increase because of deployments.

Data from prior wars are inconsistent. For example, Ruger et al. (2002) studied 3,800 veterans of World War II and the conflicts in Korea and Vietnam using data from the National Survey of Families and Households. Veterans married prior to the Vietnam War were no more likely to divorce than those married after, failing to support the stress hypothesis at least with regard to deployment-related separation. A consistent finding across wars and robust to statistical controls, however, was that exposure to combat did increase the likelihood of marital dissolution, consistent with the stress hypothesis. More recently, a large representative survey of military members (59,631) showed that deployment to Operation Desert Storm was associated with a statistically significant increase, by 4.2 percentage points, in later divorce rates of female service members (Angrist and Johnson, 2000), but no association occurred among male service members.

Contrary to the view that longer deployments raise the risk of marital dissolution, (Karney and Crown, 2007, 2011) found in a study of personnel records of over 560,000 service members who married in 2002–2005 that the longer a service member was deployed, the lower the risk of divorce or separation. Risk was lowest for individuals who would normally be thought of as the most vulnerable—those who had married younger and who had children in the home. These results were not consistent with the hypothesis that the stress of deployment undermines otherwise healthy marriages. The findings were preliminary, however, because they focused only on relatively recent marriages that were followed for only a short period.

The most recent analyses were conducted by Negrusa and Negrusa (2012), who calculated the likelihood of marital dissolution as a function of deployment, using a military longitudinal dataset spanning from 1999 to 2008. They found that deployment substantially increased the risk of divorce, with the effect being stronger for female service members and for service members who were sent on hostile deployments (typically, to Iraq and Afghanistan).

In summary, results are mixed regarding the reasons for the rise in divorce rates in the military over the past decade. Both selection effects (preexisting characteristics of couples) and stress effects (increasing operational tempo and more hostile deployments) appear to be relevant factors.

**Spousal Abuse**

Family violence, which includes spousal abuse[1] as well as child maltreatment, has become a focus of concern in the military. This section covers spousal violence in terms of prevalence, types of abuse, risk factors, health consequences of abuse, and treatment.

*Prevalence and Types*

In 2011, the rate of substantiated incidents of spousal abuse was 11.1 per 1,000 couples (DOD, 2012c). This rate extends an upward trend that began in FY 2009. Before then, from FY 2001 to FY 2008, the rate had been declining (Figure 6.1). The data are compiled annually by DOD's Family Advocacy Program (FAP), which was created in 1984 to identify, prevent, and treat family violence in the military. Because each report of spousal abuse reflects a single incident, there can be more than one report for a single victim. The abuser could have been an active-duty service member or a civilian. Finally, the data are not broken down by OEF or OIF; they are DOD-wide incidents.

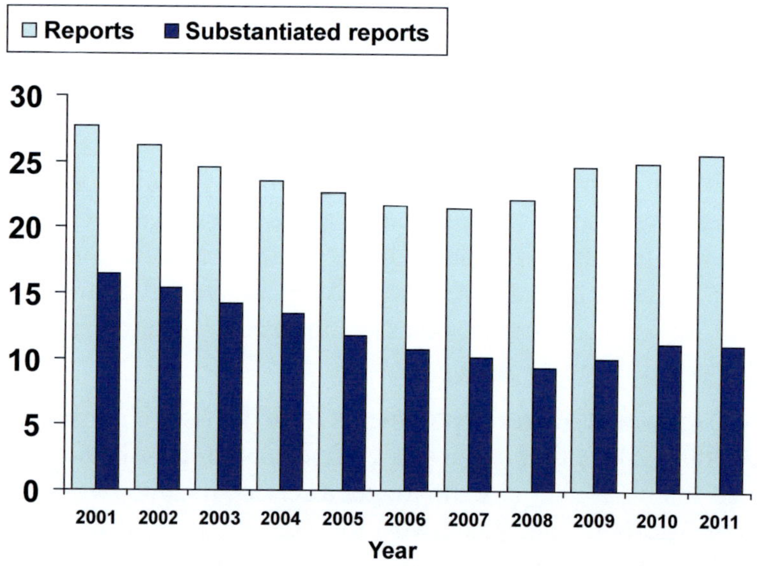


**FIGURE 6.1** Rate of spousal-abuse reports per 1,000 couples to the Family Advocacy Program, 2001–2011.
SOURCE: DOD, 2012c.

Spousal abuse is distributed as follows: physical abuse accounts for 90% of spousal-abuse cases; emotional abuse, 6–8%; sexual abuse, 0.5%; and neglect, 0.4% (Rentz et al., 2006). Two-thirds (67%) of abusers are male and one-third (33%) are female (DOD, 2012c). In FY 2011, there were 18 fatalities tied to spousal abuse (DOD, 2012c). The occurrence of spousal abuse, as compiled by the FAP, is probably an underestimate: incidents often go unreported out of concern for career implications of the active-duty service member or for victims' concerns

[1]In this chapter, spousal abuse is synonymous with intimate partner violence and domestic abuse.

about their physical safety.[2] The overall rate of spousal abuse in the military is similar to that of civilians, although the only study to address the comparison dates back to the 1990s (Heyman and Neidig, 1999).

*Risk Factors*

Deployment is perceived as the foremost stressor in the military, according to a 2005 DOD survey of some 16,000 male and female active-duty service members (Bray et al., 2006). Not surprisingly, deployment has been identified in the medical literature as a risk factor for spousal aggression in the aftermath of deployment. This finding was reported in a random sample of 26,835 deployed and nondeployed married active-duty members in the Army (McCarroll et al., 2000). The study also found that the likelihood of severe aggression rose with the length of deployment. With a short length of deployment (6 months), deployment was not found to be a risk factor in the first 10 months after return from deployment, but younger age was a risk factor (Newby et al., 2005b).

PTSD first emerged as a risk factor for intimate partner violence in Vietnam veterans. The National Vietnam Veterans Readjustment Study found that one-third of the males with PTSD exhibited violence, according to their female partners (Kulka et al., 1990). A similar rate of violence was found among veterans with PTSD seen at a Veterans Administration (VA) medical center from 2003 to 2008 (Taft et al., 2009). In a recent study of Navy recruits, PTSD also was identified as a risk factor, having an odds ratio of 2.05, compared with recruits without PTSD (Merrill et al., 2004). Having PTSD symptoms of arousal and feeling a lack of control were the most robust predictors of aggression (Taft et al., 2009).

Substance use also has been found to be a risk factor for spousal abuse, according to a study of two Army databases of offenders, the Army Central Registry and the Drug and Alcohol Management Information System. The study found that 25% of 7,424 service members were under the influence of substances during the abuse incident. They were more likely than nonsubstance abusers to be physically violent and to exert more severe spousal abuse (Martin et al., 2010). A separate study found that the odds ratios for spousal abuse were 1.90 for alcohol problems and 2.02 for drug use (Merrill et al., 2004). However, in another study, alcohol use was unrelated to intimate partner violence among 248 married enlisted female soldiers, regardless of whether they were perpetrators or victims (Forgey and Badger, 2010).

In the only study on spousal abuse specifically in OIF and OEF service members, experiential avoidance—a coping strategy that seeks to avoid emotionally painful events—was associated with physical aggression perpetration and victimization in a study of 49 male National Guard members who returned from deployment to Iraq (Reddy et al., 2011).

*Consequences and Treatment*

Although data on the consequences of spousal abuse specific to military families are not available, in civilian studies, spousal abuse has been found to be associated with numerous negative outcomes. In studies of sheltered female domestic-violence victims, PTSD prevalence ranged from 51% to 75% (Golding, 1999; Street and Arias, 2001), depression ranged from 35% to 70% (Golding, 1999; O'Leary, 1999), and substance-abuse disorders occurred in about 10% of

---

[2]The figures are also underestimated because DOD maintains another database of law-enforcement cases of abuse—the Defense Incident-Based Reporting System, which covers the minority of cases that rise to a crime.

victims (Helfrich et al., 2008). Similar findings were reported in a community sample of 94 women who were evaluated by diagnostic interviews (Nathanson et al., 2012). In the latter study, psychologic abuse was more likely to be associated with a mental disorder than with physical abuse.

The committee found little information about treatment of spousal abuse, which is a service provided by the FAP itself or in conjunction with local treatment providers. In 2010, the Government Accountability Office (GAO) concluded that, despite some improvements subsequent to the mandate to establish a DOD Task Force on Domestic Violence that was included in the National Defense Authorization Act for Fiscal Year 2000, "DOD lacks the sustained leadership and oversight of its efforts to prevent and treat domestic abuse that would enable the department to accurately assess the effectiveness of these efforts" (GAO, 2010).

The DOD monitors spousal abuse treatment by this one metric: the percentage of abusers who are not reported for spousal abuse within 1 year of program completed. As noted elsewhere in this chapter, the DOD reported that 97% of abusers who completed the program in FY 2011 were not reported (DOD, 2012b). Yet, no information is given about the content of the treatment program, how programs are evaluated, and their impact on the mental health of victims. The civilian literature indicates that many treatment programs for spousal-abuse victims or perpetrators are only minimally effective (Babcock et al., 2004; Nelson et al., 2004).

*Summary*

In summary, a service member's psychologic issues are related to increases in marital distress, divorce, and disruptions in family life. Findings also suggest that the reverse is true: family relationships, both before and after deployment, can influence how a service member experiences PTSD in terms of coping with symptoms and symptom severity. Moreover, relationship quality may have an impact on treatment seeking by a service member. A spouse's perception of a service member's psychologic health (for example, perceptions of the apparent cause for symptoms or of the service member's control over symptoms) influences the level of personal and marital distress experienced by the spouse.

Service members' deployment is associated with increases in mental-health problems, particularly depression and anxiety, among spouses. Length of deployment and cumulative months of deployment predict increases in the likelihood of distress, but the number of deployments does not. Pregnant women with deployed partners experience high levels of stress and depression, particularly if they have other children. Although overall rates of spousal abuse in the military do not appear to be higher than those in the civilian population, there is evidence that the risk of spousal physical violence is higher after deployment, the risk increasing with the length of deployment.

The impact that the presence of children has on the psychologic well-being of a parent with a deployed spouse is somewhat ambiguous. Some studies have found that a parent's worry about the well-being of their children and concerns over the logistics of providing care add to deployment-related stress. Other studies indicate that mothers and female spouses without children experience similar levels of distress. At least one study found that the presence of children is protective against depression in the stay-at-home parent. More studies are needed to understand the specific stressors faced by single parents serving in the Armed Forces.

## Single Service Members and Their Families

Little attention has been paid by researchers to single service members who have experienced deployment and the degree to which family formation processes have been delayed or disrupted as a result. However, some of the same themes relating to deployment and marital quality discussed above are evident in a study of single service members living with their parents following return from deployment. Worthen et al. (2012) conducted qualitative interviews of OEF and OIF veterans living with their parents on the basis of the finding that 60% of young people return home to live with parents at some point. In most cases, veterans described their experiences as positive, and parents were helpful in recognizing health and adjustment problems. Distinct from the experiences of couples, adult children sometimes struggled with feeling treated as a child by their parents. Some service members were motivated by conflict with their parents to pursue school, a relationship, or work with undue haste. Women veterans interviewed in the study, a substantial proportion of whom had experienced military sexual trauma, had mixed experiences in terms of parental support, some experiencing ideal support but others experiencing conflict with or "smothering" by their parents. Few programs were available to educate or support parents in their efforts to assist their adult children.

## Psychologic Health of Family Members

Among service members whose deployment experiences result in personality changes or psychologic symptoms and diagnosis, particularly PTSD, there are consequences for marital quality as well as specific psychologic effects on spouses and children. These are discussed below.

### Psychologic Health of Spouses

Several studies have examined the prevalence of psychologic symptoms among military spouses in relation to deployment-related stressors. Eaton et al. (2008) studied over 700 active-duty-component military spouses seeking primary care at military facilities. According to both broad and strict screening criteria, spouses and service members reported similar levels of major depression or generalized anxiety disorders (using broad screening criteria, 19.5% and 15.6%, respectively, for spouses and service members). Spouses were more likely than service members, however, to seek care (70% vs 40%) and less likely to be impeded in doing so by worries about stigma, although more than 25% reported one or more of the following barriers to obtaining care: arranging child care or time off from work, difficulty getting an appointment, or cost. About 20% of spouses received care only from primary care physicians rather than from mental-health specialists.

An analysis of medical records of over 250,000 military wives done by Mansfield et al. (2010) revealed similar patterns. After controlling for background characteristics (age, number of deployments, pay grade, and years of service of the military member) and mental-health history, there were 39.3 excess cases of depression per 1,000 population among spouses whose partners were deployed for longer than 11 months and 27.4 excess cases among women whose husbands had been deployed 1 to 11 months (compared with wives of nondeployed partners), and 30% of this group had higher rates of service use. Overall, wives whose husbands were deployed were significantly more likely to have diagnoses of depression, anxiety, acute stress reaction, adjustment disorders, and sleep disorders than wives whose husbands had not been deployed.

Spouses of deployed service members also used mental health services at higher rates, which increased with deployment length. The likelihood of any mental-health diagnosis was 19% higher among women whose husbands had been deployed 1 to 11 months (41.3 excess cases/1,0000) and 27% higher among women whose husbands had been deployed longer than 11 months (60.7 excess cases/1,000).

In a study by SteelFisher et al. (2008), spouses who experienced deployment extension reported increased levels of mental-health problems relative to those who did not. Half of the spouses reported frequent feelings of anxiety, and almost half reported frequent feelings of depression. In a sample of 332 National Guard members and 212 partners, Gorman et al. (2011) found that 40% and 34%, respectively, met screening criteria for one or more mental-health problems. In that group, 50% of service members and 61% of partners had attempted to obtain help. Barriers encountered by partners included cost, difficulty getting time away from work or scheduling appointments, and not knowing where to get help.

Across studies, most military spouses who reported psychologic symptoms also reported seeking care (Eaton et al., 2008; Gorman et al., 2011; Warner et al., 2009), but most encountered barriers to care, including difficulty in getting time off from work, arranging child care, difficulty getting an appointment, and cost. Barriers reported by active duty and reserve-component spouses were similar.

Two small studies focused on spouses' stress and coping with the demands of their service members' military duties. In one, spouses evaluated their partners' deployment as one of the most stressful experiences of recent years in their lives (Dimiceli et al., 2010). In turn, spouses' perceived stress was positively related to their levels of well-being (Padden et al., 2011) and psychologic symptoms (Dimiceli et al., 2010). Consistent with the broader literature on stress, coping strategies focused on problem-solving, and taking action appeared to predict better psychologic health (Dimiceli et al., 2010; Padden et al., 2011).

### Psychologic Health of Families with Children

Another topic that has received attention from researchers is the psychologic health of parents or caregivers of children in military families. Consistent with studies of civilian families (Luthar, 2006) and military families during the first Gulf War (Jensen et al., 1996), studies of military families during the current conflicts found that distress among parents and the children they care for are positively related. In addition, adults' distress was found to be a function of cumulative exposure to deployment but not to number of deployments (Lara-Cinisomo et al., 2011; Lester et al., 2010)—but note that both of these studies focused exclusively on families still in military service.

In the Lara-Cinisomo et al. (2011) study of 1,337 mothers or caregivers (children ages 11 to 17) affiliated with the active and reserve components of the military, cumulative months of deployment in the past 3 years significantly predicted difficulties related to mental health, relationship with the service member, and household management. Current deployment was significantly and positively related to caregiver mental health and relationship difficulties. Caregivers of children affiliated with the National Guard reported significantly greater difficulties than caregivers of children affiliated with the reserves or the active component.

Similarly, in another study contrasting parents with currently deployed and recently returned military spouses in the Army and Marine Corps, distress—specifically, anxiety—was significantly greater among parents whose partners were currently deployed. Emotional distress measured by global severity, depression, and anxiety scores on the Brief Symptom Inventory were significantly increased among both at-home civilians and active-duty parents. For example, global severity was 0.46 for civilians and 0.53 for active-duty parents compared with a community norm of 0.35. More than 25% of parents reported clinically significant global distress (26.4%), depression (30.1%), or anxiety (26.4%) (Lester et al., 2010).

It is not clear, however, that parenthood exacerbates stressors related to military service. Hopkins-Chadwick and Ryan-Wenger (2009) compared junior enlisted women serving in the Air Force with and without children (50 of each) younger than 5 living at home. Mothers and nonmothers reported similar levels of role strain, stress, health, and military career aspirations. Warner et al. (2009) found that the presence of children was protective in relation to depression.

**Psychologic Health of Single Parents**

The literature on stress and the military has focused primarily on two-parent families, and research on single parents is scare. What little does exist about single parents in the military was published approximately two decades ago, so it might not represent experiences from the more recent conflicts. Kelley et al. (2001) reported that, among Navy mothers, the level of separation anxiety was highest among single mothers anticipating deployment.

**Spousal Physical and Psychologic Health During Pregnancy**

A small number of studies have investigated the possible impact of deployment on the health of military spouses during pregnancy. To date, few differences in physical health have been found. For example, a cross-sectional survey of postpartum mothers at Camp LeJeune during 2003 revealed no differences in gestational age, likelihood of vaginal delivery, number of previous children, or weight gain between those with deployed or nondeployed partners. Mothers whose partners were deployed were more likely to report having changed their eating habits during pregnancy and had infants who were on average almost 300 grams heavier (Haas and Pazdernik, 2006).

Differences were found regarding the psychologic health of pregnant military spouses. For example, a survey of 525 pregnant women seeking services at the Naval Hospital at Camp LeJeune in 2005 revealed that women reported significantly higher levels of stress if their partners were deployed, if they themselves served on active duty, if they were farther along in their pregnancy, or had more than one child at home (Haas and Pazdernik, 2007). Robrecht et al. (2008) reviewed the medical records of 415 women who had recently given birth, finding that women whose spouses had been deployed during the pregnancy were 2.75 times more likely to screen positive for postnatal depression. Finally, an examination of screenings of 3,956 women with military spouses conducted at the first obstetrics visit during pregnancy, at the 28-week visit, and at 6 weeks postpartum between 2007 and 2009 revealed that mothers were significantly more likely to exceed clinical cutoffs for depression during the initial obstetrics visit if their spouses were preparing to deploy or had recently returned from deployment. At 28 weeks gestation, depression scores were higher for women whose partners were deployed or returning from deployment. Postpartum, depression scores were significantly higher for women whose partners were deployed (de Burgh et al., 2011; Smith et al., 2010). Note, however, that already having children at home was more strongly related to perceived stress among pregnant spouses than deployment of partners in most of these studies.

### Psychologic Health of Surviving Spouses

Death is an inevitable accompaniment of war, and the OEF and OIF wars have left behind thousands of spouses, children, and other family members to mourn the loss of a loved one. To date, however, there are no comprehensive studies of bereavement in US military families. To address this gap, the Center for Traumatic Stress is currently undertaking a 5-year study of bereavement in about 3,000 family members, including spouses, parents, and siblings of deceased service members—the first scientific study of the impact of US military deaths on surviving family members. The focus will be not only on combat deaths but also on homicides, suicides, and accidents (Jowers, 2011).

### Consequences of Service Members' Psychologic Symptoms for Marital Quality

The largest area of research related to deployment and families pertains to the implications of service members' combat- or deployment-related psychologic symptoms and diagnoses, particularly PTSD, for the quality and stability of relationships with intimate partners and children. Data collected from the 2004 through 2007 National Surveys on Drug Use and Health (SAMHSA, 2008), which surveyed veterans ages 21 through 39 (deployment history not known), showed that three-quarters of those who had experienced a major depressive episode the previous year reported being severely or very severely impaired in at least one of four role domains: home management, work, close relationships with others, and social life. Half reported severe or very severe impairment in role functioning with respect to close relationships with others.

Recent studies also are revealing ways in which relationship dynamics may influence vulnerability to and severity of psychologic symptoms among service members, and the likelihood of seeking treatment. In this section, we deal with the relationships between service members' psychologic symptoms and marital quality; in a later section, we consider the implications of service members' injuries for caregivers' own well-being and functioning.

According to a review by Monson et al. (2009), studies of previous conflicts repeatedly found links between PTSD and relationship problems, including divorce. Specific symptom clusters might be linked to specific types of relationship problems. For example, the arousal cluster of symptoms is found to be related to greater hostility and violence directed by service members or veterans toward their partners, while the numbing and avoidance cluster is related to difficulties with intimacy, including sharing and receiving communication about emotions, as well as general relationship satisfaction. For male service members but less so for females, the effects of combat exposure are mediated through psychologic symptoms. Other possible mechanisms of influence include secondary traumatization and caregiver burden experienced by partners, but many research questions are yet to be answered.

Almost all studies have focused on the effects of PTSD on interpersonal relationships, but there also are reasons to expect that relationships can affect the occurrence of and prognosis for PTSD (Erbes, 2011; Monson et al., 2009). For example, social support, of which family relationships are a primary source, is negatively related to PTSD symptoms. In addition, relationship patterns among intimate partners may prolong or reduce avoidant behavior or support or discourage emotional expression, each of which can affect the course of PTSD. For example, intimate-relationship partners might be helpful in keeping service members engaged with others rather than withdrawing. Conversely, strain or distance in intimate relationships might reinforce service members' negative cognitions associated with PTSD (Erbes, 2011).

Several studies from both current and previous conflicts revealed positive relationships between service members' deployment-related psychologic symptoms and disruptions in family life. Most of these studies were cross-sectional, and many were conducted with samples recruited from health clinics or hospitals. For example, Sayers (2011) studied 199 veterans of service during OEF and OIF who had been referred for behavioral health specialty care. Three of four of those who were married or living with a partner reported family problems in the past week, including feeling like a guest in their own home (40.7%). One of four reported that their children were acting afraid or distant. Among veterans who were currently or had recently separated from their partners, most reported that they had episodes of "shouting, pushing, or shoving" (54%) or that their partners were afraid of them (27.6%).

Johnson (2011) studied 60 spouses of veterans of OEF and OIF service in a mixture of branches and components, most of whom had been deployed multiple times. On average, the spouses reported significant negative change in 13 of 18 characteristics, including increases in veterans' tendencies to be quick-tempered, irritable, unhappy, cold, lifeless, mean, cruel, unreasonable, insensitive, and changeable. When service members' personalities had changed more, spouses reported higher levels of grief, which in turn were associated with more frequent arguments and less social support. These relationships appeared robust to a variety of demographic characteristics.

A group of studies using data from the Readiness and Resilience in National Guard Soldiers (RINGS) study documented interpersonal dynamics surrounding service members' PTSD symptoms. Conducted as a partnership of the Minneapolis VA, the University of Minnesota, and the Minnesota National Guard, the studies' participants were composed of members of the Minnesota Army National Guard and their partners. Erbes (2011) examined data provided by 522 RINGS participants before and after deployment, finding that 24% of the variability in postdeployment PTSD symptoms was accounted for by predeployment predictors, including psychologic symptoms at that time, prior exposure to trauma, concerns about occupational or family disruption, feeling insufficiently prepared or supported for the mission, and being younger or female.

In a factor analytic study, Erbes et al. (2011) examined the connection between specific PTSD symptom clusters and relationship adjustment. The dysphoria cluster appeared to be the most important factor explaining intimate-relationship adjustment within the 6 months following service members' return from deployment and the only significant predicting relationship adjustment 1 year later. Thus, much of the impact of PTSD on couple adjustment may be because of the generalized distress that accompanies the disorder, rather than specific symptoms related to reexperiencing or arousal. The extent to which some PTSD symptoms predicted relationship disruption was substantially greater for female soldiers. There was a trend for PTSD avoidance symptoms to have a greater impact on couple relationships among female soldiers than male soldiers.

Evidence from both the Erbes (2011) study and others suggests that spouses' attributions about their partners' symptoms influence the spouses' levels of personal and marital distress. Specifically, when spouses cannot see an obvious cause for their partners' symptoms or when they perceive their partners as being able but choosing not to exert control over symptoms, they may respond with less support and more distress. In two small studies of the OEF and OIF conflicts, wives were more distressed when they could not see an obvious cause for their husbands' symptoms, whether because wives perceived symptoms that their husbands failed to acknowledge or husbands reported more severe symptoms than their wives expected, given what was known about their combat experience (Goff et al., 2007; Renshaw and Campbell, 2011; Renshaw and Caska, 2012; Renshaw et al., 2008). Pietrzak and Southwick (2011) observed similar patterns in a sample of 272 members of the National Guard and reserves, averaging 34 years of age, in that the group who experienced high exposure to combat and high levels of PTSD symptoms also reported the most problems in psychologic and social functioning, while the group of service members who experienced high exposure to combat but reported low levels of PTSD symptoms were significantly more likely than others to report receiving support and understanding from their families and to perceive a sense of purpose and control.

Erbes (2011) and Renshaw and Campbell (2011) concluded that generalized distress was a prominent feature of couples' experiences related to PTSD. Erbes (2011) found that general dysphoria in service members, including irritability and numbing, was more strongly related to relationship adjustment than either reexperiencing or arousal, perhaps because dysphoria is less obviously connected to service members' combat experiences than other symptom clusters. Renshaw and colleagues investigated the degree to which spouses' psychologic symptoms reflected a form of secondary traumatization related to their partners' symptoms, as opposed to a more generalized form of distress, and found greater support for the generalized form of distress among most spouses (Renshaw et al., 2011).

Using data from the RINGS project, Meis et al. (2010) examined processes that could be responsible for corroding relationship quality following return from deployment. Controlling for prior exposure to trauma and prior PTSD symptoms (but not prior relationship distress), levels of negative emotionality among service members before deployment significantly predicted levels of PTSD symptoms following return. In turn, the PTSD symptoms were significantly related to lower relationship quality. Service members with probable PTSD were more than half as likely as those without to experience relationship distress (33% vs 20%).

Symptom severity of PTSD and relationship quality may interact to influence the likelihood of seeking treatment and the nature of treatment sought. Buchanan et al. (2011) conducted a qualitative study with 34 wives or partners of combat veterans to learn their strategies for encouraging service members to seek treatment, as well as the barriers spouses perceived. Partners perceived the main barriers as service members' denial, fear, and stigma about disclosing their symptoms. Partners' strategies included offering support and patience, making suggestions that treatment be sought, initiating treatment themselves, or issuing ultimatums. Meis et al. (2010), in a sample of 223 coupled RINGS participants, found that the severity of PTSD symptoms interacted with relationship quality to predict the type of treatment sought, even though symptom severity predicted greater service use overall (to the exclusion of relationship quality when both were considered together as independent variables). At higher levels of relationship adjustment, more severe PTSD symptoms predicted use of individual-oriented treatment, and relationship quality was unrelated to seeking couple or family care. At lower levels of PTSD symptoms, poorer relationship adjustment significantly predicted seeking couple or family care. These results suggest that once PTSD symptoms reach a certain (yet unknown) threshold, service members may be less willing to simultaneously deal with relationship issues and their symptoms. Or perhaps beyond this threshold, relationship difficulties are such that couple-oriented treatment does not seem possible. Researchers are only beginning to sort out these issues as they pertain to returning veterans and their families.

## MILITARY CHILDREN AND DEPLOYMENT

Children in military families have the advantage of a number of resources that help to buffer them from risks that many nonmilitary children might experience (Sheppard et al., 2010). In numerous respects, military families have a stronger socioeconomic safety net than many of their civilian contemporaries in the United States, where about 22% of children live in poverty and over a third (34%) live in a single-parent household (Annie E. Casey Foundation, 2012; Federal Interagency Forum on Child and Family Statistics, 2012). In 2010, 29% children lived in families where no parent had full-time, year-round employment (Federal Interagency Forum on Child and Family Statistics, 2012); that percentage is not a problem among military families. Although military children face the risk of traumatic events happening to their parents, so do many nonmilitary children. Military families have access to child care and health services that are often far superior to those available to civilian families at similar income levels. Housing is related to family size, and military installations tend to have good schools, good sports, and recreation facilities, and a system of support services, including ones targeted for the families of deployed or injured personnel.

On the other hand, military children may also have to cope with circumstances specific to military families, such as parents leaving for and returning from deployments (which can be unexpected, prolonged, and repeated), and the medical, psychologic, and economic consequences of deployment. The family may have to relocate frequently, either because the military member gets stationed at a new location, because the family members wish to relocate temporarily during a deployment (for example, to stay with relatives who can help with child care), or because the child of a single custodial military parent must go to live with another caretaker while the parent is deployed. Military families are more than four times as likely as civilian families to move to international locations, requiring them to adapt to unfamiliar cultures (Reinkober Drummet et al., 2003). Access to health care can also change if the family relocates during deployment, especially if they are no longer living near a military base. Relationships with peers, as well as local institutions (including schools), may also be disrupted. Parents may come back damaged, physically or psychologically. Or, tragically, they may not return at all. These contrasts are part of the lives of children in families of OEF and OIF military personnel.

### General Stressors for Military Children

Any review of military children and families dealing with deployment of a parent must take into account that these additional stressors occur against a background of exposure to the ordinary risks of daily life. Thus, before discussing the specific needs of children of parents deployed in OEF or OIF, it is useful to think about the stressors military children might experience (irrespective of whether their parent or parents have deployed) and the levels at which those stressors can occur in the general population. Stressors include parental absence, having to move multiple times, parental psychopathology, and death of a parent, as well as the effects on children of having to deal with the other parent's reactions to such events. These stressors give a sense of the ordinary level of stress and strain that military families might experience, beyond which is the need to cope with the challenges presented by deployment.

### Parental Absence

Like children in military families, children in civilian families might experience the absence of a parent. Parental absence most often refers to the absence of the father; this is certainly true in military families, where—despite the increasing number of women in the military—the deployed service member is still much more likely to be male. According to 2011 US Census Bureau data, over 20 million children under age 18 live apart from their biologic fathers[3]; that is, just over a quarter (27%) of children in America (an additional 3% live apart from their mother, and 4% live apart from both parents) (US Census Bureau, 2011b). Absence of fathers, although an expected concomitant of military life during wartime, is thus not an uncommon experience for civilian children, although the nature of that absence may be different. Examples for children are temporary absence due to deployment to a war zone of fathers in intact households or in households where custody is shared after a divorce versus the ongoing absence of noninvolved fathers with whom the children have limited or no relationship.

### Multiple Relocations

An estimated one-third of military families relocate annually, with families commonly moving every 3 years (Orthner and Rose, 2002). Just as periodic moves are an expected part of military life, it is also common for civilian families to move (NRC and IOM, 2010). From 2003 and 2004, about 14% of the US population moved—the rate for people living below the poverty level are higher (24%). Whether moving is for positive reasons (for example, relocation for a higher paying job or to be closer to family) or negative ones (for example, following eviction or foreclosure or breakup of a family), it is potentially disruptive for children. It can, for example, interrupt their learning in school, disrupt peer relationships, and disconnect children from important relationships with adults and institutions in the community (NRC and IOM, 2010). Impacts can also vary, depending on the age and developmental stage of the child, as brain development, capacities for dealing with stress, and behavior all change over time in ways that can affect a child's ability to manage a move.

National longitudinal studies that examine the impact of relocation on school achievement are sparse, and it is difficult to disentangle the effects of mobility from other factors (for example, poverty and family characteristics). However, although the impact of a single move may be negligible overall, the negative impact on achievement is cumulative and increases with the number of moves (especially above a threshold of three to four or more moves). The impact is greater for some groups of children, especially certain ethnic minority groups, those at lower socioeconomic status levels, and those whose families are downwardly mobile (NRC and IOM, 2010). In the civilian population, multiple moves are thus positively associated with social disadvantage in a way that is not the case in military families who have both stable employment and guaranteed housing.

### Parental Mental Illness and Substance Abuse

The number of children in either military or civilian families who live with a parent with a mental disorder is unknown. However, mental illness clearly occurs in both military and civilian families. Screening at the recruitment stage acts to limit the entry of individuals with serious mental illness into the military; however, mental illness can still develop later (for

---

[3]Includes children living with neither parent.

example, PTSD resulting from deployment experiences), and nonmilitary spouses may also have mental illness. National survey data on child exposure to parental mental illness are sparse, and most studies that look at children of people with mental illness focus only on clinical populations, making it difficult to estimate exposure in the general population. However, a Canadian study that extrapolated from the 2002 Canadian Community Health Survey and the 2006 Canadian census data (Bassani et al., 2009) found that approximately 12% of children under age 12 lived with a parent with a mental disorder (substance use disorder, 10.0%; mood disorder, 5.1%; and anxiety disorder, 4.6%). The National Survey on Drug Use and Health reported similar results for child exposure to parental alcohol-use disorder, finding that an average of approximately 7.5 million children each year in the United States (10.1% of all children) live with a parent with an alcohol-use disorder (Center for Behavioral Health Statistics and Quality, 2012).

### Parental Death

The death of a parent is a highly traumatic event for any child. Like military deaths, civilian deaths may be sudden, such as in the case of a suicide or a car accident, or may follow long drawn-out illness or be the eventual consequence of a serious injury. Again, like military children, civilian children lose more fathers than mothers.

Although precise figures cannot be found, about 3.5% of children experience the death of a parent by the time they are 18 years of age (Haine et al., 2008). In December 2011, more than 1.2 million children under age 18 (approximately 1.6% of all children) were receiving Old-Age, Survivors, and Disability Insurance (OASDI) benefits because of the death of a parent (US Social Security Administration, 2012), and 1.1% of children were living with an unmarried widowed parent (US Census Bureau, 2011a). According to the report of the Census Bureau's 2009 Survey of Income and Program Participation, 49,000 mothers and 36,000 fathers who were living with their children had been widowed in the previous year (Kreider and Ellis, 2011).

## The Impact of Deployment on Children of OIF or OEF Families

As of February 2007, an estimated 700,000 children had experienced a parental absence because of deployment in OEF or OIF, sometimes for multiple periods (Engel et al., 2010). Since then, the number of children affected by the deployment of a parent has increased. Many parents, service providers, and policy makers are concerned about the implications of parental deployment for children. However, research evidence remains sparse, and the use of more powerful longitudinal or quasi-experimental designs has been rare. In this section, we review the literature on children from military families, with special reference to children with one or both parents deployed in OEF or OIF. This review is limited to adequately powered studies that use sound research methods. Two main methods are used in the research to date: examination of military records and in-person studies of selected individuals.

### Deployment-Related Stressors and Children's Mental Health

Most studies of prior conflicts have suggested that deployment is associated with a variety of internalizing (such as sadness, depression, and anxiety) and externalizing (such as aggressiveness and irritability) symptoms in children that in most cases are not clinically significant (Cozza et al., 2005; Lincoln et al., 2008; Sheppard et al., 2010). Studies from the current wars have generally been consistent with that earlier research. Studies have also been consistent in finding that longer cumulative time spent deployed is associated with more problems.

Reviewing electronic medical records, Mansfield et al. (2011) compared rates of psychiatric diagnoses found in the records of over 300,000 children ages 5 to 17 of three groups of military personnel: those with up to 11 months of deployment in OIF or OEF; those with 12 or more months of deployment; and those with no deployment. Having a deployed parent was associated with an excess of all major diagnoses in comparison to being a child without a deployed parent. The excess was greater in older children and boys and those whose parent had been deployed for a year or more. As in most record-based analyses, it is not possible to conclude from this study whether children of deployed parents suffered more psychiatric disorders or whether (1) parents were more anxious or vigilant and more likely to bring their children to a medical provider and (2) medical care providers were more likely to diagnose disorders in children of deployed parents. However, the study does provide preliminary evidence that longer periods of deployment may put children at greater risk.

One of the largest studies of military parents and their children included interviews of over 1,500 caregiver-and-child pairs from military families in all branches of the military and reserve forces who were recruited from applicants for a military summer camp (Chandra et al., 2010a). Followup interviews were conducted at 6- and 12-month intervals. The study found that military children experienced significantly higher levels emotional and behavioral difficulties than those reported from the US Census Bureau's 2001 National Health Interview Survey, a large national sample. Chandra et al. (2010a) also found that more time deployed was associated with increased prevalence of adjustment difficulties (such as school problems and anxiety) in children during both deployment and reintegration. Spouses of reserve-component service members were especially likely to report that their children were experiencing difficulties. Although the study was limited by using participants from a service-seeking group, it provides valuable insight into the concerns of children of deployed service members over the course of deployment and reintegration.

A cross-sectional study of a convenience sample of 272 children ages 6 to 12 from families with a deployed or recently returned parent found that anxiety scores were higher than community norms for both deployment groups (Lester et al., 2010). No mean differences were found in depressed mood or behavioral symptoms for the children in the study compared with population norms. In multivariate analyses, mood and behavioral symptoms were higher in children whose military parent was deployed for longer periods and for whom either parent reported higher levels of psychologic symptoms; the effects of long parental deployment were seen even after the parent returned.

Using input from parents and child care providers, a study of 169 preschoolers in child development centers at a large Marine Corps installation compared children of parents deployed in OIF or OEF with other military children and with national norms and found that children of deployed parents had significantly higher scores on both internalizing (mood) and externalizing (behavior) measures (Chartrand et al., 2008). Among the small number of children who scored in the clinical range, the only significant differences were in the area of internalizing problems. Although this study was cross-sectional and did not measure change from predeployment to deployment or postdeployment, it provides some evidence for an effect of parental deployment on children's mood and behavior.

*Impact of Parental Stress on Children's Mental Health*

Another concern is the effect on children of a custodial parent's reaction to the other parent's death, injury, disability, absence, or psychopathology. Studies during the first Gulf War demonstrated that children's psychologic symptoms were more severe when their mothers' own well-being was seriously compromised (Cozza et al., 2005). Similarly, parents who reported high levels of stress were much more likely to report symptoms in their children (Flake et al., 2009).

In research focused on deployments during the current wars, Chartrand et al. (2008) found that spouses of deployed service members who had children age 3 or older had significantly higher depression scores than spouses of nondeployed personnel; their children exhibited increased behavioral symptoms compared with peers who did not have a deployed parent. Another analysis of the psychosocial effects of deployment on military children found that families experiencing deployment identified one-third of the children at "high risk" for psychosocial morbidity and that parental stress was the most significant predictor of children's psychosocial functioning (Flake et al., 2009). Lester et al. (2010) also found evidence that parental distress and length of parental deployment both increased anxiety levels in elementary-school-age children. However, the mean overall scores were not higher than those of the community samples on which the instruments were set at the norm. In another study of children of deployed parents (Chandra et al., 2011), 68% of youth reported that "helping the caregiver deal with life without deployed parent" was one of the most difficult aspects of the deployment. The study also found that youth whose nondeployed parent was doing worse emotionally reported having more difficulties during deployment; parents doing less well emotionally were likewise more likely to report that their children had greater emotional, social, and academic difficulties.

Parents who access military support services report less child psychologic morbidity. This finding suggests that use of services might ease parenting stress and underscores the necessity of providing military families with the support they need to cope with and adjust to deployment. Families considered more vulnerable to adjustment difficulties and in need of targeted outreach include families who are simultaneously undergoing other major transitions, such as relocation, pregnancy (Haas and Pazdernik, 2007), and bereavement, as well as families who have junior military personnel and families who have multiple needs and problems before deployment (Booth et al., 2007).

*Deployment and Risk for Child Maltreatment*

In FY 2011, there were 6,819 substantiated reports of child maltreatment among approximately 1,165,812 million children in military families. The number represents a rate of 5.8/1,000 children, a rate approximately half that in the US civilian population (DOD, 2012c). Still, the DOD rate is trending upward after having reached a nadir in FY 2009 (Figure 6.2).

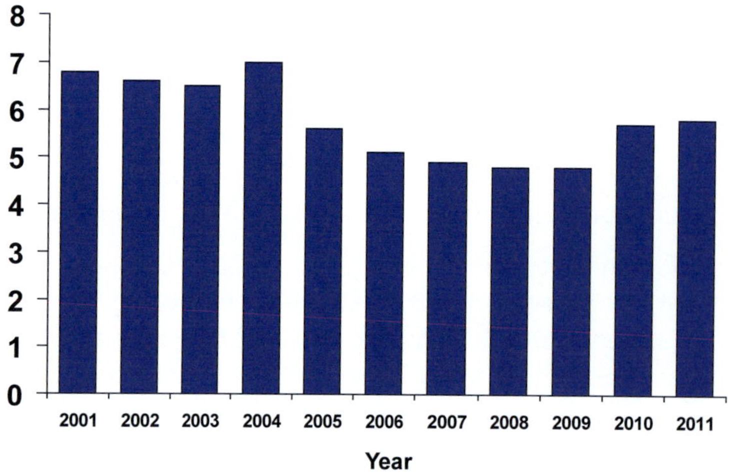


**FIGURE 6.2** Rate of substantiated child abuse and neglect reports per 1,000 children to the Family Advocacy Program, 2001–2011.
SOURCE: DOD, 2012c.

Emotional abuse and neglect account for 71% of child maltreatment cases; physical abuse for 23%; and sexual abuse for 6%. Just over half (54%) of abusers are male, 45% being female. In FY 2011, there were 33 fatalities tied to child maltreatment (DOD, 2012c).

*Risk Factors*: Parental deployment might increase children's risk for maltreatment. Although rates in general appear to be no higher than those in the civilian population, overall rates of child maltreatment (particularly neglect) by the nondeployed spouse appears to rise during deployment. A case series of substantiated child maltreatment by parents in 1,771 families of enlisted Army soldiers who were deployed at least once from September 2001 to December 2004 found that child maltreatment was more frequent during the times when the military parent was deployed than at other times, the most common perpetrators being civilian mothers (Gibbs et al., 2007). The incident records came from the Army Central Registry, which were merged with personnel records of the military parent, yielding information about entry to and exit from the Army as well as about deployment of the service member to OEF or OIF. The main type of maltreatment reported was neglect, which nearly quadrupled during deployment for civilian wives. Overall, the rate of child maltreatment was 42% higher during deployment than nondeployment; the rate of child neglect also rose during deployment, while the rate of physical abuse fell. Although information is missing in this study (for example, the psychologic status of the nondeployed parents before and during deployment), the large sample of substantiated abuse cases directs attention to the needs of the left-behind parents, especially those with preschool and grade-school-age children. This study is the only one of child maltreatment expressly in the OIF and OEF population.

Another study (Rentz et al., 2007) used time-series analysis to test the impact of operational deployments on maltreatment in military and nonmilitary families in Texas from 2000 to 2003, and the effect of deployment escalations after the September 2001 terrorist attacks in the United States. The study found that the rate of substantiated maltreatment reports for children of military families doubled, whereas the rate for civilian families was unchanged. About 90% of perpetrators were parents, with offenders being about equally divided between the military and the nonmilitary parent until October 2002, after which the nonmilitary parent was more often the offender, perhaps because more military parents were deployed. The study also found that reintegration can be a high-risk period, as the increases in rates of child maltreatment observed as service members left for deployment also occurred when they returned.

*Consequences and Treatment*: It is not surprising that child maltreatment has negative consequences. Although data from military populations are not available, child maltreatment is associated in civilian studies with the development of depression, anxiety, alcohol abuse, attempted suicide, as well as chronic health conditions, such as heart disease, cancer, and chronic lung disease (Felitti et al., 1998; McCauley et al., 1997). A longitudinal study also found that nearly half of childhood physical or sexual abuse victims developed at least two mental disorders by age 21 (Silverman et al., 1996).

The committee was unable to find any information about the treatments rendered for child maltreatment victims by DOD's Family Advocacy Program. The foremost evidence-based treatment for maltreated children is trauma-focused cognitive behavioral therapy (CBT) (Mannarino et al., 2012; Silverman et al., 2008). Trauma-focused CBT helps to alleviate posttraumatic stress, depressive symptoms, anxiety symptoms, and externalizing behavior problems.

*Impact of Parental Injury on Children's Mental Health*

There is considerable concern about the impact of parental injury on children of returning OIF and OEF military members. Injured parents might have reduced capacity to respond sensitively to their children, and noninjured parents might provide less attention to children because of the demands of caring for their injured spouses (Cozza et al., 2005; Perlesz et al., 1999).

In a study in which 41 spouses of recently injured service members were interviewed, Cozza et al. (2010) reported on the relationship of child postinjury distress to preinjury deployment-related family distress and the family postinjury disruption. The main predictor of children's distress was the emotional state of the family before deployment. As expected, children whose caregiver reported a high level of family distress before the injury were seen as having a high level of distress after the injury. This study is small and uses nonstandard measures, but it confirms a body of research showing that vulnerability to the impact of a major stressor is often influenced by the level of distress or family disruption before the stressor.

*Impact of Parental Death on Children's Mental Health*

As of March 2008, over 3,400 children had experienced the death of a parent during the OEF and OIF conflicts (US House of Representatives, 2008). Although sparse, available data indicate that bereaved children are at increased risk for psychiatric disorders or behavioral or emotional problems (Cozza et al., 2005). However, little guidance is available to help children understand and adapt to the death or life-altering injury of a parent (Cozza, 2007).

Children of service members may struggle to understand the signature rituals of a military death, including formal notification, return of remains, and military funerals (Cohen and Mannarino, 2011). Death during deployment, when there has already been a long separation, can trigger children to develop maladaptive cognitions or omens, regret, and self-blame (for example, "If daddy hadn't been so worried about me he would have been paying more attention and wouldn't have gotten shot."). Reactions to a military death can be magnified if the death is by suicide. Both children and adults can feel a mixture of guilt, confusion, rejection, anger, and shame (Cohen and Mannarino, 2011; Shear, 2012).

One of the first studies to examine childhood reactions to a combat-related death of a parent was performed by Israeli researchers examining the impact of the 1973 October War. The researchers found that 70% of the children ages 2 to 10 whose father had died in the war experienced significant emotional symptoms and behavior problems, such as fear, separation anxiety, discipline problems, learning disabilities, and social withdrawal that might today be labeled as a type of traumatic grief. In a 4-year followup of this longitudinal sample of 25 children, the likelihood of a child developing traumatic grief was enhanced by such pretraumatic risk factors as poor impulse control, emotional lability, and explosive rage. Marital discord in parents before the death also increased the likelihood of traumatic grief, as did the mother's mourning pattern. If the mother showed emotional restraint, it was difficult for children to express their feelings, and it heightened their sense of loneliness (Elizur and Kaffman, 1983). Children reacting to combat-related trauma also suffer from more conventional disorders, such as PTSD, depression, and anxiety (Smith et al., 2001), but the studies (for example, Mghir et al., 1995) focused on wartime stressors, not on the death of a parent who was a combatant.

## Use of Health Care Services for Children

Data from TRICARE, the health care program for uniformed service members, retirees, and their families, provide the primary information on the needs of children, as reflected in their use of TRICARE-related services. Researchers have merged this information with deployment data to estimate the extent to which parental deployment affects medical and mental health service use.

### *Use of Medical Services for Children*

Eide et al. (2010) used data on almost 170,000 children under the age of 2 enrolled in TRICARE and deployment data from the Defense Manpower Data Center to determine whether parental deployment influenced the rate at which parents used health care for their young children within the military health system. Overall, children made 7% more outpatient visits and 8% more well-child visits during periods of deployment. However, the increase was not consistent across marital status and age of the caregiving parent: children of younger single parents had fewer visits, and those of younger married parents had more visits. Both trends decreased as the parent's age increased. The researchers suggested that younger married parents were more able to use TRICARE as a resource for their children than were single parents of children who might have been living with other relatives or caretakers with limited knowledge of or access to the military health system while their parent was deployed (because this study only captured health care visits within the military health system, it missed visits made with caretakers of those children to civilian health care settings). Because single-parent children experienced less frequent health care visits, the authors suggested that military social services should target families with young single parents.

### *Use of Mental-Health Services for Children*

According to DOD records, military children's use of mental-health care services rose substantially from 2003 to 2008: inpatient days rose by 50% or more, and appointments for mental-health problems rose by more than 85% per capita (IOM, 2010).

In one study, researchers Gorman et al. (2010) used data on over 600,000 children ages 3 to 8 enrolled in TRICARE; these data were merged with deployment data from the Defense Manpower Data Center to determine whether parental deployment influenced the rate at which parents used either medical or mental-health care for their children within the military health system. They found that mental health was the only clinical category for which visits increased when a parent was deployed. However, this finding was true only for children whose father was deployed. When the mother was deployed, mental-health-related visits fell. The older the child, the more likely it was that mental-health care would be sought, whether the deployed parent was male or female, married or single. This study underscores how central parents are in gaining access to mental health care for children. When mothers are in charge of getting services for their children, they seem to respond to their spouse's absence with increased service-seeking. When fathers or other caregivers are in charge, help-seeking for mental and behavioral problems (but not for other areas of health care) drop.

Medicaid is an important supplement to TRICARE insurance for military children with special health care needs (CSHCN). Medicaid covers one in 9 military children with special health care needs. Among military CSHCN who are enrolled in Medicaid, 49% have low family incomes and 31% are nonwhite (Shin et al., 2005). Medicaid's capacity to mitigate the needs of military children may be reduced by state-to-state mobility of military families, variations in coverage and health care resources across states, and the location of military bases outside of metropolitan areas. In 2005, TRICARE initiated the "Extended Care Health Option" (ECHO) program, which supplements TRICARE basic benefits for qualifying disabled or special needs family members of active duty service members (Shin et al., 2005). The committee is not aware of any data about the extent to which ECHO may reduce reliance on Medicaid among lower income military CSHCN.

**Educational Achievement of Children**

There are numerous ways in which parental deployment can have negative impacts on children's school performance (Chandra et al., 2010b; Richardson et al., 2011). For example, children might have more difficulty completing homework assignments, particularly if the deployed parents were part of their children's homework routine or if their children are saddled with more household responsibilities while their parents are absent. Schooling may be disrupted if families move during deployment to be closer to supportive family members, and the children must adjust to being in a new school and having to develop new peer relationships. Sadness or distress about parents' deployment can also make it difficult for children to focus on school. Poor mental health of the nondeployed parents can likewise have a negative impact on school performance if, for example, the parents become disengaged from the school and from monitoring the children's academic performance.

Children's scores on academic achievement tests have been shown to drop slightly as a function of parental deployment. An examination of records from Texas that combined US Army personnel data with children's standardized test scores found that parental absences adversely affected children's test scores by a tenth of a standard deviation. Likewise, household relocations had modest negative effects on children's test scores (Lyle, 2006). Both parental absences and household relocations had the greatest detrimental effect on test scores of children with single parents, children with mothers in the Army, and younger children. The study highlights the finding that deployment can have many consequences, including relocations, which can mean a new school for children, the attendant risks being disrupted education and relationships. The impact on school achievement was modest overall, and no person-based analyses were carried out that could identify the children at greatest risk.

Another study, which looked at reading and math achievement for more than 44,000 students in North Carolina and Washington, found that elementary- and middle-school students with a parent who had been deployed for at least 19 months since 2001 had lower achievement scores than those of students with less or no parental deployment (Richardson et al., 2011). This association was not, however, present for high-school students. Although the total time deployed had a significant negative impact on achievement for younger students, the relationship between the number of deployments and performance was not significant.

### Summary

The findings summarized here must be taken as suggestive rather than conclusive. Military databases are not designed primarily to examine the effects of deployment on children, and most studies of families and children suffer from a range of methodologic limitations that limit their generalizability (for example, convenience samples and small sample sizes). Nonetheless, an important conclusion of the extant research is that, in normal circumstances, military children enjoy good mental health; their scores on nationally standardized scales are equal to or exceed those of the general population. Second, studies underscore the importance of parental distress as a predictor of childhood symptoms. However, the TRICARE databases, as currently analyzed, do not permit researchers to distinguish parental distress as a predictor of child problems from parental distress as a predictor of increased help-seeking behavior. Treating distressed parents might be as important to child mental health as treating the children themselves.

It is important to understand more about how parental characteristics that predict selection for deployment also predict children's response to parental deployment and parental reaction to returning home. From the viewpoint of the military-service system, it is critical to identify the small group of families at especially high risk of disruption during or after parental deployment. To answer these questions, researchers need a combination of integrated analyses of existing databases and larger, well-controlled studies of military personnel and their families, including studies that examine them over time.

## FAMILY CAREGIVERS

As Chapter 4 illustrates, physical injuries, serious mental-health diagnoses, such as PTSD, are being reported at high rates for the OEF and OIF population. Brain injuries, polytraumatic injuries, and psychologic wounds of war can have a profound impact on the injured survivors in that these injuries can often lead to long-term residual deficits and the need for ongoing care. (See Chapter 4 for more details about the incidence, prevalence, and long-term outcomes of the leading physical and psychologic injuries of the OEF and OIF conflicts.)

Family members frequently assume a significant role in caring for injured service members and veterans. In addition to providing emotional support, spouses, adult children, and parents often provide assistance with their loved ones' physical care. Family assistance, referred to as informal caregiving, is often unpaid and typically involves helping with basic self-care tasks, such as getting out of bed, dressing, and bathing—known as "activities of daily living" (ADLs)—and with "instrumental activities of daily living" (IADLs), which involve complex skills needed to live independently, such as managing finances, shopping, and housework. In addition, family members might also aid with therapies, coordinate formal health care services, and help navigate health insurance and legal systems. Given the scope of assistance, the presence of an informal caregiver is an important resource facilitating a care recipient's ability to stay at home (Griffin et al., 2012; Van Houtven et al., 2010).

This section examines research on the impact that caregiving of war-related injuries has on family caregivers. Although a significant body of research literature exists about civilian caregivers who support civilian patients with life-altering wounds and injuries, studies on caregivers of service members or veterans whose injury or illness is related to military service is sparse. Summarizing the civilian literature is beyond the scope of this report, but this section includes references to civilian literature where it is especially relevant and can possibly inform the understanding of the military population serving in OEF and OIF.

## Nature of Service Members' Injuries

In 2010, the National Alliance for Caregiving (NAC) reported findings from an online survey of 562 self-identified family caregivers, ages 19 or older, who provided care to a veteran whose injury, illness, or condition was related to military service. Of all respondents, 38% provided care to a veteran who served in the OEF or OIF conflicts. Although the report did not break out the findings separately for OEF and OIF veterans, it did show that conditions for which younger veterans (under the age of 45) needed care differed greatly from older veterans or typical civilian care recipients. Veterans under the age of 45 had mental illness, PTSD, or traumatic brain injury at rates much higher than those reported for veterans aged 65 or older (78% vs 56%, 79% vs 36%, and 61% vs 10%, respectively) or than those reported for national civilian populations, where 28% of caregivers reported that their care recipients had mental or emotional health problems. Older veterans, on the other hand, were more likely than younger veterans to have diabetes (36% vs 6%), cancer (27% vs 4%), or Parkinson's disease (13% vs 1%). One in five (20%) veterans being cared for had a spinal-cord injury (age breakdown not reported) (National Alliance for Caregiving, 2010).

Demographic data about veteran care recipients from the NAC survey revealed that veterans tend to be much younger than care recipients nationally—41% being between the ages of 18 and 54 (18% were between the ages of 18 and 34)—a reflection of the growing numbers of young veterans from the OEF and OIF conflicts.

## Nature of Care Provided by Family Caregivers

According to the 2010 NAC survey of caregivers providing assistance to veterans, the majority (64%) of caregivers reported helping the veteran with one or more ADLs, including help with getting dressed (48%), getting in and out of beds and chairs (45%), and bathing or showering (44%). Virtually all (98%) of the caregivers surveyed said they help with IADLs. Among these tasks were housework (88%), managing finances (87%), transportation (85%), grocery shopping (85%), and preparing meals (84%). Nearly three-quarters (73%) administer medications or injections, and 46% help to arrange or supervise paid services. The likelihood of helping with several IADLs increases as the veteran's age increases; those over age 65 not surprisingly need more assistance than those under age 45. Caregivers also reported that they assisted in coordinating medical care and rehabilitative services (85%) and administering physical therapy or medical or treatments (61%) (National Alliance for Caregiving, 2010).

Characterizing the level of burden experienced by caregivers on the basis of the number of ADLs and IADLs performed and the number of hours of care given, the NAC survey found that 65% of the veteran caregivers have a high burden of care, 15% have a medium burden, and 21% have a low burden (National Alliance for Caregiving, 2010). The survey also revealed that providing care for a veteran with a service-related health problem is a longer-term endeavor than family caregiving in the general population. As compared with caregivers in the general population, caregivers of veterans are twice as likely (30% vs15%) to have been in their role for 10 years or more (National Alliance for Caregiving, 2010).

Several studies involving veterans and their caregivers provided information about how much time caregivers spend supporting veterans in need of informal care. Generally, the nature and severity of the veterans' problems are factors that influence the amount of caregiving time provided. Van Houtven et al. (2010) surveyed veterans referred to home health care or home-based primary care in 2007 and their informal caregivers. Findings indicated that patients received substantially more informal than formal care from the health care system: on average, patients received 5.6 hours of VA care and 47 hours of informal care per week. The 89 veteran respondents were older and more frail, having an average age of 75 and having an average of 2.7 problems. Movement limitations and diabetes affected the largest share of respondents.

In 2009, Griffin et al. (2012) conducted a survey of 564 caregivers of service members with TBI (average age 30) who served in OEF or OIF and received care in a VA Polytrauma Rehabilitation Center from 2001 to 2009. After a median of 4 years since injury, about one in five (22%) patients still required help with ADLs and with IADLs, and nearly half (48%) required assistance with IADLs only. Nearly one-quarter (23%) of caregivers reported more than 40 hours per week of care. Among caregivers providing assistance with ADLs, half (49%) provided 80 hours or more of care per week. In addition to assisting with ADLs and IADLs, other types of tasks reported by caregivers included managing emotional issues (70%); navigating the health care (54%), benefits (53%), and legal (54%) systems; making medical appointments (44%); managing pain (36%); and aiding with therapies (37%) or assistive devices (33%) (Griffin et al., 2012).

The data provide estimates of the amount of time caregivers spend by the intensity of a care recipient's needs, as well as insight into caregiving patterns over time. Among recipients with high-intensity needs, 49% of caregivers provided 80 hours or more of help per week, and 60% of caregivers of recipients with moderate-intensity needs provided less than 20 hours of help per week. Among recipients with low-intensity needs, 73% of caregivers provided less than 5 hours. The amount of time since injury did not affect the intensity of care recipients' needs; even 7 or more years after the injuries, caregivers were still providing care (Griffin et al., 2012).

Robinson-Whelen and Rintala (2003) interviewed 348 veterans (average age 55) with a spinal-cord injury. Of the 130 participants who reported receiving informal unpaid care, 59% identified a spouse or partner as their primary caregiver; 17%, a parent; 9%, a sibling or spouse of a sibling; 8%, a child or spouse of a child; 2%, a friend; and 3%, some other person (for example, grandparent or niece). On average, informal caregivers provided all day care (11.6

hours per day)—the number of hours driven mostly by severity of injury (Robinson-Whelen and Rintala, 2003).

## Characteristics of Family Care Providers

Demographic information from the 2010 NAC survey of caregivers of veterans whose illness, injury, or condition was service-related showed that the typical caregiver is a woman (96%) who is taking care of her husband or partner (70%). The majority (61%) of the caregivers are 50 years of age or older. Of the OEF and OIF veterans in need of care, over one-quarter (26%) are being cared for by their parents. One implication of this information is that caregiving responsibilities may need to be transitioned to others as their parents grow older (National Alliance for Caregiving, 2010).

The survey of caregivers of OEF and OIF service members with TBI conducted by Griffin et al. (2012) showed that, for this type of injury, parents were more likely to be the primary caregiver (62%) than the spouses (32%). Nearly half (48%) of the caregivers were a sibling, grandparent, other relative, or friend. These caregivers tended to be women (79%) and younger than age 60 (84%). A majority of the caregivers were solely responsible for the caregiving (59%) and were balancing both work and caregiving (55%); 31% were also caring for children or other dependent adults (Griffin et al., 2012).

## Impact of Caregiving on Family Caregivers

Numerous studies of civilian populations have documented evidence that caregiving can have profound negative consequences for family caregivers in terms of burden, psychologic and physical health, emotional well-being, quality of life, employment, and financial status (for example, see Kreutzer et al., 2009; Pinquart and Sörensen, 2003; Schulz and Martire, 2004; Stenberg et al., 2010; van der Voort et al., 2007; Vitaliano et al., 2003; and Zarit, 2006). The focus of this section is on the few studies that assess caregiving effects specifically experienced by caregivers of veterans. Although there are common consequences of caregiving in the general population and those assisting veterans—for example, Griffin et al. (2009) cited evidence based on research on patients with TBI, stroke, dementia, and cancer that suggests that better functioning and supportive families are associated with improved patient outcomes—there are also differences. Even within the veteran-caregiver population, differences in caregiving are reported by type of war-related injury, for example, polytrauma versus TBI (Griffin et al., 2009).

Despite evidence for a preponderance of troublesome impacts, caregivers in the general population and caregivers of veterans also report positive aspects of caregiving. Research by Pinquart and Sörensen (2003) found that feeling useful or experiencing increases in closeness to the care recipient mitigated caregiver burden and depression. In the 2010 NAC survey of veteran caregivers, nearly all (94%) respondents reported feeling proud of the support they provide, and most felt a sense of reward from having gained new knowledge and skills from caregiving (78%) or feeling fulfilled by caregiving (67%).

The following discussion presents what is known about the impacts of caregiving, specifically experienced by caregivers of veterans.

**Psychologic and Emotional Health of Caregivers**

A study of caregivers of TBI patients who were 5 years or less postinjury found that, although about a third of the caregivers were experiencing increased levels of depression, anxiety, and somatic symptoms, most of the caregivers were coping adequately (Kreutzer et al., 2009). Higher caregiver distress was associated with caring for TBI patients who had worse functioning, who needed more supervision, who were less satisfied with life, and who abused alcohol. Respondents in the NAC survey of caregivers of veterans conveyed that providing care to their veteran took a toll on their psychologic and emotional health. Stress or anxiety was reported as the most prevalent health problem of caregivers (88%). When asked to indicate their level of emotional stress, two-thirds (68%) of caregivers reported that they were highly stressed. High emotional stress was most likely to be reported by caregivers for veterans with depression and anxiety, PTSD, or TBI. Depression was reported by 63% of the caregivers (National Alliance for Caregiving, 2010). However, caregivers also reported positive outcomes of caregiving. Nearly all (94%) agreed strongly or somewhat that they were proud of the support and assistance they provided, and 78% reported that gaining new knowledge and skills felt rewarding. Two-thirds agreed strongly or somewhat that caregiving had been fulfilling for them.

Caregiving puts strain on the caregivers' personal relationships and can contribute to social isolation. Of those who were married, separated, or divorced, three-quarters (74%) of the respondents in the NAC survey said that caregiving placed strain on their marriage. A substantial share of caregivers reported a decline in time spent with family and friends (87%). Most (76%) felt that others did not understand what they are going through; this response was especially the case for those caring for a veteran with PTSD or TBI and for those caring for a younger veteran. Among the caregivers with children in their household, over two-thirds (69%) sacrificed the amount of time they spend with their children. More than half said that their children had experienced emotional or school problems (57%) (National Alliance for Caregiving, 2010). In a review of the civilian-caregiving literature, Blais and Boisvert (2005) similarly found the effect of increased social isolation and diminished social relationships among caregivers of spouses with TBI.

In another survey of 70 caregivers, Phelan et al. (2011) found that, for caregivers of veterans with TBI who did not serve during OEF or OIF, perceived discrimination and stigma were stressors that could lead to poor caregiver mental health outcomes. Specifically, there was a relationship between caregiver strain, social isolation, depression, and anxiety and the caregivers' perceptions of being discriminated against and feelings of being stigmatized as a caregiver.

**Physical Health of Caregivers**

Caregivers are vulnerable to compromises in their physical health as a result of their caregiving responsibilities. Some of the physical effects reported by caregivers responding to the NAC survey of caregivers of veterans included sleep deprivation (77%), spending less time exercising (69%), delaying or skipping their own medical appointments (58%), poor eating habits (56%), and a high degree of physical strain (40%) (National Alliance for Caregiving, 2010). A meta-analysis of 23 studies comparing the physical health of 1,594 caregivers of family members with dementia and 1,478 demographically similar noncaregivers found that caregivers were at 9% greater risk of health problems, the size of the difference being moderated by the sex of the caregiver and the health category assessed (Vitaliano et al., 2003). This finding is especially important in light of findings that a substantial proportion of providers of informal care face important health limitations themselves. In one study, one in four veteran patients reported that they expected their care providers to no longer be able to provide "the same level of care within 5 years" (Robinson-Whelen and Rintala, 2003). In the same study, almost one-third of the caregivers reported being in only fair or poor health themselves.

**Employment and Financial Status of Caregivers**

Caregivers often must make major life decisions related to their location of residence, employment, and education as a result of their caregiving role. In a random sample of 1,730 OEF or OIF active-duty component members, reserve component members, and retired veterans in 2007, 15% to 37% reported having a family member or friend who had relocated or left a job to provide care for a veteran, either temporarily or permanently (President's Commission on Care for America's Returning Wounded Warriors, 2007).

Among the respondents to the 2010 NAC survey of veteran caregivers, 59% of the caregivers were unemployed, 27% worked full time, and 14% worked part time. Of those who worked at some point since becoming a caregiver, 69% reported taking unpaid time off from work or stopping work temporarily, 62% reported cutting back the number of hours worked per week, and 47% stopped working entirely or took early retirement. Those more likely to stop working included caregivers of a veteran with depression and anxiety, diabetes, and paralysis or a spinal-cord injury. Other caregivers were compelled to continue working because of veteran's condition and care needs. Of the caregivers aged 40 or older currently working, two-thirds (67%) said their own retirement plans were in question (National Alliance for Caregiving, 2010).

Studies examining the relationship between employment and caregiving in the general population found that caregiving affects labor-force participation and has both short-term and long-term economic consequences, particularly among women caregivers and those who are heavily involved in providing care (Lilly et al., 2007; Schulz and Martire, 2004). Other caregivers who are more likely to be out of the labor force, to work fewer hours, or to adjust their work hours to accommodate caregiving responsibilities include those in poor health, older caregivers, those with young children at home, those heavily involved in caregiving, those with less education or income, and those caring for persons with greater health limitations (Lilly et al., 2007).

The employment consequences reported by caregivers of veterans are also likely to be a major contributing factor to the serious financial strain experienced by families caring for veterans. Half (50%) of all caregivers responding to the 2010 NAC survey reported that caring for their veteran caused them a high degree of financial hardship. This percentage is a much higher proportion than the 13% of family caregivers nationwide reporting the same level of financial hardship (National Alliance for Caregiving, 2010). A survey of seriously wounded, ill, and injured service members about the economic impact of caregiving on their caregivers revealed that 37% of caregivers had unmet financial obligations, and 41% had new financial obligations. Those who provided more hours of assistance were more likely to have higher financial burdens (Christensen et al., 2009). The researchers estimated that the average loss in income and benefits for caregivers of seriously wounded, ill, and injured service members (assuming that care is needed for 19 months) is $60,300.

## Factors Influencing Caregiver Experiences

Caregivers' experiences vary considerably, and several variables, such as characteristics of the caregiver and the care recipient, are associated with the burden that caregivers experience. The following discussion largely reflects findings from the civilian literature but is not an exhaustive review.

Time since injury is not necessarily predictive of the need for care (Griffin et al., 2012; National Alliance for Caregiving, 2010; Vitaliano et al., 2003). In other words, care needs appear not to decline over time for some kinds of injuries. For example, Griffin et al. (2012) found that nearly a quarter (22%) of service members with TBI who had previously received inpatient rehabilitation care still required help with activities of daily living and instrumental activities of daily living about 4 years after injury; nearly half (48%) needed help only with instrumental ADLs. In addition, over half (56%) of caregivers in the 2010 National Alliance for Caregiving (2010) survey reported that they had been providing care to their veteran for 5 or more years; nearly a third (30%) had been providing care for a decade or longer.

Several characteristics of the care recipient were found to have an impact on caregiver burden. These included the presence of behavior problems (for example, aggression, agitation, and nighttime wandering) or dementia (Etters et al., 2008; Pinquart and Sörensen, 2003), as well as the severity of the care recipient's symptoms, frequency of relapse, and hospitalization (van der Voort et al., 2007).

Characteristics of caregivers also were found to have an effect on caregiver burden. As reported in research with civilians, burden was positively related to living with the patient, difficulties in the relationship with the patient, an inability to cope with difficult behavior, stigma, and the caregiver's belief that the patient was not making an effort to influence his or her symptoms (van der Voort et al., 2007). Caregivers who reported more self-efficacy, took time for themselves, and those who used more effective coping strategies had less burden (Etters et al., 2008). Ethnicity also plays a role; minority caregivers reported worse physical health than white caregivers, but findings were mixed for psychologic health (Pinquart and Sörensen, 2005).

The nature of the caregiver–recipient relationship was also associated with caregiver burden. Partners experienced more stress than parents, and young families with little social, financial, and psychiatric support or with medical problems were found to be the most vulnerable (Verhaeghe et al., 2005). Burden was higher for spouses who became caregivers than it was for adult children (Pinquart and Sörensen, 2011). There is also some research with the veteran population that informs understanding of caregiver burden. As discussed in the previous section, Psychologic Health of Family Members, research with spouses of combat veterans of OEF and OIF suggested that, in addition to the service members' symptoms, spouses' individual characteristics and perceptions of their partners' symptoms might influence their levels of personal distress (Goff et al., 2007; Renshaw and Campbell, 2011; Renshaw and Caska, 2012; Renshaw et al., 2008). In particular, spouses might respond with less support and experience more distress when they cannot identify an obvious cause for their partners' symptoms (for example, such as attributing their spouses' emotional withdrawal to traumatic experiences during deployment) or when they perceive their partners as choosing not to exert control over symptoms.

### Department of Veterans Affairs Caregiver Support Program

In recognition of the significant burden caregiving places on families, Congress passed and President Obama signed into law the Caregivers and Veterans Omnibus Health Services Act of 2010 (PL 111-163; 124 Stat. 1130), which authorizes the VA to provide new support services and benefits to caregivers of eligible veterans and service members seriously injured in the line of duty on or after September 11, 2001. Caregivers who qualify for the program are eligible to receive a monthly financial stipend, averaging about $1,600 a month, after completing a comprehensive caregiver training program. Other benefits available to caregivers include travel expenses associated with caregiving, access to health insurance (for caregivers not already entitled to health-plan coverage), mental-health services and counseling, and respite care that can help care for the veteran for a short time when the caregiver needs relief. As of August 30, 2012, nearly 6,000 primary family caregivers are receiving the monthly caregiver stipend (Gould, 2012).

### Summary

In summary, although studies with civilian populations are helping to inform the understanding of the experiences of family caregivers, there is a paucity of evidence on the challenges and needs faced by families caring for patients with serious war-related injuries. The war-related care experience is complex, in part because of the severity of the injuries, the changing role from military to civilian family, and the stigma attached to disability and injuries (Griffin et al., 2009). Griffin et al. (2009) discussed the existence of "huge gaps in our understanding of the information, resources, and services families need to cope and function as their injured loved one recovers, rehabilitates, and reintegrates into the community." Evidence suggested that providing caregivers with information they seek is an effective coping mechanism that can help reduce stress, anxiety, and uncertainty (Griffin et al., 2009).

## PROGRAMS AND SERVICES FOR MILITARY FAMILIES

On the basis of the rationale that a well-served family is essential for retaining service members and force readiness, the DOD increased its support for military families with an ever-evolving catalog of programs aimed at meeting the needs of service members and their families. The wide-ranging programs cover such areas as psychologic health, child care, education, and personal finance. In this section, the discussion centers on programs and services for which there are data on implementation, utilization, or outcome research with military populations.

### Programs and Services

#### Child Care

DOD has provided child care services to more than 200,000 military children from birth to age 12 at more than 900 child-development centers in over 300 locations worldwide and at 5,000 Family Child Care homes (DOD, 2012b). On the basis of demographic data, DOD estimated that an additional 37,000 military children still need child care but are not receiving it (DOD, 2010b). DOD (2012a) reported that it is continuing to build new child care facilities, both on and off base, to accommodate child care needs, concentrating on 13 states to expand availability and the quality of child care services (DOD, 2012b). DOD also reported that 97% of its child care services are accredited by national accreditation agencies, thereby meeting standards for quality, and 100% are certified internally by DOD (2012b). All programs are inspected, unannounced, four times annually.

Regarding deployment-specific problems, in a 2009 survey of 802 spouses of active-duty Air Force airmen, the majority of respondents reported that their child care problems worsened following their spouses' deployment. Parents who lived within 30 minutes of the base reported more problems finding child care than those who lived more than 30 minutes away, as did parents who were part of a dual-military family as compared with parents who were civilians. Spouses of enlisted airmen also reported more problems finding child care than did spouses of officers (Miller et al., 2011a).

## Education

### *DOD Schools*

Approximately 86,000 children of service members or DOD civilians attend 194 Department of Defense Education Activity (DODEA) schools in 14 school districts, 12 countries, 7 states, plus Guam and Puerto Rico. DODEA employs approximately 8,700 educators (DOD, 2012b). All DODEA schools are accredited by AdvancED (DOD, 2011a), an accreditation organization responsible for accrediting more than 30,000 public and private schools and districts in the United States (AdvancED, 2012).

DODEA tracks school performance with two standardized tests, the TerraNova and the Scholastic Aptitude Test (SAT). Both tests allow the DODEA to compare their students' performance with national samples. For 2011, the DODEA's goal was to have 75% of social-studies students, 73% of students in reading and science, 72% of language arts students, and 70% of math students score at or above the 51st percentile on the TerraNova. The DODEA nearly met this goal; however, targets were missed by 1 percentage point in reading, science, and social studies, 2 percentage points in language arts, and 5 percentage points in math. In all subjects, DODEA schools failed to meet the goal of having no more than 7% of all students score below the 25th percentile (DOD, 2012b), rates for most subjects being 1 to 4 percentage points above the 7% benchmark (the highest rates were for math—11% of students scoring in the bottom 25%). For 2012, the DODEA goal is for 75% of students to score above the 51st percentile in all subjects, having no more than 7% fall into the bottom 25%.

On the SAT, the 2011 average critical reading score was 503, six points above the national average. In writing, the average was 489, the same as the national average. In math, the DODEA average was 495, which is 19 points below the national average (DOD, 2012b). When ethnicity was stratified, African American and Hispanic students scored significantly higher on the SAT in all three subjects in 2010 than was scored by African American and Hispanic students nationwide (DOD, 2011a).

To help improve student performance, DODEA has begun reducing class size in kindergarten to achieve a student-to-teacher ratio of 18:1 or better (DOD, 2011a). The DODEA has also launched an initiative to improve SAT math scores, which are lower than the national average. Program leaders reviewed and revised mathematics standards at all levels throughout the DODEA school system; the initiative also includes an extensive math program evaluation. In the 2010–2011 school year, the DODEA began implementation of the new standards, which received top ratings from the Mid-continent Regional Educational Laboratory (DOD, 2011a).

In 2011, the DODEA announced plans to adopt the Common Core State Standards (CCSS), a research and evidence-based curriculum to replace its own curriculum standards in math and language arts. The new curriculum includes more progress assessments designed to help schools identify student achievement gaps. The CCSS is currently used in 46 states, so its use by the DODEA school system is expected not only to improve student performance but also to relieve problems arising from out-of-state school transfers (DOD, 2012b).

*Disruptions in Children's Education*

Children from military families must relocate and change schools when a parent receives an order for what is called a "Permanent Change of Station" (PCS). A military child will attend, on average, six to nine schools from kindergarten to 12th grade (DOD, 2010b). Aside from the social disruptions associated with frequently switching schools, educational standards and requirements vary from state to state, creating administrative problems and delaying graduation and advancement. In response to problems with interstate school transfers, DOD developed the "Interstate Compact on Educational Opportunity for Military Children." States that adopt the compact agree to provide uniform eligibility, enrollment, placement, and graduation policies with regard to military children. As of 2012, 40 states have adopted the compact, eliminating many of the problems associated with transferring from one state to another for 93% of all military children (DOD Education Activity, 2012). The DOD's goal is for the compact to cover 100% of military school children by FY 2013 (DOD, 2012b).

**Exceptional Family Member Program**

Each military department has an "Exceptional Family Member Program" to work with the 120,000 enrolled military families with special-needs members (DOD, 2011a). DOD estimated that there are many more families with exceptional family members who have not enrolled, but it offered no estimate of how many (DOD, 2012b). The DOD provides, through TRICARE, basic medical services to exceptional family members at military installations within the United States. DOD will also provide in-home care and respite care when needed. However, the Government Accountability Office (GAO) found that DOD is not always equipped with the needed specialists, forcing some families to seek specialist services from neighboring installations or civilian providers (GAO, 2007). The GAO could not determine the scope and extent of the problem.

The National Defense Authorization Act FY 2010 established the Office of Community Support for Military Families with Special Needs (OSN) and requires military branches to expand community support for families with special-needs members to include referral assistance, assistance in obtaining services, and providing oversight (DOD, 2011a). The Act also requires DOD to report annually on gaps in service and to recommend ways to help fill those gaps (DOD, 2012b).

The OSN is currently collaborating with land-grant university faculty to complete several studies related to improving support for exceptional family members. A benchmark study will establish a uniform family support policy across the four services. The autism review study, conducted in two phases, is examining access in 15 states to evidence-based educational services for military children with autism. A Medicaid study—a collaboration with West Virginia

University—will assess the accessibility of Medicaid to military families with exceptional family members and assess how interstate relocation may be a barrier to receipt of Medicaid benefits. Finally, a functional analysis study will look at the support and services that each military service provides to families with exceptional family members. The findings are expected to help inform recommendations for a DOD-wide policy (DOD, 2012b).

**Financial Readiness**

DOD offers an array of financial management education programs, available both online and in person, aimed at all military personnel. The "Financial Readiness Campaign," launched in 2003, is a DOD-wide program designed to provide additional financial readiness education and resources to complement existing efforts by individual services (DOD, 2010b).

The Status of Forces Survey, conducted by the Defense Manpower Data Center, provided a portrait of financial issues from junior enlisted soldiers in pay grades E1–E4. In general, respondents indicated fewer problems today than in 2002. About 15% of respondents in 2011, compared with about 26% in 2002, reported that it was "tough to make ends meet, but keeping your head above water" or "in over your head" (DOD, 2012b). Likewise, about 25% of respondents in 2010, compared with 47% in 2002, reported "one or more bill paying problems in the previous 12 months" (DOD, 2011a). In a separate 2010 survey of military spouses, however, 41% reported concerns about their personal finances (Defense Manpower Data Center, 2011). DOD did not undertake an assessment of its own financial readiness programs, so the disparity across surveys cannot be reconciled. Regarding deployment and its effect on finances, 29% of Air Force spouses surveyed reported that their financial problems worsened during the last deployment (Miller et al., 2011a). The committee was unable to find examples of DOD targeting financial problems specifically associated with deployment. Metrics to assess financial readiness programs are "currently being considered," but no other information was provided over 3 consecutive years (DOD, 2010b).

**Nonmedical Counseling**

Nonmedical counseling refers to short-term, problem-focused counseling designed to address general conditions of living; it addresses such issues as stress management, marital problems, parenting issues, grief, and crisis intervention. (Medical counseling, on the other hand, is designed to address long-term, medically diagnosable issues, such as substance abuse, mental illness, or PTSD.) DOD offers confidential, free nonmedical counseling sessions to all active-duty, National Guard, and reserve members and their families. Services are available through Military OneSource and the Military and Family Life Counselor (MFLC) program. In FY 2009, Military OneSource provided over 133,000 in-person counseling sessions (DOD, 2010b). In FY 2010, it provided nearly 270,000 in-person counseling sessions (DOD, 2011a) and nearly 313,000 in 2011 (DOD, 2012b). Data regarding the number of telephone or online counseling sessions completed by Military OneSource were not reported. The MFLC program provides services to active-duty service members and families on or off military installations. Support is provided to the reserve components for mobilization, deployment, and reunion activities as requested by reserve unit commands. In FY 2009, the MFLC program completed almost 470,000 face-to-face contacts with military children and adults (DOD, 2010b). The number rose dramatically in FY 2010 to 5.5 million face-to-face contacts (DOD, 2011a) and 6.9 million face-to-face contacts in FY 2011 (DOD, 2012b). DOD sources did not give an explanation for the striking rise in contacts from FY 2009 to FY 2010 and FY 2011, although it might be explained in part by some base commanders requiring returning troops to complete counseling with a Military and Family Life Counselor, additional staffing to increase capacity, expanded services for units returning from combat ("surge support"), and enhanced outreach capabilities (DOD, 2010b, 2012b).

DOD sponsored two evaluation and assessment studies to improve effectiveness measures of the counseling (DOD, 2012b). In one study, conducted in collaboration with Virginia Polytechnic University in 2010, researchers collected data from an assessment tool completed by counseling participants to measure the impact of counseling through the MFLC program. The study found that 98% of respondents reported the counseling sessions helped them deal more effectively with their problems and that they would use the service again. Virtually all (99%) reported that they received the kind of counseling service they wanted and that they would recommend MFLC services to a friend (DOD, 2012b). In the second study, DOD included questions on the use of nonmedical counseling in the May 2010 "Military Family Life Survey" for military spouses and a paired subset of active-duty personnel. Spouses reported that MilitaryOne Source counseling is the second most utilized source of counseling. Over half found it to be "very useful" (Defense Manpower Data Center, 2011). (The most utilized source is medical counseling sponsored under TRICARE.)

Despite the positive reviews from individuals using available counseling, the 2010 Military Family Life Survey found that many military spouses had concerns that deterred them from seeking counseling. Concerns included the following: "it would be difficult to get time off work or child care for counseling" (47%), "it would harm my spouse's career" (45%), "don't know where to get help" (40%), and "it is difficult to get help" (43%). In all, 78% of spouses surveyed reported that they had at least some concern discouraging them from seeking counseling. More than half of spouses reported they were more stressed than usual at the time of the survey, and 17% reported that they had talked to a counselor in the previous 6 months (Defense Manpower Data Center, 2011).

**Couples Education**

The "Prevention and Relationship Enhancement Program (PREP) for Strong Bonds" is a scientifically based education-program manual for couples designed to address the stress on military couples posed by long separations, frequent relocations, and deployment. Its goal is to strengthen the family and prevent divorce by teaching couples skills, principles, and strategies associated with healthy relationships. The program, which is led by trained Army chaplains, includes a 1-day weekday training on post, followed by a weekend retreat at a hotel off post. Program modules address such topics as communication and effective management skills, deployment and reintegration issues, fun and friendship, and relationship dynamics. A randomized controlled trial found that the divorce rate for Army couples assigned to participate in PREP for Strong Bonds was one-third of that for control couples (2.03% for Army couples vs 6.2% for the control group) when assessed 1 year after the intervention. The study authors concluded that couples education—at least in the short run—can reduce the risk of divorce (Stanley et al., 2010).

**Health Care**

TRICARE is the health care plan that serves approximately 9.7 million beneficiaries, including active-duty personnel, their families, eligible reserve-component populations, and retirees (DOD, 2012b). User satisfaction is captured through two questions on the Health Care Survey of Department of Defense Beneficiaries (HCSDB). The questions are based on the Consumer Assessment of Healthcare Providers and Systems (CAHPS), a widely used tool to measure client satisfaction with health care. In 2011, 62% of eligible beneficiaries (active-duty, families, and retirees) rated their care an 8, 9, or 10 of 10 (10 being the best). When stratified by group, retirees and their families were most satisfied (72%), followed by active-duty families (62%), and then active-duty personnel (50%) (DOD, 2012b). Respondents reported similar levels of satisfaction for their military health care plan (as opposed to actual care). Overall, 65% of eligible beneficiaries were satisfied with their plan. Retirees and their families were most satisfied (72%); 69% of active-duty families were satisfied, and 56% of active-duty personnel were satisfied. However, no information was provided about HCSDB's response rates or the survey population (DOD, 2012b).

In September 2009, DOD adopted the Patient-Centered Medical Home (PCMH) model for implementation throughout its health care system. The model is designed to lower hospital visits and admissions and lower the cost of care by fostering a stronger relationship between a patient and primary care provider. Early data from the PCMH within the military health system indicated improved access to care, higher-quality health outcomes, better patient satisfaction, and reduced health costs per patient (DOD, 2011a).

DOD recognizes the shortage of mental-health providers that accept TRICARE and that the shortfall must be addressed in the next 5 years to meet the demand (DOD, 2010b). DOD is working through TRICARE but also with the US Department of Health and Human Services to help increase community capacity for mental-health care for military families. DOD does not offer specifics regarding these activities in the "family readiness" reports to Congress.

DOD also established the Office of Wounded Warrior Care and Transition Policy to help streamline care coordination for wounded service members and their families as they receive care (DOD, 2010b).

**Family Advocacy**

Every military installation has a Family Advocacy Program (FAP) in place to provide an array of services dealing with sexual, physical, or emotional abuse of a family member (DOD, 2010b). One prominent service, the New Parent Support Program (NPSP), is a voluntary home visitation program targeting active-duty parents with children under age 3 identified as being at risk for family violence. Families can self-refer or be referred by a health provider. From 2005, when the program assessment began, to 2011, at least 85% of families who received intensive NPSP services for at least 6 months were not reported for child abuse or neglect within 1 year of completing the program (DOD, 2011a, 2012b). No control group data were presented.

In regard to spousal abuse in FY 2009, 90% of service members who completed FAP treatment were not reported for spousal abuse (physical, sexual, or emotional) within 1 year of program completion (DOD, 2010b). In FY 2010, the figure rose to 96% of service members who completed a FAP treatment program and were not reported for spousal abuse within 1 year (DOD, 2011a). In FY 2011, the figure rose to 97% of participating service members (DOD,

2012b). Again, no control group data were presented, but DOD cited evidence indicating that abusers who complete a treatment program are less likely to repeat abuse compared with those who drop out of the program (DOD, 2012b). DOD noted, however, that spousal abusers are a heterogeneous group (for example, men or women who are emotional or physical abusers) and that treatment for each type of abuser differs greatly. The outcome data do not stratify by treatment type, so some treatments may be more effective than others (DOD, 2010b). The FAP is working toward capturing treatment-specific outcome data, but DOD did not report on the specifics of those efforts (DOD, 2010b).

### Family Caregivers

As described above in the section about family caregivers, the Comprehensive Assistance for Family Caregivers program provides support for severely injured post-9/11 veterans and their family caregivers (VA, 2011). Although the program is designed to provide some economic relief to family caregivers of injured veterans, the committee is unaware of any plans to evaluate program outcomes or participant satisfaction.

### Bereavement

There are a variety of interventions to help families cope with their grief, ranging from counseling by military chaplains to trauma-focused CBT. Trauma-focused CBT is an evidence-based treatment for children and parents that often includes a mixture of psychoeducation to help patients understand and cope with their loss, relaxation skills, cognitive coping, trauma narration, and emotional processing (Cohen and Mannarino, 2011). Despite many DOD-sponsored programs serving bereaved military families, such as the Army's Survivors Outreach Services, a DOD (2010a) Task Force on the Prevention of Suicide by Members of the Armed Forces found that no programs expressly meet the needs of family members whose loved one died by suicide.

## Program Evaluation

The committee was unable to find evidence of evaluation efforts of DOD programs beyond what is presented above. The evidence base for understanding the needs of military families is thus lacking, as is the evidence base for measuring the performance of military family readiness programs (Miller et al., 2011b). The committee is aware of an evaluation tool developed by Miller and her colleagues at the RAND Corporation and sponsored by the Under Secretary of Defense for Personnel and Readiness (Miller et al., 2011b). Rather than develop program-specific evaluation instruments, they developed an adaptable survey instrument to measure (1) the problems and needs of service members and their families; (2) the actions families take to address their needs; (3) their satisfaction with the resources they use to meet their needs; (4) why certain resources were used and others were not (either military, civilian, formal, or informal resources); and (5) the effectiveness of the resources on retention and readiness. The authors noted that, by measuring these issues rather than focusing on the individual programs, service providers and military leadership at all levels can better understand the needs of their service members, identify unmet needs among specific demographic groups and locations, and adjust service provision as needed to more effectively meet their needs (Miller et al., 2011b). The committee is unaware if the DOD has used or plans to use the survey instrument in any capacity.

The RAND Corporation compiled a list of about 200 DOD programs that address psychologic health and traumatic brain injury, of which 120 serve families. RAND likewise concluded that there is no centralized mechanism to catalog these programs and track which are effective, whether they meet the needs of families, whether there are any gaps, and whether programs need more resources (Weinick et al., 2011). It is possible that greater attention will be paid to evaluate family needs and program effectiveness in response to an initiative by President Obama on "Strengthening Our Military Families: Meeting America's Commitment," which strives to improve the quality of life among service members and their families. Although the initiative seeks to have a monitoring and evaluation component (Interagency Policy Committee et al., 2011), the committee could not find any descriptions of performance measures or any information regarding evaluation schedules for the initiative's outlined activities.

What little program information is available is largely contained in DOD's annual reports to Congress on "Plans for the Department of Defense for Support of Military Family Readiness" (DOD, 2011a, 2012b). However, what is reported there focuses primarily on program capacity, frequency of delivery, and utilization rather than on program performance and effectiveness in meeting the needs of families. It is important to emphasize, however, that the majority of programs compiled by RAND are not mentioned in the reports to Congress.

### Summary

Assuring the health and welfare of military families is both an obligation for DOD and a necessity for retaining and supporting service members. DOD thus has in place hundreds of programs to support military families that address a wide range of needs—from child care and financial readiness to counseling and health care services. Despite the growth in programs that serve families, the committee found that DOD does not maintain a complete list of programs, describe their scope, or assess whether they have been evaluated, and if evaluated, by what metrics. As a consequence, a comprehensive catalog of programs for which there is empirical evidence of effectiveness cannot be compiled.

## TREATMENT AND MEDICAL COUNSELING FOR FAMILIES

In 2006, family participation in treatment and other mental-health services was declared to be a national priority for veterans (VA, 2006) and active-duty military members (Interagency Policy Committee et al., 2011). Their mental-health problems not only deserve treatment in their own right, but family-based care also carries the advantage of ameliorating psychiatric illness in the service member (Makin-Byrd et al., 2011). Further, service members wisely prefer and express the desire for family participation in treatment (Batten et al., 2009; Khaylis et al., 2011). This preference is no surprise for personal reasons, but for complex mental-health problems, family participation leads to better outcomes. Mental-health-service needs for military family members span a broad continuum—from education about mental illness to inpatient and resident treatment services. There is also a need for a range of additional services, including behavioral management services, psychopharmacologic management, and family and individual psychotherapy. Many evidence-based treatments for individuals and families have been developed in civilian communities, and mental-health providers often adapt these services to the special needs of a military or veteran population, whether informally or formally. These treatments often take the form of "new programs" that might or might not be as effective for military families as they are for civilians.

Many of the family programs are psychoeducational, a generic term for evidence-based interventions aimed at teaching problem solving and other crucial skills families need to deal with serious mental illness. More than 30 randomized trials in the civilian literature attest to its capacity to enhance psychosocial and family outcomes, in addition to reducing relapse and improving symptoms in the ill family member (Murray-Swank and Dixon, 2004).

## Family Education

Understanding the symptoms, diagnosis, causes, and treatments for a particular condition can help to improve family selection of and adherence to treatment programs. There are a number of models of family educational programs, most of which are intended to assist families of individuals who have a serious psychiatric illness, such as severe depression, schizophrenia, or PTSD.

The Support and Family Education (SAFE) program was developed at the Oklahoma City Veterans Affairs Medical Center (Sherman, 2006). It works with groups of families to provide them with information about the symptoms, causes, and treatment of mental illness, and about various resources available to them. They also receive information to help them better understand what their family member with mental illness is experiencing, and skills that they can use to work more effectively with their family member, such as how to set boundaries or manage violent behavior. The SAFE program also helps families to cope with their own stresses related to the illness, while teaching them how to relate more effectively to other family members, friends, community resources, and professionals. SAFE consists of a series of 18 90-minute confidential workshops that include didactic presentations and group discussions. Workshops are scheduled to take place once or twice a month and are facilitated by two mental-health professionals, such as a psychologist and a social worker or psychiatric nurse; a psychiatrist also attends at the end of the workshop to address questions about medications. A 5-year evaluation that gathered information from participants in the SAFE program found that attending more sessions was associated with lower levels of caregiver distress, having a better understanding of mental illness, being more aware of VA resources, and being better able to engage in self-care activities. The evaluation also reported high levels of participant satisfaction and retention (Sherman, 2006).

The Family-to-Family Education Program (FFEP) is similar to SAFE but uses trained family members rather than mental-health professionals as group leaders. FFEP, which was developed by the National Alliance on Mental Illness (NAMI), consists of 12 weekly group sessions designed to help families address the challenges they face in dealing with an ill family member. Sessions teach problem solving, listening, and communication skills to enhance relationships with the family member as well as service providers. FFEP also focuses on addressing issues related to the mental-health service systems and on dealing with problems related to social or financial support. The goal of FFEP is to teach family members to become better advocates for the care of their ill family member. The VA offers FFEP in at least one Veterans Health Administration (VHA) facility in each state; the program is also provided by NAMI chapters around the country (Makin-Byrd et al., 2011).

The VA has trained a number of VHA clinicians in both behavioral family therapy (BFT) and multifamily group therapy (Makin-Byrd et al., 2011). BFT is a form of behavior therapy in which a clinician meets with one patient and his or her family members to change specific maladaptive behavior patterns. This process is done by enhancing awareness and then teaching specific skills to enhance communication and problem solving. In the VHA, BFT is tailored to veterans with PTSD and their families. After initial orientation and assessment sessions, the program offers two sessions on education, three on communication training, two on anger management, and the remaining six to eight sessions on problem solving that is specific to the veteran and his or her family (Glynn et al., 1995).

In contrast to BFT, multifamily group therapy (MFGT) operates in a large group setting with several families who typically meet biweekly in 90-minute sessions that can continue for 12 months or longer. A therapist uses a structured problem-solving format to discuss relapse prevention, provide support for social and vocational rehabilitation, build relationship skills, and foster interdependence among the families. Targeted areas for intervention include increasing family coping skills and providing education about the course of illness and its treatment. The sessions also provide an opportunity to meet other families with similar struggles, thus helping families to feel less isolated (Sherman et al., 2012). Families are typically invited to participate in the MFGT sessions after participating in two to three individual family sessions and an educational session about the family member's illness. In the civilian literature, MFGT has been demonstrated to increase family-member quality of life and lessen family-member burden (McFarlane et al., 1995).

A version of MFGT adapted for veterans with PTSD includes additional education in an extended family workshop and more attention to relationship building, which focuses on the common problems that veterans with PTSD have with trust, intimacy, and communication. The problem-solving component of this form of MFGT also focuses on the specific PTSD symptoms of avoidance and emotional numbing (Sherman et al., 2012). MFGT has been adapted for veterans with TBI (Perlick et al., 2011) by adding information about the military experience and the pathophysiology and treatment of TBI and comorbid conditions, such as depression and PTSD. The workshop is divided over 2 days to minimize overload for veterans with TBI who have memory impairment. The group therapy phase is modified in three ways: (1) it addresses reduced or impaired communication, parenting conflicts, and partner frustration associated with cognitive deficits of TBI; (2) it includes problem solving related to forgetfulness; and (3) it focuses on loss of identity and difficulty accepting cognitive limitations. No information is available regarding efficacy for OIF and OEF veterans, but a pilot study has shown that TBI-adapted MFGT is helpful for civilians and families with spinal-cord injury and TBI. Reduced family burden was also reported in a pilot study of civilians (Rodgers et al., 2007).

## Couples Therapy

Couples therapy can be useful for various problems, such as communication, marital-stability, sexuality, and joint-parenting issues. Couples therapy does not preclude the use of other forms of therapy, including group and individual therapies.

Behavioral couples therapy (BCT) has been adapted for a variety of purposes, including work with veterans who have PTSD and their partners. BCT encourages acceptance, tolerance, and expression of emotions, such as fear and sadness, both of which characterize PTSD. Adaptations for PTSD include a shorter length of treatment, incorporation of motivational interviewing, trauma education, and emphasis on scheduling activities during treatment that increase couples' shared experiences (Erbes et al., 2008). The VHA is also training its clinicians to add parenting and domestic violence to their content (Makin-Byrd et al., 2011). No evaluation of PTSD-adapted BCT has been reported.

Cognitive behavioral conjoint therapy (CBCT) is another form of couples therapy directed at PTSD and associated disruptions in the functioning of couples. CBCT is a 15-session structured treatment that includes family psychoeducation, behavioral interventions to enhance approach behaviors and communication, and cognitive interventions aimed at the maladaptive cognitions that are associated with PTSD and that create relationship distress. Glynn et al. (1999) compared a version of CBCT along with exposure therapy in a controlled clinical trial of 42 combat-exposed Vietnam veterans and their partners. As compared with wait-list controls, veterans and partners who received both therapies experienced improved interpersonal problem-solving and reduced symptoms of PTSD, such as reexperiencing and hyperarousal. A subsequent uncontrolled clinical trial of CBCT alone in veterans found posttreatment reductions in PTSD symptoms and partner reports of improved relationship satisfaction and mental-health functioning (Monson et al., 2005). Another small uncontrolled trial yielded similar findings (Monson et al., 2011).

A related couples therapy, strategic approach therapy, is designed to ameliorate PTSD symptoms, specifically avoidance and emotional numbing. One study found reductions in self-reported, clinician-rated, and partner-rated avoidance, emotional numbing, and overall PTSD symptoms; however, there were no measures for its effect on relationship functioning (Sautter et al., 2009).

## Alcohol and Substance-Abuse Treatment for Dependents

The TRICARE benefit pays for certain SUD services for military dependents, including assessment and diagnosis by SUD professionals. In addition, there are a few programs that provide SUD screening, diagnosis, or treatment for military spouses or children in the direct care system, but data on the effectiveness of these programs is scarce. "Military Pathways" includes a self-assessment/self-screening component that can serve as a secondary prevention mechanism for military members or spouses who self-identify as being at personal risk for SUD and subsequently seek help. This intervention reaches more than 305,000 active-duty service members and their families each year and appears to follow evidence-based principles (IOM, 2012). The Adolescent Substance Abuse Counseling Program is focused on children of military families in grades 6–12 who are considered at risk for substance use and who are authorized to use military treatment facilities. Services include treatment, identification and referral, and prevention education in community settings. The effectiveness of the program is unknown as no formal outcome evaluations have been conducted with the target population (IOM, 2012). Military OneSource provides a confidential means for service members and their families to be screened for SUDs and referred to resources; however, the program is not designed to provide actual treatment for SUD or other mental health issues (IOM, 2012).

## Prevention Interventions for Families

Although effective treatments are essential for military families with mental-health, behavioral, and marital problems, preventing the initiation of such problems is ideal. Many prevention programs for military populations are adaptations of preventive interventions designed for civilian populations. There is a need for preventive intervention strategies addressing the needs of military families facing deployment. Of special note is the Families Over Coming Under Stress (FOCUS) intervention, which shows great promise for prevention. This treatment is a relatively new family-centered resiliency training program developed for military families by the University of California, Los Angeles (UCLA), and Harvard researchers. FOCUS has been delivered since 2008 to thousands of military families who experienced stress associated with multiple deployments. Designed to enhance resiliency (defined as "engagement in adaptive behaviors and achieving developmental milestones in the face of stressful or traumatic life events"), FOCUS involves eight structured family-training sessions that are targeted at increasing resiliency skills in the domains of communication, emotional regulation, managing trauma or loss, problem solving, and goal setting (Lester et al., 2011). A program evaluation that examined 331 families with a mean of 4.5 service-member deployments found improved family function and adaptation for those who participated in FOCUS. Parents reported that they had fewer symptoms of anxiety and depression, as well as healthier family functioning; lower than expected behavioral and emotional problems were also reported for children (Lester et al., 2012).

After Deployment: Adaptive Parenting Tools (ADAPT) is a relatively new program for returning military parents that focuses on preventing behavioral and adjustment problems among children, using role-playing exercises and audiovisual materials to teach parenting skills. It is based on the well-validated program known as the Parent Management Training Oregon-Model (PMTO); however, materials and curriculum were modified to make them more applicable to military and veteran families. The program focuses on providing parents with specific skills in five distinct areas: (1) contingency management, (2) limit setting, (3) positive involvement, (4) monitoring children's activities, and (5) effective family problem solving. ADAPT is currently undergoing evaluation (Gewirtz et al., 2011).

### Summary

In summary, although there are many family-based interventions for individuals who have or are at risk for psychiatric disorders, few are adapted or readily available for use with military and veteran families. When they are available, trained clinicians who can provide the interventions are not always accessible. There is clearly a need for new evidence-based programs, including prevention interventions, that are specifically designed to meet the needs of military families. Evaluation of these programs must be multifaceted and multimodal so that not only individual psychopathology and marital relationships are studied but also overall family function, parent–child interactions, and child functioning are studied.

## CONCLUSIONS

Military service members are also members of families, and their families can provide essential support to them as well as—at times—be a source of stress and concern. Families have a crucial, although sometimes unrecognized, role to play in military readiness, helping to ensure the well-being and functioning of service members so that they can be effective in their jobs. Family members are an essential asset to the military; they help to prepare service members for their deployments, provide emotional support and motivation, assist with readjustment and reintegration after deployment, and provide hands-on informal care and management for service members who return from war with physical or psychologic injuries. When families are doing poorly, service members also function worse. Quite simply, it is in the best interests of the military to work to ensure that families are also doing well, including before, during, and after deployments. The demographics of the military have changed, however, and it is important that the military consider the full spectrum of family configurations instead of limiting its focus to married heterosexual couples and their children; excluding the nontraditional families misses key opportunities to enhance military readiness. Although a wide array of services are available to families, few have been evaluated for effectiveness, and most are focused solely on married couples and their children—a family configuration that no longer captures the full diversity of military families.

## FUTURE RESEARCH DIRECTIONS

The committee identified a number of areas for future research and direction based on its reviews of the literature and the federally funded research on military families with service members who had deployed with OEF or OIF (see Appendix D). Although the committee found that research attention to military families (including the impact of deployments) is growing, many of the findings are limited by poor sampling strategies (for example, the use of nonrandom convenience samples) and small sample sizes. Certain populations, including women, reserve, and National Guard families, are also understudied. Few studies have examined military families over time, and none of those reviewed by the committee used inclusive definitions of family beyond traditional marriage. The committee recommends that research be supported to increase understanding of the following:

- Research is needed to better understand the nature of deployment. Although several emotional stages of adjustment to deployment have been proposed and are widely used, they have not been empirically validated longitudinally. Furthermore, the interaction between chronic military challenges and deployment-related stressors is not well understood and should be studied. More knowledge is needed about the impact of different characteristics of deployment, such as timing, duration, and frequency. Research should also be done on the impact of multiple short (for example, under 30 days) deployments on families; these deployments are usually not included in research, and better understanding is needed particularly of the impact of multiple parental departures on children.
- Although healthy and stable marital and other romantic partner relationships provide important supports for service members, there are many knowledge gaps regarding how these relationships influence military readiness and how they are affected by deployments. There is evidence, for example, that deployment erodes marital quality, but the factors that moderate these processes are not well understood; therefore, knowledge is insufficient about the best way to prevent such erosion in association with military service. Although patterns of marital formation and dissolution in the military have been studied repeatedly, little information is available about the accumulation of marital transitions among military members and the implications of such accumulation for family needs. Young military members marry at much higher rates than civilians of similar age, and such marriages have been demonstrated to be susceptible to divorce; military policies might unintentionally promote such marriages. Studies should be undertaken to determine how best to minimize both the threats to marital

stability posed by military service and the likelihood of premature marriage. Finally, in the context of relationships, deployment-related wounds and injuries and PTSD, particularly with regard to the impact on prognoses and recovery, is not well understood. Social isolation is, however, a risk factor for poor outcomes. Therefore, greater understanding of relationship dynamics is needed in regard to wounds and injuries in both nuclear and extended families.
- Research is needed to improve understanding of which children in military families are at highest risk, whether their mental-health needs are different from those of nonmilitary children, and of effective treatments that work within the context of military life.
- Despite now representing a significant minority of the armed forces, female military members are understudied. Studies should be conducted that focus on the specific characteristics, needs, and experiences of female service members and their families (including single female heads of households, members of dual-military couples, and military women with civilian partners). There is a need for better understanding of dual-military families, particularly as they relate to the needs of female service members and their ability to pursue their military careers.

In addition, the committee calls for the following to improve the quality of research and to increase the availability of research findings on military service members and their families:

- Although there are important longitudinal studies under way that examine the impact of deployments on service members and their families, they do not fully represent the diversity of military families. DOD should conduct longitudinal studies that include the full range of family configurations and support systems (for example, grandparents and unmarried partners). Studies are especially needed to quantify the value and impact of families on military readiness, including helping to prepare service members for deployment, supporting them during deployment, and providing physical and psychologic care for them upon their return.
- DOD collects large amounts of data about military members and families. However, most of these data remain unanalyzed. Large military data sets should be anonymized and made publicly available to researchers. Such availability will greatly increase the capacity of DOD to reap benefits from the vast amount of data it already collects. Access to unpublished DOD data is needed to identify current trends in child maltreatment; the last data were published in 2007.
- Many large, nationally representative population studies deliberately exclude individuals living in institutions, including military installations (for example, the National Longitudinal Survey of Youth). Service members and their families should be included in these large national surveys wherever feasible, both to expand knowledge about them and to allow comparisons of comparable population groups within studies.

## RECOMMENDATIONS

The committee found that DOD has many programs and policies to support families. However, DOD policies, programs, and practices typically do not take into consideration the full spectrum of military families. By focusing almost exclusively on traditional families (married heterosexual spouses and their children), DOD is missing critical opportunities to support the readjustment needs of many service members' nontraditional families. To be able to support all families, DOD will need data on the full constellation of service members' families.

**The committee recommends that the Department of Defense ensure that policies, programs, and practices aim to support and strengthen all military families, including nontraditional ones.**

Healthy families help service members to do their jobs effectively and readjust after deployment. The demands placed on military family members call for support in the areas of relationship building, family and individual function, and reduction of risk of psychologic and physical-health problems. The committee found that little information is available on the potential effectiveness of broad-based, universal prevention efforts aimed at military children and their families. In addition, most treatment interventions for family members have been developed and tested in civilian communities and lack evidence of their effectiveness for military families. The committee concludes that military families would benefit from increased efforts to identify, develop, and test new prevention and treatment interventions targeted toward military families, including interventions directed at children and adolescents.

**The committee recommends that the Department of Defense use evidence-based primary prevention programs and treatments that have been specifically evaluated in service members and their families and that are focused on preventing and treating mental-health and relationship problems.**

The committee concludes that there are substantial gaps in knowledge about the effects of deployment on military families that hinder DOD's ability to meet the needs of military service members and their families effectively. The committee found that—although some important large-scale, well-designed studies are under way—much of the research heretofore has been methodologically flawed, suffering, for example, from the use of small convenience samples, use of cross-sectional designs, and the like. The committee concludes that well-designed studies that use rigorous and diverse methods (both qualitative and quantitative) are needed to increase understanding of the challenges faced by military service members and their families.

**The committee recommends that the Department of Defense and other relevant federal agencies fund methodologically rigorous research on the social, psychologic, and economic effects of deployments on families, including nontraditional families.**

Studies of families of service members deployed to OEF and OIF have documented a rise in domestic violence (typically including abuse of spouses or neglect of children). In the FY 2000 National Defense Authorization Act (PL 106-65, Section 591), Congress directed the secretary of defense to establish a Defense Task Force on Domestic Violence to make recommendations for reducing the prevalence of domestic violence in military families. The task force submitted a report in 2003 that identified multiple shortcomings in the current systems and recommended many improvements. The Government Accountability Office, in 2006 and 2010, issued reports concerning progress in implementing the nearly 200 recommendations made by the task force. Both reports described progress on some recommendations but little on others, including a recommendation for reliable documentation of violent events.

**The committee recommends that the Department of Defense place high priority on reducing domestic violence because it degrades force readiness and the well-being of military family members.**

## REFERENCES


Adams, G. A., S. M. Jex, and C. J. L. Cunningham. 2006. Work-family conflict among military personnel. In *Military Life: The Psychology of Serving in Peace and Combat*, Vol. 3. Edited by C. A. Castro, A. B. Adler and T. W. Britt. Westport, CT: Praeger. Pp. 169-192.

Adler-Baeder, F., J. F. Pittman, and L. Taylor. 2006. The prevalence of marital transitions in military families. *Journal of Divorce and Remarriage* 44(1-2):91-106.

AdvancED. 2012. *Advanced Company Overview*. http://www.advanc-ed.org/company-overview (accessed July 9, 2012).

Allen, E. S., G. K. Rhoades, S. M. Stanley, and H. J. Markman. 2010. Hitting home: Relationships between recent deployment, posttraumatic stress symptoms, and marital functioning for Army couples. *Journal of Family Psychology* 24(3):280-288.

Allen, E. S., S. M. Stanley, G. K. Rhoades, H. J. Markman, and B. A. Loew. 2011. Marriage education in the Army: Results of a randomized clinical trial. *Journal of Couple and Relationship Therapy* 10(4):309-326.

Alvarez, L. 2007. Long Iraq tours can make home a trying front. *New York Times*, February 23.

Angrist, J. D., and J. H. Johnson. 2000. Effects of work-related absences on families: Evidence from the Gulf War. *Industrial and Labor Relations Review* 54(1):41-58.

Annie E. Casey Foundation. 2012. *Kids Count Data Book: State Trends in Child Well-Being.* Baltimore, MD: Annie E. Casey Foundation.

Babcock, J. C., C. E. Green, and C. Robie. 2004. Does batterers' treatment work? A meta-analytic review of domestic violence treatment. *Clinical Psychology Review* 23(8):1023-1053.

Baptist, J. A., Y. Amanor-Boadu, K. Garrett, B. S. Goff, J. Collum, P. Gamble, H. Gurss, E. Sanders-Hahs, L. Strader, and S. Wick. 2011. Military marriages: The aftermath of Operation Iraqi Freedom (OIF) and Operation Enduring Freedom (OEF) deployments. *Contemporary Family Therapy: An International Journal* 33(3):199-214.

Bassani, D. G., C. V. Padoin, D. Philipp, and S. Veldhuizen. 2009. Estimating the number of children exposed to parental psychiatric disorders through a national health survey. *Child and Adolescent Psychiatry and Mental Health* 3(1):6.

Batten, S. V., A. L. Drapalski, M. L. Decker, J. C. DeViva, L. J. Morris, M. A. Mann, and L. B. Dixon. 2009. Veteran interest in family involvement in PTSD treatment. *Psychological Services* 6(3):184-189.

Bethea, M. C. 2007. *Long War and the Forgotten Families: Dual-Military Couples.* Carlisle Barracks, PA: US Army War College.

Blais, M. C., and J. M. Boisvert. 2005. Psychological and marital adjustment in couples following a traumatic brain injury (TBI): A critical review. *Brain Injury* 19(14):1223-1235.

Booth, B., M. W. Segal, and D. B. Bell. 2007. *What We Know About Army Families: 2007 Update.* Arlington, VA: Department of the Army, Family and Morale, Welfare and Recreation Command.

Bowen, G. L., and J. A. Martin. 2011. The resiliency model of role performance for service members, veterans, and their families: A focus on social connections and individual assets. *Journal of Human Behavior in the Social Environment* 21(2):162-178.

Bowling, U. B., and M. D. Sherman. 2008. Welcoming them home: Supporting service members and their families in navigating the tasks of reintegration. *Professional Psychology: Research and Practice* 39(4):451-458.

Bray, R. M., L. L. Hourani, K. L. Rae Olmsted, M. Witt, J. M. Brown, M. R. Pemberton, M. E. Marsden, B. Marriott, S. Scheffler, R. Vandermaas-Peeler, B. Weimer, S. Calvin, M. Bradshaw, K. Close, and D. Hayden. 2006. *2005 Department of Defense Survey of Health Related Behaviors Among Military Personnel.* Research Triangle Park, NC: RTI international.

Bray, R. M., M. R. Pemberton, M. E. Lane, L. L. Hourani, M. J. Mattiko, and L. A. Babeu. 2010. Substance use and mental health trends among US military active duty personnel: Key findings from the 2008 DOD health behavior survey. *Military Medicine* 175(6):390-399.

Buchanan, C., J. Kemppainen, S. Smith, S. MacKain, and C. W. Cox. 2011. Awareness of posttraumatic stress disorder in veterans: A female spouse/intimate partner perspective. *Military Medicine* 176(7):743-751.

Buckman, J. E. J., J. Sundin, T. Greene, N. T. Fear, C. Dandeker, N. Greenberg, and S. Wessely. 2011. The impact of deployment length on the health and well-being of military personnel: A systematic review of the literature. *Occupational and Environmental Medicine* 68(1):69-76.

Burrell, L. M., G. A. Adams, D. B. Durand, and C. A. Castro. 2006. The impact of military lifestyle demands on well-being, army, and family outcomes. *Armed Forces and Society* 33(1):43-58.

Carter, S., B. Loew, E. Allen, S. Stanley, G. Rhoades, and H. Markman. 2011. Relationships between soldiers' PTSD symptoms and spousal communication during deployment. *Journal of Traumatic Stress* 24(3):352-355.

Castro, C. A., A. B. Adler, and T. W. Britt. 2006. Future directions. In *Military Life: The Psychology of Serving in Peace and Combat.* Edited by C. A. Castro, A. B. Adler and T. W. Britt. Westport, CT: Praeger. Pp. 245-248.

Center for Behavioral Health Statistics and Quality. 2012. *National Survey on Drug Use and Health (NSDUH) Data Spotlight: More Than 7 Million Children Live with a Parent with Alcohol Problems.* Rockville, MD: Substance Abuse and Mental Health Services Administration.

Chandra, A., S. Lara-Cinisomo, L. H. Jaycox, T. Tanielian, R. M. Burns, T. Ruder, and B. Han. 2010a. Children on the homefront: The experience of children from military families. *Pediatrics* 125(1):16-25.

Chandra, A., L. T. Martin, S. A. Hawkins, and A. Richardson. 2010b. The impact of parental deployment on child social and emotional functioning: Perspectives of school staff. *Journal of Adolescent Health* 46(3):218-223.

Chandra, A., S. Lara-Cinisomo, L. H. Jaycox, T. Tanielian, B. Han, R. M. Burns, and T. Ruder. 2011. *Views from the Homefront: The Experiences of Youth and Spouses from Military Families.* Santa Monica, CA: RAND Corporation.

Chartrand, M. M., D. A. Frank, L. F. White, and T. R. Shope. 2008. Effect of parents' wartime deployment on the behavior of young children in military families. *Archives of Pediatrics and Adolescent Medicine* 162(11):1009-1014.

Christensen, E., P. Netzer, E. Schaefer, C. Hill, D. Farr, and J. McMahon. 2009. *Economic Impact on Caregivers of the Seriously Wounded, Ill, and Injured.* Alexandria, VA: Center for Naval Analyses.

Cohen, J. A., and A. P. Mannarino. 2011. Trauma-focused CBT for traumatic grief in military children. *Journal of Contemporary Psychotherapy* 41(4):219-227.

Copen, C. E., K. Daniels, J. Vespa, and W. D. Mosher. 2012. First marriages in the United States: Data from the 2006–2010 National Survey of Family Growth. *National Health Statistics Reports* 49:1-21.

Cozza, S. J. 2007. Proceedings: Workgroup on intervention with combat injured families. Paper read at *Workgroup on Intervention with Combat Injured Families*, December 11–12, 2007, Bethesda, MD.

Cozza, S. J., R. S. Chun, and J. A. Polo. 2005. Military families and children during Operation Iraqi Freedom. *Psychiatric Quarterly* 76(4):371-378.

Cozza, S. J., J. M. Guimond, J. B. A. McKibben, R. S. Chun, T. L. Arata-Maiers, B. Schneider, A. Maiers, C. S. Fullerton, and R. J. Ursano. 2010. Combat-injured service members and their families: The relationship of child distress and spouse-perceived family distress and disruption. *Journal of Traumatic Stress* 23(1):112-115.

Crary, D. 2005. As deployments increase, so does Army's divorce rate. *USA Today.* http://usatoday30.usatoday.com/news/nation/2005-06-29-army-divorces_x.htm (accessed April 20, 2011).

Crum-Cianflone, N. F., J. Fairbank, C. Marmar, W. Schlenger, and H. McMaster. 2012. Millennium Cohort Family Study. Paper presented at *Annual Review Meeting, Military Operational Medicine Research Program*, Fort Detrich, MD.

de Burgh, H. T., C. J. White, N. T. Fear, and A. C. Iversen. 2011. The impact of deployment to Iraq or Afghanistan on partners and wives of military personnel. *Internal Review of Psychiatry* 23(2):192-200.

Defense Manpower Data Center. 2011. *2010 Military Family Life Project.* Arlington, VA: Department of Defense.

Department of the Army. 2012. *Army 2020: Generating Health and Discipline in the Force.* Washington, DC: Department of Defense.

Dimiceli, E. E., M. A. Steinhardt, and S. E. Smith. 2010. Stressful experiences, coping strategies, and predictors of health-related outcomes among wives of deployed military servicemen. *Armed Forces and Society* 36(2):351-373.

DOD (Department of Defense). 1998. *Selected Manpower Statistics, MO1 (Directorate for Information, Operations, and Reports).* Washington, DC: US Government Printing Office.

———. 2010a. *The Challenge and the Promise: Strengthening the Force, Preventing Suicide and Saving Lives.* Washington, DC: Department of Defense.

———. 2010b. *Plans for the Department of Defense for the Support of Military Family Readiness: Report to the Congressional Defense Committees Pursuant to Section 1782b of Title 10, United States Code.* Washington, DC: Department of Defense.

———. 2011a. *Annual Report to Congress on Plans for the Department of Defense for the Support of Military Family Readiness.* Washington, DC: Department of Defense.

———. 2011b. *Demographics 2010: Profile of the Military Community.* Washington, DC: Department of Defense.

———. 2012a. *2011 Demographics Profile of the Military Community.* Washington, DC: Department of Defense.

———. 2012b. *Annual Report to Congress on Plans for the Department of Defense for the Support of Military Family Readiness.* Washington, DC: Department of Defense.

———. 2012c. *Department of Defense Family Advocacy Program Child Abuse/Neglect (CAN) Data FY11 Report.* Washington, DC: Department of Defense.

———. 2012d. *TRICARE.* http://www.tricare.mil/mybenefit/ProfileFilter.do;jsessionid=
PQ2hM96Jx9ybGG8xnbhCwqnvK331Lxql3d5vQgcLjC1pNv21J2ND!349025571?puri=%2Fhome (accessed March 2, 2012).

DOD Education Activity. 2012. *Interstate Compact on Educational Opportunity for Military Children.* http://www.dodea.edu/teachers/interstate.cfm (accessed June 28, 2012).

Eaton, K. M., C. W. Hoge, S. C. Messer, A. A. Whitt, O. A. Cabrera, D. McGurk, A. Cox, and C. A. Castro. 2008. Prevalence of mental health problems, treatment need, and barriers to care among primary care-seeking spouses of military service members involved in Iraq and Afghanistan deployments. *Military Medicine* 173(11):1051-1056.

Eby, L. T., J. S. DeMatteo, and J. E. A. Russell. 1997. Employment assistance needs of accompanying spouses following relocation. *Journal of Vocational Behavior* 50(2):291-307.

Eide, M., G. Gorman, and E. Hisle-Gorman. 2010. Effects of parental military deployment on pediatric outpatient and well-child visit rates. *Pediatrics* 126(1):22-27.

Elizur, E., and M. Kaffman. 1983. Factors influencing the severity of childhood bereavement reactions. *American Journal of Orthopsychiatry* 53(4):668-676.

Engel, R. C., L. B. Gallagher, and D. S. Lyle. 2010. Military deployments and children's academic achievement: Evidence from Department of Defense Education Activity schools. *Economics of Education Review* 29(1):73-82.

Erbes, C. R. 2011. Couple functioning and PTSD in returning OIF soldiers: Preliminary findings from the readiness and resilience in National Guard soldiers project. In *Risk and Resilience in US Military Families*, edited by S. MacDermid Wadsworth and D. Riggs. New York: Springer. Pp. 47-67.

Erbes, C. R., M. A. Polusny, S. Macdermid, and J. S. Compton. 2008. Couple therapy with combat veterans and their partners. *Journal of Clinical Psychology* 64(8):972-983.

Erbes, C. R., L. A. Meis, M. A. Polusny, and J. S. Compton. 2011. Couple adjustment and posttraumatic stress disorder symptoms in National Guard veterans of the Iraq war. *Journal of Family Psychology* 25(4):479-487.

Etters, L., D. Goodall, and B. E. Harrison. 2008. Caregiver burden among dementia patient caregivers: A review of the literature. *Journal of the American Academy of Nurse Practitioners* 20(8):423-428.

Faber, A. J., E. Willerton, S. R. Clymer, S. M. MacDermid, and H. M. Weiss. 2008. Ambiguous absence, ambiguous presence: A qualitative study of military reserve families in wartime. *Journal of Family Psychology* 22(2):222-230.

Federal Interagency Forum on Child and Family Statistics. 2012. *America's Children in Brief: Key National Indicators of Well-Being.* Washington, DC: US Government Printing Office.

Felitti, V. J., R. F. Anda, D. Nordenberg, D. F. Williamson, A. M. Spitz, V. Edwards, M. P. Koss, and J. S. Marks. 1998. Relationship of childhood abuse and household dysfunction to many of the leading causes of death in adults. *American Journal of Preventive Medicine* 14(4):245-258.

Flake, E. M., B. E. Davis, P. L. Johnson, and L. S. Middleton. 2009. The psychosocial effects of deployment on military children. *Journal of Developmental and Behavioral Pediatrics* 30(4):271-278.

Forgey, M. A., and L. Badger. 2010. Patterns of intimate partner violence and associated risk factors among married enlisted female soldiers. *Violence and Victims* 25(1):45-61.

Franklin, K. 2011. The impact of deployment and psychological well-being on family relationships: A secondary analysis of Air Force community assessment data. *Dissertation Abstracts International Section A: Humanities and Social Sciences* 72(4-A):1441.

GAO (US Government Accountability Office). 2001. *Military Personnel: Longer Time Between Moves Related to Higher Satisfaction and Retention.* Washington, DC: US Government Accountability Office.

———. 2007. *Military Personnel: Medical, Family Support, and Educational Services Are Available for Exceptional Family Members.* Washington, DC: US Government Accountability Office.

———. 2010. *Sustained Leadership and Oversight Needed to Improve DOD's Prevention and Treatment of Domestic Abuse.* Washington, DC: US Government Accountability Office.

Gewirtz, A. H., C. R. Erbes, M. A. Polusny, M. S. Forgatch, and D. S. Degarmo. 2011. Helping military families through the deployment process: Strategies to support parenting. *Professional Psychology Research and Practice* 42(1):56-62.

Gibbs, D. A., S. L. Martin, L. L. Kupper, and R. E. Johnson. 2007. Child maltreatment in enlisted soldiers' families during combat-related deployments. *Journal of the American Medical Association* 298(5):528-535.

Glynn, S. M., S. Eth, E. T. Randolph, D. W. Foy, G. B. Leong, G. G. Paz, J. D. Salk, G. Firman, and J. W. Katzman. 1995. Behavioral family therapy for Vietnam combat veterans with posttraumatic stress disorder. *Journal of Psychotherapy Practice and Research* 4(3):214-223.

Glynn, S. M., S. Eth, E. T. Randolph, D. W. Foy, M. Urbaitis, L. Boxer, G. G. Paz, G. B. Leong, G. Firman, J. D. Salk, J. W. Katzman, and J. Crothers. 1999. A test of behavioral family therapy to augment exposure for combat-related posttraumatic stress disorder. *Journal of Consulting and Clinical Psychology* 67(2):243-251.

Goff, B. S. N., J. R. Crow, A. M. J. Reisbig, and S. Hamilton. 2007. The impact of individual trauma symptoms of deployed soldiers on relationship satisfaction. *Journal of Family Psychology* 21(3):344-353.

Golding, J. M. 1999. Intimate partner violence as a risk factor for mental disorders: A meta-analysis. *Journal of Family Violence* 14(2):99-132.

Gorman, G. H., M. Eide, and E. Hisle-Gorman. 2010. Wartime military deployment and increased pediatric mental and behavioral health complaints. *Pediatrics* 126(6).

Gorman, L. A., A. J. Blow, B. D. Ames, and P. L. Reed. 2011. National Guard families after combat: Mental health, use of mental health services, and perceived treatment barriers. *Psychiatric Services* 62(1):28-34.

Gould, M., House Committee on Veterans Affairs. 2012. *Veterans Affairs in the 112th Congress: Reviewing VA's Performance and Accountability*. September 20, 2012.

Griffin, J. M., G. Friedemann-Sanchez, C. Hall, S. Phelan, and M. van Ryn. 2009. Families of patients with polytrauma: Understanding the evidence and charting a new research agenda. *Journal of Rehabilitation Research and Development* 46(6):879-892.

Griffin, J. M., G. Friedemann-Sanchez, A. C. Jensen, B. C. Taylor, A. Gravely, B. Clothier, A. B. Simon, A. Bangerter, T. Pickett, C. Thors, S. Ceperich, J. Poole, and M. van Ryn. 2012. The invisible side of war: Families caring for US service members with traumatic brain injuries and polytrauma. *Journal of Head Trauma Rehabilitation* 27(1):3-13.

Haas, D. M., and L. A. Pazdernik. 2006. A cross-sectional survey of stressors for postpartum women during wartime in a military medical facility. *Military Medicine* 171(10):1020-1023.

———. 2007. Partner deployment and stress in pregnant women. *Journal of Reproductive Medicine* 52(10):901-906.

Haine, R. A., T. S. Ayers, I. N. Sandler, and S. A. Wolchik. 2008. Evidence-based practices for parentally bereaved children and their families. *Professional Psychology: Research and Practice* 39(2):113.

Harrell, M. C., N. Lim, L. Werber Castaneda, and D. Golinelli. 2004. *Working Around the Military: Challenges to Military Spouse Employment and Education.* Santa Monica, CA: RAND Corporation.

Helfrich, C. A., G. T. Fujiura, and V. Rutkowski-Kmitta. 2008. Mental health disorders and functioning of women in domestic violence shelters. *Journal of Interpersonal Violence* 23(4):437-453.

Heyman, R. E., and P. H. Neidig. 1999. A comparison of spousal aggression prevalence rates in US Army and civilian representative samples. *Journal of Consulting and Clinical Psychology* 67(2):239.

Hill, R. 1949. *Families Under Stress.* New York: Harper and Brothers.

Hinojosa, R., M. S. Hinojosa, and R. S. Hognas. 2012. Problems with veteran-family communication during Operation Enduring Freedom/Operation Iraqi Freedom military deployment. *Military Medicine* 177(2):191-197.

Hopkins-Chadwick, D. L., and N. Ryan-Wenger. 2009. Stress in junior enlisted Air Force women with and without children. *Western Journal of Nursing Research* 31(3):409-427.

Hosek, J., B. Asch, C. C. Fair, C. Martin, and M. Mattock. 2002. *Married to the Military: The Employment and Earnings of Military Wives Compared with Those of Civilian Wives.* Santa Monica, CA: RAND Corporation.

Hosek, J., J. Kavanagh, and L. Miller. 2006. *How Deployments Affect Service Members.* Santa Monica, CA: RAND Corporation.

Huebner, A. J., J. A. Mancini, G. L. Bowen, and D. K. Orthner. 2009. Shadowed by war: Building community capacity to support military families. *Family Relations* 58(2):216-228.

Huffman, A. H., and S. C. Payne. 2006. The challenges and benefits of dual-military marriages. In *Military Life: The Psychology of Serving in Peace and Combat (Vol 3): The Military Family.* Westport, CT: Praeger Security International. Pp. 115-137.

Hurley, E. C. 2011. Rejection sensitivity as a predictor of marital adjustment among military spouses during military deployments. *Dissertation Abstracts International: Section B: The Sciences and Engineering* 72(5-B):3096.

Interagency Policy Committee, Presidential Study Directive, and The White House. 2011. *Strengthening Our Military Families.* Washington, DC: The White House.

IOM (Institute of Medicine). 2008. *Gulf War and Health: Volume 6. Physiologic, Psychologic, and Psychosocial Effects of Deployment-related Stress.* Washington, DC: The National Academies Press.

———. 2010. *Returning Home from Iraq and Afghanistan: Preliminary Assessment of Readjustment Needs of Veterans, Service Members, and Their Families.* Washington, DC: The National Academies Press.

———. 2012. *Substance Use Disorders in the US Armed Forces.* Washington, DC: The National Academies Press.

Jensen, P. S., D. Martin, and H. Watanabe. 1996. Children's response to parental separation during Operation Desert Storm. *Journal of the American Academy of Child and Adolescent Psychiatry* 35(4):433-441.

Johnson, A. J. 2011. Examining partner experiences of returning Operation Enduring Freedom and Iraqi Freedom Veterans. *Dissertation Abstracts International: Section B: The Sciences and Engineering* 71(11-B):7118.

Jowers, K. 2011. *Bereavement Study to Focus on 3,000 Survivors.* http://militarytimes.com/news/2011/10/military-ausa-bereavement-study-3000-survivors-101111w (accessed October 25, 2012).

Karney, B. R., and T. N. Bradbury. 1995. The longitudinal course of marital quality and stability: A review of theory, method, and research. *Psychological Bulletin* 118(1):3-34.

Karney, B. R., and J. S. Crown. 2007. *Families Under Stress: An Assessment of Data, Theory, and Research on Marriage and Divorce in the Military.* Santa Monica, CA: RAND Corporation.

———. 2011. Does deployment keep military marriages together or break them apart? Evidence from Afghanistan and Iraq. In *Risk and Resilience in US Military Families.* New York: Springer. Pp. 23-45.

Karney, B. R., D. S. Loughran, and M. S. Pollard. 2012. Comparing marital status and divorce status in civilian and military populations. *Journal of Family Issues* 33(12):1572-1594.

Kavanagh, J. 2005. *Stress and Performance: A Review of the Literature and Its Applicability to the Military.* Santa Monica, CA: RAND Corporation.

Kelley, M. L., E. Hock, J. F. Bonney, M. S. Jarvis, K. M. Smith, and M. A. Gaffney. 2001. Navy mothers experiencing and not experiencing deployment: Reasons for staying in or leaving the military. *Military Psychology* 13(1):55-71.

Kelley, M. L., E. Hock, M. S. Jarvis, K. M. Smith, M. A. Gaffney, and J. F. Bonney. 2002. Psychological adjustment of Navy mothers experiencing deployment. *Military Psychology* 14(3):199-216.

Khaylis, A., M. A. Polusny, C. R. Erbes, A. Gewirtz, and C. M. Rath. 2011. Posttraumatic stress, family adjustment, and treatment preferences among National Guard soldiers deployed to OEF/OIF. *Military Medicine* 176:126-131.

Knapp, S. J., and B. Lott. 2010. Forming the central framework for a science of marital quality: An interpretive alternative to marital satisfaction as a proxy for marital quality. *Journal of Family Theory and Review* 2(4):316-333.

Knobloch, L. K., and J. A. Theiss. 2011. Depressive symptoms and mechanisms of relational turbulence as predictors of relationship satisfaction among returning service members. *Journal of Family Psychology* 25(4):470-478.

Kreider, R. M., and R. Ellis. 2011. Living arrangements of children: 2009. *Current Population Reports* (June):P70-126.

Kreutzer, J. S., L. J. Rapport, J. H. Marwitz, C. Harrison-Felix, T. Hart, M. Glenn, and F. Hammond. 2009. Caregivers' well-being after traumatic brain injury: A multicenter prospective investigation. *Archives of Physical Medicine and Rehabilitation* 90(6):939-946.

Kulka, R. A., W. E. Schlenger, J. A. Fairbank, R. L. Hough, B. K. Jordan, C. R. Marmar, D. S. Weiss, and D. A. Grady. 1990. *Trauma and the Vietnam War Generation: Report of Findings from the National Vietnam Veterans Readjustment Study*. New York: Routledge.

Lara-Cinisomo, S., A. Chandra, R. Burns, L. Jaycox, T. Tanielian, T. Ruder, and B. Han. 2011. A mixed-method approach to understanding the experiences of non-deployed military caregivers. *Maternal and Child Health Journal* 16(2):374-384.

Lester, P., K. Peterson, J. Reeves, L. Knauss, D. Glover, C. Mogil, N. Duan, W. Saltzman, R. Pynoos, K. Wilt, and W. Beardslee. 2010. The long war and parental combat deployment: Effects on military children and at-home spouses. *Journal of the American Academy of Child and Adolescent Psychiatry* 49(4):310-320.

Lester, P., C. Mogil, W. Saltzman, K. Woodward, W. Nash, G. Leskin, B. Bursch, S. Green, R. Pynoos, and W. Beardslee. 2011. Families overcoming under stress: Implementing family-centered prevention for military families facing wartime deployments and combat operational stress. *Military Medicine* 176(1):19-25.

Lester, P., W. R. Saltzman, K. Woodward, D. Glover, G. A. Leskin, B. Bursch, R. Pynoos, and W. Beardslee. 2012. Evaluation of a family-centered prevention intervention for military children and families facing wartime deployments. *American Journal of Public Health* 102(Suppl1):S48-S54.

Lilly, M. B., A. Laporte, and P. C. Coyte. 2007. Labor market work and home care's unpaid caregivers: A systematic review of labor force participation rates, predictors of labor market withdrawal, and hours of work. *Milbank Quarterly* 85(4):641-690.

Lim, N., and D. Schulker. 2010. *Measuring Underemployment Among Military Spouses.* Santa Monica, CA: RAND Corporation.

Lincoln, A., E. Swift, and M. Shorteno-Fraser. 2008. Psychological adjustment and treatment of children and families with parents deployed in military combat. *Journal of Clinical Psychology* 64(8):984-992.

Lundquist, J. H. 2004. When race makes no difference: Marriage and the military. *Social Forces* 83(2):731-757.

———. 2006. The black-white gap in marital dissolution among young adults: What can a counterfactual scenario tell us? *Social Problems* 53(3):421-441.

Luthar, S. S. 2006. Resilience in development: A synthesis of research across five decades. In *Developmental Psychopathology: Risk, Disorder, and Adaptation*, edited by D. Cicchetti and D. J. Cohen. New York: Wiley. Pp. 740-795.

Lyle, D. S. 2006. Using military deployments and job assignments to estimate the effect of parental absences and household relocations on children's academic achievement. *Journal of Labor Economics* 24(2):319-350.

MacDermid Wadsworth, S., and K. Southwell. 2011. Military families: Extreme work and extreme "work-family." *Annals of the American Academy of Political and Social Science* 638(1):163-183.

MacLean, A., and G. H. Elder. 2007. Military service in the life course. *Annual Review of Sociology* 33:175-196.

Makin-Byrd, K., E. Gifford, S. McCutcheon, and S. Glynn. 2011. Family and couples treatment for newly returning veterans. *Professional Psychology—Research and Practice* 42(1):47-55.

Mannarino, A. P., J. A. Cohen, E. Deblinger, M. K. Runyon, and R. A. Steer. 2012. Trauma-focused cognitive-behavioral therapy for children sustained impact of treatment 6 and 12 months later. *Child Maltreatment* 17(3):231-241.

Mansfield, A. J., J. S. Kaufman, S. W. Marshall, B. N. Gaynes, J. P. Morrissey, and C. C. Engel. 2010. Deployment and the use of mental health services among US Army wives. *New England Journal of Medicine* 362(2):101-109.

Mansfield, A. J., J. S. Kaufman, C. C. Engel, and B. N. Gaynes. 2011. Deployment and mental health diagnoses among children of US Army personnel. *Archives of Pediatrics and Adolescent Medicine* 165(11):999-1005.

Martin, S. L., D. A. Gibbs, R. E. Johnson, K. Sullivan, M. Clinton-Sherrod, J. L. Walters, and E. D. Rentz. 2010. Substance use by soldiers who abuse their spouses. *Violence Against Women* 16(11):1295-1310.

Mateczun, J. M., and E. K. Holmes. 1996. Return, readjustment, and reintegration: The three R's of family reunion. In *Emotional Aftermath of the Persian Gulf War: Veterans, Families, Communities and Nations*, edited by R. J. Ursano and A. E. Norwood. Washington, DC: American Psychiatric Press, Inc. Pp. 250-282.

McCarroll, J. E., R. J. Ursano, X. Liu, L. E. Thayer, J. H. Newby, A. E. Norwood, and C. S. Fullerton. 2000. Deployment and the probability of spousal aggression by US Army soldiers. *Military Medicine* 165(1):41-44.

McCarroll, J. E., K. J. Hoffman, A. Grieger, and H. C. Holloway. 2005. Psychological aspects of deployment and reunion. In *Military Preventive Medicine: Mobilization and Deployment Vol. 2*, edited by P. W. Kelley. Washington, DC: Office of the Surgeon General, Department of the Army and Borden Institute. Pp. 1395-1426.

McCauley, J., D. E. Kern, K. Kolodner, L. Dill, A. F. Schroeder, H. K. DeChant, J. Ryden, L. R. Derogatis, and E. B. Bass. 1997. Clinical characteristics of women with a history of childhood abuse. *Journal of the American Medical Association* 277(17):1362-1368.

McCreary, D. R., M. M. Thompson, and L. Pasto. 2003. Predeployment family concerns and soldier well-being: The impact of family concerns on the predeployment well-being of Canadian forces personnel. *Canadian Journal of Police and Security Services* 1:33-40.

McCubbin, H. I. 1979. Integrating coping behavior in family stress theory. *Journal of Marriage and the Family* 41(2):237-244.

McCubbin, H. I., and C. R. Figley. 1983. Bridging normative and catastrophic family stress. In *Stress and the Family, Volume I: Coping with Normative Transitions*, edited by H. I. McCubbin and C. R. Figley. New York: Brunner/Mazel. Pp. 218-228.

McCubbin, H. I., B. B. Dahl, G. R. Lester, and B. A. Ross. 1975. The returned prisoner of war: Factors in family reintegration. *Journal of Marriage and the Family* 37(3):471-478.

McFarlane, W. R., B. Link, R. Dushay, J. Marchal, and J. Crilly. 1995. Psychoeducational multiple family groups: Four-year relapse outcome in schizophrenia. *Family Process* 34(2):127-144.

McKean, D., J. Goodman, B. Bodnar, H. Warden, E. Shirey, Z. Stokes, A. Scheideberg, and A. Searvis. 2011. *Freedom to Serve: The Definitive Guide to LGBT Military Service.* Washington, DC: Servicemembers Legal Defense Network.

McNulty, P. A. F. 2005. Reported stressors and health care needs of active duty Navy personnel during three phases of deployment in support of the war in Iraq. *Military Medicine* 170(6):530-535.

Meis, L. A., C. R. Erbes, M. A. Polusny, and J. S. Compton. 2010. Intimate relationships among returning soldiers: The mediating and moderating roles of negative emotionality, PTSD symptoms, and alcohol problems. *Journal of Traumatic Stress* 23(5):564-572.

Merrill, L. L., J. L. Crouch, C. J. Thomsen, and J. M. Guimond. 2004. Risk for intimate partner violence and child physical abuse: Psychosocial characteristics of multirisk male and female Navy recruits. *Child Maltreatment* 9(1):18-29.

Mghir, R., W. Freed, A. Raskin, and W. Katon. 1995. Depression and posttraumatic stress disorder among a community sample of adolescent and young adult Afghan refugees. *Journal of Nervous and Mental Disease* 183(1):24-30.

MHAT-IV. 2006. *Mental Health Advisory Team IV (MHAT- IV): Operation Iraqi Freedom 05-07 Final Report.* Washington, DC: Office of the Surgeon General, United States Army Medical Command, Office of the Surgeon Multinational Force-Iraq.

MHAT-V. 2008. *Mental Health Advisory Team V (MHAT-V) Operation Iraqi Freedom 06-08: Iraq; Operation Enduring Freedom 8: Afghanistan.* Washington, DC: Office of the Surgeon General, United States Army Medical Command, Office of the Surgeon Multinational Force-Iraq.

MHAT-VII. 2011. *Joint Mental Health Advisory Team 7 (J-MHAT 7) Operation Enduring Freedom 2010.* Washington, DC: Office of the Surgeon General, United States Army Medical Command, Office of the Command Surgeon HQ, USCENTCOM, Office of the Command Surgeon U.S. Forces Afghanistan.

Miller, L. L., S. O. Meadows, L. M. Hanser, and S. L. Taylor. 2011a. *Year of the Air Force Family: 2009 Survey of Active-Duty Spouses.* Santa Monica, CA: RAND Corporation.

Miller, L. L., B. D. Rostker, R. M. Burns, D. Barnes-Proby, S. Lara-Cinisomo, and T. R. West. 2011b. *A New Approach for Assessing the Needs of Service Members and Their Families.* Santa Monica, CA: RAND Corporation.

Milliken, C. S., J. L. Auchterlonie, and C. W. Hoge. 2007. Longitudinal assessment of mental health problems among active and reserve component soldiers returning from the Iraq war. *Journal of the American Medical Association* 298(18):2141-2148.

Monson, C. M., S. P. Stevens, and P. P. Schnurr. 2005. Cognitive-behavioral couple's treatment for posttraumatic stress disorder. In *Focus on Posttraumatic Stress Disorder Research*, edited by T. A. Corales. Hauppauge, NY: Nova Science Publishers, Inc. Pp. 250-274.

Monson, C. M., C. T. Taft, and S. J. Fredman. 2009. Military-related PTSD and intimate relationships: From description to theory-driven research and intervention development. *Clinical Psychology Review* 29(8):707-714.

Monson, C. M., S. J. Fredman, K. C. Adair, S. P. Stevens, P. A. Resick, P. P. Schnurr, H. Z. MacDonald, and A. Macdonald. 2011. Cognitive-behavioral conjoint therapy for PTSD: Pilot results from a community sample. *Journal of Traumatic Stress* 24(1):97-101.

Mulligan, K., N. Jones, M. Davies, P. McAllister, N. T. Fear, S. Wessely, and N. Greenberg. 2012. Effects of home on the mental health of British forces serving in Iraq and Afghanistan. *British Journal of Psychiatry*.

Murray-Swank, A. B., and L. Dixon. 2004. Family psychoeducation as an evidence-based practice. *CNS Spectrums* 9(12):905-912.

Nathanson, A. M., R. C. Shorey, V. Tirone, and D. L. Rhatigan. 2012. The prevalence of mental health disorders in a community sample of female victims of intimate partner violence. *Partner Abuse* 3(1):59.

National Alliance for Caregiving. 2010. *Caregivers of Veterans—Serving on the Homefront*. Bethesda, MD: National Alliance for Caregiving.

Negrusa, B., and S. Negrusa. 2012. *Home Front: Post-Deployment Mental Health and Divorces*. Santa Monica, CA: RAND Corporation.

Nelson, H. D., P. Nygren, Y. McInerney, and J. Klein. 2004. Screening women and elderly adults for family and intimate partner violence: A review of the evidence for the US Preventive Services Task Force. *Annals of Internal Medicine* 140(5):387-396.

Nelson Goff, B. S., and B. D. Smith. 2005. Systemic traumatic stress: The couple adaption to traumatic stress model. *Journal of Marital and Family Therapy* 31(2):145-157.

Newby, J. H., J. E. McCarroll, R. J. Ursano, Z. Fan, J. Shigemura, and Y. Tucker-Harris. 2005a. Positive and negative consequences of a military deployment. *Military Medicine* 170(10):815-819.

Newby, J. H., R. J. Ursano, J. E. McCarroll, X. Liu, C. S. Fullerton, and A. E. Norwood. 2005b. Postdeployment domestic violence by US Army soldiers. *Military Medicine* 170(8):643-647.

NRC (National Research Council) and IOM. 2010. *Student Mobility: Exploring the Impact of Frequent Moves on Achievement: Summary of a Workshop*. Washington, DC: The National Academies Press.

O'Leary, K. D. 1999. Psychological abuse: A variable deserving critical attention in domestic violence. *Violence and Victims* 14(1):3-23.

Orthner, D. K., and R. Rose. 2002. *Relocation Adjustment Among Army Civilian Spouses*. Washington, DC: Army Research Institute for the Behavioral and Social Sciences.

Padden, D. L., R. A. Connors, and J. G. Agazio. 2011. Stress, coping, and well-being in military spouses during deployment separation. *Western Journal of Nursing Research* 33(2):247-267.

Parsons, C. 2008. *US Military Marriages Strained by Long Deployments*. http://www.reuters.com/article/2008/05/06/us-usa-military-marriage-idUSN2228946820080506 (accessed August 22, 2012).

Patterson, J. M. 2002. Integrating family resilience and family stress theory. *Journal of Marriage and Family* 64(2):349-360.

Peebles-Kleiger, M. J., and J. H. Kleiger. 1994. Re-integration stress for Desert Storm families: Wartime deployments and family trauma. *Journal of Traumatic Stress* 7(2):173-194.

Perlesz, A., G. Kinsella, and S. Crowe. 1999. Impact of traumatic brain injury on the family: A critical review. *Rehabilitation Psychology* 44(1):6-35.

Perlick, D. A., K. Straits-Troster, D. G. Dyck, D. M. Norell, J. L. Strauss, C. Henderson, J. Close, N. Berger, E. R. Bonuck, K. H. Taber, C. Kalvin, T. Dolber, and A. Cristian. 2011. Multifamily group treatment for veterans with traumatic brain injury. *Professional Psychology—Research and Practice* 42(1):70-78.

Phelan, S. M., J. M. Griffin, W. L. Hellerstedt, N. A. Sayer, A. C. Jensen, D. J. Burgess, and M. van Ryn. 2011. Perceived stigma, strain, and mental health among caregivers of veterans with traumatic brain injury. *Disability and Health Journal* 4(3):177-184.

Pietrzak, R. H., and S. M. Southwick. 2011. Psychological resilience in OEF-OIF veterans: Application of a novel classification approach and examination of demographic and psychosocial correlates. *Journal of Affective Disorders* 133(3):560-568.

Pincus, S. H., R. House, and J. Christenson. 2001. The emotional cycle of deployment: A military family perspective. *Army Medical Department Journal* 4/5/6:15-23.

Pinquart, M., and S. Sörensen. 2003. Differences between caregivers and non-caregivers in psychological health and physical health: A meta-analysis. *Psychology and Aging* 18:250-267.

———. 2005. Ethnic differences in stressors, resources, and psychological outcomes of family caregiving: A meta-analysis. *Gerontologist* 45(1):90-106.

———. 2011. Spouses, adult children, and children-in-law as caregivers of older adults: A meta-analytic comparison. *Psychology and Aging* 26(1):1-14.

Polusny, M. A., C. R. Erbes, P. A. Arbisi, P. Thuras, S. M. Kehle, M. Rath, C. Courage, M. K. Reddy, and C. Duffy. 2009. Impact of prior Operation Enduring Freedom/Operation Iraqi Freedom combat duty on mental health in a predeployment cohort of National Guard soldiers. *Military Medicine* 174(4):353-357.

President's Commission on Care for America's Returning Wounded Warriors. 2007. *Serve, Support, Simplify: Report of the President's Commission on Care for America's Returning Wounded Warriors.* Washington, DC.

RAND Center for Military Health Policy. 2012. *The Deployment Life Study.* http://www.rand.org/multi/military/deployment-life.html (accessed October 17, 2012).

Reddy, M. K., L. A. Meis, C. R. Erbes, M. A. Polusny, and J. S. Compton. 2011. Associations among experiential avoidance, couple adjustment, and interpersonal aggression in returning Iraqi war veterans and their partners. *Journal of Consulting and Clinical Psychology* 79(4):515-520.

Reinkober Drummet, A., M. Coleman, and S. Cable. 2003. Military families under stress: Implications for family life education. *Family Relations* 52(3):279-287.

Renshaw, K. D., and S. B. Campbell. 2011. Combat veterans' symptoms of PTSD and partners' distress: The role of partners' perceptions of veterans' deployment experiences. *Journal of Family Psychology* 25(6):953-962.

Renshaw, K. D., and C. M. Caska. 2012. Relationship distress in partners of combat veterans: The role of partners' perceptions of posttraumatic stress symptoms. *Behavior Therapy* 43(2):416-426.

Renshaw, K. D., C. S. Rodrigues, and D. H. Jones. 2008. Psychological symptoms and marital satisfaction in spouses of Operation Iraqi Freedom veterans: Relationships with spouses' perceptions of veterans' experiences and symptoms. *Journal of Family Psychology* 22(4):586-594.

Renshaw, K. D., E. S. Allen, G. K. Rhoades, R. K. Blais, H. J. Markman, and S. M. Stanley. 2011. Distress in spouses of service members with symptoms of combat-related PTSD: Secondary traumatic stress or general psychological distress? *Journal of Family Psychology* 25(4):461-469.

Rentz, E. D., S. L. Martin, D. A. Gibbs, M. Clinton-Sherrod, J. Hardison, and S. W. Marshall. 2006. Family violence in the military: A review of the literature. *Trauma Violence and Abuse* 7(2):93-108.

Rentz, E. D., S. W. Marshall, D. Loomis, C. Casteel, S. L. Martin, and D. A. Gibbs. 2007. Effect of deployment on the occurrence of child maltreatment in military and nonmilitary families. *American Journal of Epidemiology* 165(10):1199-1206.

Richardson, A., A. Chandra, L. T. Martin, C. M. Setodji, B. W. Hallmark, N. F. Campbell, S. Hawkins, and P. Grady. 2011. *Effects of Soldiers' Deployment on Children's Academic Performance and Behavioral Health.* Santa Monica, CA: RAND Corporation.

Riggs, S. A., and D. S. Riggs. 2011. Risk and resilience in military families experiencing deployment: The role of the family attachment network. *Journal of Family Psychology* 25(5):675-687.

Robinson-Whelen, S., and D. H. Rintala. 2003. Informal care providers for veterans with SCI: Who are they and how are they doing? *Journal of Rehabilitation Research and Development* 40(6):511-516.

Robrecht, D. T., J. Millegan, L. L. Leventis, J. B. Crescitelli, and R. N. McLay. 2008. Spousal military deployment as a risk factor for postpartum depression. *Journal of Reproductive Medicine* 53(11):860-864.

Rodgers, M. L., A. D. Strode, D. M. Norell, R. A. Short, D. G. Dyck, and B. Becker. 2007. Adapting multiple-family group treatment for brain and spinal cord injury intervention development and preliminary outcomes. *American Journal of Physical Medicine and Rehabilitation* 86(6):482-492.

Rosen, L. N., D. Durand, D. J. Westhuis, and J. M. Teitelbaum. 1995. Marital adjustment of Army spouses one year after Operation Desert Storm. *Journal of Applied Social Psychology* 25(8):677-692.

Ruger, W., S. E. Wilson, and S. L. Waddoups. 2002. Warfare and welfare: Military service, combat, and marital dissolution. *Armed Forces and Society* 29(1):85-107.

Sahlstein, E., K. C. Maguire, and L. Timmerman. 2009. Contradictions and praxis contextualized by wartime deployment: Wives' perspectives revealed through relational dialectics. *Communication Monographs* 76(4):421-442.

Saltzman, W. R., P. Lester, W. R. Beardslee, C. M. Layne, K. Woodward, and W. P. Nash. 2011. Mechanisms of risk and resilience in military families: Theoretical and empirical basis of a family-focused resilience enhancement program. *Clinical Child and Family Psychology Review* 14(3):213-230.

SAMHSA (Substance Abuse and Mental Health Services Administration). 2008. *Results from the 2007 National Survey on Drug Use and Health: National Findings: Major Depressive Episode and Treatment for Depression Among Veterans Aged 21 to 39.* Rockville, MD: Substance Abuse and Mental Health Services Administration.

Sautter, F. J., S. M. Glynn, K. E. Thompson, L. Franklin, and X. Han. 2009. A couple-based approach to the reduction of PTSD avoidance symptoms: Preliminary findings. *Journal of Marital and Family Therapy* 35(3):343-349.

Sayers, S. L. 2011. Family reintegration difficulties and couples therapy for military veterans and their spouses. *Cognitive and Behavioral Practice* 18(1):108-119.

Schok, M. L., R. J. Kleber, M. Elands, and J. M. P. Weerts. 2008. Meaning as a mission: A review of empirical studies on appraisals of war and peacekeeping experiences. *Clinical Psychology Review* 28(3):357-365.

Schulz, R., and L. M. Martire. 2004. Family caregiving of persons with dementia: Prevalence, health effects, and support strategies. *American Journal of Geriatric Psychiatry* 12(3):240-249.

Segal, M. W. 1986. The military and the family as greedy institutions. *Armed Forces and Society* 13(1):9-38.

Shear, M. K. 2012. Grief and mourning gone awry: Pathway and course of complicated grief. *Dialogues in Clinical Neuroscience* 14(2):119-128.

Sheppard, S. C., J. W. Malatras, and A. C. Israel. 2010. The impact of deployment on US military families. *American Psychologist* 65(6):599-609.

Sherman, M. D. 2006. Updates and five-year evaluation of the S.A.F.E. Program: A family psychoeducational program for serious mental illness. *Community Mental Health Journal* 42(2):213-219.

Sherman, M. D., D. A. Perlick, and K. Straits-Troster. 2012. Adapting the multifamily group model for treating veterans with posttraumatic stress disorder. *Psychological Services* 9(4):349-360.

Shin, P., S. Rosenbaum, and D. R. Mauery. 2005. *Medicaid's Role in Treating Children in Military Families.* Washington, DC: George Washington University SPHHS Center for Health Services Research and Policy.

Silverman, A. B., H. Z. Reinherz, and R. M. Giaconia. 1996. The long-term sequelae of child and adolescent abuse: A longitudinal community study. *Child Abuse and Neglect* 20(8):709-723.

Silverman, W. K., C. D. Ortiz, C. Viswesvaran, B. J. Burns, D. J. Kolko, F. W. Putnam, and L. Amaya-Jackson. 2008. Evidence-based psychosocial treatments for children and adolescents exposed to traumatic events. *Journal of Clinical Child and Adolescent Psychology* 37(1):156-183.

Skopp, N. A., M. A. Reger, G. M. Reger, M. C. Mishkind, M. Raskind, and G. A. Gahm. 2011. The role of intimate relationships, appraisals of military service, and gender on the development of posttraumatic stress symptoms following Iraq deployment. *Journal of Traumatic Stress* 24(3):277-286.

Smith, D. C., M. L. Munroe, L. M. Foglia, P. E. Nielsen, and S. H. Deering. 2010. Effects of deployment on depression screening scores in pregnancy at an Army military treatment facility. *Obstetrics and Gynecology* 116(3):679-684.

Smith, P., S. Perrin, W. Yule, and S. Rabe-Hesketh. 2001. War exposure and maternal reactions in the psychological adjustment of children from Bosnia-Herzegovina. *Journal of Child Psychology and Psychiatry* 42(3):395-404.

Spera, C. 2009. Spouses' ability to cope with deployment and adjust to Air Force family demands. *Armed Forces and Society* 35(2):286-306.

Stanley, S. M., E. S. Allen, H. J. Markman, G. K. Rhoades, and D. L. Prentice. 2010. Decreasing divorce in Army couples: Results from a randomized controlled trial using prep for strong bonds. *Journal of Couple and Relationship Therapy* 9(2):149-160.

SteelFisher, G. K., A. M. Zaslavsky, and R. J. Blendon. 2008. Health-related impact of deployment extensions on spouses of active duty Army personnel. *Military Medicine* 173(3):221-229.

Stenberg, U., C. M. Ruland, and C. Miaskowski. 2010. Review of the literature on the effects of caring for a patient with cancer. *Psycho-Oncology* 19(10):1013-1025.

Street, A. E., and I. Arias. 2001. Psychological abuse and posttraumatic stress disorder in battered women: Examining the roles of shame and guilt. *Violence and Victims* 16(1):65-78.

Taft, C. T., R. P. Weatherill, H. E. Woodward, L. A. Pinto, L. E. Watkins, M. W. Miller, and R. Dekel. 2009. Intimate partner and general aggression perpetration among combat veterans presenting to a posttraumatic stress disorder clinic. *American Journal of Orthopsychiatry* 79(4):461-468.

US Census Bureau. 2011a. *America's Families and Living Arrangements: 2011, Table C2: Household Relationship and Living Arrangements of Children Under 18 Years, by Age and Sex: 2011.* http://www.census.gov/population/www/socdemo/hh-fam/cps2011.html (accessed October 25, 2012).

———. 2011b. *America's Families and Living Arrangements: 2011, Table C3: Living Arrangements of Children Under 18 Years and Marital Status of Parents, by Age, Sex, Race, and Hispanic Origin and Selected Characteristics of the Child for all Children: 2011.* http://www.census.gov/population/www/socdemo/hh-fam/cps2011.html (accessed October 25, 2012).

———. 2011c. *Current Population Survey, 2010 Annual Social and Economic Supplement.* www.census.gov/hhes/migration/files/cps/cps2010/tab02.xls (accessed June 1, 2012).

US House of Representatives. 2008. *National Month of the Military Child.* H. Res. 265. 110th Congress.

US Social Security Administration. 2012. *Office of Retirement and Disability Policy.* http://www.ssa.gov/policy/docs/statcomps/supplement/2012/5f.html#table5.f4 (accessed October 25, 2012).

VA (Department of Veterans Affairs). 2006. *VHA directive 2006-041: Veterans Health Care Service Standards.* Washington, DC: Veterans Health Administration, Department of Veterans Affairs.

———. 2011. *New Services for Family Caregivers of Post-9/11 Veterans.* http://www.caregiver.va.gov/support_benefits.asp (accessed July 9, 2012).

van der Voort, T. Y., P. J. Goossens, and J. J. van der Bijl. 2007. Burden, coping and needs for support of caregivers for patients with a bipolar disorder: A systematic review. *Journal of Psychiatric and Mental Health Nursing* 14(7):679-687.

Van Houtven, C. H., E. Z. Oddone, and M. Weinberger. 2010. Informal and formal care infrastructure and perceived need for caregiver training for frail US veterans referred to home and community-based services. *Chronic Illness* 6(1):57-66.

van Steenbergen, E. F., N. Ellemers, S. A. Haslam, and F. Urlings. 2008. There is nothing either good or bad but thinking makes it so: Informational support and cognitive appraisal of the work-family interface. *Journal of Occupational and Organizational Psychology* 81(3):349-367.

Verhaeghe, S., T. Defloor, and M. Grypdonck. 2005. Stress and coping among families of patients with traumatic brain injury: A review of the literature. *Journal of Clinical Nursing* 14(8):1004-1012.

Vitaliano, P. P., J. Zhang, and J. M. Scanlan. 2003. Is caregiving hazardous to one's physical health? A meta-analysis. *Psychological Bulletin* 129(6):946-972.

Vormbrock, J. K. 1993. Attachment theory as applied to wartime and job-related marital separation. *Psychological Bulletin* 114(1):122-144.

Walsh, F. 2006. *Strengthening Family Resilience*, 2nd ed. New York: Guilford.

Warner, C., G. N. Appenzeller, C. Warner, and T. Grieger. 2009. Psychological effects of deployments on military families. *Psychiatric Annals* 39(2):56-63.

Weinick, R. M., E. B. Beckjord, C. M. Farmer, L. T. Martin, E. M. Gillen, J. D. Acosta, M. P. Fisher, J. Garnett, G. C. Gonzalez, T. C. Helmus, L. H. Jaycox, K. A. Reynolds, N. Salcedo, and D. M. Scharf. 2011. *Programs Addressing Psychological Health and Traumatic Brain Injury Among US Military Servicemembers and Their Families.* Santa Monica, CA: RAND Corporation.

Werber, L., M. C. Harrell, D. M. Varda, K. Curry Hall, and M. K. Beckett. 2008. *Deployment Experiences of Guard and Reserve Families: Implications for Support and Retention.* Santa Monica, CA: RAND Corporation.

Wiens, T. W., and P. Boss. 2006. Maintaining family resiliency before, during, and after military separation. In *Military Life: The Psychology of Serving in Peace and Combat, Volume 3: The Family*, edited by C. A. Castro, A. B. Adler, and T. W. Britt. Westport, CT: Praeger.

Worthen, M., R. Moos, and J. Ahern. 2012. Iraq and Afghanistan veterans' experiences living with their parents after separation from the military. *Contemporary Family Therapy*:1-14.

Wright, K. M., L. M. Burrell, E. D. Schroeder, and J. L. Thomas. 2006. Military spouses: Coping with the fear and the reality of service member injury and death. In *Military Life: The Psychology of Serving in Peace and Combat. Volume 3: The Family*, edited by C. A. Castro, A. B. Adler, and T. W. Britt. Westport, CT: Praeger.

Zarit, S. 2006. Assessment of family caregivers: A research perspective. In *Caregiver Assessment: Voices and Views from the Field. Report from a National Consensus Development Conference (Vol. II)*, edited by Family Caregiver Alliance. San Francisco, CA: Family Caregiver Alliance. Pp. 12-37.

# 7

# COMMUNITY IMPACTS OF DEPLOYMENT

This chapter examines the effects of deployments to Operation Enduring Freedom (OEF) and Operation Iraqi Freedom (OIF) on communities. The committee studied the effects in two ways: First, it conducted an extensive review of the literature. Second, it commissioned ethnographic studies to illustrate the effects of the deployments on six communities either located near major military installations (Jacksonville, North Carolina; El Paso, Texas; Watertown, New York; Lakewood and Lacey, Washington) or having relatively large, recently deployed National Guard populations (Georgetown and Andrews, South Carolina; Little Falls, Minnesota).

## REVIEW OF THE LITERATURE

The body of literature documenting the effects of OEF and OIF deployment on communities is scant. The committee found no community-wide assessments of the effects of OEF and OIF deployment. In an effort to find related research, the committee expanded its literature search to cover the community effects of any military deployment. The committee broadly defined the term *community effect* to refer to any impact on local public or private providers of goods and services.

### Community-Wide Economic Effects of Deployments

The committee found no studies that examined the community-wide economic effects of OEF and OIF deployments. It did identify one study, published in 1994, that quantified, over a seven-county region, the economic effects of troops deploying from Fort Stewart and Hunter Airfield in Georgia (Kriesel and Gilbreath, 1994). At the time of the study, Fort Stewart held 25,000 Army troops and had had recent deployments—to the First Gulf War, and to Florida in response to Hurricane Andrew. Fort Stewart is a major employer in the surrounding rural communities. For the economic analysis, the investigators focused on the consequences of a 1,000-troop deployment for 1 year. That unit was selected so that study results could be extrapolated to future deployments of varying lengths and sizes. The investigators found that such a deployment is associated with decreased expenditures in sectors of the local economy including food, housing, retail, transportation, health care, and entertainment. In all, the authors estimated that the 1,000-troop deployment for 1 year reduced direct local spending by $10.56

million (in 1991 dollars) in the seven-county region. Reduced expenditures were made by the Army itself ($2.71 million) and by individual troops ($7.85 million).

Kriesel and Gilbreath (1994) applied those estimates to a software model for input-output analysis that contained county-level economic data. With the model, they were able to forecast the economic consequences of the deployment within the seven-county study area. The model showed that 240 economic sectors were affected by troop deployments from Fort Stewart; however, only 101 of the sectors were present in the seven-county study region, meaning that many of the economic effects associated with deployments from Fort Stewart were felt outside the immediate region. The results of the model are summarized in Table 7.1.

"Direct impact" as shown in Table 7.1 includes, for example, decreased sales at restaurants as a result of fewer patrons. "Indirect impact" includes the decreased purchases that restaurants in turn would make from wholesalers, as well as the ensuing chain of decreased economic activity (for example, wholesalers purchasing less produce from farmers, who in response might decrease their production the following year). "Induced impact" considers the broader economic fallout from the deployments—for example, reduced overall consumer spending caused by lower wages as a consequence of less revenue at local businesses. "Direct impact plus indirect impact plus induced impact" equals the total economic impact in the region for each of the categories in Table 7.1.

The column labeled "Total Gross Output" in Table 7.1 quantifies the impact that deploying 1,000 troops for 1 year has on the output of goods and services in the region. In 1991 dollars, such a deployment from Fort Stewart would reduce the total gross output in the seven counties by $13.87 million. Wages and salaries paid to employees of local vendors would be reduced by $4.15 million over the year, and total income (wages plus interest, profits, rental income) would be reduced by $7.05 million. Value added (employee compensation plus indirect business taxes and property income) would be reduced by $7.77 million, and a total of 266 jobs would be lost.

Although this type of analysis is geographically specific, it does shed light on how a deployment might affect local economies with heavy reliance on military installations. The Kriesel and Gilbreath study suggests that there are significant economic losses to communities that deploy a relatively high concentration of service members.

**TABLE 7.1** Local Economic Impacts from Deploying 1,000 Troops for 1 Year, Fort Stewart and Hunter Army Airfield (in 1991 USD)

| | Total Gross Output ($ in millions) | Wages and Salaries ($ in millions) | Total Income ($ in millions) | Value Added ($ in millions) | Jobs |
|---|---|---|---|---|---|
| Direct Impact | −8.3097 | −2.5900 | −4.1870 | −4.5845 | −172 |
| Indirect Impact | −1.8761 | −0.4982 | −0.9299 | −1.0339 | −27 |
| Induced Impact | −3.6811 | −1.0636 | −1.9380 | −2.1513 | −65 |
| Direct + Indirect + Induced Impact | −13.8669 | −4.1519 | −7.0548 | −7.7697 | −266 |

SOURCE: Kriesel and Gilbreath, 1994 (with permission).

## Impact of Deployment on Employers

The majority of reservists and National Guard soldiers hold private-sector jobs in the community (CBO, 2005). They are often activated for deployment with little warning, which can be disruptive and costly to employers. The effects of activation vary greatly among businesses that employ reservists, depending on the size of the business and the nature of the position vacated by the deploying employee. The most adverse effects of deployment are borne by small businesses that lose essential employees, businesses that rely on employees with highly specialized skills, and self-employed businesses owned by reservists (CBO, 2005; Hope et al., 2009).

Small businesses (fewer than 100 employees) employed about 18% of reservists in 2004 (CBO, 2005). Approximately 8,000–30,000 of 860,000 reservists in the Selected Reserves[1] were estimated to hold key positions in small businesses in 2004. About 55,000 reservists (9% of total reservists in 2004) were self-employed or employed by a family business. Self-employed reservists were more likely to be in construction, legal, health care, and building-maintenance fields than were reservists who were not self-employed.

### Types of Deployment Effects

The committee reviewed the limited literature documenting the effects of National Guard and reserve activation on civilian employers. According to the Congressional Budget Office (CBO), only 6% of businesses employ reservists. However, in communities with a higher concentration of National Guard and reservists, the effect of deployments can be more profound. That is particularly true among businesses that employ reservists in key positions or those with specialized skills (CBO, 2005).

Allison-Aipa et al. (2005) interviewed 28 private-sector employers of reservists to measure problems following the activation of the reservists. The employers were a convenience sample identified by a unit of the Maryland National Guard. The 28 employers, 39% of which were in law enforcement, reported that reserve activation had a negative impact on work scheduling (61%), product delivery (50%), coworker workload (68%), morale (29%), and the hiring and training of replacements (57%). Many reported that reserve call-ups came with too little notice (72%), at an inconvenient time (50%), and with an unclear length of assignment (61%). Most employers (71%) reassigned the responsibilities of the activated employee to his or her coworkers. Forty-two percent of employers stated that 2 weeks was the maximum that a reservist could be away before the workplace was negatively affected.

A CBO survey found that about 15,000 small businesses reported experiencing financial loss or difficulty operating their businesses in 2001–2004 (CBO, 2005). Reservists notified their civilian employers, on average, 13 days ahead of activation. Sixty percent of reservists gave their employers notice of 1 week or less. Unclear length of deployment further complicated employers' responses to the reservists' activation. In many cases it was not known how long a reservist would be away, making it difficult for employers to decide how to respond to the temporary vacancy.

---

[1]The Selected Reserve is a subset of reservists who are required to be available for mobilization within 24 hours. They are drawn from all services: the Air National Guard, Air Force Reserve, Army National Guard, Army Reserve, Coast Guard Reserve, Marine Corps Reserve, and Navy Reserve.

**Economic Impact on Employers**

Call-ups of reservists have direct financial impact on their employers largely because the reservists' jobs and some benefits are guaranteed to them by law when they return. The Uniformed Services Employment and Reemployment Rights Act of 1994 (USERRA; PL 103-353) requires employers to reemploy reservist employees after their service is completed; the act also prohibits employment discrimination based on past, present, or future military service. Returning reservists are entitled to continued pension benefits as if they had not been activated, and they have the right to retain their health coverage. When they return from activation, reservists are also entitled to career advancement and seniority benefits as if they had been continuously employed. USERRA does not require employers to pay salaries for reservists during mobilization, but some employers elect to supplement military pay.

The Institute for Defense Analysis attempted to quantify the cost to employers resulting from reserve activation (Doyle et al., 2004). On the basis of published civilian age-group and firm-size data, Doyle et al. estimated that 50–58% of employed reservists participate in an employer-provided retirement plan and that employers' costs for reservists' retirement plans average $372 per month. In addition, using published civilian age-group and firm-size data, Doyle et al. estimated that about 65% of reservists participate in employer-provided health-insurance plans and that the monthly employer cost averages $215 for a single individual and $550 for a family.

Small businesses are disproportionately affected by the loss of reservists who are ordered to active duty, because an employee at a small firm accounts for a greater share of output than that of an employee at a large firm. Doyle et al. (2004) interviewed a small number of recipients of Small Business Administration Military Reservist Economic Injury Disaster Loans, which are given to companies that are unable to meet their operating expenses after an essential employee has been called to active duty. The findings indicate that the most common effect of activation is lost business and that losses are experienced even after reservists return from active duty. Furthermore, replacing a reservist, even if it is feasible, does not necessarily offset lost business; in some cases the long-term effect of activation might result in permanent harm to the business (Doyle et al., 2004).

The CBO study found financial effects similar to those cited above (CBO, 2005). Health care coverage for activated reservists who elect to keep their employer's health coverage costs about $260 per month for individual coverage and about $600 per month for family coverage, regardless of how long the activation lasts. If the employer offers a matched contribution to the reservist's retirement plan and the reservist continues to contribute while activated, the employer is required to continue to match the contribution for the duration of the activation. The CBO estimates that paying this benefit costs employers about $175 a month, or $2,100 for a 1-year activation, for each participating reservist. Some employers voluntarily pay benefits that exceed those required by USERRA. For example, CBO reports that 16% of recently activated reservists continued to receive either partial or full salaries for the duration of their activation.

**Effect on the Workforce**

A study conducted by the RAND Corporation found that the overall effect of reservist activation on the workforce was minimal (Loughran et al., 2006). The study found that, at most, activated reservists or deployed active-duty service members constituted 0.2% of the workforce nationwide in 2001–2004. The study notes, however, that active-duty service members and reservists are geographically concentrated, and thus the effect of their deployment is likely far greater in some communities than in others.

For active-duty deployments, the authors found that for every 10 service members deployed, about one civilian is hired and enters the workforce. It is unclear why this occurs, although the authors speculate that it might be due to the entering of the workforce by spouses of deployed service members while their husbands or wives are away (Loughran et al., 2006). For every reservist activated, the authors found a corresponding short-term decline in the workforce; after 4 months, however, employment levels return to preactivation levels, which is likely due to employers simply taking time to hire replacement workers. The authors acknowledge that although in the aggregate, activations and deployment are not likely to have any long-term effect on the US economy, certain communities and businesses with relatively large concentrations of reservist employees might feel the brunt of deployment more significantly. Police departments, for example, are often staffed by reservists and might have difficulty restaffing in the short term following activations. This is especially true in smaller communities where the pool of eligible trained officers looking for work is likely minimal.

Hickman (2006) examined the effect of reserve activation expressly on police forces. The analysis, covering a 12-month period, found that about 2% of the police workforce nationwide was activated in 2003. However, the rate of activation varied greatly depending on the size of the force and community. For example, in the 362 law-enforcement agencies supporting larger communities (250,000 or more), 1.6% of the workforce was activated. The 4,178 law-enforcement agencies serving small-to-medium-sized communities (10,000–49,000) lost 3.7% of the workforce to activation. However, the 9,941 agencies serving small communities (10,000 or less) lost 11.4% of the workforce. Costs associated with those losses are mostly attributable to the increased overtime needed to compensate for the lost workforce. Using the Department of Justice's Law Enforcement Management and Administrative Statistics (LEMAS) survey data, the author calculated that the total cost per activated officer was $650–$2,000 per week. Hickman estimated the total cost per law-enforcement agency was $2,050–$6,020 per week.

The Small Business Administration looked at revenue loss in small businesses related to reserve activation (Hope et al., 2009). The authors found that among small firms (100 or fewer employees), for every reservist activated there was a 0.30% decrease in sales. In large firms, a 0.02% decrease in sales was associated with every employee activated. This 15-fold difference in sales impact demonstrates the heavier toll experienced by small businesses. The authors also found that for every 10% increase in activations of 30 days or more, small firms face a 3.7% decrease in sales.

**Programs to Assist Employers**

The committee is aware of programs and federal laws designed to lessen the financial burden that employers of reservists or self-employed reservists face when reservists are activated and deployed. The Veterans Entrepreneurship and Small Business Development Act of 1999 (PL 106-50) allows small businesses that lose essential employees or owners to active duty to defer payment of preexisting direct loans from the Small Business Administration. The law also requires the Small Business Administration to lower the borrower's interest rate. This law helps many activated reservists who are self-employed, considering that they are generally essential employees or owners.

The Servicemembers Civil Relief Act of 2003 (H.R. 100) can also help relieve the effects of activation on self-employed reservists by allowing them to reduce certain business-debt interest costs and, under certain circumstances, to terminate business leases before a call-up. Finally, the Military Reservist Economic Injury Disaster Loan (MREIDL) program under the Small Business Administration provides funds to help an eligible small business meet the ordinary and necessary operating expenses that it is unable to meet because an essential employee was called up for active duty (US Small Business Administration, 2011).

## Employment of the Returning Veteran in the Community

When veterans return to their communities, they need to readjust to the civilian workforce. Recently separated reservists have the opportunity to return to their previous positions because employers are required by law to hold the reservists' jobs open. But recently separated veterans who enlisted in the military at a young age might be entering the civilian workforce for the first time. As discussed in Chapter 8, among those in the labor force, veterans who served after 2001 have higher rates of unemployment than do their civilian counterparts. One reason might be that approximately 20–25% of returning veterans have psychiatric symptoms or diagnoses (Hoge et al., 2006; Jacobson et al., 2008; Seal et al., 2007; Tanielian and Jaycox, 2008).

Burnett-Zeigler et al. looked at employment status among 585 National Guard service members recently separated (45–60 days), returning from OIF and OEF (Burnett-Zeigler et al., 2011). Less than half (41%) of the participants were employed at the time of the survey. Those who reported recent combat exposure were more likely to be employed (46%) compared with those who did not report recent combat (36%). Physical- and mental-health status, posttraumatic stress disorder (PTSD), depression, alcohol use, and anxiety did not affect the participants' employment status. Among the employed, 79% were employed full time. Service members below age 30 were less likely to be employed than those 31 or older (29% and 57%, respectively). In the adjusted analyses, those with better mental-health status and poorer physical-health status were more likely to be employed full time vs part time. The authors note that more time might be required for the negative effects of mental-health status, alcohol use, recent combat exposure, and PTSD to affect employment rates. Additionally, Burnett-Zeigler et al. suspect that having a psychiatric illness or combat trauma might affect the maintaining of employment more than it affects the obtaining of employment. The authors also note that selection bias should be considered, as only 60% of those approached chose to participate in the study.

Erbes et al. (2011) studied 262 National Guard and reserve service members who returned from OIF after a 16-month deployment. The authors conducted structured diagnostic interviews with these individuals on their reentry into civilian life and sent out a questionnaire 1 year later. In total, 5% had PTSD, 6% had subthreshold PTSD, 11% had major depressive disorders, and 11% were experiencing alcohol abuse or dependence. The study found that the rates of employment of the study participants at both time points did not differ from the rates of employment in veterans without a psychiatric diagnosis, but those with psychiatric diagnoses reported functioning, at both time points, at a lower level of work performance.

Smith et al. (2005) looked at PTSD-symptom severity and its effect on employment outcomes. Researchers used the Clinician-Administered PTSD Scale (CAPS) to measure PTSD-symptom severity in the 325 Vietnam-era veterans participating in the study. All participants had either severe or very severe symptoms. For every 10-point rise in the CAPS score, indicating a meaningful increase in PTSD symptoms, the likelihood of no employment increased 5.9 percentage points ($p < 0.01$). Correspondingly, the probability of part-time work decreased 2.1 percentage points ($p < 0.01$), and the probability of full-time work decreased 3.8 percentage points ($p < 0.01$). CAPS scores did not have any significant association with earnings for full-time workers or all workers (full-time and part-time combined).

Taken together, studies of employment show that veterans who have psychiatric illness are at a disadvantage in obtaining or maintaining employment. When they are employed, it might only be part time rather than full time, or they might be functioning at lower levels. PTSD appears to be the strongest risk factor for occupational impairment.

**Community Interventions to Assist Employment**

There are many Department of Veterans Affairs (VA) and other public- and private-sector programs and interventions designed to help veterans enter the workforce. The question is: What types of vocational services are most effective for veterans with psychiatric illness? Resnick and Rosenheck looked at the relationship between PTSD and employment among 5,862 veterans in Veterans Health Administration Compensated Work Therapy, a vocational rehabilitation program (Resnick and Rosenheck, 2008). This program, dating back to the 1930s, aids veterans with disabilities in obtaining competitive employment in the community, working in jobs they choose, and receiving compensation. The VA employs them, finds work for them at other federal agencies, or enters into contracts with private providers that employ them. Resnick et al. found that veterans who had received a diagnosis of PTSD were 19% less likely to be employed on completion of the program (odds ratio [OR] = 0.81, 95% confidence interval [CI] = 0.69–0.96, $p = 0.02$) compared with veterans who had not received a diagnosis of PTSD. Mood disorders and substance-use disorders were unrelated to employment. Compared with unemployed veterans, employed veterans were more likely to be younger, to receive less public financial support, and to have fewer medical conditions. Veterans with severe mental illness were less likely to be employed. Those who had served in a theater of operations had higher rates of employment, a finding that the authors assert was anomalous. In terms of program efficacy, 30% of veterans who had received a diagnosis of PTSD were employed on completion of the program vs 36% of veterans who had not received a diagnosis of PTSD—rates that the authors considered to be low.

Rosenheck and Mares (2007) examined the individual placement and support (IPS) approach to job training for veterans who had a diagnosis of mental illness. IPS is an evidence-based practice that stresses rapid job placement, choice of jobs, emphasis on obtaining competitive jobs, ongoing support without a time limit, and integration of vocational support and clinical care (Bond et al., 2001). The Rosenheck and Mares (2007) study compared employment outcomes between two cohorts: the Phase 1 cohort of 308 veterans participated in the VA program before the IPS was established in 2001, and the Phase 2 cohort of 321 veterans received IPS. Both cohorts were followed and interviewed quarterly for 2 years. Because the cohorts were not assigned randomly, the analyses were adjusted for characteristics that were significantly different between the two groups. Veterans were eligible if they were homeless, were not receiving VA health services, sought competitive employment (a non-VA job in the community), had received a diagnosis for a psychiatric or substance-use disorder, and had been unemployed for the previous 30 days or longer. The Phase 2 group had 15% more days per month of competitive employment (8.4 days compared with 7.3 days; $p < 0.001$) and 32% fewer days of noncompetitive employment (a job through the compensated work therapy program, for example). Overall, days of combined employment (competitive and noncompetitive) were not significantly different between the groups; however, the difference in the number of competitive work days was significant at eight of the nine study sites.

Davis et al. (2012) were the first to perform a randomized controlled clinical trial of IPS in veterans who had received a diagnosis of PTSD. Veterans were randomly assigned to receive IPS (n = 42) vs standard vocational services (n = 43) sponsored by the VA. Over the course of 12 months, 76% of IPS recipients gained competitive work vs 28% of controls—that is, the IPS group was 2.7 times more likely to gain competitive employment. Further, the IPS recipients worked substantially more weeks and earned higher income. Taken as a whole, the evidence supports IPS as a preferred type of vocational rehabilitation service. Communities serving veterans can utilize this model to deliver vocational assistance for veterans who do not qualify for VA services.

## Homelessness and Community Impacts

Among veterans, those who are homeless have the greatest needs for community-based services—not only for shelter but also for identification and amelioration of the risk factors for homelessness, including psychiatric and substance-use disorders. Consequently, the community-based services needed by the homeless are wide ranging. They include housing, employment, health care, social services, education, and outreach, among others.

### Epidemiology of Homelessness Among Veterans

By January 2009, only 916 veterans of OEF and OIF had formally sought VA homeless services (Perl, 2010). However, the VA has classified an additional 2,986 OEF and OIF veterans at risk for homelessness. Those numbers are relatively low at present, but the risk of homelessness can continue for many years after separation, and the current numbers might well not be indicative of lifetime incidence. For example, 76% of homeless Vietnam combat veterans reported that they had not been homeless for at least the first 10 years after separation (Perl, 2010).

The committee is not aware of any studies examining the population-based prevalence of homelessness among those deployed to OEF and OIF. There is one study of the prevalence of homelessness in a national sample of 1.1 million recipients of VA mental-health services: it found that of 124,471 OEF and OIF veterans, 4,478, or 3.8%, were homeless in 2009 (Edens et al., 2011). That figure is likely to be an underestimate because it only examined recipients of VA mental-health services. The only other estimate, made by the VA and the Department of Housing and Urban Development (HUD), pertains to *all* homeless veterans—irrespective of deployment. The most recent estimate by the VA and HUD is that 75,609 veterans were homeless in January 2009. Of those, 57% were in shelters or transitional housing, and 43% were either on the street or in a place not intended for human habitation, such as in an abandoned building (US Department of Housing and Urban Development and VA, 2011).

From 2008 to 2009, 1 of every 168 veterans, or 136,334 veterans, spent at least one night in an emergency shelter or in transitional housing. Veterans are about three times more likely than are nonveterans to be homeless. Veterans make up less than 8% of the general population, but they comprise about 12% of the overall homeless population and, more specifically, 16% of the homeless adult population (US Department of Housing and Urban Development and VA, 2011).

Minorities are overrepresented among homeless veterans. African Americans constitute 34% of homeless veterans but are only 10.5% of the overall veteran population. Similarly, Latinos are 8.3% of homeless veterans but comprise only 3.6% of the overall veteran population. Native Americans make up 3.4% of the homeless veteran population but are only 0.7% of the overall veteran population. Homeless veterans are generally older, with only 7% of homeless veterans being younger than 30 years of age, compared with 26% of homeless nonveterans (US Department of Housing and Urban Development and VA, 2011). Males who are 45–54 years of age and women who are 18–29 years of age are at higher risk of homelessness compared with those of other ages (Fargo et al., 2012).

Similar demographic data are contained in a report from the Congressional Research Service (Perl, 2010). Homeless veteran men are generally older and better educated as compared with nonveteran homeless men. Homeless veteran women are also more educated than their nonveteran homeless counterparts, and homeless veteran men have more physical-health problems than those of nonveteran homeless men. Examined separately, female veterans, of all ages, are two to four times more likely to be homeless than their nonveteran counterparts (Perl, 2010).

**Risk Factors for Homelessness in Veterans**

Veterans and nonveterans share many of the same risk factors associated with homelessness (Balshem et al., 2011). These include childhood risk factors (absent or negligent parenting), living in foster care, and prolonged episodes away from home (as a runaway). The homeless, regardless of veteran status, tend to have similar rates of substance abuse, but it is unclear whether homeless veterans compared with the nonveteran homeless have comparable rates of mental illness and different overall health status. Certain veteran-specific exposures, including combat injury, intense combat exposure, and military sexual trauma, are associated with future mental illness and unstable income and employment, all of which are risk factors for homelessness in veteran and nonveteran populations.

Prolonged or intense combat exposure can negatively affect long-term employment, mental health, and other social outcomes, all of which can increase the risk of homelessness (Jacobson et al., 2008). Substance-use problems and weak social networks often emerge during active-duty service or during readjustment to civilian life. Alcohol abuse, a known risk factor for homelessness, is generally higher among male and female veterans as compared with the general population. Additionally, National Guard and reserve soldiers are at increased risk of new problem drinking in the postdeployment period after combat exposure. Among persons who are homeless, alcohol abuse is more prevalent among veterans than among nonveterans, but veterans and nonveterans had similar rates of other substance abuse.

Homeless individuals are more likely to engage in survival criminal behaviors, such as theft and prostitution, which can lead to incarceration (Balshem et al., 2011). Likewise, legal restrictions and other readjustment difficulties following incarceration increase the risk for homelessness. Adjusted for age, about 1,253 of every 100,000 veterans, or 1.3%, are incarcerated, which is about 10% lower than the rate in the nonveteran population. Among incarcerated veterans in state prisons, 57% committed violent crimes, compared with 47% of incarcerated nonveterans who committed violent crimes. Legal and regulatory restrictions previously limited homeless veterans with criminal records and untreated drug abuse from accessing some public services. Recent policy changes by the VA and HUD under the Obama administration have relaxed these restrictions and established subsidized housing vouchers in an effort intended to end veteran homelessness by 2015 (VA National Center on Homelessness Among Veterans; Vogel, 2011).

War-zone stress among Vietnam-era veterans led to difficulties in readjusting to civilian life, to social isolation, and homelessness among white male veterans, according to the landmark National Vietnam Veterans Readjustment Study (NVVRS) (Kulka et al., 1990). In a followup study involving 1,460 male veterans from the NVVRS, Rosenheck and Fontana (1994) found that postmilitary social isolation, psychiatric disorder, and substance abuse were the strongest risk factors for homelessness. Several premilitary factors also increased risk, including childhood physical or sexual abuse, other childhood traumas, and placement in foster care during childhood.

The committee identified two studies on homelessness among OEF and OIF veterans. Tsai et al. (2012) characterized the homeless OEF and OIF veteran population, comparing it with the homeless veteran population overall. Investigators identified 994 OEF and OIF veterans among the 44,577 homeless veterans referred to the Housing and Urban Development–Veterans Affairs Supportive Housing (HUD–VASH) program between 2008 and 2011. OEF and OIF veterans were underrepresented in the homeless population in comparison with the overall veteran population (3% vs 12%). Naturally, however, OEF and OIF veterans are younger than veterans having served prior to OEF and OIF, and more time might be needed before the full extent of homelessness among OEF and OIF veterans is realized. The authors also found that OEF and OIF homeless veterans were much more likely to have received a diagnosis of PTSD compared with homeless veterans from prior conflicts (67% vs 8–13%). Among OEF and OIF veterans, 38% had a substance-use disorder. The authors point out that most homelessness services focus on substance-abuse problems, which is appropriate given the number of homeless with substance-abuse issues. However, they point out that among OEF and OIF homeless veterans, it might be more appropriate to focus on treating PTSD, given the very large number of homeless OEF and OIF veterans with the condition.

Edens et al. (2011) studied a national sample of veterans (1.1 million) who used mental-health services at the VA in FY 2009. The authors performed a nested case control study of OEF and OIF veterans, who constituted 11% of the national sample. Consistent with the findings involving Vietnam veterans, almost all psychiatric and substance-use disorders increased the risk of homelessness (Table 7.2). The major exception was PTSD, which neither increased the risk of, nor protected against, homelessness. The authors point out that this finding might be explained by increased outreach by the VA to aid OIF and OEF veterans to access services. The following factors protected against homelessness in this sample: receiving a service-connected disability rating, having income greater than $25,000, and living in a rural location. For reasons unclear, having an anxiety disorder was also mildly protective (OR = 0.9, $p < 0.001$).

**TABLE 7.2** Multivariate Comparison of Recently Homeless vs Nonhomeless Department of Veterans Affairs Mental-Health Service Users, FY 2009

| Diagnosis | Odds Ratio for Homelessness |
|---|---|
| Schizophrenia | 3.3[c] |
| Bipolar disorder | 1.7[c] |
| Major depression | 1.4[c] |
| Anxiety disorder | 0.9[b] |
| Posttraumatic stress disorder | 1.0 |
| Alcohol-use disorder | 1.8[c] |
| Drug-use disorder | 4.4[c] |
| Pathological gambling | 2.4[a] |
| Personality disorder | 2.2[c] |

[a]$p < 0.01$.
[b]$p < 0.001$.
[c]$p < 0.0001$.
SOURCE: Edens et al., 2011 (with permission).

Female veterans, as noted above, are at two- to fourfold increased risk for homelessness (Perl, 2010). Washington et al. (2010) looked at risk factors among female homeless veterans in Los Angeles, California. They matched 33 homeless women veterans with 165 housed women veterans on age, geographic region, and period of service. Significant risk factors for homelessness included unemployment (adjusted odds ratio [AOR] = 13.1; 95% CI = 2.7, 63.0); being disabled (AOR = 12.5; 95% CI = 3.5, 45.0); having a positive PTSD screen (AOR = 4.9; 95% CI = 1.9, 12.7); having been sexually assaulted during military service (AOR = 4.4; 95% CI = 1.4, 14.0); having a positive anxiety disorder screen (AOR = 4.1; 95% CI = 1.3, 13.2); and having overall fair or poor health (AOR = 3.2; 95% CI 1.3, 7.9). Having at least a college degree and being married were protective, lowering the odds of homelessness 5 and 10 times, respectively.

**Community Services Needed by Homeless Veterans**

The Congressional Research Service identified three needs that will have to be met to minimize homelessness among OEF and OIF veterans (Perl, 2010):

1. Permanent and supportive housing for homeless and low-income veterans,
2. Adequate transition assistance for recently returned veterans to help identify and mitigate issues that put them at increased risk of homelessness, and
3. Specific services for women veterans, such as treatment for physical and sexual trauma and child care for dependent children (North and Smith, 1993; Wenzel et al., 2000).

A more comprehensive range of services was identified by nearly 20,000 consumers and providers of homeless services who were surveyed by the VA (Kuhn and Nakashima, 2010). The consumer sample consisted of three groups of homeless veterans: those who are homeless, those in transitional housing, and those in permanent housing. The top 10 list of needs varies among the three types of homeless veterans and the providers, but there are many overlapping service needs, such as long-term permanent housing, welfare payments, child care, dental care, job training, and legal assistance (Table 7.3).

**TABLE 7.3** Top 10 Unmet Needs Perceived by Veteran Consumer Respondents and Providers, FY 2010

| | Veterans Literally Homeless | Veterans in Transitional Housing | Veterans in Permanent Housing | Providers |
|---|---|---|---|---|
| 1. | Long-term permanent housing | Welfare payments | Dental care | Child care |
| 2. | Welfare payments | Child care | Legal assistance for child-support issues | Legal assistance for child-support issues |
| 3. | Dental care | Legal assistance for child-support issues | Welfare payments | Legal assistance for outstanding warrants and/or fines |
| 4. | Guardianship (financial) | Family reconciliation assistance | Child care | Family reconciliation assistance |
| 5. | Legal assistance for child-support issues | Guardianship (financial) | Legal assistance for outstanding warrants and/or fines | Legal assistance to help restore driver's license |
| 6. | Job training | SSI/SSD process | Family reconciliation assistance | Credit counseling |
| 7. | Legal assistance for outstanding warrants/ fines | Long-term permanent housing | Credit counseling | Long-term permanent housing |
| 8. | SSI/SSD Process | Legal assistance for outstanding warrants and/or fines | Reentry services for incarcerated veterans | Dental care |
| 9. | Family reconciliation assistance | Discharge upgrade | Legal assistance to help restore driver's license | Help managing money |
| 10. | Job finding | Women's health care | Job training | Guardianship (financial) |

SOURCE: Kuhn and Nakashima, 2010 (adapted from Table 7 on p. 13 and Table 8 on p. 17).

The VA survey was conducted by Project CHALENG (Community Homelessness Assessment, Local Education and Networking Groups). Launched in 1994, this VA program is designed to enhance the continuum of care for homeless veterans provided by the local VA and its surrounding community service agencies. The concept behind Project CHALENG is that no single agency is capable of providing the full spectrum of services required to reduce homelessness. Project CHALENG enhances coordinated services by bringing the VA together with community agencies and other federal, state, and local governments that provide services to the homeless to raise awareness of homeless veterans' needs and to plan to meet those needs (VA, 2012a).

### Community-Based Homelessness Programs

Communities that strive to provide services to homeless veterans need to be aware of (1) the federal housing and related social service programs sponsored by the VA and other federal agencies and (2) the research on the effectiveness of these programs. To implement their programs, the VA and other federal agencies often enter into contracts with local providers of community-based services.

*Federal Programs and Their Effectiveness*

The VA, HUD, and Department of Labor (DOL) have a number of programs for mitigating homelessness among veterans (Table 7.4; GAO, 2010). One of the most high-profile programs is the VA initiative to end homelessness by 2015. Under this initiative, community organizations can apply for grants for purposes including the following: to assist homeless veterans in obtaining housing and other federal benefits and to offer them temporary financial assistance toward rent, utility payments, security deposits, and moving costs. The initiative, begun in the summer of 2012, is expected to dispense $100 million to VA programs and community-based service providers nationwide (VA, 2012b). The initiative to end homelessness is affiliated with the joint federal program HUD–VASH, which provides homeless veterans with housing vouchers and VA case-management services. Voucher recipients pay no more than 30% of their income on rent. For FY 2012, Congress appropriated $75 million to the HUD–VASH program, with which HUD–VASH plans to house an additional 11,000 veterans. By the end of FY 2012, HUD–VASH will have issued 49,000 housing vouchers to chronically homeless veterans—80% of the administration's target of 60,000 by 2015 to end chronic homelessness among veterans (National Coalition for Homeless Veterans, 2011).

**TABLE 7.4** Targeted Homelessness Programs for Veterans

| Federal Agency | Program | Description | Funding, FY 2009 ($ in thousands) |
|---|---|---|---|
| VA | Initiative to End Homelessness by 2015 | Make grants to community organizations to provide services to very-low-income veteran families living in, or transitioning to, permanent housing | $100,000 |
| HUD–VA | HUD- and VA-Supported Housing (HUD–VASH) | Provide subsidized housing and services for homeless veterans | (HUD) $75,000<br>(VA) $54,218 |
| VA | Healthcare for Homeless Veterans | Perform outreach to identify homeless veterans for VA services and assist them in accessing appropriate health-care and benefits | $80,219 |
| | Compensated Work Therapy Transitional Residence Program | Provide vocational opportunities in residential setting for veterans recovering from chronic mental illness, chemical dependency, and homelessness | $22,206 |
| | Homeless Providers Grants and per Diem Program | Promote the development and provision of supportive housing and supportive services to help homeless veterans achieve residential stability, increase skill levels, and obtain greater self-determination | $130,000 |
| | Domiciliary Care for Homeless Veterans | Provide services to economically disadvantaged veterans | $98,789 |
| | Loan Guarantee for Transitional Housing for Homeless Veterans | Increase the amount of housing available, and provide services | $45 |

| Federal Agency | Program | Description | Funding, FY 2009 ($ in thousands) |
|---|---|---|---|
| | Supportive Services for Veteran Families | Provide supportive services to very-low-income veteran families in or transitioning to permanent housing | $218 |
| DOL | Homeless Veterans Reintegration Program | Provide services to assist in reintegrating homeless veterans into meaningful employment and stimulate the development of effective service delivery systems to address problems facing homeless veterans | $26,330 |

SOURCE: GAO, 2010.

*Research on the Efficacy of the Housing and Urban Development–Veterans Affairs Supportive Housing (HUD–VASH) Program*

Researchers have studied the cost-effectiveness of HUD–VASH housing programs for veterans (Rosenheck et al., 2003). During a 3-year prospective study, the authors compared the cost-effectiveness of three different housing programs for veterans. Study participants included a total of 460 veterans: 107 veterans in San Francisco, California; 165 veterans in New Orleans, Louisiana; 91 veterans in San Diego, California; and 97 veterans in Cleveland, Ohio. Eligible veterans had to have been homeless at enrollment for 1 month or longer and had to have received a major psychiatric diagnosis (schizophrenia, bipolar disorder, major affective disorder, or posttraumatic stress disorder) or a substance-abuse disorder diagnosis. Participants were randomly assigned to one of three programs: (1) HUD–VASH, which included case management plus Section 8 housing vouchers[2] (n = 182), (2) case management without special access to Section 8 vouchers (n = 90), or (3) standard VA homeless services (n = 188). Researchers followed up with participants every 3 months for 3 years in order to ascertain housing outcomes and the cost-effectiveness of supported housing.

Overall, the HUD–VASH participants had 36.2% fewer homeless days than those experienced by the standard treatment group and 35.8% fewer homeless days than those experienced by the case-management group. The case-management group was not significantly different from the standard treatment group. Veterans in the HUD–VASH program reported greater satisfaction with housing and reported fewer problems than were reported by the other groups. HUD–VASH participants also reported larger social networks and better relationships with family and friends. Researchers calculated cost-effectiveness acceptability curves which illustrate that the benefits outweigh the costs, depending on the societal value of a day of housing. If a day of housing is valued at $50, the researchers calculated a 56% probability that the benefits outweigh the costs. The probability goes up to 80% if a day of housing is worth $75.

---

[2]Section 8 housing vouchers are so named by virtue of the authorizing legislation: Section 8 of the Housing Act of 1937 (42 U.S.C. § 1437f). The law allows voucher recipients to choose any housing that meets the requirements of the program and is not limited to units located in subsidized housing projects. The administration of the housing vouchers is accomplished locally by public housing agencies. These agencies receive federal funds from the U.S. Department of Housing and Urban Development. See http://portal.hud.gov/hudportal/HUD?src=/topics/housing_choice_voucher_program_section_8 (accessed July 20, 2012).

If it is worth $100, then the probability of benefits exceeding costs is 92%; it is 97% if housing is worth more than $125 (Rosenheck et al., 2003).

O'Connell et al. (2010) conducted a 5-year longitudinal study that examined the housing and care provided to HUD–VASH participants. The study was a real-world analysis as opposed to the clinical trial of Rosenheck et al. (2003). HUD and local housing authorities, between 1992 and 2006, handed out more than 4,000 Section 8 vouchers to HUD–VASH participants. The VA, in turn, provided case management for the delivery of health and social services. O'Connell et al. studied 2,925 (71%) of the 4,125 veteran participants in the HUD–VASH program between August 1992 and July 2006. Most were recruited through the Health Care for Homeless Veterans (HCHV) program. About one-third of participants were homeless 1–6 months before they enrolled in the program, and nearly 20% had been homeless for 2 or more years. The investigators found that entry into the program was slow, taking an average of 161 days (Standard deviation [SD] = 213 days) after initial intake. Eighty-two percent of the sample was housed through HUD–VASH, and housing lasted 2.6 years, but not the 5 years advertised by the program. Only a small fraction of participants received rehabilitation (6%) or employment (17%) services. The investigators concluded that housing programs did not adhere to the stated aims of the program, either because of implementation failure or because the needs and preferences of veterans differed from those suggested by the program.

**Residential Treatment Programs**

McGuire et al. (2010) studied homeless veterans who participated in residential treatment programs of three different types. The authors sought to determine which type of program was responsible for housing and several other outcomes 1 year after the time-limited program ended. Three forms of residential care services, funded by the VA, were available:

1. Health Care for Homeless Veterans, which utilizes locally contracted halfway-house and substance-abuse treatment programs to provide residentially based treatment;
2. Grant and Per Diem (G&PD) program, which provides services and housing per diem payments to community-based grant recipients that also work with local VA medical centers to provide physical- and mental-health services; and
3. Domiciliary Care for Homeless Veterans (DCHV) program, which provides physical- and mental-health treatment, substance-abuse treatment, and sobriety maintenance, rehabilitation services, and work-for-pay programs at 35 locations, mostly at VA medical centers.

Nearly all 1,003 participants in the McGuire et al. (2010) study reported substance-use problems, a mental-health problem, or a serious medical condition, in addition to homelessness. One year after the residential treatment program ended, the investigators found improvement across eight outcome measures, including income, mental and physical health, quality of life, and independent housing. The outcomes did not differ by program type or diagnosis. Across each of the three programs evaluated, roughly 78% of all participants maintained housing at the 12-month followup. The investigators concluded that the benefits of the three programs were substantial. The type of program and diagnoses of participants had no differential impact on the salutary outcomes; the only factor that emerged as a positive predictor of program efficacy was length of stay. The longer the stay in the residential program, the stronger the gains were 1 year later. In other words, all three program types succeeded in improving the health and housing status of homeless veterans, with the greatest effects being tied not to program type but rather to length of stay.

### Employment Assistance for Homeless Veterans

The Homeless Veterans Reintegration Program (HVRP) is the only federal program that provides dedicated employment assistance to homeless veterans (National Coalition for Homeless Veterans, 2008). The program serves veterans who are ineligible for other assistance programs because of severe PTSD, long histories of substance abuse, serious mental-health problems, legal problems, and other health issues. Veterans with these issues require more rigorous attention and counseling to prepare them for the workforce than most employment programs other than HVRP can provide. After the emergency needs (shelter, food, substance-use treatment) of the veteran are met, HRVP assists in the finding and sustaining of employment for homeless veterans. The program then allocates the funding to community-based organizations and government agencies to provide job training, employment services, and other support. In 2007, 16,000 homeless veterans received these services through the program. In 2006, HRVP reported a 72.8% job-placement success rate. In 2007, the Government Accountability Office (GAO) named HRVP one of the most effective veteran homeless assistance programs in the country (National Coalition for Homeless Veterans, 2008).

## Community-Based Mental-Health Care

Although the VA and the Department of Defense (DOD) provide a significant amount of mental-health care to returning service members, those agencies' eligibility rules or limited capacity leave many service members and families with unmet needs for mental- and physical-health care. Communities often seek to fill such gaps by funding services of their own or by obtaining grant and contract funds from federal and state agencies to fund community-based services.

### Federal Programs

Although the DOD and the Veterans Health Administration (VHA; a component of the VA) are the primary sources of physical- and mental-health care for veterans and active-duty personnel, veterans and active-duty personnel have the option of receiving outside care if they are unable to access needed services. The VA and DOD contract with a myriad of community-based providers, but there is no central inventory of such providers that receive funding.

Apart from the VA and DOD, no other federal programs are dedicated to funding physical- and mental-health care for veterans. However, some federal grant programs are encouraged for use by veterans. One pertinent example is Access to Recovery, a $379 million discretionary grant program administered by the Substance Abuse and Mental Health Services Administration (HHS and SAMHSA, 2010). Grant recipients at the local level, which are often community-based service providers, distribute vouchers for substance-abuse treatment and recovery services. The latter includes family services (including marriage education, parenting, and child-development services), employment services, transportation, housing support, relapse prevention, and self-help and support groups. The vouchers can be used to obtain any kind of eligible care from any service provider in the community. Even though the program is not explicitly for veterans, grantees are encouraged to place special emphasis on directing vouchers to veterans.

**Colocation of Health Services for Homeless Veterans**

In the 1990s, service fragmentation was recognized as a barrier to care in the VA Greater Los Angeles Healthcare System (GLA) (Blue-Howells et al., 2008). Before improvements to the program, GLA services were housed in several different buildings, requiring veterans (homeless and otherwise) to make multiple appointments and trips to receive all of the services (housing, mental health, ambulatory care) that were provided. Under this fragmented system, wait times of several months were typical, for both specialty and routine care. The wait time led to severe service underutilization, especially among the homeless with severe medical or cognitive disabilities. Based on a model at the West Haven, Connecticut, VA facility that consolidated physical- and mental-health services into one location (Druss et al., 2001), the VA funded a plan to integrate services for homeless veterans within a single building. Local funds were also used to finance the project.

The GLA designed the clinic, which opened in July 2002, to be a "one-stop shop" for VA services (Blue-Howells et al., 2008). When a veteran first arrives at the facility, he or she is assessed by the Access Center (intake office), which directs the patient to the appropriate providers that same day. Primary care, mental-health, substance-abuse, and housing services are offered. A monitoring and evaluation program was in place to help address any need for program adjustments.

For homeless veterans requiring specialty services (optometry or dentistry, for example) that operate outside the new integrated system, the GLA program established a system enabling homeless veterans to fill same-day cancellations and "no-shows" at the specialty clinics. This arrangement helps to ensure that veterans receive same-day service even when they require specialized attention. By 2007, some staff restructuring adjustments aside, the program was mostly unchanged from what it had been at its initial launch. Partially based on its success, the VA continues to mandate integrated mental-health and primary care for VA medical centers servicing 10,000 unique veterans or more (VA, 2008).

**State Programs**

In recognition of barriers to the accessing of services, several states have taken the initiative to offer community-based services by entering into contracts with local providers. Washington state offers free PTSD counseling services through contracts with community-based providers (Washington State VA, 2012). One of the unique components of this arrangement is to educate teachers and school counselors with respect to the potential needs of school-age children of war-exposed parents. The State of New York offers mental-health screening and a host of other services under its New York National Guard Yellow Ribbon Reintegration program (State of New York, 2012). Colorado has established the Civilians for Veterans Fund, which offers free community-based mental-health and substance-abuse services (Colorado Behavioral Healthcare Council, 2012). California has a well-developed portal for providing veterans' services, ranging from suicide prevention to treatment and recovery (California Department of Mental Health, 2012). It has an inventory of county-based offices where veterans can obtain care. Maryland has forged a Maryland Veterans Resilience Initiative, the purpose of which is to identify gaps in veterans' services and to train mental-health professionals, primary care doctors, and clergy to deal with veterans' unique needs (University of Maryland School of Public Health, 2012). The Maryland initiative is also tasked with developing peer-support networks to help veterans reintegrate into civilian life. Other states might sponsor programs, but there is no central inventory of them.

## Veterans and the Criminal Justice System

### Demographics

There is a dearth of information regarding crime, incarceration rates, and risk factors expressly for OEF and OIF veterans. The only study that included information on OEF and OIF veterans found that they constituted only 4% of the entire veteran population in federal and state prisons in 2004 (Noonan and Mumola, 2007). Overall, in that same year, there were about 140,000 veterans in federal and state prisons, according to the Bureau of Justice Statistics (Noonan and Mumola, 2007). The bureau reports that the age-adjusted incarceration rate for veterans was about 10% lower than that in nonveterans in 2004 (1,253 per 100,000 vs 1,390 per 100,000, respectively). Veterans were, however, more likely to be serving sentences for violent or sexual crimes and more likely to victimize women or minors than were the nonveteran prisoners. Of incarcerated veterans in state prisons, 57% committed violent crimes, compared with 47% of incarcerated nonveterans (Noonan and Mumola, 2007).

One of the risk factors for incarceration among Vietnam veterans is combat exposure. Egendorf et al. (1981) found that 24% of those over age 23 with heavy combat exposure were arrested after service, compared with 10% of veterans with light or no combat exposure and 14% of comparable nonveterans. Other risk factors for incarceration include homelessness, mental illness, substance-use disorder, being a member of a minority group, and not being married (Balshem et al., 2011; Noonan and Mumola, 2007). These risk factors also apply to the general population (Hawthorne et al., 2012). One difference, however, is that veterans, most typically Vietnam veterans, are likely to be older than their nonveteran counterparts in jails and prisons (Greenberg and Rosenheck, 2011; Noonan and Mumola, 2007).

### Needs for Services in the Criminal Justice System

Although veterans are not overrepresented in the criminal justice system relative to their representation in the general population, the US Center for Mental Health Services (CMHS) recognized the importance of satisfying unmet mental-health needs of combat veterans in the criminal justice system. Through one of its programs, in 2008 CMHS convened a consensus panel made up of 30 participants—representing community health providers, law enforcement, the courts, veteran service organizations (VSOs), veterans' health programs, and federal agencies—to develop recommendations for criminal justice and community-based mental-health systems to connect justice-involved combat veterans with mental-health services (CMHS National GAINS Center, 2008). The five major recommendations of this group are as follows:

1. Screen for military service and traumatic experience (use an existing instrument).
2. Train law enforcement, probation and parole, and corrections officers to identify signs of combat-related trauma and the role of adaptive behaviors in justice-system involvement. Although such training is already occurring in some locations, it should be expanded.
3. Help connect veterans to VHA health care services for which they are eligible, either through a community-based benefits specialist or a transition planner, the VA's OEF and OIF coordinators, or through a local Vet Center.
4. Expand community-based veteran-specific peer-supported services.

5. Beyond meeting mental-health needs, service providers should be ready to meet substance-use, physical-health, employment, and housing needs. Because many of these conditions are co-occurring, comprehensive services should be available.

*Veterans Treatment Courts*

Veterans Treatment Courts (VTCs) are modeled after drug and mental-health treatment courts that emerged in the US judicial system in the 1990s. These courts, typically geared for lower-level criminal offenses, offer mandatory mental-health and substance-use treatment in lieu of incarceration (Clark et al., 2010). The courts, in other words, treat veterans not as criminals in need of punishment but rather as patients in need of treatment and rehabilitation. Defendants are closely monitored and held accountable for their continued treatment and sobriety (Office of National Drug Control Policy, 2010). There are currently at least 95 VTCs in 30 states (Justice for Vets, 2012). Funding for some of them comes from the Substance Abuse and Mental Health Services Administration, which seeks to address the behavioral-health service needs of justice-involved veterans.

The VA offers its full range of services to eligible veterans in VTCs (Holt, 2011). These include inpatient and outpatient treatment services and mental-health and substance-use treatment. This arrangement allows a veteran in a VTC to access his or her court-supervised treatment plan through a single point of service. Although the VA's involvement varies depending on the jurisdiction, the VA typically works with the court to develop a court-approved treatment plan for the offender. In nearly all operating VTCs, VA staff is present during proceedings. Veteran eligibility for consideration in a VTC varies by jurisdiction; most VTCs consider all individuals with prior military service, but a few only see defendants eligible for VHA services. Some require a specific mental-health or substance-use-disorder diagnosis, and some require the diagnosis to be linked to the veteran's military service.

VTCs vary regarding the types of charges that they will hear. Some courts, for example, will only hear misdemeanors, whereas others will hear certain felony charges. Some will hear only nonviolent charges, but others will consider certain violent charges, such as assault. Some states have legislatively mandated the eligibility criteria that the VTC must follow. In other states, courts often review defendants on a case-by-case basis when no laws have dictated the type of charge that triggers referral to a VTC.

Several states have passed legislation that either encourages or requires their judicial systems to establish VTCs. States and communities with preexisting drug treatment courts have led the charge. Federal legislation (111th Congress, S. 902) introduced to create a grant program to fund VTCs died in committee in 2009. The legislation would have required all federally funded VTCs to assign a veteran peer mentor for each defendant. It also would have barred from VTCs violent offenders or offenders with prior convictions for violent crimes.

Because VTCs are relatively new, studies have yet to examine their effectiveness in treating veterans and reducing or preventing recidivism. But the evidence is strong that comparable civilian programs are effective. Huddleston et al. (2008) examined drug courts (not specifically for veterans) in the United States in 2008. The authors reported that individuals who participate in drug courts are re-arrested at a lower rate than the rate of re-arrest of those that have committed similar offenses but proceed through traditional criminal courts. Additionally, drug courts were found to be more cost-effective than the traditional judicial process for drug offenders, saving $4,700–$11,000 per defendant that might otherwise have been spent on future judicial proceedings and law-enforcement efforts. A related finding by McNiel and Binder (2007) pointed to salutary effects of mental-health courts: they lower the rates of recidivism and violence by individuals with mental illness.

**Care After Release from Prison**

Because of a constellation of social and legal barriers to reintegration, veterans released from prison are at high risk for homelessness (Balshem et al., 2011). Homeless veterans are, in turn, at increased risk for recidivism as a result of engaging in such activities as theft and prostitution to survive on the street. The authors note that there has yet to be widespread awareness of this problem, but, as described below, one administrative change has already occurred.

The VA has found that when veterans are released from transitional housing or halfway houses after incarceration, they become ineligible for the medical care that they need, which can often lead to homelessness. An administrative change announced in the Federal Register authorizes the VA to provide outpatient and hospital care to veterans recently released from prison and enrolled in a temporary housing program (VA, 2011). The VA is permitted to work with the veterans after they are released from the temporary housing program in an effort to prevent them from becoming homeless. This changes a previous rule that barred the VA from providing "hospital and outpatient care for a veteran who is either a patient or inmate in an institution of another government agency if that agency has a duty to give the care or services" (17.38(c)(5)).

## Summary of the Review of Existing Literature

In summary, the existing literature is sparse on the effects of OEF and OIF deployments on communities. However, by examining the limited literature on OEF and OIF deployments and other surrogate markers, the committee finds significant economic losses to communities that deploy a relatively high concentration of service members. The most adverse effects of these deployments are borne by small businesses that lose essential employees, businesses that rely on employees with highly specialized skills, and self-employed businesses owned by reservists. Homelessness has been identified as an area that affects veterans and communities. Homeless and low-income veterans need a supply of permanent and supportive housing; recently returned veterans need adequate transition assistance to help identify and mitigate issues that put them at increased risk of homelessness; and women veterans need specific services, such as treatment for physical and sexual trauma and child care for dependent children. Communities also must address the mental-health issues that affect returning veterans and seek to fill gaps in the available services by funding services of their own or by obtaining grant and contract funds from federal and state agencies to fund community-based services. Finally, incarceration of returning service members is another area of concern for communities. Although there are very limited data on incarceration, one study noted that OEF and OIF veterans constituted only 4% of the entire veteran population in federal and state prisons in 2004; the age-adjusted incarceration rate for veterans was about 10% lower than that in nonveterans in 2004. Veterans released from prison are at high risk for homelessness.

## ETHNOGRAPHIC ASSESSMENT

As noted in Chapter 2, ethnographic assessments were undertaken in an effort to gain an understanding of the effects of deployments on communities. The committee directed Westat to conduct ethnographic research in six military-dense communities to determine the ways in which multiple deployments have interacted with five community domains:

- The economy, including overall commerce, housing, and labor;
- Information and communication about deployments and available resources;
- Community health;
- Formal services and supports in the community ("community competence"); and
- Informal services and supports ("social capital").

Additionally, the committee sought information about areas of continued need within each community, and Westat study teams solicited from community members suggestions of additional supports and services for mitigating the effects of multiple deployments (see Chapter 2).

### Description of the Study Site Communities

The primary basis for the selection of study sites was that a community had to have experienced multiple deployments of service members in support of the wars in OEF and OIF. Additional factors taken into consideration included the size of the community (which needed to be small enough to accommodate a 1-week ethnographic visit) and the study's objective that the sites selected represent diverse geographic regions of the country. The locations of the six sites[3] selected for the study are depicted in Figure 7.1.

The six study sites vary significantly in population size: Little Falls, Minnesota, and Georgetown, South Carolina—which are the two National Guard sites—have the smallest populations, at approximately 8,400 and 9,000, respectively. Of the active-duty sites, the one with the smallest population is Watertown, New York (27,000); followed by Lacey, Washington (42,000); Lakewood, Washington (58,000); and Jacksonville, North Carolina, which has slightly more than 70,000 residents. By far the largest study site is El Paso, Texas, which has an estimated 650,000 residents. As a whole, El Paso is too large to accommodate a 1-week site visit, but telephone calls made to key informants prior to the visit indicated that the two districts (Districts 2 and 4) adjacent to Fort Bliss, Texas, are the areas of El Paso that are most affected by military processes. Those districts were the focus of the study team's visit; each of them contains approximately 81,000 residents (Ramirez, 2012).

The sites also show some demographic variability, as indicated in Figure 7.2.

Four of the communities have a majority white population, but with some racial and ethnic diversity. Of note, however, are El Paso, in which 80% of the residents self-identify as

[3]Although "six sites" are referred to throughout the report, the study teams explored two communities in Washington. Unless otherwise indicated, Lakewood and Lacey, Washington, will be combined in this report as a single site. For descriptions about the ways in which these two communities differ from each other, please see Appendix E.

Hispanic; Georgetown, South Carolina, where 58% of community residents are African American; and Little Falls, Minnesota, in which 96% of the residents are white.

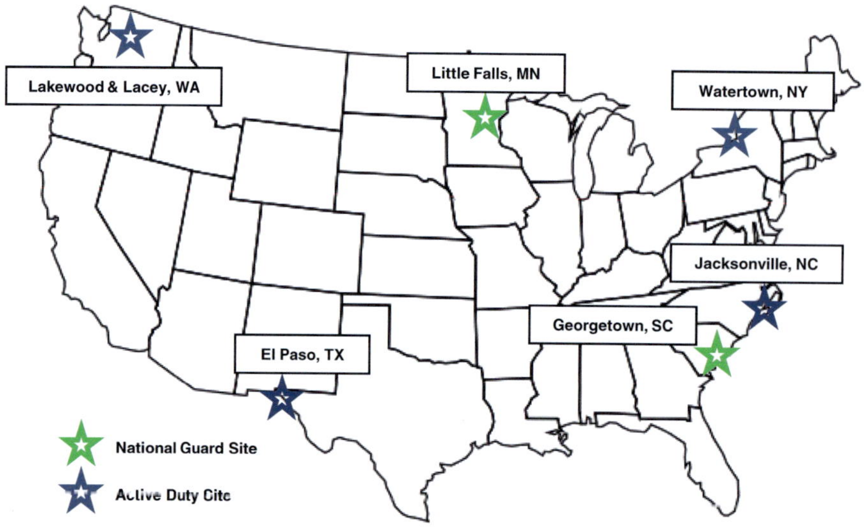


**FIGURE 7.1** Geographic locations of the six study sites.

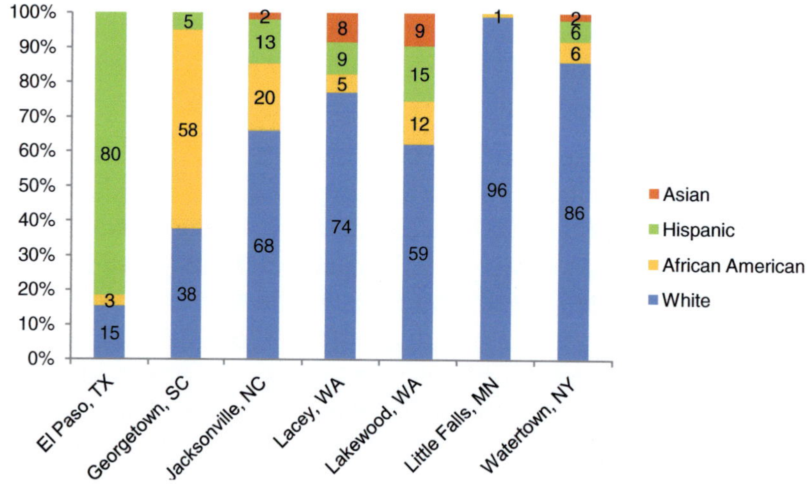


**FIGURE 7.2** Race and Hispanic ethnicity, by study site.

Georgetown, which has only a local National Guard armory rather than a nearby military installation, reportedly has experienced no economic boost from the presence of the military. Key employers include the Georgetown county government, the local hospital, and the International Paper plant that is located on the southern edge of town. As discussed throughout this section, this South Carolina community is an outlier, which might be the result of the absence of a nearby military installation.

Interviewees in the five communities with nearby installations, however, said that the military is an important economic contributor to their regions. That was particularly noticeable in Little Falls, Watertown, and Jacksonville, where the military is the key economic driver.

Although there are numerous economic engines in the state of Washington and in El Paso, both Fort Bliss in Texas and Joint Base Lewis-McChord (JBLM) in Washington have gained local economic prominence in recent years because of net gains resulting from the Base Realignment and Closure (BRAC) process.

The Army has deployed the greatest number of service members in support of OEF and OIF, and the Army was represented in five of the six study sites: Fort Drum (New York), Camp Ripley (Minnesota), Fort Bliss (Texas), Joint Base Lewis-McChord (formerly Fort Lewis; Washington), and the National Guard unit in Georgetown (South Carolina). The Air Force was represented at both Camp Ripley (Air National Guard unit) and Joint Base Lewis-McChord (formerly Airbase McChord). The Marines are represented by Camp LeJeune (North Carolina), one of only a few Marine training installations in the country.

All five installations that are nearby five of the study sites are very active military bases that have experienced large-scale troop movements since OIF began in 2003. Because OEF began in the fall of 2001, OIF opened up a second combat theater, requiring a greater number of active-duty service members. In Georgetown, the local National Guard unit saw its first deployment to OIF in 2004. At the other sites, interviewees reported noticing an increase in activity starting around 2005.

### Relationship Between Communities and the Military

As noted previously, the military is an important economic contributor to each of the five communities located near a military installation. In many respects, the local economies have been shielded from the recession as a result both of the activity associated with war being waged on two fronts and of the two installations benefiting from the BRAC process. One unanticipated characteristic shared by all of the communities, however, is the extent to which the towns have a military identity. At all six sites, interviewees repeatedly described their communities as "military towns" and pointed to the rich military history in their respective regions. Citizens of these communities pay attention to military issues and to their neighbors' service to the country, thus creating a context in which service members and their families can feel understood and appreciated. Equally important, at five of the sites, the civilian "side" of the community has a long-standing symbiotic relationship with the nearby military installation and has learned to adjust to the installation's ever-changing dynamics,[4] including the multiple deployments associated with the wars in Iraq and Afghanistan. Although all six study sites have been affected by multiple deployments to some degree, each town's support for the military might have helped mitigate some of the potential effects of these deployments. It is possible that such effects might be more pronounced in communities in which military ties are not so strong.

### Findings of the Ethnographic Assessment

Overall, it was difficult to ascertain the degree to which multiple deployments have had an effect on the economies of the six study sites. Interviewees from these communities frequently talked about local economic *growth* resulting from expansion of the military

---

[4]One might view a university town as an interesting point of comparison and contrast. In an academic community, citizens are likely to be attuned to and conversant about the accomplishments of the school's athletic teams or faculty (such as a winner of the Nobel Prize in literature). The town will also have long since adapted itself to the annual rhythms of students coming and going.

installations generally, and there was some talk of a *shift from home ownership to apartment rentals* because so many service members were increasingly single, young, and mobile. But when pressed, interviewees were unable to tie either of those community trends to multiple deployments. The exception to that pattern was Little Falls, Minnesota, where interviewees suggested that multiple deployments were taking a toll on local family-owned and family-operated small businesses. Interviewees in Georgetown, South Carolina, talked about the effects of deployments on small businesses or agencies (such as fire and police departments), but they described the deployments as an "inconvenience" rather than as events resulting in long-term adverse consequences for the employers. In two of the four active-duty locations, interviewees did not identify any major effects on the labor force from multiple deployments. In El Paso and Washington, however, interviewees reported efforts by the local military installations to increase on-base mental-health-service capacity in response to the demand resulting from multiple deployments. In both of those locations, community members said that the installation was actively and successfully recruiting mental-health providers to work on base, thus diminishing the supply of providers available to meet community needs.

In terms of information and communication, community-level discussions about the military are quite common, a not unexpected finding given the military orientation of the study site towns. However, interviewees expressed a need for a more *formal* flow of information from the military to the civilian community about troop deployments and reintegration. In the five sites with installations nearby, communication about resources for service members and their families reportedly occurred through both formal and informal, word-of-mouth channels. In Georgetown, interviewees said that although formal communication about resources had "improved" between the local unit's first and second deployments, additional steps could be taken to ensure that information, particularly about military benefits, is more readily available to National Guard members and their families.

Mental-health concerns were a primary topic of conversation with interviewees at the five installation sites.[5] First, residents and behavioral-health providers alike said that they worried about service members who have been deployed multiple times returning home with posttraumatic stress disorder and other behavioral-health issues such as drug and alcohol abuse. This was a particular concern in Washington, where a couple of negative high-profile events focused media attention on PTSD among service members at JBLM. Similar concerns about increasing violence were expressed by community members in Jacksonville, North Carolina. Community members at the other sites mentioned isolated disturbing incidents, but their major concerns were about increased substance use by service members and an increase in drunk- and reckless-driving accidents. Consequently, interviewees perceived the need for additional services and supports for service members who are currently struggling with the stresses of multiple deployments and for individuals whose stress responses might be delayed by months, or even years, postdeployment. Community-based providers also emphasized the importance of increasing community service capacity because of service members' reluctance to seek help on the installation, where the information might get back to their commands, and because of a perception that such information could jeopardize service members' careers.

---

[5]Georgetown community members acknowledged that many of the local National Guard members had returned home with symptoms of PTSD, but none of the interviewees perceived the symptoms to have risen to a level of community concern.

A second and related issue raised by interviewees at the five installation sites was their expressed concern about the spouses and children of service members who have been deployed multiple times. They noted that the steady pace of deployment and reintegration can exact a toll on young families, creating stress on the nondeployed spouses and potential attachment issues among the children. Interviewees noted the need for additional mental-health services for young people to help them cope with the strains of having a parent—or parents—deployed multiple times.

Findings with respect to supports and social services were consistent across the sites. Behavioral-health services, although available at all six sites, were widely described as being insufficient to meet the needs of civilians, much less military-affiliated individuals. In Georgetown, South Carolina, for example, interviewees reported that there were virtually no private-sector mental-health providers in town. Moreover, state budget cuts were said to have put an enormous strain on county services, resulting in more stringent eligibility criteria. In El Paso, the service-delivery system was struggling to address the trauma of women and children fleeing the drug violence in Juarez, Mexico, yet interviewees expressed significant concerns about the mental health of military youth. With reportedly only one child psychiatrist in town, the system was already stretched to capacity. Both Little Falls, Minnesota, and Georgetown, South Carolina, have community hospitals, but neither has any dedicated emergency psychiatric beds. Individuals in crisis must be held in the hospitals' emergency rooms (reportedly up to a couple of days) until an inpatient slot opens up elsewhere in these states. And, as indicated previously, interviewees both in Washington and in El Paso reported a move by the military to increase mental-health service capacity on the installation, but at the expense of the community. Because the military can offer much higher salaries than those offered by community-based providers, clinicians reportedly were leaving their community positions for the better-paying government civilian jobs serving the military.

Finally, at all sites, interviewees said that not only are the local systems insufficient at the present time, but that they are also unprepared to handle any delayed onset of symptoms associated with multiple deployments. The interviewees worried about various issues—about the possibility that service members might develop symptoms of PTSD some years after their combat experience; about families, whose struggles with multiple deployments might finally take a toll on marriages; and about children, who might have dealt with a parent's—or parents'—deployments by detaching, a coping mechanism that many believed might have long-term effects on those youths' ability to form healthy relationships.

Despite challenges to the formal service-delivery systems, informal services and supports were quite robust at all of the study sites. Examples of such supports include face-to-face and online peer supports, services provided through the faith community (including faith-based counseling), military discounts offered by local businesses, neighbors helping neighbors, and family members pitching in to assist a nondeployed spouse. Those bonds appeared particularly strong in the smallest communities (Little Falls, Georgetown, and Watertown), but they were also widely present in the three other self-declared "military towns." The following sections provide more detailed information about each of the five areas targeted for study, including economic health, information and communication, community health, formal services and supports in the community (community competence), and informal services and supports (social capital).

**Economic Health**

The measures of economic health studied include general commerce, housing, and the labor market.

*General Commerce*

It did not appear that multiple deployments had had large-scale economic effects on the communities at the six sites visited. In the four active-duty sites, interviewees described economies that were reasonably robust—infrastructure was growing and new businesses were being created. In El Paso and in Washington, the growth had been spurred by BRAC; in Watertown, New York, and Jacksonville, North Carolina, interviewees said that the changes were related to a sheer increase in the number of active-duty service members and their families coming into the communities. In any event, they believed, the growth had masked any potential financial effects of multiple deployments.

An additional factor that likely has mitigated the effects of multiple deployments is the civilian–military partnership that has been established in all four communities, partly as a result of lessons learned from previous military conflicts. In Jacksonville during the First Gulf War, for example, the town experienced a substantial drop in its population when military spouses and their children left to return to their families of origin for support during deployments. One city official said:

> In the first Gulf War . . . a lot of people broke their leases because they thought that war was going to be an incredibly long period of time . . . they picked up and went back home to be with their loved ones.

In an effort to prevent this type of flight from recurring, in 2003 the Onslow County (North Carolina) Chamber of Commerce put in place an innovative program called Project CARE (Jacksonville-Onslow Chamber of Commerce, 2012). That program, which has been activated several times since 2003, combines the efforts of various local government, military, Chamber of Commerce, and community organizations to provide support to families of deployed service members, assist businesses in dealing with the deployments, and increase community spirit toward the troops. Project CARE was cited by many interviewees as a successful strategy for mitigating the potential negative effects of multiple deployments:

> I think the community as a whole . . . made it important to let the dependents know during the second Gulf War that they could stay here, that people in the community cared about them and were going to take care of them. It made a very big difference. Jacksonville certainly didn't clear out. [City official]

That intervention has helped create a social and economic stability in Jacksonville throughout the OEF and OIF engagements. The El Paso Chamber of Commerce has similarly worked to stem the outflow of military families during a large deployment. A local business leader explained:

> It used to be where we would see a deployment, then we would feel the impact because the families would go home and so all of a sudden the grocery stores weren't as busy, clothing stores, the shopping centers . . . we don't see that so much anymore because a lot of families stay here. . . . Part of the reason for that is

> the community is extremely welcoming. Soldiers with families who actively engage in the community, they see a genuine, a sincere approach towards, "You're part of our community and you're welcome here and we want to support you."

The El Paso Chamber of Commerce has an Armed Services Division that serves as the liaison between Fort Bliss and the business community. In addition, the garrison commander attends the monthly Chamber of Commerce meetings and discusses any needs of the installation or its constituents. Although BRAC-related growth has perhaps overshadowed the effects of this partnership, community leaders anticipate that the relationship will curtail any potential deployment-related instability affecting the city in the future.

In Washington, the South Sound Military and Communities Partnership (SSMCP) was established in an effort to coordinate growth and planning between Lakewood and Joint Base Lewis-McChord. Although the SSMCP was intended to identify a broad scale of community needs related to growth at JBLM, lessons learned from the needs assessment and the resulting action plans have helped to mitigate the impacts of multiple deployments on this region. In Watertown, New York, the community has formed two nonprofit organizations to identify and address military–civilian challenges: the Fort Drum Regional Liaison Organization (FDRLO), which grew out of a committee formed in the 1980s and addresses community planning in general and any specific issues as they arise; and the Fort Drum Regional Health Planning Organization (FDRHPO), which focuses on meeting physical- and behavioral-health needs of Fort Drum soldiers and their families. The boards of both organizations represent the local civilian and military communities.

All four partnerships described above reflect not only the civilian communities' commitment to the military, but also their desire for service members and their families to see themselves as part of the larger civilian community. When these efforts are successful, spouses of deployed service members will view the community as "home," thus mitigating the potential economic effects of a large exodus of community members.

No large-scale economic effects were reported in the two National Guard sites of Little Falls, Minnesota, and Georgetown, South Carolina; however, the limited opportunity afforded by the local economies appeared to contribute to National Guard members' volunteering to go on additional deployments. Limited local employment opportunities and low-wage jobs reportedly have prompted some National Guard members to return to active-duty status, in part because of the potential earnings. Thus, although the Georgetown National Guard unit deployed as a unit twice, several members have volunteered for additional deployments with other nearby units.

Some Jacksonville respondents also reported that the economy has contributed to changing the dynamics among military families in that town. Many family members of deployed Marines, they said, have moved to Jacksonville to help the nondeployed spouse because they themselves are unemployed and thus able to relocate:

> We've been seeing a lot of family members relocate here . . . to help them take care of the kids . . . and once they've been here for 3 or 4 months, they start getting into the job market. . . . It's not a short-term thing, it's a long-term thing. [Chamber of Commerce member]

The surplus of local labor reportedly has left many of those relocated family members chronically underemployed, which interviewees said often creates additional strains in the household of the nondeployed spouse. This phenomenon was not mentioned at any of the other study sites.

*Housing*

Overall, it did not appear that multiple deployments had had a noticeable effect on the local housing market at the six sites. Both in Washington and in El Paso, interviewees said that service members had been moving away from owning homes to occupying rental housing, but plausible explanations other than multiple deployments were offered. For instance, many of the incoming service members are young, single males who, interviewees said, are much more likely than are their older counterparts to rent an apartment. Many of the families coming into town are also young and simply lack the capital to invest in a home. The fact that permanent change of station (PCS) rotations might occur every 3 years also discourages home ownership. It is important to note that the national recession might also be playing a significant role in this trend. With banks now tightening up their lending practices, mortgage loans are no longer easy to obtain.

*Labor Market*

There were no obvious markers directly tying multiple deployments and the general labor supply. In Jacksonville, North Carolina, the many families moving into the area were creating a surplus labor situation, but their arrival could not be clearly tied to multiple deployments. At both National Guard sites (Little Falls, Minnesota, and Georgetown, South Carolina), interviewees did talk about how multiple deployments of local National Guard members had affected small businesses or departments. Emergency-services agencies, for example, reported having to adjust their staffing to accommodate the loss of one or two employees, but managers in Georgetown mostly described these adjustments merely as an "inconvenience."

In contrast, some individuals in Little Falls believed that small, family-owned businesses had "taken a hit." One interviewee said, "It's tough, it's really tough, especially in a small town because it's a lot of small businesses." When a business only has a couple of employees, she said, and one or two of them deploy, there is no redundancy to keep the business going. She concluded, "I would say a lot of small companies are closing their doors because of deployments."

**Information and Communication**

Study findings indicate that at all six sites, communities pay great attention to military issues. Local media outlets extensively cover the local military installation or National Guard unit, and community members pay close attention to the wars overseas. Yet, interviewees reported that formal communication about deployments and demobilizations is confined to a few, very specific areas, such as communication with the business community and with local schools. Citizens reported that they often found out about local service members leaving or returning home by word of mouth. Interviewees also offered a mixed assessment of how information about available supports and services is communicated to service members and their families. Although some official channels exist and are used by military-affiliated individuals (for example, Army One Source), interviewees suggested that word of mouth continues to be the most common way for individuals to learn about resources that are available to them. These findings are discussed below.

*The Military as a Topic of Conversation*

In all communities with a military installation nearby, attention is clearly being paid not only to the local installation but also to the military more generally. Jacksonville, North Carolina, and Lacey and Lakewood, Washington, for example, all have statues in town honoring the military and their families; signs have been put up in business windows throughout these communities expressing thanks to the troops; and advertisements for military discounts were seen in business windows and in local newspapers in those communities. And, at all six study sites, substantial coverage appears in the local media, including newspapers (for example, *Jacksonville Daily News, El Paso Times, Watertown Daily Times*) and television news (for example, *Watertown News* and all three El Paso television stations, which covered the presence in town of the Westat study team. These findings are consistent with interviewees' expressed views that "we are a military town." Not only is there a large population of active-duty service members and their families at these locations, but interviewees noted that many retired military members have settled in their communities. This level of attention to the military clearly reflects the composition of the communities as well as the fact that the military is such a strong economic contributor in the study site regions.

*Communication About Deployments and Deployment-Related Issues*

Despite the widespread attention of the study site communities to the military as described above, study findings suggest that, in general, communication about the challenges and needs associated with multiple deployments is occurring only in specific areas (such as commerce and education). Local residents report learning about troop movements either by word of mouth or from local media outlets (such as newspapers and television news). Indeed, Georgetown interviewees reported that for the local National Guard unit's first deployment, the rumor mill outpaced even the local media's efforts to get official confirmation from South Carolina National Guard Headquarters in Columbia. A local newspaper reporter described being puzzled by the reticence of the Headquarters office to confirm news of the deployment: "It's going to be common knowledge amongst the community, so why not [give us information]?"

In the active-duty sites, the lack of timely communications was not described by civilians as being particularly troublesome. At both National Guard sites, however, interviewees said that the lack of information has affected their communities' ability to support their local National Guard members. Citizens in Georgetown reported being wholly unprepared for their local unit's first deployment, indicating that many citizens were even unaware that the deployment was happening. As a result, interviewees said, the community was not prepared to send their citizen soldiers off to war. Improved communications thereafter helped the community come together to welcome service members home from Iraq and, 4 years later, to send them back to the combat theater.

Interviewees in Little Falls described a similar scenario—civilians wanting to engage in community ceremonies honoring the local National Guard unit but being reluctant to do so because they were uncertain about whether the events were "for family members only." Interviewees attributed this uncertainty to weak communication between the National Guard leadership and the broader community and suggested that more open lines of communication would rectify that concern.

*Communication About Deployments with Government and Business Leaders*

As previously described, the economies of five of the six study communities are strongly tied to the local military installation. As a result, ongoing channels of communication have been established between the local business community and the local installation to facilitate joint strategies for addressing any potential adverse effects of multiple deployments. In Jacksonville, North Carolina, for example, city officials and the Chamber of Commerce receive biweekly reports from the installation on the number of Marines to be deployed and the number to return from deployments; they then disseminate that information to aid local businesses in planning. According to one Chamber of Commerce member, those updates "are well received and help our businesses not be taken by surprise by a large influx of people." The Chamber of Commerce in El Paso and that of Watertown, New York, serve as liaison between their respective communities and local installations so as to ensure timely communication of deployment-related information; and the South Sound Military and Communities Partnership serves a similar function between Lakewood, Washington, and JBLM.

*Communication About Deployments with School District Officials*

Strong communication channels also have been established between the local military installations and several of the local school districts. In El Paso, for example, all nine school districts participate in the Fort Bliss Process Action Team together with military leadership and military parents. This team serves as a conduit of information between the community and the installation, addresses questions with changes of command on base, and gives the incoming command information about the school districts and their activities. A school administrator in El Paso offered the following perspective:

> Communication is critical, whether it be what's happening at the school, construction on the base, new families coming in, dates when they anticipate growth to happen, deployments, reintegrations, all those things . . . and we'll continue to accommodate them. . . . We feel like it's part of our community and so we'll continue to work with them.

Such communications channels have been particularly important in both Watertown, New York (Indian River Central School District), and Lakewood, Washington (Clover Park School District), where the public school districts operate the schools located on the installation. One program implemented in schools in Lakewood and Watertown to help those affected by multiple deployments is the Military Family Life Consultants (MFLC) program. Military Family Life Consultants have been trained to address family issues related to multiple deployments confidentially, and they are available to provide information, support, and guidance to all students, parents, teachers, and school staff, regardless of military affiliation. A similar liaison program has been instituted in El Paso; school liaison officers (SLOs) interface with the installation, military families, and the teachers and counselors. The SLOs help school staff understand military culture, notify them about upcoming deployments or returns, and help defuse challenges that arise—for example, when children transition to a new school or their parents are deployed.[6] The school liaison program is regarded as being highly successful and has been adopted by DOD schools in Germany as a best practice.

Despite programs such as those described above and other efforts implemented to help children and schools affected by multiple deployments, several respondents emphasized that more is needed, both in schools and throughout the community. In Watertown, for example, although most large public schools in the area have MFLC programs, the study team was told that parochial schools and smaller school districts either have no MFLCs or too few to address deployment-related issues. And in Washington, the SSMCP report indicated that regional schools are affected negatively by multiple deployments that result in either overburdened or underused classrooms. The report also indicated that district schools receive short notice of population changes that will affect staffing and budgets.

*Communication About Deployments with Law-Enforcement Agencies*

Study results indicate that communication is rare between the military and local law-enforcement agencies regarding the potential behavioral-health effects of multiple deployments. In El Paso, Fort Bliss has worked with the El Paso Police Department to train officers to recognize situations that might have a mental-health component and to try to stabilize potentially explosive situations long enough for the department's crisis-management team to arrive on the scene. Such situations involving the police could range from a traffic citation that might rapidly escalate out of control to a crisis situation, such as a service member who takes someone hostage or threatens to commit suicide. The impetus for the training reportedly stemmed not solely from the department's concerns about the soldiers stationed at Fort Bliss, but also from officers having numerous encounters with traumatized citizens fleeing the drug violence in Juarez. The Westat study team heard from an emergency-services provider about a similar effort to provide needed skills to local law-enforcement officers in Watertown, New York:

> We routinely have meetings between state police, the sheriffs, and myself and military police. When there is a soldier they're worried about, they share that with us. . . . We had a PhD from the Fort Drum Behavioral Science come and talk to a group of 40 people in law enforcement and medical staff about posttraumatic stress . . . to help us basically understand it and to try to defuse it.

Yet not all emergency personnel in Watertown appeared to have the same kind of communication with the installation. One respondent noted:

> I don't have any specific contacts with the military . . . at Drum. And like I said, the only way I know that there's people deployed or people coming home is by watching the news. So we don't get any special bulletin. [Emergency services provider no. 1]

In contrast, another respondent reported regular communication between him and his military counterpart:

---

[6]More information about the El Paso Independent School District Military Family Liaison Program is available at http://www.episd.org/_schools/mil.php?KeepThis=true&TB_iframe=true&height=290&width=350.

> As far as Fort Drum, my interactions with them is sometimes several times a week. . . . We communicate via phone and email on a regular basis—3 to 4 times a week, and more if necessary. He does alert me to times that they are expecting deployed troops home. We have discussed posttraumatic stress syndrome at length. [Emergency services provider no. 2]

Those findings suggest that communication in Watertown could be more systematic. And in Washington, although law-enforcement officials noted a strong relationship with their counterparts at JBLM, they said that they learn about deployments and demobilizations by word of mouth. Interviewees also told the Westat study team that there is relatively poor communication between JBLM and local police departments about services available for managing deployment-related disorders such as PTSD.

*Information About Resources*

The many resources available to service members and their families at all six study sites include peer-support groups, recreational activities for youth, pastoral counseling, therapy dogs, financial planning services, food banks, and numerous others. Information about the services and supports is communicated both formally and informally. At most sites, interviewees reported that information about military resources is available through various official military channels: for example, pre- and postdeployment briefings; Morale, Welfare, and Recreation (MWR) activities; Army One Source; and Family Readiness Groups (FRGs). Also, in Jacksonville, North Carolina, and El Paso, interviewees described collaborative efforts between the community and the military installation to link military members and their families with community resources. For example, and as noted previously, Jacksonville's Project CARE has been activated at times of high deployments to make a community-wide effort to inform military families of the resources available to them. El Paso is served by the Northeast Coalition, an organization of approximately 200 schools, elected officials, agencies, community organizations, and Fort Bliss, that is responsible for identifying existing service capacity and helping to link individuals to the services and supports that they need.

Although formal channels reportedly worked well at the study sites with military installations nearby, some channels were less effective at the National Guard sites. Interviewees in Georgetown, South Carolina, said that official communication channels were not well formed at the time of the initial deployment. For example, interviewees reported that up until that time, the existing FRG had served primarily to build social connections among Guard members' families, not to provide information about resources and supports. Information flow reportedly was poor throughout the first deployment but had improved by the second one.

Following the first deployment, a National Guard member noted that he thought the state and the National Guard realized:

> Wait, we need to get something going here where we actually train these volunteers to kind of know what to do at an FRG meeting and to anticipate what questions are going to be asked and how to answer them. . . . And so they put together basically a training program for the volunteers. . . . At the end of it, you've got an FRG leader who has contacts across the state [and] has a list of resources.

Noting that communications are much improved, the current FRG leader in Georgetown was still worried that important information (relating, for example, to benefits) might not be reaching National Guard members and their families in a timely fashion. In addition, community members from schools and emergency services expressed concern about communications still being too sparse between National Guard leaders and their agencies.

In Little Falls, Minnesota, interviewees identified FRGs as a potential but limited source of information because members of deployed units come from such a broad geographic area. One FRG leader said that the geographic distance "is hard. You send emails to these people, but very seldom will they travel 100 miles to attend a 2- or 3-hour FRG meeting." In part because soldiers attach and reattach to multiple units, FRGs were said to be less active or even "dormant" when the unit was not deployed. Consequently, families of deployed National Guard members reportedly relied more on the Family Assistance Center (FAC) at Camp Ripley, Minnesota, for information.

At all sites, interviewees said that informal, word-of-mouth communications continue to be one of the most consistent ways in which information is exchanged about available resources. Individuals might learn about or obtain supports through their participation in shared interest organizations (such as church congregations) or by attending community events. Westat study team members who attended the Armed Forces Day event in Washington said they saw little information about community services at that event, whereas team members in Jacksonville, North Carolina, saw booths at the Jacksonville Jamboree for community-wide organizations and for organizations specifically dedicated to military-related issues. Services advertised at the Jamboree included P.S. Charities, which was raising money to build an accessible home for a veteran with triple amputations and severe burns sustained from an improvised explosive device (IED) blast in Afghanistan; Paws for Veterans, which was promoting its efforts to provide therapy dogs for veterans with PTSD, traumatic brain injury, or mobility issues; and a chiropractic practice at which military members could discuss their medical and chiropractic needs with the clinic's staff. Interviewees also said that they use established community networks to ensure that the needs of service members and their families are addressed. In Georgetown, for example, a community member described how these networks are used:

> If it ever comes [up] that something needs to be done [for the Guard unit], then the community is right behind it. Nobody steps back from that. Just go to one council meeting, say what's gonna happen; before you know it, whoever they're having breakfast with downtown . . . the old men sit there, and all you gotta do is tell them once and the whole street knows. . . . They're like the fathers in this little city here, and if there's issues going on, every business knows about it because they'll be talking fast and personal to them [the businesses].

In addition to those "live" communications, interviewees often mentioned the importance of online networking, particularly through Facebook. Team members learned about Facebook pages set up by FRGs, unit spouses, veterans' organizations (for example, Veterans of Foreign Wars [VFW], American Legion), church congregations, and other mutual-interest groups at all six study sites. Service providers and community leaders also recognized the importance of online networks for this generation. For example, in Jacksonville a mental-health care provider said, "Brochures don't work for 18 to 20-year-olds; we have stopped printing them." At Fort Bliss, the now-former Garrison Commander Colonel Joseph Simonelli established a Facebook page called "Colonel Joe Wants to Know." He said that his initial intention in setting up the site was to allow him to address problems faced by service members and their families quickly and efficiently. Over time, the colonel said, visitors to the site started to help each other by directing people to appropriate resources either in the installation or in the community. He also noted that the page was open to community service providers so that these organizations could respond to emerging needs within the military community. The new garrison commander, Colonel Brant Dayley, has continued the practice by setting up his own Facebook page, "Tell It to Col. D."

**Community Health**

Traumatic brain injuries and limb amputations caused by IEDs are often called the "signature" physical wounds of the wars in Iraq and Afghanistan. However, community members did not indicate that there are challenges presented by physically injured service members. Inasmuch as those wounds are being treated within military medical facilities, such injuries might not be seen in the broader community. What interviewees did express concern about is how the wars' "hidden wounds," such as behavioral-health problems brought on by multiple deployments, are affecting their communities. Community members' concerns went beyond just the service members and included service members' families as well. These health issues are explored in the following subsection.

*Health of Service Members*

The current presentation of deployment-related behavioral-health challenges by service members was reported to be quite different among the six study sites. In Georgetown, South Carolina, for example, interviewees stated consistently that they were unaware of any community-level challenges posed by service members. At the other five sites, community members described behavioral-health challenges that varied in degree of severity. Interviewees from Little Falls, Minnesota, said that they believe that there has been an increase in drug and alcohol use by formerly deployed service members, as well as an increase in suicidal behaviors. They noted, however, that those issues had always plagued the community, and many were reluctant to attribute those behaviors strictly to multiple deployments.

In Watertown, New York, behavioral-health issues, such as depression, anxiety, substance abuse, PTSD, and suicide, were identified by multiple community members as being among the most serious negative effects of multiple deployments. Suicide of soldiers was mentioned by several interviewees as a particular issue of concern associated with multiple deployments. According to the Watertown TV news station, "Fort Drum saw its highest level of active-duty suicides in almost a decade . . . seven Fort Drum soldiers took their own lives in 2011 . . . that makes 31 suicides among Fort Drum soldiers since 2003" (Fox 28 News WNYF, 2012). Although suicide is a concern for the community of Watertown, it seems as if most, if not all, military-related suicides are confined to the post. The Westat study team found no evidence of deployment-related suicides in the city of Watertown. One emergency-service provider said, "I have read in the paper that military suicides are up. [But] I don't know of any in the city of Watertown . . . in the last 6 years."

Several interviewees in El Paso expressed concern about the potential effects on the community of service-related PTSD, but they did not report any events specifically linked to multiple deployments. Community members believed that both alcohol use and reckless driving were more prominent within the military community, but the interviewees generally attributed those behaviors to the young age of the service members and not to the number of deployments that they might have experienced. A city police representative said that his department had anticipated having to deal with large numbers of service members returning from theater with behavioral-health problems, but that this had not occurred. The officer also reported no noticeable increase in violent crime in the community committed by service members.

Community members in Jacksonville, North Carolina, described numerous behaviors that were attributed to the deployment patterns and to possible PTSD. The behaviors included an increase in automobile accidents originating from reckless driving, driving under the influence, and substance use, according to representatives from Onslow County Emergency Medical Services (EMS), the Jacksonville Police Department, and the Health Department. A representative from Onslow County EMS noted that the area has North Carolina's highest rate of accidents related to substance use, and the second-highest crash rate in the state. Another interviewee noted:

> In 2002 we went from 10 or 11 DUIs to . . . 484 last year . . . that was one thing we did see, prior to a deployment, people would get intoxicated. A lot of times we would take them straight to the base. [Police Department representative]

Also in Jacksonville, both Onslow County EMS employees and police discussed the rise in suicide attempts, and a Health Department representative described an increase in gun accidents:

> We had two officer-assisted suicides where the people charged the officer with guns, and we've seen some other suicides. [Police Department representative]

> We've had a lot of fatalities from gun accidents . . . you've got military guys . . . and it's really hard to always know what exactly is going on in those situations. . . he was cleaning his gun, but was he? [Health Department representative]

And an emergency-services representative spoke about recent acts of violence by Marines, including a man stabbing dogs in his house. The representative added:

> We've seen some other things that are quite disturbing. . . We had another Marine who was intoxicated, sitting on top of his roof with an M4 pointing it at people. . . those kinds of things we have seen on an occasional basis.

The greatest focus on deployment-related behavioral-health issues was in Washington as a result of several high-profile events involving deployed service members from Joint Base Lewis-McChord. In March 2012, Sergeant Robert Bales, who was deployed with a Stryker brigade out of JBLM, was accused of gunning down 17 Afghanistan civilians during a "rogue" shooting spree. In an interview with the local news, a community member linked Bales's behavior to the deployment cycles:

> The problems keep happening on this base, and that's why it was no surprise when I heard he was from Joint Base Lewis-McChord. Soldiers [are] being redeployed over and over and [are] not being given the time to [be] adequately taken care of, physically or mentally (Kiro 7 News, 2012).

The Bales incident and other troubling events tied to JBLM-based service members had led to a heightened awareness within the community about potential mental-health problems among service members. During the Westat study team visits, interviewees talked about several recent incidents, two of which involved suicide attempts by service members: one necessitated a response from a Special Weapons and Tactics (SWAT) team; the second involved the fatal shooting of a service member who had a gun pointed at police. Interviewees also cited two hostage situations involving active-duty service members, one of whom was an officer. Interviewees from both Washington communities—Lakewood and Lacey—expressed the opinion that there has been an increase in violent crimes locally involving service members. They added, however, that because these events are being sensationalized in the press, the association between local crime and PTSD might be an unfounded perception.

Although interviewees regularly expressed concerns that multiple deployments are leading service members in their communities to display negative behaviors, it was not always clear when those behaviors could be attributed to multiple deployments, to one individual's particularly violent single deployment, or simply to youthful fascination with fast cars and motorcycles and a tendency to engage in risk-taking behaviors. An interviewee in Watertown, New York, suggested that the duration of deployment in combination with the level of associated risk is a better indicator of the extent to which deployments affect service members and their families and in what ways. Regardless of the actual cause, community members' concerns are quite real and might be having an adverse effect on their perception of local service members. A mental-health counselor in El Paso said,

> I think there's also a community perception that what's coming to Fort Bliss now . . . are a lot of men and women who've been in Afghanistan and Iraq and that they may be coming with a whole range of problems. And there's a little bit of fear, I think, in the community at large about that. . . . There's this kind of stereotype that everybody coming back is coming back with this raft of problems, when in fact they may not be coming back with any such thing.

A longer-term worry, brought up by interviewees at all six study sites, is that there might be a delayed onset of symptoms related to multiple deployments. Service members might be fine right now, interviewees said, but what will happen in these communities if PTSD symptoms begin to emerge en masse 2 years from now? Community members perceive their *current* mental-health-service delivery systems to be inadequate to meet the present needs of both civilians and service members; they are concerned about how would they manage in the face of a sudden rise in demand (see the subsection below entitled "Community Competence").

*Health of Military Families*

Interviewees at multiple study sites did not focus solely on the issues facing the service members themselves, but also reported the "ungodly amount of stress" that the deployments place on military families. One issue that some families have to face is trying to cope with a returned service member's PTSD. Respondents from multiple study sites noted the tendency for young couples to get married just before the service member's first deployment or immediately after his or her return from combat. With the quick turnaround time between deployments, they said, the couple barely gets a chance to become reacquainted before the service member is deployed again. Immaturity, combined with the individuals' limited familiarity with each other, can contribute to the challenge of coping with PTSD:

> We've been hearing about people getting married without knowing the other person. [One soldier on leave for 2 weeks in the United States] met a girl in a bar, fell in love . . . they were married, he went back to Afghanistan, they had a baby . . . and now they're getting divorced. And this is [soldier is suffering from] PTSD issues, shrapnel from IEDs, he's been blown up three times in IED incidents, he's had horrible [experiences, such as] stuffing intestines back into the guy that was driving . . . And so he comes home . . . he drinks all the time. She doesn't know him; his personality is such that he just blows up. And it scares . . . her. Well, of course—she doesn't know him! [El Paso divorce lawyer]

A long-term relationship does not necessarily serve as a protective factor for the family, however. A mental-health provider in Jacksonville, North Carolina, reported to the study team that she had been getting more calls from senior members of the military and officers: "They're tired and never thought they'd need counseling," she said, "but now their families are falling apart."

PTSD is not the only issue challenging service members' families. Numerous interviewees described the strain that the rhythm of multiple deployments appears to be placing on the family as a unit. They pointed particularly to the stress associated with the separation created by deployment, the difficulties of postdeployment reintegration, and the toll that this rhythm takes on a family when it occurs numerous times. First is the strain placed on the service member. Interviewees in Jacksonville said that returning Marines might not be able to reintegrate into the family easily; they are "trained to wake at a pin-drop, and come back to 2-year-olds jumping on [the] bed in the middle of the night." According to a service provider in Washington, multiple deployments only exacerbate the challenge:

> They [service members] don't have enough time to shut it off [constant state of vigilance] before they go out again.

Interviewees also pointed to the stress that the pattern of repeated deployments places on children in these families, who must try to adjust to the changing dynamics of the household and, potentially, the altered behavior of the deployed parent. The following story, from the spouse of a service member in Watertown, New York, illustrates the concerns that interviewees expressed:

> Previous to this particular deployment, I didn't notice it [signs of PTSD] because of the jobs that he had previous to this one. His first tour out . . . was a civil affairs thing, and they were . . . not really in the line of fire. . . . They were helping with the infrastructure. . . . His second tour . . . he never fired his weapon one time. . . . I talked to him three and four times a day. . . . This [third] time . . . was scary. I was definitely on the edge pretty much every day. His job was to take a bullet before the colonel did. . . . So this time, I've really noticed quite a bit . . . noises get him. We were just in Washington, DC . . . and we got out of the car and he's doing one of these things—looking [and] scanning constantly. . . . He's tense and I could feel it in his body and I could see it in his arms and I said, "Sweetheart, calm down. It's ok. Nobody is trying to kill us." . . . He had to sit down on a

> bench. He's like, "I can't do this . . . I don't know what's wrong. I don't know if it's the smells. I don't if it's the number of people. I don't know if it's all the faces. I don't know, but I can't do this" and he was unglued for the rest of the day. . . . My kids had never seen this. My 15-year-old was just like, "Dad, what's wrong?" My 11-year-old was just beside himself. He was like, "Daddy, did we do something wrong? You didn't want to go to the zoo with us?" [His father responded], "No buddy. I wanted to. I just couldn't do it." That was really hard because that's never happened before. That was really difficult.

Several interviewees in El Paso said that the deployments are particularly difficult for young children, who, they believe, are having trouble attaching to the deployed parent because of the repeated separations. A counselor explained:

> It's very hard, and when there are multiple deployments . . . there's not even time for the soldier to recoup, much less the family, and when the kids know this they don't even have the opportunity to think, "Let's get comfortable" because they're on their guard—"I want to be prepared, I don't want to get hurt again."

In addition to having near-term adverse effects on the children, parents and mental-health counselors in El Paso expressed worry about how children will be affected by those experiences over the long term, such as their possibly developing an inability to form healthy attachments and relationships as adults.

How children handle those issues was a point of debate among interviewees. Some suggested that youth "act out" in response to their family situations, and pointed particularly to behaviors (including fighting, talking back to adults) that are exhibited in the schools. Others argued that the youth are "detached" and tend to "internalize" their feelings—that is, an affected youth might become more withdrawn. Still other interviews described these youth as "resilient" and "strong" and perceived these early hardships as being character building. Undoubtedly all such perceptions are based in fact: some youth act out, some become withdrawn, and some handle the situation effortlessly. Nevertheless, most site interviewees believed that some youth are adversely affected by the stresses of having a parent deploy multiple times and that this stress is rising to the level of a community concern.

Finally, but certainly not least important, interviewees pointed out the strains that the deployments place on the nondeployed spouse. That individual takes on the role of a single parent during deployment and then relinquishes some of the responsibilities when the service member returns. And as one military spouse said, multiple deployments only add to the struggle:

> Here you are as a spouse, you have control of your kids and the household and the yard and the bills and everything, and here comes the soldier who's supposed to be the king of the castle and you're wanting to give it back to him, but you're not. How much do you keep? How much are you wanting to give back knowing that he's going to be gone in a few months again?

> We're sort of missing a piece of our population to some degree in that the spouses have this emotional burden that is this bubble that is beyond comprehension right now. . . . And that's a whole other piece that I don't know if you guys have looked

> at . . . the extent to which a huge piece of the population that—it's sort of this "stuck" situation that we as the spouse are in because we have to always tell our soldier, "Don't worry, we got it, Honey, you go. We got it." And no matter what's happening we're not allowed to talk about that because he has to be safe downrange. And to our kids—"Don't worry, we got it! We got you, we got me, we got Dad, we got it all!" And it's affecting our spousal population to a huge, huge degree. And although the resources are out to get the counseling and things like that, right now we're so busy being stellar . . . that we're not going after it. We're not seeking the support that *we* need right now because we don't have time to seek that. We're too busy being stable . . . we're [so] busy [keeping] our feet on the ground that we don't have the chance to crumble.

The next two subsections include descriptions of the formal and informal resources that are available to help service members, their families, and the communities cope with these many challenges.

**Community Competence**

For the purposes of this study, "community competence" refers to the formal services and supports that might be available in a community, such as emergency care or behavioral-health services offered by licensed clinicians. The committee asked Westat to assess the formal service-delivery capacity in each community, including what services are (or are not) available, and what the barriers are that interviewees believe keep individuals from accessing services. Additionally, Westat was requested to assess what the mechanisms are in each community that might help mitigate barriers to care.

In the four active-duty communities, it was learned that many services are available to address the challenges presented by multiple deployments both on the bases and in their respective surrounding communities. With regard to education, for example, and as noted earlier, efforts are being made to ensure that educators have sufficient training and knowledge about military life so that they can be aware of and attend to issues presented by military children. Specific programs that interviewees said have been successful include the use of school-based military liaisons, such as Military Family Life Consultants in both Watertown, New York, and Lakewood, Washington; school liaison officers in El Paso; and military transition counselors in Jacksonville, North Carolina, schools. Also, training efforts are under way at those four sites to increase teacher and counselor awareness about behavioral issues that might arise in children of service members experiencing multiple deployments.

Some services are targeted specifically for families dealing with the strains of multiple deployments. In Little Falls, Minnesota, interviewees mentioned the Lutheran Social Service (LSS), a Minnesota not-for-profit organization that provides services for veterans. LSS Case Management, Outreach, Referral, and Education (LSS C.O.R.E.) is a statewide program for military members, veterans, and family members. LSS C.O.R.E. provides, by telephone, mental-health counseling and referrals and also offers financial counseling services. The Families OverComing Under Stress (FOCUS) project is an on-base program that provides resiliency-training and skill-building resources to military families and children. The program is not offered at all US military installations, but it does exist at both Camp LeJeune, North Carolina, and Joint Base Lewis-McChord, Washington, and was mentioned in Jacksonville as an important resource.

Interviews with off-base mental-health clinicians suggested some interface with military families, but it was often said that the family might be reluctant to seek counseling because of the perceived possible adverse effect on the service member's career. That particular barrier is discussed in greater detail below and in Chapter 9.

Interviewees frequently mentioned the high divorce rate among military families. Two programs were mentioned that attempt to mitigate the additional strain that divorce places on the children of the families involved: the Help Establishing Responsive Orders and Ensuring Support for Children in Military Families (HEROES) program, run through the Texas Attorney General's office, helps parents navigate custody disputes that might arise across state lines; and the El Paso County Domestic Relations Office has been working with the Office of the Judge Advocate General (JAG) at Fort Bliss, Texas, to train JAG lawyers on Texas child custody law and pro se divorce (that is, representing oneself in court). They also reported working with the Fort Bliss Morale, Welfare, and Recreation office to provide seminars on issues that might emerge between military and civilian law.

With regard to supporting military youth in these communities, a common strategy is employed, operating through the provision of various recreational opportunities. Interviewees mentioned activities sponsored by Boys and Girls Clubs, community athletic leagues, and common-interest clubs. Also mentioned were Department of Defense grants to school districts that provided additional monies for recreational activities. One of the most unique youth outlets was described to the Westat study team in Watertown, New York, where military and civilian youth got together to create a "docudrama" play, *In My Shoes*, in which young people described their experiences in trying to cope with multiple deployments. As reported by several respondents, the play served as an important opportunity for teens in the community to "voice what their experiences are." Interviewees also reported that the performance of the play has opened up the conversation between military children and their parents in Watertown about the deployment-related stresses that youth undergo.

Despite the programs described above and related efforts, at all six study sites interviewees described significant challenges with the behavioral-health service-delivery system, primarily with respect to insufficient service capacity. Interviewees regularly described community-based systems that are underfunded and strained and installation-based mental-health services that are also insufficient to meet the needs of service members and their families. Examples of such insufficiency were profound: all four active-duty sites have hospitals that offer inpatient psychiatric beds, but capacity is limited. In Watertown, New York, for example, all behavioral-health care for military families is provided in the civilian community, but there is only one hospital that has an inpatient behavioral-health care unit (Samaritan Medical Center). In Georgetown, South Carolina, and Little Falls, Minnesota, local inpatient services are not available at all. In both communities, interviewees said, an individual in acute psychiatric distress will not receive mental-health treatment at the hospital, but will be held in the facility's emergency room for a couple of days until a bed becomes available elsewhere in the state. In Little Falls, a Mobile Crisis Outreach (MCO) and stabilization team from Northern Pines Mental Health Center provides support for these emergency-room admissions. Nevertheless, that stop-gap approach to managing acute psychiatric crises potentially affects those emergency rooms' capacity to treat others coming into the facility, not to mention the delay in treating service members and/or their family members.

In addition, interviewees reported a dearth of psychiatrists in these communities. El Paso respondents said that there is only one child psychiatrist in town, Watertown interviewees described a lack of mental-health providers for children, and an interviewee in Georgetown said that there is only one full-time psychiatrist (for both adults and children) in the community. "Temporary" psychiatrists rotate through the local County Mental Health Department, she said, but at the expense of continuity of care for the patient. Challenges in the capacity of community-based mental-health services have reportedly been exacerbated on occasion by the military's efforts to increase service capacity on the installations. In both El Paso and Washington, mental-health clinicians reported that, a couple of years ago, they received calls from officials at Fort Bliss and JBLM, respectively, requesting their community provider agencies' assistance in providing counseling to service members. According to a provider in El Paso:

> Last summer, Fort Bliss called us and said, "We have a whole brigade of people coming back from Iraq; there's no way we can handle them; can you help us?" So at that time we had an influx of military families come in.

Interviewees said that they did offer assistance, although military-affiliated individuals never made up a large proportion of their client population (3–5%, according to one interviewee). Nevertheless, the arrangement proved to be a "win–win": service members, they said, developed therapeutic rapport with their assigned counselors at the community provider agency, and the agency benefited from the additional revenues. More recently, however, and at both the El Paso and Washington sites, interviewees noted that not only are installations expanding on-base capacity, but that the military reportedly is requiring service members to receive services on base. That requirement has potential negative effects, as agency staff noted that some service members are concerned that the receipt of services on base will affect their careers and thus are not continuing with counseling on base even if they need it. Interviewees said that the concern extends to the individual's entire family—that spouses might also be reluctant to seek care for themselves or their children because of the potential adverse effects on the military spouse's career. This perception was pervasive at the study sites:

> If you are an officer or an officer's wife, you don't want to be seen walking into the building where everyone knows it is where the mental health providers are. For enlisted, you don't want to be seen as showing any weakness. [Washington study site interviewee]

> With the rapid succession, there has been no time to debrief, or to reintegrate with your family, . . . or [with regard to] seeking services . . . it continues to be a double-edged sword for that service member, fearful that their career will inadvertently be harmed. [Jacksonville, North Carolina, study site interviewee]

> If your husband's looking to get promoted, and you as the wife goes and gets help with some mental health issues—for your husband that could affect his promotion. They'd like to say it doesn't, but it does. [Watertown, New York, study site interviewee]

Although the expansion of on-base services was intended to be a positive response to a growing need, interviewees said, the concomitant "requirement" was likely to reduce the use of mental-health services by service members and their families. Stigma is still a very important issue that has to be addressed (see Chapter 9).

It is noteworthy, however, that not everyone supported the perception addressed above. Several interviewees firmly believe that the military has changed its view on those seeking treatment for symptoms of PTSD. In El Paso, a high-ranking service member said, "We've all got PTSD when we come back from combat," a comment that the study team perceived as an attempt to normalize the experience. An interviewee in Georgetown similarly suggested that many unit members had PTSD symptoms when they came back from their first deployment, and that the "appropriate" response was to seek help. In Watertown, the spouse of an officer reported that her husband openly sought counseling to address combat stress so that the soldiers under his command would feel comfortable seeking assistance if they needed help. However, that was not the predominant view expressed by interviewees, which suggests that the military still needs to do more to counter the prevailing opinion that counseling will upend a service member's career.

Another issue raised by community-based providers was that individuals who do receive mental-health services through the military reportedly see a different therapist at each visit, and those visits might be more than a month apart. The protocol for effective counseling, they believed, was for a client to see the same therapist at each weekly (not monthly) appointment. Interviewees worried that the services provided on the installations are not intensive enough to address the needs of service members and their families effectively.

Finally, interviewees reported that the military's increased service capacity was not augmenting overall service availability in the region, but instead it was occurring at the expense of community capacity. Because the military can pay a higher salary than the community provider agencies, interviewees said, their agencies are losing staff to the installations. That movement, from the community to the military installation, places additional stress on community systems that already lack the capacity to meet the needs of the civilian population.

Despite the challenges, interviewees described an array of efforts being made to reach out to service members and their families and to ensure timely delivery of services. In Texas, for example, in 2007–2010, the San Antonio Federation partnered with the Dallas Foundation and the Permian Basin Area Foundation to establish the Texas Resources for Iraq-Afghanistan Deployment (TRIAD) Fund. The goal of the TRIAD grants was to support Texas-based military families affected by deployment to OEF or OIF. More than $11.9 million in grants were made to Texas community organizations, including mental-health providers, food banks, and children's services. Fourteen agencies in El Paso received grants, which interviewees reported were important in building behavioral-health capacity and expanding the availability of community resources to military families.

Similarly, in Jacksonville, North Carolina, there are numerous grant-based services designed to help military families and individuals during deployments. For example, the military transition counselors in the school system are funded through a Department of Defense Education Activity (DoDEA) grant that started in 2009. The counselor positions were initially funded to help students deal with deployments, but they now assist children with reintegration challenges, such as a parent's altered behavior. Interviewees reported that those staff positions filled a major gap in services.

Both Lacey and Lakewood, Washington, have also been able to put programs in place through grant funding. In the Clover Park School District (CPSD), schools located on base, in partnership with JBLM, can access a school-based mental-health program that provides psychiatric care, if requested, to all students in the schools. The administration of this program is being piloted through CPSD, which is the second district in the country[7] to use it. CPSD has also benefited by receiving several DoDEA grants, one for academic support and professional development and another for providing school-based mental-health counselors in three of the secondary schools off base that have large populations of military-dependent students. At the time of the site visit, this grant program was in its second year, and was cited as being very successful. The counselors' presence in the school was described as providing support either informally, such as talking with students in the hallway between classes, or by formal counseling sessions with children and family members, or by both types of support. At the time of the site visit, the CPSD also was waiting to hear about an award of a $2.5 million grant to fund mental-health services.

The North Thurston Public School (NTPS) District, which serves the city of Lacey, Washington, also has programs in place to support the estimated 20% of the district's student population who are from military families. The NTPS District secured a DoDEA grant to provide children in 6 of the district's 13 elementary schools with positive behavioral, social, and emotional supports. These include support groups for children with parents who have been deployed that allow the children an opportunity to share with others who are in similar situation at home. Those lunch-time groups also have engaged parents, including nondeployed spouses, to talk about what it is like to adjust to being the only parent at home. Returning service members also might attend, and describe what it was like to be separated from the family.

Interviewees did indicate that although these grant-funded programs have been invaluable in helping the communities meet the needs of service members and their families, the drawdown in troops and the end of funding will not mean an end to the needs. The TRIAD grants in El Paso, for example, ended in 2010. However, providers who were seeing clients with the assistance of those monies said that they continue to serve those clients, but that the agencies are no longer being compensated for the care. Jacksonville interviewees also expressed concern about how to continue to provide school-based services in the future.

Finally, interviewees at five of the six sites stressed the importance of having behavioral-health service providers who understand the military, both from the service member's perspective and from that of the spouse and children. A clinician in Little Falls, Minnesota, noted that it is the shared experience that increases the credibility of the provider and makes service members more willing to confide in a mental-health professional. To address that concern, Jefferson Community College (JCC) in Watertown, New York, is working to train more health care professionals, both to meet local service needs and to provide career opportunities for military and nonmilitary residents; the college reportedly provides courses at Fort Drum. And, in El Paso, interviewees described training efforts to increase teacher and counselor awareness of deployment-related issues with children in their schools. Fort Bliss also is working with the University of Texas at El Paso to develop a curriculum to train teachers about working with military children. The goal of the program is to ensure that teachers will be prepared to understand the ways in which deployments—indeed, multiple deployments—might adversely affect children in military families.

---

[7]The program is modeled after a successful program administered in on-base schools in Hawaii.

**Social Capital**

For the purposes of this study, "social capital" refers to the range of informal supports and services that are available in a community. In all six sites, study teams found strong informal support networks that helped to mitigate the impact of multiple deployments on these communities.

*Military Towns*

As noted earlier in this report, interviewees at all sites expressed the sentiment that their towns are "military communities." Common bases for that claim include the long-standing presence of a military installation in or near the community, a community history deeply rooted in patriotism, support for citizens who enlist in the active-duty military or join the National Guard, and large populations of retired service members living in the community. The sentiment expressed by interviewees that their towns are military communities likely has an impact in the communities: service members and their families do not have to explain their experiences and needs continually, but have a social nexus in which many friends and neighbors understand and empathize with what the family is going through. Shared experience, as Little Falls, Minnesota, mental-health providers explained, goes a long way toward creating an environment in which military-affiliated individuals can feel comfortable and supported. Additionally, because these communities have decades of experience with the military, they have had to make only slight adjustments to existing processes or programs in an effort to mitigate potential community-level effects of multiple deployments. Partnerships between the military installations and city entities such as the Chamber of Commerce or school districts offer excellent examples of ways in which communities have continually modified their programs to accommodate the ever-changing dynamics with their military neighbors.

Georgetown, South Carolina, stands as an exception to this rule, both because there is no nearby installation and because the role of the National Guard effectively changed (from strategic to operational) as a result of the wars in Iraq and Afghanistan. Interviewees' descriptions of problematic communications with National Guard leaders about the logistics of the unit's first deployment are therefore not surprising. Nevertheless, citizens' support for the unit reportedly never wavered, thereby reinforcing the importance of affective supports in helping a community cope with the potential effects of multiple deployments.

*Peer Supports*

Numerous community-based peer-support groups were reported or observed at each of the six study sites. These groups included mental-health peer-support groups, community-sponsored programs for families with a deployed service member (for example, Hearts Apart in El Paso, Project New Hope Military Family Retreats, a program sponsored by the Lions Club in Washington), several opportunities in each community for children in military families to come together and talk about their experiences, and countless virtual support groups through Facebook or other online resources.

Outreach was also being conducted by several military-focused organizations, including Family Readiness Groups, the VFW, American Legion posts, other local veterans' groups, and the VFW Ladies Auxiliary. Outreach efforts described by interviewees included FRG meetings and newsletters, VFW membership drives oriented toward OIF and OEF veterans, and, in Georgetown, a baby shower for National Guard wives sponsored by the VFW Ladies Auxiliary.

Community members described the response to these outreach efforts as "mixed." The FRG, for example, reportedly is not the best venue for everyone. In Little Falls, participation is said to be severely limited by the geographic dispersal of unit members. And Georgetown's FRG was said by interviewees to have struggled through the first deployment to move beyond its traditional social function to become a source of information and support for families of deployed National Guard members. Enthusiasm for the FRG was mixed in the active-duty sites as well, with one El Paso interviewee saying, "The FRG is helpful to many and for many it's their worst nightmare," as the rank of the deployed appears to influence whose issues are addressed. A Marine wife in Jacksonville, North Carolina, expressed a similar concern, noting that wives of Marines might have difficulty talking to each other about their problems when their spouses are of different rank.

Traditional veterans groups, such as the VFW and the American Legion, also reported a mixed response from OEF and OIF veterans. Several Vietnam-era interviewees said that they made a concerted effort to reach out to this group to ensure that "they didn't have to go through what we went through" (experiences like being spat on or yelled at by civilians). They reported numerous efforts by their veterans' groups to engage the younger generation of service members, including "Welcome Home" picnics for returning service members and their families and membership outreach targeted specifically to this cohort. Yet interviewees expressed dismay over what they perceived to be "lean" participation by OEF and OIF veterans. When a Vietnam-era veteran in Georgetown was asked why he thought that engagement with OEF and OIF veterans was so hard, he responded:

> It's hard to take, it really is. We've opened the posts and we just can't get them. I do know we got two members at the VFW out of it, but that's about all we picked up. . . . We welcomed them back and tried to do everything we can. Hopefully they'd want to come join us, but there's a separation there for some reason or another, I don't know. We even tried to give them a free membership, we opened that door, and then finally we had to make a decision, we just can't leave it open like that.

Other Vietnam-era veterans in Georgetown and at the rest of the study sites offered various explanations for this phenomenon. One veteran in El Paso, for example, said, "They feel they can take care of whatever issues emerge on their own." Others concluded that between work obligations and responsibilities to their families (especially young children), many of the OEF and OIF generation simply lack sufficient free time to be able to participate fully in various organizations engaged in outreach efforts. Despite the limited response, veterans interviewed maintained they would continue their outreach to those younger service members.

*Faith Community*

At all of the sites except for Washington and Little Falls, Minnesota,[8] the Westat study teams learned that the faith community offers a wide array of supports and services for service members and their families, some in direct response to the challenges caused by multiple deployments. A pastor in El Paso said:

---

[8]This is not to suggest that the faith community at those two sites is not supportive of the military, but simply that study visit teams heard little about such efforts from interviewees at those locations.

> We consciously 3.5 years ago, as a staff, saw the deployments and what they were doing to the families. So, on a staff planning meeting for the next year we said, We're going to do everything we can to reach out to our military community and meet them where their need is.

A Jacksonville, North Carolina, minister noted that the church can offer immediate supports "without the red tape," that is, without the bureaucratic overlay that might occur within the military. He also pointed out that for families or service members who are worried about how seeking help might affect the service member's career, church-based assistance is confidential and lies completely outside of the chain of command. Specific faith-based support services that were reported to study teams include pastoral counseling for individuals and couples, men's PTSD support groups, spouses' support groups, military luncheons, support for single service members, care packages for deployed units, and financial respite and household support. Equally important, interviewees said that families and service members benefit from the comfort of both faith and prayer.

*Family, Friends, and Neighbors*

At all six study sites, interviewees described an array of supports offered by family, friends, and neighbors. At both National Guard sites, which are small, rural communities, interviewees frequently commented that extended families live in the area and help pick up the children from school, provide child care while the nondeployed spouse is at work, and offer emotional support to the service member, spouse, or children as needed. In Georgetown, South Carolina, in a telephone conversation with a study team member, a National Guard member about to leave on his third deployment was asked where his wife finds support during his extended absences. He described a social geography of support, including his wife's sister and brother who live on either side of his and his wife's home, and his relatives who live very close by. "She has plenty of support when I'm gone." Similar support networks were described in Jacksonville, North Carolina, where the national recession left some family members unemployed and reportedly prompted them to move into the community to help the nondeployed spouse. Families were foremost in people's minds at the other sites as well, such as in El Paso, where business leaders said that they intentionally sought to create a service-rich environment so that nondeployed spouses might stay in the city rather than "return home to their families."

Friendships were also described by service-member interviewees as providing valuable support. In the four active-duty sites, however, because so many service members and their families live outside of the military installation, interviewees often reported having only one or two close friends in their neighborhoods or apartment buildings. Although these friendships are strong, they also leave individuals vulnerable to the vagaries of military life. In El Paso, for example, a young woman described the kinds of supports that she and her best friend, a neighbor, provided to each other while their husbands were deployed. Recently, however, her friend's husband had been severely wounded in an IED attack and the woman was spending all of her free time at Beaumont Medical Center. The interviewee said that she was continuing to support her friend, but she also realized that the mutual nature of their relationship had changed. And with no other military-affiliated individuals in her apartment complex, this young woman's "network" had diminished considerably.

Finally, interviewees routinely described different ways in which neighbors and community members take care of each other, including "Welcome Home" parades, community fundraisers, neighbors' shoveling snow or cleaning someone's gutters, a random patron picking up the restaurant tab for a service member, and a Little League coach who provides rides to and from practices and games. Unfortunately, not all military-affiliated individuals described feeling so supported by their communities. For example, two spouses of service members interviewed in El Paso perceived the community to be "disingenuous" about their support for the military and mentioned various frustrations with the schools, landlords, and business community. For the most part, however, interviewees recognized community members' good intentions and appreciated the efforts people were making on behalf of the military.

## Conclusions Related to the Ethnographic Assessment

It is clear from a review of the case study reports from the six communities visited that multiple deployments have notable effects—both positive and negative—on the communities visited.

### Formal Partnerships Between the Community and the Installation

In each of the four active-duty sites, community leaders have worked closely with the local installation command to establish formal, named partnerships that promote the timely flow of information between the two entities and facilitate joint planning efforts. The partnerships include the following:

- The South Sound Military and Communities Partnership established between the city of Lakewood, Washington, and JBLM. The SSMCP was developed in response to BRAC and the resultant growth of the installation and aims to foster collaboration around community development projects.
- The Armed Services Division within the Greater El Paso Chamber of Commerce that integrates directly with Fort Bliss. The Chamber of Commerce has made a concerted effort to reach out to Fort Bliss leaders, service members, and their families to try to discourage military families from leaving the area when the service member deploys. This communication channel also allows local businesses to prepare for upcoming deployments or demobilizations that might affect their business patterns.
- In North Carolina, Project CARE, developed by the Onslow County Chamber of Commerce. Project CARE combines the efforts of various local government, military, and community organizations to provide support to families of deployed services members, assist businesses in dealing with the deployments, and increase community spirit toward the military.
- In Watertown, New York, two "homegrown" nonprofit organizations formed by the community to identify and address military-civilian challenges. One of these organizations, the Fort Drum Regional Liaison Organization, which grew out of a committee formed in the 1980s, addresses community planning in general and any specific issues as they arise. The other organization, the Fort Drum Regional Health Planning Organization, focuses on meeting physical and behavioral-health needs. The boards of both organizations represent the local civilian and military communities.

Those partnerships reinforce the symbiotic relationship between the military installation and the local community and help to ensure that the needs of all local citizens—whether military or civilian—are acknowledged and addressed. The open channels of communication also promote the timely discussion and resolution of any emerging problems.

### Liaisons Between the Military and Civilian Schools

In Lakewood, Washington, Watertown, New York, and El Paso, Texas, the local public schools have implemented programs to assist school-age children of military parents through School Liaison Officers. In all instances, the SLOs have been trained to address family issues related to multiple deployments confidentially and are available to provide information, support, and guidance to all students, parents, teachers, and school staff, regardless of military affiliation. The SLOs help school staff understand military culture, notify them about upcoming deployments or returns, and help defuse challenges that arise, such as when children transition to a new school or their parents are deployed. Interviewees commented that the liaisons have been instrumental in helping address the challenges of multiple deployments because faculty are apprised of events (such as deployments or combat casualties) that might adversely affect one or more of their students.

### Training of Law-Enforcement Officers in Posttraumatic Stress Disorder Symptoms and Crisis Management

At each of the active-duty sites, representatives of the city police departments described fairly open lines of communication with their military counterparts. But only in El Paso and in Watertown, New York, did the study teams learn that law-enforcement officers are being trained in how to recognize the symptoms of PTSD and how to respond appropriately to a mental-health crisis. Communities with large populations of service members who have experienced multiple deployments might consider the value of training all law-enforcement personnel in crisis prevention and intervention techniques.

### Social Capital

As noted elsewhere in this report, interviewees at all six study sites said that their communities were "military towns" and that they both recognized and valued the sacrifices made by service members and their families. With rare exceptions, military spouses who were interviewed by study team members acknowledged the importance to them of living in a community where they felt they were "understood."

In addition, the Westat study teams discovered a vast array of community-based supports and services in these locations, including faith-based efforts, outreach conducted by traditional veterans' organizations, and virtual support groups that make use of Facebook and other social networking technologies. The reader will find accounts of numerous other such efforts in Appendix E containing the detailed case study reports.

### Continued Needs and Challenges

Interviewees enumerated a fairly consistent set of challenges that their communities continue to face with respect to the effects of multiple deployments. Many of these challenges are tied to formal service-delivery systems that lack adequate capacity to meet the demand.

#### *Community-Based Behavioral-Health Services*

None of the six study communities reportedly has sufficient behavioral-health service capacity to meet the needs of its civilian clientele, much less the needs of service members and their families. Fiscal challenges at the state level have only added to financial strains on these agencies. Yet community provider agencies believe that it is important to maintain a robust community system because they are aware of the issues related to stigma in the military. In the absence of community services, those individuals in need of treatment might forgo counseling altogether. Targeted grants, such as the TRIAD grants in Texas, have provided an important funding bridge for the military population, but interviewees expressed concern that these funding streams will dry up as the US military continues its drawdown in the Middle East. Interviewees pointed out that some service members might need support for years, whereas others might not show symptoms for years after returning from deployment. Community-based services need to be augmented, interviewees said, in order to properly address the continued and potentially growing demand.

*Supports and Services for Military Youth*

With the exception of Georgetown, South Carolina, where youth distress was not reported, interviewees at all sites said that they are worried about the well-being of youth from families in which one or both parents have been deployed multiple times. Interviewees described the availability of numerous resources for military youth, but still expressed the belief that not enough is being done to support that vulnerable population. Commonly mentioned was the need to increase the availability of counseling services that are age-appropriate in order to address issues that arise from deployments and that might have a developmental component.

*Attention to the Needs of Underserved Populations*

Interviewees described several populations of service members who, they believe, have unique needs, but who are receiving scant attention from both military and community service agencies. Community members often pointed to single service members, whose social networks were deemed to be leaner and thus less supportive than those of their married counterparts. Some worried that single service members might not receive needed services while deployed, but most expressed concern about the level of social safety nets for these single individuals when they return home from deployment. In the absence of strong supports and social activities, interviewees were worried about a rise in behavioral-health symptoms in the young single population. Community members also mentioned concern for single parents who deploy and for families in which both parents are deployed simultaneously; in those two cases, however, the concerns expressed were primarily for the well-being of the children. Finally, a very few interviewees argued for special attention for the needs of women service members returning home from combat. In particular, they believe that those women might have symptoms of PTSD associated with combat as well as potential sexual trauma from fellow service members. A peer-support network for female service members was being initiated by a community provider in El Paso that might serve as a model for other communities.

*Communication*

Despite numerous efforts to establish lines of communication between military installations or National Guard leaders and the local community, interviewees continued to note the need for more formal channels of information exchange. Although much information—including deployment dates, details about resources, and recommendations for useful service and supports—was being communicated by word of mouth, interviewees indicated that informal channels are not always timely or accurate. Areas of particular concern include better communication with school administrators and faculty about deployments and which of their students might be affected, need for the development of a central point of information at which individuals could learn about both formal and informal community-based supports, and better dissemination of information about PTSD to nonmilitary community members.

## CONCLUSIONS

Local communities are affected by OEF and OIF deployments as troops depart from military installations, return to base, and return home after separation. However, the peer-reviewed literature that has systematically assessed the consequences of deployments and reintegration on communities is sparse. The data that were available to the committee did not have sufficient specificity to allow for a rigorous quantitative analysis of the impact of deployments on local communities that have military installations nearby. Although the committee found no sectorwide economic assessments of communities during the OEF and OIF conflicts, the one study available (Kriesel and Gilbreath, 1994) suggests that there are significant economic losses to communities that deploy a relatively high concentration of service members. Another study from the Congressional Budget Office (CBO, 2005) noted that reservists and National Guard members are often activated for deployment with little forewarning a practice that can be disruptive and costly to employers. The most adverse effects of deployment are borne by small businesses that lose essential employees, businesses that rely on employees with highly specialized skills, and self-employed businesses owned by reservists. Another study reviewed found that for every 10% increase in activations of 30 days or more, small firms face a 3.7% decrease in sales (Hope et al., 2009). Additionally, among those in the labor force, veterans serving after 2001 have higher rates of unemployment than those of their civilian counterparts (see Chapter 8).

The findings from the ethnographic analyses that the committee undertook did not necessarily agree with economic findings from national studies; however, in the communities visited, a clear need for communication between local installations and community leaders was highlighted. Additionally, the perceived shortfall of behavioral-health resources available to returning veterans has also been emphasized. With regard to the community impact of veterans returning home after separation from the service, there is good evidence from past conflicts indicating that communities which receive a substantial number of returning veterans contend with homelessness and behavioral disorders. However, interviewees in the five communities with nearby installations noted that the military is an important economic contributor to their regions. In many respects, the local economies have been shielded from the recession as a result of activity associated with war being waged on two fronts and two installations benefiting from the BRAC process.

Finally, a persistent theme in the ethnographic assessment was that clear communication between installations and surrounding communities is important for reducing potential adverse effect of deployments on local communities. Open formal channels of information exchange between base commanders and National Guard leaders with local community leaders, including business leaders, school administrators, law enforcement, and local social service agencies, regarding expected deployments and returns from theater appear to be useful in mitigating some adverse effects on communities.

## FUTURE RESEARCH DIRECTIONS

As the committee reviewed the sparse literature on community effects of OEF and OIF deployments and examined the range of federally funded research on outcomes for those deployed in OEF and OIF (Appendix D), it identified several areas for future research and direction:

- Studies are needed to quantify the effects of deployment and the return of active duty service members and recently separated veterans on military families and civilians living in the affected communities. Such studies should be a priority for a future comprehensive research agenda that aims to understand readjustment after OEF and OIF deployments.
- Studies designed to comprehensively address the questions around readjustment after OEF and OIF deployment should include geographic identifiers that indicate where each service member was residing when deployed, the location to which the service member/veteran returned, and where the veteran went after separation. In addition, such studies should include a systematic set of currently collected indicators of community well-being, including measures of economic performance, availability of social and support services, law-enforcement activity, and school and educational functioning. Those data are available, but data linkages are needed to allow for specific analyses that can more clearly illuminate opportunities to mitigate potential adverse community consequences after service members deploy, return, and separate.
- Longitudinal studies of veterans returning from overseas deployment are needed to assess the risk factors for homelessness. Future studies of homelessness should focus on the entire population of veterans and not only on those who enroll in VA health care.

## RECOMMENDATION

There has been too little research on community effects of deployments to OEF and OIF. To supplement the published research, the committee completed ethnographic assessments in six communities that are near large military installations or that have recently deployed National Guard populations. Those efforts provided some insight, but the lack of community-wide assessments of the effects of OEF and OIF deployments on communities made it difficult to respond to this aspect of the committee's charge.

**The committee recommends that the Department of Defense, the Department of Veterans Affairs, and other relevant federal agencies fund research on the effects of Operation Enduring Freedom and Operation Iraqi Freedom deployments on communities. Such research should include current indicators of community well-being, such as measures of economic performance, availability of social and support services, law-enforcement activity, and school and educational functioning.**

Relevant data are available, but data linkages are needed to allow specific analyses that can more clearly illuminate opportunities to mitigate potential adverse community consequences after service members deploy, return, and separate.

## REFERENCES


Allison-Aipa, T. S., G. M. De La Rosa, M. C. Stetz, and C. A. Castro. 2005. The impact of National Guard activation for homeland defense: Employers' perspective. *Military Medicine* 170(10):846-850.

Balshem, H., V. Christensen, A. Tuepker, and D. Kansagara. 2011. *A Critical Review of the Literature Regarding Homelessness Among Veterans.* Portland, OR: Department of Veterans Affairs, Evidence Based Sythesis Program.

Blue-Howells, J., J. McGuire, and J. Nakashima. 2008. Co-location of health care services for homeless veterans: A case study of innovation in program implementation. *Social Work in Health Care* 47(3):219-231.

Bond, G. R., D. R. Becker, R. E. Drake, C. A. Rapp, N. Meisler, A. F. Lehman, M. D. Bell, and C. R. Blyler. 2001. Implementing supported employment as an evidence-based practice. *Psychiatric Services* 52(3):313-322.

Burnett-Zeigler, I., M. Valenstein, M. Ilgen, A. J. Blow, L. A. Gorman, and K. Zivin. 2011. Civilian employment among recently returning Afghanistan and Iraq National Guard veterans. *Military Medicine* 176(6):639-646.

California Department of Mental Health. 2012. *Services for Veterans.* http://www.dmh.ca.gov/services_and_programs/VeteransResources/default.asp#services (accessed July 24, 2012).

CBO (Congressional Budget Office). 2005. *The Effects of Reserve Call-Ups on Civilian Employers.* Washington, DC: CBO.

Clark, S., J. McGuire, and J. Blue-Howells. 2010. Development of veterans treatment courts: Local and legislative initiatives. *Drug Court Review* 7(1).

CMHS National GAINS Center. 2008. *Responding to the Needs of Justice-Involved Combat Veterans with Service-Related Trauma and Mental Health Conditions: A Consensus Report of the CMHS National Gains Center's Forum on Combat Veterans, Trauma, and the Justice System.* Delmar, NY: CMHS National GAINS Center.

Colorado Behavioral Healthcare Council. 2012. *Resources for Veterans and Families Through CVF.* http://www.cbhc.org/cvf/resources-for-veterans-and-families (accessed July 24, 2012).

Davis, L. L., A. C. Leon, R. Toscano, C. E. Drebing, L. C. Ward, P. E. Parker, T. M. Kashner, and R. E. Drake. 2012. A randomized controlled trial of supported employment among veterans with posttraumatic stress disorder. *Psychiatric Services* 63(5):464-470.

Doyle, C. M., G. A. Gotz, N. M. Singer, and K. W. Tyson. 2004. *Analysis of Employer Costs from Reserve Component Mobilization.* Alexandria, VA: Institute for Defense Analyses.

Druss, B. G., R. M. Rohrbaugh, C. M. Levinson, and R. A. Rosenheck. 2001. Integrated medical care for patients with serious psychiatric illness: A randomized trial. *Archives of General Psychiatry* 58(9):861-868.

Edens, E. L., W. Kasprow, J. Tsai, and R. A. Rosenheck. 2011. Association of substance use and VA service-connected disability benefits with risk of homelessness among veterans. *American Journal on Addictions* 20(5):412-419.

Egendorf, A., C. Kadushin, and R. Laufer. 1981. *Legecies of Vietnam: Comparative Adjustment of Veterans and Their Peers, vol 1-5.* Washington, DC: US Government Printing Office.

Erbes, C. R., M. E. Kaler, T. Schult, M. A. Polusny, and P. A. Arbisi. 2011. Mental health diagnosis and occupational functioning in National Guard/reserve veterans returning from Iraq. *Journal of Rehabilitation Research and Development* 48(10):1159-1170.

Fargo, J., S. Metraux, T. Byrne, E. Munley, A. E. Montgomery, H. Jones, G. Sheldon, V. Kane, and D. Culhane. 2012. Prevalence and risk of homelessness among US veterans. *Preventing Chronic Disease* 9:E45.

Fox 28 News WNYF. 2012. *Fort Drum Sees Highest Level of Active Duty Suicides.* http://www.wwnytv.com/news/local/Fort-Drum-Sees-Highest-Level-Of-Active-Duty-Suicides-137775573.html (accessed July 25, 2012).

GAO (US Government Accountability Office). 2010. *Homelessness: A Common Vocabulary Could Help Agencies Collaborate and Collect More Consistent Data.* Washington, DC: GAO.

Greenberg, G. A., and R. A. Rosenheck. 2011. Incarceration among male veterans: Relative risk of imprisonment and differences between veteran and nonveteran inmates. *International Journal of Offender Therapy and Comparative Criminology* 56(4):646-667.

Hawthorne, W. B., D. P. Folsom, D. H. Sommerfeld, N. M. Lanouette, M. Lewis, G. A. Aarons, R. M. Conklin, E. Solorzano, L. A. Lindamer, and D. V. Jeste. 2012. Incarceration among adults who are in the public mental health system: Rates, risk factors, and short-term outcomes. *Psychiatric Services* 63(1):26-32.

HHS (Department of Health and Human Services) and SAMHSA (Substance Abuse and Mental Health Services Administration). 2010. *SAMHSA Awards $379 Million for Access to Recovery Grants.* http://www.samhsa.gov/newsroom/advisories/1010081330.aspx (accessed July 23, 2012).

Hickman, M. J. 2006. Impact of the military reserve activation on police staffing. *Police Chief Magazine.* http://www.policechiefmagazine.org/magazine/index.cfm?fuseaction=display_arch&article_id=1021&issue_id=102006 (accessed April 2, 2011).

Hoge, C. W., J. L. Auchterlonie, and C. S. Milliken. 2006. Mental health problems, use of mental health services, and attrition from military service after returning from deployment to Iraq or Afghanistan. *Journal of the American Medical Association* 295(9):1023-1032.

Holt, K. 2011. *A Second Change: Veterans Treatment Courts.* http://www.blogs.va.gov/VAntage/2018/a-second-chance-veterans-treatment-courts (accessed July 23, 2012).

Hope, J. B., D. B. Christman, and P. C. Mackin. 2009. *An Analysis of the Effect of Reserve Activation on Small Business.* Annandale, VA: SAG Corporation.

Huddleston, C. W., B. M. Douglas, and R. Casebolt. 2008. *Painting the Current Picture: A National Report Card on Drug Courts and Other Problem Solving Court Programs in the United States.* Alexandria, VA: National Drug Court Insititute.

Jacksonville-Onslow Chamber of Commerce. 2012. *Project Care Jacksonville.* http://www.projectcarejacksonville.com (accessed July 25, 2012).

Jacobson, I. G., M. A. Ryan, T. J. Hooper, T. C. Smith, P. J. Amoroso, E. J. Boyko, G. D. Gackstetter, T. S. Wells, and N. S. Bell. 2008. Alcohol use and alcohol-related problems before and after military combat deployment. *Journal of the American Medical Association* 300(6):663-675.

Justice for Vets. 2012. *Justice for Vets.* http://www.justiceforvets.org/veterans-treatment-court-locations (accessed May 24, 2012).

Kiro 7 News. 2012. *Afghan Shooter Was Sniper from JBLM Stryker Brigade.* http://www.kirotv.com/news/news/local-military/afghan-shooter-was-stryker-brigade/nLQ87 (accessed July 25, 2012).

Kriesel, W., and G. L. Gilbreath. 1994. Community impacts from a temporary military deployment: The case of Fort Stewart, GA. *Southern Journal of Rural Society* 10(1):37-54.

Kuhn, J. H., and J. Nakashima. 2010. *The Sixteenth Annual Progress Report Community Homelessness Assessment, Local Education and Networking Group (CHALENG) for Veterans (FY 2009).* Washington, DC: VA National Center on Homelessness Among Veterans.

Kulka, R. A., W. E. Schlenger, J. A. Fairbank, R. L. Hough, B. K. Jordan, C. R. Marmar, D. S. Weiss, and D. A. Grady. 1990. *Trauma and the Vietnam War Generation: Report of Findings from the National Vietnam Veterans Readjustment Study*. New York: Routledge.

Loughran, D. S., J. A. Klerman, and B. Savych. 2006. *The Effect of Reserve Activations and Active-Duty Deployments on Local Employment During the Global War on Terrorism.* Santa Monica, CA: RAND Corporation.

McGuire, J., R. A. Rosenheck, and W. J. Kasprow. 2010. Patient and program predictors of 12-month outcomes for homeless veterans following discharge from time-limited residential treatment. *Administration and Policy in Mental Health* 38(3):142-54.

McNiel, D. E., and R. L. Binder. 2007. Effectiveness of a mental health court in reducing criminal recidivism and violence. *American Journal of Psychiatry* 164(9):1395-1403.

National Coalition for Homeless Veterans. 2008. *Homeless Veterans Reintegration Program: Best Practices Profiles of Employment Assistance Programs.* Washington, DC: National Coalition for Homeless Veterans.

———. 2011. *11,000 New Permanent Supportive Housing Vouchers for Veterans Signed into Law.* http://nchv.org/content.cfm?id=110 (accessed May 24, 2012).

Noonan, M. E., and C. J. Mumola. 2007. *Veterans in State and Federal Prison, 2004.* Washington, DC: Bureau of Justice Statistics.

North, C. S., and E. M. Smith. 1993. A comparison of homeless men and women: Different populations, different needs. *Journal of Community Mental Health* 29(5):423-431.

O'Connell, M., W. Kasprow, and R. A. Rosenheck. 2010. National dissemination of supported housing in the VA: Model adherence versus model modification. *Psychiatric Rehabilitation Journal* 33(4):308-319.

Office of National Drug Control Policy. 2010. *Veterans Treatment Courts Fact Sheet.* http://www.whitehouse.gov/sites/default/files/ondcp/Fact_Sheets/veterans_treatment_courts_fact_sheet_12-13-10.pdf (accessed April 23, 2012).

Perl, L. 2010. *Veterans and Homelessness.* Washington, DC: Congressional Research Service.

Ramirez, C. 2012. *Redistricting: El Paso City Council Oks New Map, Some Neighborhoods Affected.* http://www.elpasotimes.com/news/ci_21143061/redistricting-city-representative-districts-boundaries-shift (accessed July 30, 2012).

Resnick, S. G., and R. A. Rosenheck. 2008. Posttraumatic stress disorder and employment in veterans participating in Veterans Health Administration compensated work therapy. *Journal of Rehabilitation Research & Development* 45(3):427-435.

Rosenheck, R., and A. Fontana. 1994. A model of homelessness among male veterans of the Vietnam War generation. *American Journal of Psychiatry* 151(3):421-427.

Rosenheck, R., W. Kasprow, L. Frisman, and W. Liu-Mares. 2003. Cost-effectiveness of supported housing for homeless persons with mental illness. *Archives of General Psychiatry* 60(9):940-951.

Rosenheck, R. A., and A. S. Mares. 2007. Implementation of supported employment for homeless veterans with psychiatric or addiction disorders: Two-year outcomes. *Psychiatric Services* 58(3):325-333.

Seal, K. H., D. Bertenthal, C. R. Miner, S. Sen, and C. Marmar. 2007. Bringing the war back home: Mental health disorders among 103,788 US veterans returning from Iraq and Afghanistan seen at Department of Veterans Affairs facilities. *Archives of Internal Medicine* 167(5):476-482.

Smith, M. W., P. P. Schnurr, and R. A. Rosenheck. 2005. Employment outcomes and PTSD symptom severity. *Mental Health Services Research* 7(2):89-101.

State of New York, DMNA. 2012. *New York Army National Guard Yellow Ribbon Events.* http://dmna.ny.gov/family/reintegration.php (accessed July 24, 2012).

Tanielian, T., and L. H. Jaycox. 2008. *Invisible Wounds of War: Psychological and Cognitive Injuries, Their Consequences, and Services to Assist Recovery*. Santa Monica, CA: RAND Corporation.

Tsai, J., R. H. Pietrzak, and R. A. Rosenheck. 2012. Homeless veterans who served in Iraq and Afghanistan: Gender differences, combat exposure, and comparisons with previous cohorts of homeless veterans. *Administration and Policy in Mental Health* July 24[Epub ahead of print].

University of Maryland School of Public Health. 2012. *New Partnership Targets Maryland Veterans' Mental Health*. http://sph.umd.edu/index.cfm (accessed July 24, 2012).

US Department of Housing and Urban Development and VA (Department of Veterans Affairs). 2011. *Veteran Homelessness: A Supplemental Report to the 2009 Annual Homeless Assessment Report to Congress.* Washington, DC: US Department of Housing and Urban Development and VA.

US Small Business Administration. 2011. *Military Reservists Economic Injury Loans*. http://www.sba.gov/content/military-reservists-economic-injury-loans (accessed August 25, 2011).

VA (Department of Veterans Affairs). 2008. *Uniform Mental Health Services in VA Medical Centers and Clinics.* Washington, DC: VA.

———. 2011. *Hospital and Outpatient Care for Veterans Released from Incarceration to Transitional Housing*. RIN 2900-AN41 Federal Register.

———. 2012a. *Project CHALENG*. http://www.va.gov/homeless/chaleng.asp (accessed January 25, 2012).

———. 2012b. *VA Announces New Grants to Help End Veterans Homelessness.* http://www.va.gov/opa/pressrel/pressrelease.cfm?id=2355 (accessed July 20, 2012).

VA National Center on Homelessness Among Veterans. *HUD-VASH Resource Guide on Permanent Housing and Clinical Care.* Washington, DC: VA.

Vogel, S. 2011. Veterans Affairs claims progress in ending homelessness among vets. *Washington Post*, December 26, 2011.

Washington, D. L., E. M. Yano, J. McGuire, V. Hines, M. Lee, and L. Gelberg. 2010. Risk factors for homelessness among women veterans. *Journal of Health Care for the Poor and Underserved* 21(1):82-91.

Washington State VA. 2012. *PTSD Counseling Services*. http://www.dva.wa.gov/ptsd_counseling.html (accessed July 24, 2012).

Wenzel, S. L., P. Koegel, and L. Gelberg. 2000. Antecedents of physical and sexual victimization among homeless women: A comparison to homeless men. *American Journal of Community Psychology* 28(3):367-390.

# 8

# SOCIOECONOMIC IMPACTS OF DEPLOYMENT ON SERVICE MEMBERS AND SPOUSES

This chapter examines the social and economic impacts of deployment to Operation Enduring Freedom (OEF), Operation Iraqi Freedom (OIF), and Operation New Dawn (OND) on individual service members and their spouses. It also assesses estimates of the long-term costs associated with deployment and the signature wounds of the conflicts, posttraumatic stress disorder (PTSD), traumatic brain injury (TBI), and depression. Costs of those and other injuries can be borne by many individuals beyond the afflicted service member. The chapter presents those assessments based on the current state of knowledge in these areas, which continues to evolve rapidly. The chapter's main findings are the following:

- Veterans of the post-9/11 period suffer higher rates of unemployment than nonveterans, but veterans who are employed appear to earn higher wages than their nonveteran counterparts, after adjusting for demographic characteristics.
- Long deployments, PTSD, and disability are associated with unemployment.
- Activated reservists may have lower earnings when they return from active duty if they have PTSD.
- Studies of veterans from earlier periods suggest that negative impacts of deployment to OEF, OIF, and OND and combat exposure may be revealed later in the life cycles of today's veterans and service members. Surveillance systems should be in place.
- The budgetary costs of providing care for injured veterans are significant and will rise over time. The uncompensated socioeconomic costs of war injuries may be large. Planning for the funding and provision of care should take a long-term perspective.
- Spouses of service members face an array of challenges that are often made more acute by deployment, and their socioeconomic well-being can suffer. Spouses of veterans face similar issues and impacts, about which less is known.

To examine socioeconomic impacts, the committee sought to measure the impact of deployment to OEF, OIF, and OND on several outcomes: veterans' civilian employment if separated from the military; service members' earnings and other income both during and following service; their household wealth and finances; their acquired education and access to further education; the incidence of homelessness among separated veterans; the incidence of criminal behavior; and spousal employment, earnings, and education. The committee first reviewed extant studies of deployment-related outcomes along these dimensions. Because there are relatively few population-based studies of socioeconomic well-being among veterans of

OEF, OIF, and OND, the committee also examined other studies whose findings seemed likely to generalize to OEF, OIF, and OND population.

The committee also reviewed recent studies of the short- and long-term budgetary and socioeconomic costs of war-related injuries and trauma. Budgetary costs include the costs of health care treatments and disability benefits paid by the Department of Veterans Affairs (VA), which reflect the direct cost of caring for injured veterans. The socioeconomic costs of injuries consist of all other negative impacts stemming from injuries that could have been avoided had the injury not occurred. There is agreement in the literature that short-run budgetary costs of caring for wounded veterans are large but affordable. If past trends continue, the long-run budgetary costs are likely to be much larger, although specific predictions of long-term costs associated with PTSD, and especially TBI, are highly uncertain. The socioeconomic costs of injury are controversial but deserving of more study given the nature of psychological wounds and their prevalence in the recent conflicts.

In the following sections, the committee first presents its assessments of the social and economic impacts of deployment on individual service members. Second, the committee discusses socioeconomic impacts of deployment on military spouses and speculates about the impacts on spouses of veterans. Third, the committee discusses estimates of short- and long-term costs associated with war injuries. Fourth and finally, the committee highlights gaps in knowledge and articulates a research plan for increasing understanding of the impacts and costs of deployment.

## SOCIOECONOMIC IMPACTS OF DEPLOYMENT ON SERVICE MEMBERS

This section presents what is known about how deployment to OEF, OIF, and/or OND has affected the socioeconomic well-being of service members and veterans. There are a number of reasons why deployment might have affected outcomes, and, in particular, the earnings and employment status of veterans, their level of education, and their wealth and risk of homelessness (see Chapter 7). Military service of any kind represents a break in civilian labor force participation, which may carry an earnings penalty if military experience is less rewarded in the labor market than civilian experience. For enlistees, time spent in the military could postpone or preclude further schooling. The psychological and physical wounds associated with deployment to a combat or war zone might directly reduce human capital, impair veterans' ability to work, and generate psychosocial impediments to functioning in civilian society. Unreimbursed medical expenses associated with mental or physical injuries may absorb wealth, and household finances might be strained by long and frequent absences of deployed service members. It also is possible that military service could positively affect socioeconomic outcomes. Deployment to a war zone raises military compensation, and Congress has also authorized generous education subsidies for certain cohorts, including post-9/11 veterans. The net effect of deployment on socioeconomic outcomes could therefore be either positive or negative, and it could change over the life cycles of surviving veterans.

Readjusting to civilian life is the first challenge faced by separated service members, and several conditions associated with combat or deployment-related stress may impact their socioeconomic well-being in the near term. Sayer et al. present a snapshot of readjustment problems faced by a sample of OEF and OIF combat veterans who had sought and received VA medical care (Sayer et al., 2010). Respondents were home from their most recent deployment for a median of 42 months, and 22% reported more than one deployment to Iraq or Afghanistan. About one-quarter (27%) reported a formal PTSD diagnosis, while 7% had a substance use disorder diagnosis, but a screening tool used in the survey estimated higher incidences of PTSD (41%) and substance abuse (38%). More than one-third (40%) reported at least some difficulty readjusting to civilian life within the last 30 days, and many reported at least some difficulty getting along with a spouse or partner (42%), or with relatives (34%), or with finding meaning in life (42%). Roughly a third reported at least some productivity problems, including difficulty keeping a job and problems completing the tasks needed for home, work, or school.

Perhaps the most visible indicator of socioeconomic well-being among recent veterans is their employment status, which is measured and reported monthly in the Current Population Survey (CPS) of the Bureau of Labor Statistics (BLS). The CPS does not ask about deployment, so little can be said about the specific impacts of deployment to OEF, OIF, and OND based on these data, but the available literature has produced some useful insights. Others studies using different data have also evaluated the effect of military service and deployment on earnings. For those on active duty, earnings rise mechanically with deployment through the combat zone tax exclusion and the additions of imminent danger pay or hostile fire pay. For National Guard and reserves, deployment could raise or lower earnings depending on how military pay compares to the civilian pay that is foregone during deployment. For all service members, deployment-related injuries may reduce future earnings ability, although the VA disability system is designed to replace such losses. The committee found little research that had explicitly examined the impact of deployment to these recent wars on educational attainment, wealth, homelessness, or crime, but this chapter presents some related findings that are related and plausibly relevant. For example, earlier research has suggested that veterans may obtain education that is less valuable than that obtained by nonveterans. Patterns of homelessness among all US veterans suggest that younger veterans are relatively more at risk, which suggests that veterans who deployed to OEF, OIF, and OND might be at greater risk of being homeless (see Chapter 7).

## Employment

When recent veterans or recently separated reserve component soldiers return to their communities, in addition to readjusting to family life and personal relationships, they also must readjust to the civilian workforce. Recently separated veterans, who probably enlisted at a young age, may be entering the civilian workforce for the first time following separation. Of those returning, 20% or more have psychiatric symptoms, and nearly as many (18%) have problems with steady employment (Tanielian and Jaycox, 2008). The Uniformed Services Employment and Reemployment Rights Act (USERRA) requires that employers accept recently separated reserve component service members back into their previously held positions, but that does not necessarily guarantee seamless readjustment.

As described in the committee's Phase 1 report, reserve service members who have been activated are more likely to be unemployed after they have returned from their deployments, a relationship that appears to strengthen as the term of deployment lengthens (Loughran and Klerman, 2008). Other researchers have shown that job loss was associated with PTSD and poorer mental health among National Guard troops who had deployed in 2005–2007 (Riviere et al., 2011). To what extent that relationship represents a causal effect of deployment-related trauma on employment status or reverse causality of poor mental health by job loss is technically unclear. But it seems likely that deployed veterans have difficulties finding and keeping jobs because they suffer combat-related disabilities. Adler et al. showed that disabled OEF and OIF veterans have difficulties with work-related tasks, for example (Adler et al., 2011).

Burnett-Zeigler et al. looked at employment status among 585 recently separated (45–60 days) National Guard service members (Burnett-Zeigler et al., 2011). Less than half (41%) of the participants were employed at the time of the survey. Service members below age 30 were much less likely to be employed (29%) than those aged 31 or older (57%). Those that reported recent combat exposure were more likely to be employed (46%) compared to those that did not (36%). Surprisingly, physical- and mental-health status, PTSD, depression, alcohol use, and anxiety were not significantly associated with employment status, although those with either better mental health or poorer physical health were more likely to be employed full rather than part time. As those authors noted, negative effects of mental health status, alcohol use, recent combat exposure, and PTSD might require more time before they measurably affect employment, because many of those characteristics are themselves unobservable to employers and probably affect maintaining employment more than obtaining it.

How employers might perceive veterans in the hiring pool is the subject of research by Kleykamp (2009). The author examined how prior military experience might influence a potential employer's interest in an employee candidate in New York City. Fabricated resumes were faxed in response to classified job listings in an effort to record callback rates for veteran vs nonveteran applicants, where military experience was classified as either combat or administrative. Resumes were matched on education, work experience, race (based on name), sex, and approximate age and were submitted in matched pairs. The researchers measured differences between veterans and their nonveteran peers in call backs or emails from the potential employers. There was no significant difference in callback rates among white, black, or Hispanic applicants with clerical (noncombat) experience in veterans vs nonveterans. Among combat veterans, there was no significant difference in callback rates for white and Hispanic applicants. However, 13 black civilian applicants (10%) received callbacks while black combat veterans did not receive any callbacks, a statistically significant difference that may represent biased perceptions. Combat-related trauma such as PTSD appears to affect employability and/or productivity, and some research suggests there may have been differential effects of combat exposure by race in the Vietnam era (Rohlfs, 2010). If employers in fact perceive recent veterans as more likely to suffer from invisible war wounds, they might discriminate in hiring.

Resnick and Rosenheck (2008) looked at the relationship between PTSD and employment among veterans in Veterans Health Administration Compensated Work Therapy, a vocational rehabilitation program. They found that veterans with PTSD were 19% less likely to be employed upon completion of the program compared to veterans without a PTSD diagnosis. Smith et al. (2005) examined the effect of PTSD symptom severity on employment outcomes among 325 Vietnam veterans. For every 10-point rise in Clinician-Administered PTSD Scale (CAPS) score, which is considered a meaningful increase in PTSD symptoms, the likelihood of no work increased 5.9 percentage points, the probability of part-time work decreased 2.1 percentage points, and the probability of full-time work decreased 3.8 percentage points. Interestingly, CAPS scores had no significant association with earnings once hired.

Although PTSD diagnosis among OEF, OIF, and OND veterans hovers around 10–20% (Hoge et al., 2004), there is little to no direct evidence of latent effects of deployment on employment. In an unpublished working paper, Edwards (2012) examines patterns of socioeconomic well-being among 753 veterans of the post-9/11 period surveyed in the 2010

National Survey of Veterans (NSV). The 2010 NSV sampled a nationally representative cross section of all living veterans between late 2009 and early 2010. Among the 453 veterans who self-reported being deployed in support of OEF and/or OIF, rates of employment and unemployment were both about 1 percentage point higher than among post-9/11 veterans who had not deployed, but the differences were statistically indistinguishable. Correcting for different underlying propensities of deployment across demographic groups revealed some limited evidence of greater employment rates among the deployed. Adjusting for differences in demographic characteristics switched the sign of the association but left the result statistically insignificant.

There are clear gaps in research concerning how deployment and physical or mental trauma may affect later employment. One key shortcoming is that there are few studies examining how prevention or treatment programs early in the postdeployment period may differentially affect later employment. Tanielian and Jaycox (2008) and related studies by the RAND Corporation have addressed employment and health dynamics over a 2-year window, but further research is needed. A second issue concerns questions of preexisting robustness or predisposition among service members prior to deployment. Military service might attract resilient individuals, or it might reflect difficulties maintaining civilian employment, or both might be true for different service members. Analysis of pre-service screening information linked to post-service outcomes, to disentangle causes and effects, should be a top research priority.

Employment patterns among veterans relative to nonveterans or to all civilians are reported in the monthly CPS of the BLS and in the annual August supplement to the CPS, which asks detailed questions about disability ratings and membership in the National Guard or reserve. Those data reveal the challenges that are broadly faced by veterans of the post-9/11 era and particularly by young veterans. In 2011, the unemployment rate among all post-9/11 veterans aged 18 and over was one-third higher than among equivalent nonveterans, 12.1% compared to 8.7%. Among young veterans aged 18–24, the rate was almost twice as high, 30.2% compared to 16.1% (BLS, 2012a). Monthly statistics on veterans' employment are reported without seasonal adjustment and tend to fluctuate.

Part of the observed differences in employment rates may be driven by basic demographic differences between veterans and nonveterans beyond age and sex, such as educational attainment and race or ethnicity. After controlling for all demographic differences and other compositional factors in the CPS data, Kleykamp (2012) reveals that male veterans of the post-9/11 era between the ages of 18 and 40 faced a 2.6 percentage point disadvantage in unemployment rates, 10.6% compared to 8% for comparable nonveterans, over the period 2005–2010. For female veterans in the same age group, the difference was even more stark: 11.5% compared to 7%, a difference of 4.5 percentage points.

A recent RAND study examines the effects on employment of the 2007 expansion of the Work Opportunity Tax Credit (WOTC) (Heaton, 2012). The expansion provided a maximum credit of $4,800 toward the hiring of any veteran drawing VA disability benefits who had been discharged within the previous 12 months or unemployed for 6 or more of those months. In contrast with standard employment tax credits targeting disadvantaged workers whose effectiveness at raising employment has often been empirically ambiguous (Heaton, 2012; Katz, 1998; Neumark, 2011), the 2007 WOTC expansion appears to have raised employment by some 2 percentage points, on average, among disabled veterans above what it would have been, with robustness across specifications. Impacts on veterans younger than 40 or on female veterans were not statistically significant. The effects of a 2009 extension of the WOTC to cover unemployed veterans more broadly and a related extension and expansion under the Vow to Hire Heroes Act of 2011 remain unclear and await future research efforts.

## Earnings

Researchers at RAND have found that reserve service members benefited in the short and long runs from being activated, but they also suffered lower earnings in the year immediately after returning from active duty during the OEF and OIF era. As described in the Phase 1 report, those researchers have demonstrated that reserve service members likely earned more after they were activated in the OEF or OIF era than they did before. The researchers have begun more recently to assess how the earnings of activated reservists change over time when they return to civilian life (Loughran and Klerman, 2010). According to that research, reservists earn less in the first year after they return from active duty than do reservists who were not activated. Over time, however, they earn more. Taken together, these findings suggest that deployment negatively affects earnings only in the year immediately after the end of active duty.

RAND researchers have also explored how the earnings of activated reservists are affected by PTSD symptoms, suggesting that deployed reservists have lower earnings after deployment if they have those mental health symptoms (Heaton and Loughran, 2010). The researchers combine information derived from the postdeployment health assessment reports with administrative data on earnings for approximately 300,000 reservists who served between 2003 and 2006. They compare results from cross-sectional analyses with those from regressions that employ fixed effects and instrumental variables methods to take account of nonrandom selection. According to that research, reservists with PTSD had slightly lower earnings than those who did not have the disorder in the year immediately after they returned from active duty. In subsequent years, they were more likely to leave the armed forces, and thus also experienced a drop in their military earnings, which meant that they earned less overall (Heaton and Loughran, 2010).

The 2010 NSV asked about household income but not earnings per se. Edwards (2012) found that household income was lower among veterans who deployed to OEF and/or OIF, but that the penalty was due to demographic differences associated with deployment, such as age and sex. Household income would also include any lost earnings replaced by disability benefits, making it difficult to tell what might have happened to earnings as a result of deployment-related mental or physical trauma. But the 2010 NSV data indicates lower VA disability among post-9/11 veterans who deployed to OEF and/or OIF, or essentially a healthy warrior effect.

A more recent RAND study (Heaton et al., 2012) used a causal estimation approach to analyze whether veteran's disability compensation was sufficient to cover lost productivity among returning service members with combat-related injuries, measured as life-altering or life-threatening combat injuries on the Post-Deployment Health Assessment. The analysis found that while lost earnings due to combat-related injuries were substantial, disability payments more than replaced lost earnings for the average wounded veteran. But disability payments did not quite replace household earnings losses among those with less severe injuries, although lost earnings were also lower for those with less severe injuries. The RAND study did not isolate the effects for veterans with PTSD or other mental health disabilities. However, a 2007 Center for

Naval Analysis study (Christensen et al., 2007) found that disability compensation for veterans classified with a primary physical disability adequately replaced expected lifetime earnings, while disability compensation for veterans with a primary mental disability compensated for only about 80–90% of expected lifetime earnings.

In CPS data, male and female veterans of the post-9/11 era had higher wages than observationally equivalent nonveterans, 6% in the case of males and 5% for females, during 2005–2010 (Kleykamp, 2012). This result is notable in light of reduced employment among the same veterans during the same period, and it could represent the effects of heterogeneity among veterans, with employers selecting healthy veterans with transferrable skills.

Loughran et al. (2011) present a new look at the causal effect of military service on the earnings and education of individuals who applied for active-component enlistment between 1989 and 2003. They compare subsequent outcomes among enlistees with outcomes among applicants who chose not to enlist, an extension of the method proposed by Angrist (1998), and they reveal sustained increases in earnings associated with military service that are concentrated among enlistees who are still serving in the military and among enlistees with lower AFQT scores. Those effects could represent a compensating wage differential paid for military service, the value added of skills imparted during military service, or a combination of both.

The rise in the use of private contractors by the US government to provide security and other services during recent overseas engagements may be important for veterans' earnings, but the committee is unaware of any systematic study of this issue. Earnings may be high for such occupations, but presumably so are the risks. To the extent they include such individuals, labor market surveys may be providing measures of average earnings that present a skewed picture of the typical experience among separated veterans.

## Educational and Vocational Needs

Veterans who served during the OEF and OIF period might have greater educational attainment than they might otherwise because of the educational benefits that are available to veterans under the different forms of the GI Bill. Until September 2009, such veterans could draw on funding from the Montgomery GI Bill. After that, they have had access to the more generous funding available through the Post-9/11 GI Bill era. Yet apparently no research has systematically examined how these benefits may have affected veterans' education. A recent story published in the *Chronicle of Higher Education* suggests that approximately 270,000 students used benefits from the Post-9/11 GI Bill in 2009–2010. The same article reports that among the top 15 institutions receiving GI Bill benefits, 7 were for-profit organizations and 5 were community colleges (Sewall, 2010). According to focus groups conducted by RAND, veterans credit the more generous benefits of the Post-9/11 GI Bill with inspiring them to obtain higher education (Steele et al., 2011). One congressional study, however, points out that veterans have disproportionately used the funding to obtain education from private for-profit educational institutions, which have significantly lower retention rates than do nonprofit institutions (Senate Health Education Labor and Pension Committee, 2011). Recently, President Obama issued an Executive Order (April 27, 2012) intended to provide mechanisms for "oversight, enforcement and accountability" of the GI Bill and other training and education benefits. Such mechanisms should provide meaningful information about the cost and quality of educational programs.

We know of relatively little research that explicitly examines the effects of serving or being deployed during the OEF and OIF period on educational attainment. One study has, however, assessed the effects of service in a sample that includes veterans who served during the first years of the OEF and OIF period and suggests that the effects might be negative. Among comparable military applicants between 1989 and 2003, those who ultimately enlisted were more likely to get associate's degrees, and less likely to get bachelor's degrees following military service than those who did not enlist. Enlistees also finished their education at older ages than did nonenlistees (Loughran et al., 2011). Similarly, Wang et al. (2012) found that military service appears to increase attainment of associate's degrees. Furthermore, Elman and O'Rand (2004) have demonstrated that people benefit less from earning associate's degrees than they do from earning bachelor's degrees. They have also shown that people who earn degrees when they are older also do not benefit as much from their education as do people who earn their degrees when they are younger. Thus, more recent veterans may suffer in general from two features of their education: the type of degree and the age at which they receive it.

The 2010 NSV asked about educational attainment and use of VA educational benefits, including among deployed and nondeployed veterans of the post-9/11 era. Edwards (2012) reports that veterans who deployed had fewer years of education than the nondeployed, but that the difference vanishes after controlling for demographic differences. Veterans who deployed were more likely to report using VA educational benefits and more likely to report having completed VA-subsidized education or training programs.

According to CPS data from 2005–2010, post-9/11 veterans were more likely to be enrolled in college than their civilian counterparts after controlling for other observable differences (Kleykamp, 2012). Male veterans between ages 18 and 40 were more likely (31.4% vs 22.8%) to be enrolled in college as were nonveterans, and there were similar findings for female veterans (39.2% vs 27.7%), although the latter differences were statistically insignificant, possibly because of a stronger effect of marital status or other covariates.

Veterans have access to vocational training through the VA and through a variety of individual veterans service organizations, although the efficacy of these programs is unclear. The Veterans Opportunity to Work (VOW) to Hire Heroes Act (2011) included provisions for additional training assistance to long-term unemployed veterans between the ages 35 and 60 who may not be eligible for the GI Bill, through the Veterans Retraining Assistance Program. This program was only recently implemented, and no evaluation of its efficacy is available. Veterans with at least a 10% service-connected disability rating may be eligible for the Vocational Rehabilitation and Employment (VR&E, also called VetSuccess) program. The program connects veterans with counselors to develop a plan under one of five tracks (self-employment, reemployment, rapid access to employment, independent living, and employment through long-term services) and to identify and coordinate services to achieve success in that track. The committee is not aware of any research that systematically identifies the vocational training needs of OEF, OIF, and OND veterans and their families, or of research evaluating the efficacy of such education and training programs. However, the GAO has raised concerns that the VR&E program has emphasized training programs over actual employment. In particular, veterans in training programs received subsistence payments while in training and for 2 months during an employment search, while those seeking direct employment did not receive any subsistence payments. Unsurprisingly, given these incentives, 80% of VR&E enrollees were in training programs, while only 7% were in the rapid access to employment program (GAO, 2009).

Further, the GAO highlighted the opacity of VR&E performance measures and a recent change in how rehabilitation outcomes were measured, with the new measures increasing the rate of rehabilitation (GAO, 2009).

Legislation passed in 2008 (Veterans' Benefits Improvement Act of 2008 in October of 2008, section 334) mandated a 20-year longitudinal study of three cohorts of participants in the VA vocational rehabilitation programs. A baseline report on a cohort of vocational rehabilitation participants in 2010 found that approximately 75% of the 10,793 participants served from the Gulf War era (1990) onward but did not report on OEF and OIF veterans separately. Of the 10,793 participants, 42 were between ages 17 and 21 (0.4%), 1,501 were between ages 22 and 29 (14.4%), and 2,719 were between ages 30 and 39 (26.0%), suggesting that many veterans in the VA vocation rehabilitation program may have served in OEF and/or OIF. The report does not report statistics for OEF or OIF or deployment and does not identify the vocational needs or outcomes of the population of interest in that report.

In the fall of 2012, the military announced a revamping of the transition assistance program (TAP) planned for November that was to focus on enhancing flexibility and guidance for service members in planning their post-service careers (Sheftick, 2012). The reconfiguration is meant to help establish a new model of the military life cycle in which service members start planning earlier in their military careers for separation and post-service employment or entrepreneurship. The committee believes this is a wise endeavor and calls on the DOD to conduct cost-effectiveness studies of the new TAP. Providing earlier advising regarding educational and occupational goals could be a relatively inexpensive way to improve post-separation employment and earnings outcomes.

## Household Wealth and Finances

As reported in the committee's Phase 1 report, the challenges posed by overseas deployment for the finances of military families can be significant. Although deployment typically raises military compensation, the absence of a key family member alone can create liquidity problems for families. To combat predatory lending practices targeting military families short on liquidity, the National Defense Authorization Act for Fiscal Year 2007 implemented new regulations on payday loans made to active duty service members and their families.

The committee is aware of few subsequent studies of the financial well-being of military families or of veterans who deployed to OEF, OIF, and/or OND. Elbogen et al. (2012) examine how positive screenings for major depression, PTSD, and TBI were associated with self-reported measures of financial well-being or stress among 1,388 veterans of the post-9/11 era who responded to the 2009 National Post-Deployment Adjustment Survey. While it remains unclear how veterans with mental health trauma may compare with nonveterans, this study shows they suffer significantly reduced financial well-being compared to other post-9/11 veterans, possibly because of impeded decision-making capabilities. The study also showed that veterans without financial stresses were less likely to report readjustment difficulties like criminal arrest or homelessness.

The 2010 NSV asked veterans of all periods about a few limited aspects of financial well-being, including homeownership, the presence of capital income (i.e., interest or dividends), and Internet access at home. As discussed by Edwards (2012), none of those indicators varied significantly across deployment status. That is consistent with the negligible association between deployment and household income among post-9/11 veterans in those data.

## Crime

The committee found no studies reviewing veteran status and criminal behavior among OEF and OIF veterans. However, homelessness, poverty, mental illness, and substance abuse are all predisposing factors for criminal behavior. While the committee is not aware of any studies associating OEF and/or OIF combat exposure with criminal behavior, Egendorf et al. (1981) found that among a sample of noninstitutionalized Vietnam veterans over age 23, 24% of those with heavy combat exposure were arrested after service compared to 10% of those with light or no combat exposure and 14% of comparable nonveterans. Only about 10% of arrests among veterans led to a conviction, but this is likely an underestimate because incarcerated veterans were not included in the study.

Despite the link between combat exposure and subsequent criminal behavior found in some veteran subpopulations (Rohlfs, 2010), veterans as a group are less likely to be incarcerated than nonveterans. The Bureau of Justice Statistics reports that, in 2004, the age-adjusted incarceration rate for veterans was about 10% lower than that for nonveterans (1,253 per 100,000 vs 1,390 per 100,000 respectively) (Noonan and Mumola, 2007). According to that same study, veterans were also somewhat more likely than nonveterans to be serving sentences for violent or sexual crimes, and veterans were more likely than other violent offenders to have victimized women or minors.

The only statistic concerning crime among veterans of OEF and OIF that the committee found was also reported by Noonan and Mumola (2007) and was based on incarceration data for 2004. Given that the conflicts extended well into the following decade, those patterns are unlikely to be broadly informative of criminal behavior among the OEF, OIF, and OND cohort. The study revealed that in 2004, 4% of the veteran population in state and federal prison were veterans of OEF and OIF. Data from the 2004 American Community Survey (Ruggles et al., 2010) indicated that about 8% of all US veterans or resident military in 2004 had served in the post-9/11 era. Although far from a perfect comparison, because one should at a minimum adjust for age-related differences between these subpopulations, this quick look suggests that by 2004, criminal behavior was not disproportionately prevalent among veterans of OEF or OIF.

The dearth of research on saving behavior and finances among service members, recent veterans, and their spouses is noteworthy given the well-known connection between financial planning earlier in life and later-life outcomes. While the short-run financial stresses faced by military families are relatively unique and important, a comprehensive evaluation of their financial planning and well-being is essential for understanding whether differences in later-life well-being may be linked to military service and deployment.

## Summary

The existing literature has identified a few impacts of deployment on average socioeconomic outcomes among service members and veterans, but in general the committee finds limited evidence of impacts on outcomes among deployed post-9/11 veterans at this stage of their life cycles. Based on findings in the committee's Phase 1 report, there are reasons to suspect the true effects may remain latent for some time. In it, the committee showed how the numbers of war veterans receiving disability benefits has tended to rise strongly with age among all previous war cohorts. Part of that could be attributable to any trend toward more generous disability rating, but the pattern also suggests latent need that unfolds during the course of aging. In the analysis of the 2010 NSV, Edwards (2012) also examines combat exposure and outcomes among post-9/11 veterans and older veterans. The author shows that deployment to OEF and/or OIF is a strong predictor of combat exposure and that combat exposure strongly predicts poorer self-reported health, although not household income, among post-9/11 veterans. Among older veterans of previous conflicts, combat exposure strongly predicts poorer self-reported health, disability, and poorer marital outcomes, although the impact on household income remains insignificant. Altogether, the limited evidence from the 2010 NSV suggests that overseas deployment increases combat exposure, which has had lifelong impacts on socioeconomic well-being among older cohorts of war veterans. Whether and how today's war veterans might differ from earlier cohorts in their resilience are important questions that may be unanswerable until later in their life cycles. The evidence motivates continued vigilance and development of effective surveillance systems.

## SOCIOECONOMIC IMPACTS OF DEPLOYMENT ON SPOUSES

As the committee reported in Phase 1, 55–60% of military service members are married (IOM, 2010), and about 60% of post-9/11 veterans in the 2010 NSV were married (Edwards, 2012). Spouses of active-duty service members face frequent relocations and deployment-related absences, and they may be affected by combat-related trauma if it alters the service member's roles or relationships in the household. Spouses of veterans may face heightened caregiving responsibilities, earnings requirements, or both, if the veteran is wounded or unemployed. Those multiple effects of deployments can impact the employment, earnings, and educational attainment of spouses. There are likely to be similar consequences for other family members, such as parents or siblings.

There are few studies to date that have assessed the specific impacts of deployment to OEF, OIF, and OND on those spousal outcomes. The 2010 NSV included separate questionnaires sent to spouses of active duty service members, veterans, and deceased veterans, but as of 2012 none of the spouse data are publicly available. The Defense Manpower Data Center (DMDC) has conducted several waves of Active Duty Spouse Surveys (ADSS) that might be informative, but there is controversy regarding sampling and weighting techniques in those data and thus the quality of statistical inference (Al Nassir et al., 2012; Losinger, 2010).

Deployments have been cited by military spouses as key factors affecting their employment. Based on a survey of over 1,000 military spouses, Harrell et al. (2004) report that spouses perceive deployments as likely causing interruptions in work, because time must be reallocated to household matters during the absence of the service member. Furthermore, military spouses in the survey believed potential employers were wary of hiring them because of the probability of absences. That could partially explain why military spouses are less likely to be employed than observationally equivalent civilian counterparts (Hosek et al., 2002). They also earn less, possibly because more frequent relocations reduce job search time and the inability to move nearer to a higher wage job. Accelerated and lengthened deployments to OEF, OIF, and OND might thus have reduced employment among military spouses but seem less likely to have affected their earnings. Concerning spousal education, deployments are likely to have impeded outcomes to the extent they force a reallocation of time away from studies and toward the household (Harrell et al., 2004). Relocations are probably a larger threat to spousal education because of the difficulties inherent in transferring course credit and variation in curricula across educational institutions.

What we know about spousal socioeconomic outcomes specifically associated with deployment to OEF, OIF, and/or OND is limited to observational inference from self-reports in recent waves of the ADSS. The 2009 Quadrennial Quality of Life Review (DOD, 2009) summarizes the characteristics of military spouses in these surveys and provides some perspectives on the effects of accelerated overseas deployments to OEF, OIF, and/or OND. Data from the 2006 ADSS revealed that 19% of all spouses had lost their jobs during their spouse's most recent deployment, while among spouses of lowest rank enlisted service members, the share was 27%. More than half (55%) said the deployment had an effect on their jobs, and 31% reported a reduction in earnings due to deployment. The causal effects of deployment on those outcomes may be substantially different.

## THE COSTS OF WAR-RELATED INJURIES PAID BY GOVERNMENTS AND INDIVIDUALS

Like medical treatment costs associated with war-related injuries, socioeconomic impacts of injuries or deployment such as those considered in this chapter can also be conceptualized as costs. If deployment causes mental or physical trauma that reduces the ability to work, for example, the lost earnings are a cost borne by the afflicted service member. The system of VA disability benefits is designed to replace those lost earnings. Provided that disabled veterans are reimbursed, such costs will be measured as a traditionally recognized cost of war-related injury: federally provided VA disability benefits. In addition, any Veterans Health Administration (VHA) treatment costs associated with that injury and with other ailments treated by the VA will be measured as federally provided VA benefits. Death and survivor benefits are also budgetary costs of war-related fatalities that are measured in government statistics.

But there are other types of costs of war-related injuries that will not be captured in the VA budget but that are arguably still relevant for policy and well-being. Health economists believe that optimal medical decisions should take into account the complete range of costs associated with ailments regardless of who pays and that a good measure of the cost of an injury is the willingness to pay to avoid it. According to this framework, the cost of a statistical injury, like a lost limb, for example, is the willingness to pay to avoid the risk of losing a limb. The willingness to pay will include the present value of lost earnings attributable to losing a limb, but it will also include the present value of any lost enjoyment associated with losing a limb, such as the inability to type with both hands, or any residual pain and suffering that treatment cannot reverse. In principle, the willingness to pay is the maximum amount an individual would pay for a medical procedure that could completely reverse the ailment. When choosing among a set of treatments that vary in terms of unit price and effectiveness, patients and care providers seeking to maximize the net benefits to the patient should measure the costs of ailments according to this broader definition. The extra cost associated with an injury above and beyond the present value of lost earnings and treatments, which are typically paid by the VA, can be termed the "socioeconomic cost."

Those distinctions are important for understanding fundamental differences in scope across cost estimates in the literature. Broadly speaking, most studies either measure just the direct treatment costs that are paid by the VA or, less frequently, treatment costs borne by other payers. Fewer studies attempt to measure the indirect costs associated with injury such as lost productivity, emotional costs, family hardship, and other related factors. Measuring the indirect costs is typically more difficult and thus also more controversial, but it provides answers to an important question. Tallying the direct treatment cost reveals how much the government should set aside to care for wounded veterans. Measuring the full costs helps inform optimal treatment strategies for wounded veterans.

In this section, the committee first reviews the literature on total budgetary costs, or the spending by the VA on disability benefits and health care for injured veterans of OEF, OIF, and OND. Then it explores the broader literature on costs of treatment before examining studies of the full costs of injuries and the cost effectiveness of various treatment interventions.

### Budgetary Costs of VHA Treatments

Several studies published since the committee's Phase 1 report have assessed the budgetary costs of caring for service members injured in OEF, OIF, and/or OND, with special emphasis on the cost of medical care provided through VHA. In late 2010, the Congressional Budget Office (CBO, 2010) provided a 10-year projection of VHA spending associated with OEF, OIF, and/or OND deployments based on current policies. In two scenarios that differed by the assumed rate of medical price inflation and force drawdowns, 10-year cumulative costs were $40 billion and $54 billion. Those forecasts assumed the number of treated veterans was 382,000 in 2010 and that treatments that year cost $5,170 per veteran and would rise either at the rate of Medicare price inflation or 30% faster.

By comparison, Stiglitz and Bilmes (2008) had predicted annual medical costs per treated veteran of OEF, OIF, and/or OND of either $3,500 or $5,765 starting in 2007. In a contemporaneous CBO estimate, the average cost was $2,740 that year (CBO, 2007), which had since been revised upward to $3,176 (CBO, 2010), after adjusting for inflation. Today, the estimates of Stiglitz and Bilmes and CBO are broadly consistent because the average cost per enrolled veteran rose at an average annual rate of 16% between 2007 and 2010 according to the CBO statistics. That was much faster than the 6% rate of medical price inflation assumed by Stiglitz and Bilmes and also faster than the 5.5% rate in the current CBO forecast. Short-term aggregate VHA cost forecasts by CBO and Stiglitz and Bilmes are thus now broadly in agreement. Stiglitz and Bilmes also predicted the present value of total lifetime VHA costs associated with OEF and OIF at between $121 billion and $285 billion. The CBO does not produce detailed long-term forecasts of this type, but the rough agreement between current levels and their predicted rates of growth suggests they would not diverge were they produced.

Early in 2012, the CBO released results from a new study of longitudinal data obtained from the VHA on the treatment of PTSD and TBI among OEF, OIF, and OND service members (CBO, 2012). To preserve confidentiality, the data were coded in a way that scrambled effects associated with calendar year, such as medical price inflation or changing eligibility, with effects associated with time in treatment. As a result, it is difficult to be certain about the sources of change in average costs or enrollment through time or during treatment. For example, the average cost of treating TBI rose strongly during the 4 years of treatment in the study, but the

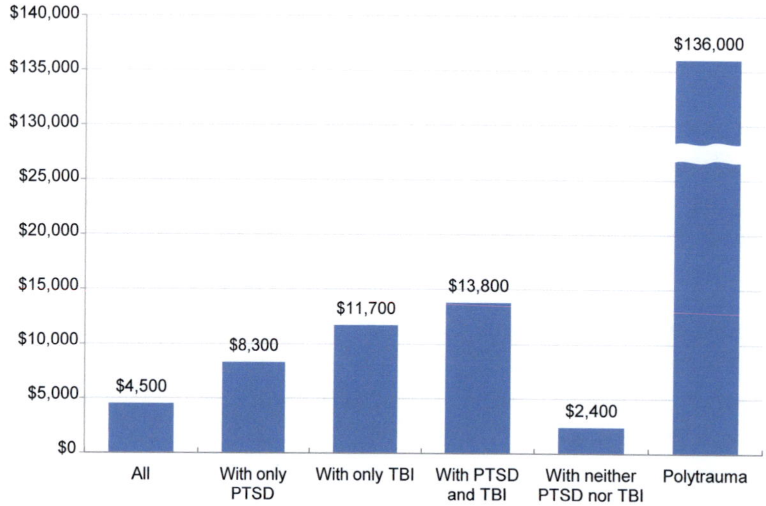


**FIGURE 8.1** Average cost per OEF/OIF/OND veteran treated in VHA, 2007.
SOURCE: CBO, 2012.

CBO argued that was primarily a data artifact reflecting an expansion of the definition of TBI to include milder cases following the shift toward comprehensive screening in 2007.

Cost and prevalence estimates are, therefore, rough measures, but the results of this study are illuminating (see Figure 8.1). The CBO reported average costs and number of treated OEF, OIF, and OND veterans in the first year of treatment by condition. The implicit average cost for the 497,300 treated veterans was roughly $4,500 in the year 2007, slightly higher than previous CBO estimates. The difference likely reflects the data construction, in which statistics were averaged across several years. Average costs in the first year for the 103,500 veterans with only PTSD were $8,300; for the 8,700 with only TBI was $11,700; and for the 26,600 with both PTSD and TBI, $13,800. Average costs for the 358,000 veterans with neither PTSD nor TBI were $2,400. For the 500 veterans with polytrauma, costs were $136,000 (CBO, 2012).

The CBO study also offers a glimpse into the dynamics of these illnesses over time. Among veterans without PTSD or TBI, only about 40% remained in treatment after 4 years, with almost the entire reduction coming after the first year. Continuation of treatment was highest among patients with PTSD and TBI, more than 90% of whom remained in treatment for all 4 years. Roughly 80% of patients with only PTSD remained in treatment all 4 years, while about 70% of patients with only TBI remained. Although imperfect, those utilization statistics suggest a relatively long right tail of medical expenditures for veterans with psychological ailments and especially among those with multiple diagnoses (CBO, 2012). That could represent lingering trauma, the structure of health and disability benefits, or some combination of these.

Trends in average treatment costs offered no clear evidence about the intensity of treatments. When measured over the entire veteran cohort, which includes those who remain in treatment and those who leave treatment, average treatment costs typically fell over time because patients left treatment, lowering the numerator (costs). When measured over the veterans who remained in treatment, average costs showed no clear trend.

## Other Cost Estimates

The committee also reviewed literature in the medical sciences that explored costs of war-related injuries, most of which focused on treatment costs. Topic areas covered in these articles included mental health trauma such as PTSD and depression; loss of limb; suicide; TBI; and a variety of miscellaneous topics such as cost measurement techniques, costs relative to length of deployment, and overall health care utilization among returning veterans.

Relatively few studies report actual cost estimates rather than offering commentary or discussing costs in a general sense. Among those that estimate costs, most typically consider treatment costs only and do not assess effects of injuries or treatments on quality of life, productivity, or other secondary outcomes. Most studies also focus on annual costs in the short run, rather than long-term or lifetime costs. Given knowledge about lifetime impacts of combat exposure, such a singular focus seems misplaced.

Studies that make longer-term projections tend to focus on the impacts of physical injuries. Blough et al. (2010) estimate the lifetime costs of prosthetics and assistive devices for amputees. Their per-person lifetime estimates range from $0.8 million to $3 million, depending on the type of amputation. Those are likely to be lower bounds because they do not incorporate the cost of repairs or the costs of new technological developments that might improve the quality of prosthetics but also increase their cost. Another key limitation is that Blough et al. do not explore effects on quality of life or work productivity.

Masini et al. (2009) estimate inpatient costs and disability benefits for injured service members, both overall and by type of injury. For the 31,708 injured patients as of May 2008, they found that total inpatient costs for initial hospitalization were $718 million and projected disability benefits were $1.9 billion. Their estimates might be too low because they do not account for inflation or cost-of-living adjustments, nor do they consider outpatient visits, rehabilitation, and prosthetics. In their study, the majority of costs accrue to patients with extremity injuries such as loss of limb, as opposed to injuries to the head and neck, thorax, and abdomen.

Studies that estimate treatment costs are also limited because they typically only consider VHA care. In some and perhaps many cases, patients who use the VA for health care might be only partially reliant on the VA. They might receive health insurance coverage through an employer or through the employer of a spouse or other family member. Care delivered outside the VA is relevant in assessing the total costs of injury, and the case could be made that it is more relevant than VHA care in understanding the burden on veterans and their families. However, it is more difficult to measure care received outside of the VHA, since federal agencies do not routinely track veteran's provider visits if they are paid for by private sources.

Another notable limitation of existing studies is that they often do not consider the association between deployment to OEF, OIF, and OND and costs, perhaps because they cannot measure deployment. For example, Leslie et al. (2011) estimate total health care utilization costs for a sample of veterans after their first year back from OEF and OIF. They found that average costs were $2,185 for men and $1,847 for women. But it is impossible to attribute these costs to deployment to OEF, OIF, and OND without knowing what veterans' health care costs would have been in the absence of deployment. Furthermore, those are estimates for all returning veterans, regardless of their health status. In a separate study, Chan et al. (2009) estimated that annual average VHA costs are $5,860 for veterans with depression and $7,300 for veterans with depression and PTSD symptoms. Both of those statistics are broadly consistent with the results of the recent CBO study of VHA data (CBO, 2012), but Chan et al. did not limit their study to OEF, OIF, and OND veterans. The average age of their sample is 55, suggesting that it contains a mix of Vietnam, OEF, OIF, and OND, and other veterans.

One way in which existing studies are helpful is that they highlight the importance of ancillary costs of well-known deployment-related conditions, above and beyond the direct treatment costs associated with the conditions themselves. Although the literature often does not actually measure these ancillary costs, at least it itemizes them. Examples include consequences of TBI, such as personality changes and aggression; infections stemming from TBI; and increased general medical use among those with PTSD. Formulating long-term policy responses to war injuries requires a better understanding of their ancillary impacts.

**Costs of Treating or Not Treating Mental-Health Disorders**

Some of the more successful omnibus studies of the full costs of mental-health trauma associated with deployment and cost-effective treatment interventions include the ongoing Invisible Wounds research project developed by the RAND Corporation (Taniclian and Jaycox, 2008). To estimate the costs of PTSD and major depression among service members deployed to OEF, OIF, and OND, RAND conducted its own telephone-based survey of prevalence in the population and then modeled a broad array of outcomes over a 2-year period based on other research regarding probabilities of remission and relapse and intervention cost and effectiveness. RAND then published a followup study with some updated statistics (Kilmer et al., 2011). The contributions of the RAND studies are manifold. They measure the total costs over 2 years of mental health trauma associated with PTSD and major depression, including treatment costs, lost earnings, reductions in quality of life, and the value of lives lost to potential suicides. By estimating changes in the total costs across changes in treatment regimen, these studies also inform the optimal choice of treatments.

As reported by Kilmer et al. (2011), estimates suggest that more than 20% of service members returning from OEF, OIF, and OND would experience major depression or PTSD within 2 years, or more than 58,000 out of a deployed cohort of 261,827. They project aggregated 2-year costs of major depression or PTSD totaling $923 million in their baseline forecast, or about $16,000 per case. The cost of suicide is considerable at about $5,000 or 32% of the total, but the largest element is lost productivity, at about $10,200 per case or 64% of the total. Treatment costs over 2 years accounted for only 4–5% of the total. If the afflicted service member successfully obtained a VA disability rating that covered lost earnings, the government rather than the service member would bear that cost. In the case of suicide, although there are military and VA death gratuities, the contribution to total cost is large in those estimates because they are based on a large estimate of the private value of a statistical life, $7 million per life lost. Although that estimate is commonly used in the health economics literature and by government agencies, it is an order of magnitude larger than official death gratuities. Thus, the cost of suicides primarily represents a privately borne cost, which may be viewed as controversial.

The great utility of the RAND studies is that they help inform optimal treatment policies. In their simulations, Kilmer et al. (2011) found that expanding evidence-based treatments to all afflicted service members, rather than the half they expect will receive them in the baseline, would significantly reduce the total costs of major depression and PTSD, even though it would raise treatment and thus budgetary costs paid by the VHA. Expanding evidence-based treatments to all, which in this study primarily involves increases in the frequency and intensity of psychotherapy sessions and increases in the frequency of selective serotonin reuptake inhibitors, would more than quadruple treatment costs per case, from $706 to $3,206, but it would actually reduce total costs per case by about 15%, from $16,000 to $13,551. This is because the RAND model suggests that universal evidence-based treatments would reduce average lost productivity and the chance of suicide by about 30% each, reducing those cost components by a total of almost $5,000 per case. The broad-based accounting of the RAND study suggests that expanding evidence-based treatment of major depression and PTSD in this way would be a socially desirable outcome that veterans would themselves choose if they could determine VHA treatment strategies. But VHA treatment costs rise. Still, the net effect of this change in policy could be to reduce total VA spending if disability benefits were reduced by the amount of the gained productivity, $3,320, which exceeds the increase in VHA treatment costs.

Although those studies have been groundbreaking in their discussion of mental-health trauma and the costs and benefits of treatments, the studies have not been able to assess the costs of TBI as thoroughly because the state of knowledge about TBI is not as advanced. In addition, the studies have not been able to fully address all costs that could be attributed to combat-related mental health trauma, such as homelessness, family strain, and the costs of pain and suffering. Going forward, these types of studies, and the basic science describing the dynamics of ailments, are critical focal points for future research efforts and funding.

## CONCLUSIONS

Veterans of the post-9/11 period suffer higher rates of unemployment than nonveterans, but veterans who are employed appear to earn higher wages than their nonveteran counterparts. Using nationally representative data, researchers have shown that the average OEF/OIF veteran is more likely to be unemployed than comparable nonveterans (BLS, 2012b; Kleykamp, 2012). But employed veterans also appear to have higher earnings than their nonveteran counterparts after adjusting for observable differences (Kleykamp, 2012). Others have found that reservists earn less at first when they are activated, but over time they appear to earn more than comparable reservists who were not activated (Loughran and Klerman, 2010). A recent study suggests that hiring tax credits may be an effective tool for increasing employment rates of disabled veterans (Heaton et al., 2012), but there is no direct evidence yet that such policies can increase employment among younger veterans of the post-9/11 era.

Long deployments, PTSD, and disability are associated with unemployment, and activated reservists may have lower earnings when they return from active duty if they have PTSD. Some researchers have found that OEF and OIF veterans were more likely to be unemployed if they had PTSD, poor mental health, or if they were deployed for longer time periods than those without those symptoms or who were deployed for shorter time periods (Loughran and Klerman, 2010; Riviere et al., 2011). One study showed that veterans also appeared to earn less if they had PTSD symptoms (Heaton and Loughran, 2010). Another study reported that combat exposure among National Guard members who deployed to OEF and OIF seemed to increase the odds of employment, and that there was no simple association between mental health symptoms and employment (Burnett-Zeigler et al., 2011).

Studies of veterans from earlier periods suggest that negative impacts of deployment to OEF, OIF, and OND and combat exposure may be revealed later in the life cycles of today's veterans and service members. Surveillance systems should be in place. As the committee noted in its Phase 1 report, the number of veterans from past war cohorts who are observed drawing disability benefits tends to rise over time before ultimately falling as the cohort reaches old age and dies. The pioneering work of Hearst et al. (1986) on the Vietnam draft lottery suggested that elevated mortality due to suicide and motor vehicle accidents was plausibly caused by prior military service. Patterns also suggest that rising disability compensation among Vietnam veterans may reflect the program's implicit work disincentives (Angrist et al., 2010).

The budgetary costs of providing care for injured veterans are significant and are likely to rise over time. Uncompensated socioeconomic costs of war injuries may be large. Planning for the funding and provision of care should take a long-term perspective. Academic researchers and the nonpartisan Congressional Budget Office now tend to agree on short- and medium-term forecasts of budgetary costs associated with medical treatment. If past trends continue, these costs will continue to rise over the remaining lifetimes of OEF and OIF veterans and present a clear motivation for long-term planning. In the short term, research suggests that spending more now to implement evidence-based treatments of mental health trauma will generate significant cost savings in the future, most significantly by reducing suicides, which impose enormous costs on families (Kilmer et al., 2011; Tanielian and Jaycox, 2008).

Spouses of service members face an array of challenges that are often made more acute by deployment, and their socioeconomic well-being can suffer. Spouses of veterans face similar issues and impacts, about which less is known. Researchers have shown that spouses of service members are less likely to be employed than nonmilitary spouses, and they appear to earn less than their nonmilitary counterparts (Hosek et al., 2002). Spouses of service members deployed to OEF, OIF, and OND have likely faced the same challenges that confront military spouses generally, such as potential job loss, earnings losses, and other costs of household reorganization (DOD, 2009).

## STUDIES OF SOCIOECONOMIC OUTCOMES CURRENTLY UNDER WAY

As was made clear in the committee's Phase 1 report and in the responses of VA and Department of Defense (DOD) to that report, there are several studies currently under way that can address socioeconomic outcomes associated with deployment to OEF, OIF, and OND. But the number of these studies is very small relative to the broader array of inquiries focused on specific health impacts of military deployments.

In particular, the list of currently federally funded studies given in Appendix D of this report contains very few studies that address the social and economic outcomes discussed in this chapter. These studies, highlighted in Appendix D, are being conducted by VA researchers on VA populations and might not be representative of the overall veteran population, many of whom are not enrolled in such services. Veterans of OEF and OIF who do not interface regularly with the VA are unlikely to be the subjects of current funded research, a major shortcoming in the committee's view.

But as the committee mentioned in its Phase 1 report (p. 156), and as the responses of VA and DOD discussed, two ongoing studies are likely to shed light on the socioeconomic impacts of deployment: the Millennium Cohort Study (McSally, 2007) and RAND's Deployment Life Study (DLS). As of this writing, the committee is unaware of research based on those data-collection efforts that specifically addresses socioeconomic outcomes.

The committee remains concerned that socioeconomic outcomes for separated veterans and their families will not be suitably measured by existing studies, which do not explicitly focus on separated military service members and thus may not measure them in large enough numbers. There was no indication in VA's response to the committee's Phase 1 report that it has plans to assess socioeconomic well-being among the population of OEF and OIF veterans in any systematic way. The only analysis tool the committee found for such purposes is the 2010 NSV, which offers limited insights (Edwards, 2012).

In addition to the DLS and other concurrent RAND studies, the committee is aware of ongoing inquiries into the effects of military service in the National Longitudinal Study of Adolescent Health (Add Health), which follows a nationally representative sample of individuals born between 1976 and 1984. Data collection is funded by the National Institute of Child Health and Human Development. Cesur et al. (2013) use those data to assess the impact of deployment to combat zones on mental health and medical costs. Wang et al. (2012) use the Add Health to explore military service, preservice social status, and educational attainment. Some of these efforts are being funded by a grant from the Army Research Institute for the Behavioral and Social Sciences. While datasets that sample individuals from the population are sometimes limited in their power to describe military and veteran subsamples, the committee believes these efforts will produce important new insights because the data are more representative of all veterans than studies of individuals who have entered the VA system.

## FUTURE RESEARCH DIRECTIONS

The committee's statement of task requested information about gaps in care and opportunities for research. For many social and economic outcomes, the committee does not know enough to definitively describe the gaps associated with deployment that might exist between deployed and nondeployed service members and veterans and their families. Furthermore, where gaps can be identified, the mechanisms for those gaps, or why those gaps might exist, are often unknown. Measuring gaps and understanding mechanisms are important first steps in recommending changes in policies. As a result, the committee's recommendations for future research directions on socioeconomic outcomes focus primarily on enhancing data collection and analysis and surveillance efforts. But some readjustment needs associated with deployment are already clear, and the committee begins by discussing their nature and implications.

The committee believes there are several clear policy implications regarding the lifelong costs associated with deployment-related mental health trauma, such as major depression and PTSD, and TBI. Studies suggest that expanding evidence-based treatment regimens for those disorders, which emphasize more frequent use of psychotherapy and pharmacologic interventions, might increase short-term treatment costs but would strongly reduce the broader costs paid by governments and individuals by improving outcomes. These insights have been gleaned from decades of basic research into mental health trauma; the same efforts must now be directed toward understanding TBI and its sequelae to inform policy with a similar degree of certitude.

- Studies on cost-effectiveness focusing on the signature wounds of TBI, PTSD, and major depression should continue to be funded and conducted; the implications of prior cost effectiveness studies, where knowledge is sufficiently developed, guide the evolution of policy inside the VA and elsewhere.
- Because much current evidence is equivocal on the issue of socioeconomic impacts of deployment to OEF, OIF, and OND, the committee believes that more analysis with improved data is needed. Much statistical evidence cannot support rejection of the hypothesis that there is no effect of deployment on the average service member, nor can it strongly support accepting that the precise effect is zero. But given current patterns connecting overseas deployment with combat exposure, and past patterns of need among older cohorts of war veterans, the committee believes that socioeconomic impacts of deployment may reveal themselves later in the life cycles of today's service members returning from overseas deployments.
- Enhanced surveillance efforts and data collection to measure the socioeconomic and other impacts of deployment among aging veterans that may potentially emerge with time should be considered. An expanded set of questions about military service in Census data products such as the American Community Survey or the Current Population Survey of the BLS would be examples of such efforts, as would an expanded and more frequently fielded National Survey of Veterans, or new linkages between VA and military records and existing data collection efforts such as the Health and Retirement Study, Panel Study of Income Dynamics, or the National Longitudinal Study of Adolescent Health.

Isolating causality is a cross-cutting concern for understanding the socioeconomic impacts of military service, overseas deployment, and combat exposure. It is difficult to disentangle the impacts of deployment on outcomes from the effects of other characteristics that may affect deployment and outcomes alike. Military readiness precludes the conducting of randomized control trials, but there are statistical strategies available to deal with nonrandom selection into treatment and control: instrumental variables; limited comparison groups, such as comparing activated to nonactivated reservists; and fixed effects models, in which researchers compare outcomes before and after deployment across different groups or individuals using longitudinal data. All of these would require that enhanced data be made available to researchers.

- Future research and funding efforts seeking to enhance the ability of independent researchers to explore causal relationships between military service and outcomes. One type of approach identifies so-called "instrumental variables" associated with service that are exogenous to an individual's characteristics but that affect outcomes. Publishing rates of deployment by year or quarter of birth, measurable characteristics that inform without compromising privacy and thus minimizing harm to human subjects, are one such strategy that might prove illuminating, and there might be others. Establishing restricted data centers with longitudinal service records containing detailed characteristics that determine the propensity to deploy would be another strategy.

While there is much successful research on socioeconomic outcomes among older cohorts of veterans, who are measured in publicly available Census data products, there is very little research on the socioeconomic impacts of OEF, OIF, and OND. This is likely because the relevant data are not publicly unavailable.

- To facilitate effective social science research on the impacts of overseas deployment in the near past on outcomes, the VA and DOD should provide new publicly available databases of de-identified data on individuals over time.

Previous research has focused on employment and earnings primarily among reservists, but less is known about employment and earnings among separated veterans.

- The committee suggests that future researchers address the impact of deployment on earnings and employment among all veterans, not just National Guard and reservists. Researchers could link DMDC payroll data on service members to Social Security records to examine earnings and employment. To assess the causal impact of deployment on these outcomes, instrumental variables or other approaches should be used.
- Research on previous generations of veterans identified important gains in educational attainment resulting from military educational benefits like the GI Bill. Little is understood about how or why the new Post-9/11 GI Bill is affecting educational attainment among veterans and among the family members to whom benefits may now be transferred. Future research efforts and funding should explicitly target how overseas deployment to OEF, OIF, and OND might have affected educational attainment among service members or their eligible family members. In particular:
- Research should examine how deployment relates to the use of educational benefits. Are deployed veterans more or less likely to use their educational benefits than are nondeployed veterans? This research should be feasible using existing administrative data, but it should ideally also address issues of causality; veterans may have other characteristics that are associated with both their use of benefits and their deployment.
- Research should examine how deployment relates to overall educational attainment. Do deployed veterans ultimately obtain more or fewer years of schooling than nondeployed veterans? Do they attend different types of institutions, and does that matter for graduation rates? This research likely cannot rely solely on government administrative data, but a partnering with institutions of higher learning could produce data linkages that reveal key patterns.

The committee is unaware of systematic efforts to assess how wealth and household finances are affected by military service or deployment. The committee is also unaware of preexisting datasets that could be used to assess this outcome in large samples; most surveys of finances are either not large to begin with, have small veteran subsamples, or both, which raises acute problems of statistical power.

- Future research and funding efforts should seek to address the impact of deployment on household finances and wealth. Partnering with firms in the private sector, such as USAA or regional banks, might be the easiest way forward short of launching new data collection efforts.

The state of knowledge regarding the tolls of accelerated and lengthened deployment on the socioeconomic status of military spouses is poor, and thus it is difficult to assess needs or recommend policies. Even less is known about the current impacts of past deployments on the spouses of veterans.

- Future studies should attempt to measure the impacts of deployments on spousal well-being in a more systematic way.

## RECOMMENDATIONS

Problems of unemployment and underemployment, which are broadly felt by the US civilian population today, appear to be more acute for veterans of the post-9/11 era, particularly young veterans. In 2011, the unemployment rate among all post-9/11 veterans 18 years old and older was more than one-third higher than that among equivalent nonveterans—12.1% compared with 8.7%. Among veterans 18–24 years old, the rate was almost twice as high—30.2% compared with 16.1%. The sources of those disparities remain unclear and could include skills mismatch, impeded ability to maintain or obtain employment because of physical or mental-health trauma, stigma or discrimination, or some combination of those factors or other elements. Successful readjustment depends on reentry into the civilian workforce, and the available evidence suggests that this is an important gap for policy to address. The committee found that the literature assessing the effectiveness of DOD's and VA's transition-assistance programs is relatively thin, even though reentry into the labor force is one of the most important readjustment challenges. One study suggests that recent expansions of hiring tax credits might have been effective in raising rates of employment of older veterans who have disabilities. But OEF, OIF, and OND veterans did not appear to benefit from the expansions.

**The committee recommends that the Department of Defense and the Department of Veterans Affairs evaluate the effectiveness of transition-assistance programs to ensure that they are effective in reducing unemployment among returning veterans of Operation Enduring Freedom, Operation Iraqi Freedom, and Operation New Dawn.**

Evaluation of the effectiveness of transition-assistance programs, with research that examines employment patterns after separation from the military over time, will provide data to ensure that scarce resources can be allocated to effective programs. Further study might focus on whether employment tax credits are a cost-effective means of expanding employment for Operation Enduring Freedom and Operation Iraqi Freedom veterans and whether programs to counsel and prepare service members for long-term postservice careers are effectively implemented.

The Post-9/11 GI Bill is one of the largest expansions of educational subsidies to veterans and their families on record, but its effectiveness is difficult to gauge. The committee is aware of no studies that have explicitly evaluated the effects of deployment to OEF and OIF on the use of the Post-9/11 GI Bill or the effects of the Post-9/11 GI Bill.

**The committee recommends a comprehensive evaluation of the effects of the Post-9/11 GI Bill on the educational attainment of veterans and eligible family members.**

The committee views the current evidence on the costs of caring for injured veterans as an overwhelming challenge. There is a need to assess the costs of caring for injured veterans systematically and publicly. The Congressional Budget Office publicly assesses short-term and medium-term costs, and, as the VA stated in response to the committee's Phase 1 report, it already produces some forecasts of health and disability spending. But the committee continues to believe that long-term planning for veterans' care requires public long-term cost forecasts in the same way that Social Security and Medicare require them, and these forecasts should take a similar form to be internally and externally useful.

**The committee reiterates its call for comprehensive long-term forecasts of the costs of the Veterans Health Administration's medical care and the Veterans Benefits Administration's disability benefits associated with combat deployments; these forecasts should be conducted annually and should be released publicly by the Department of Veterans Affairs and confirmed by an independent external authority.**

## REFERENCES

Adler, D. A., K. Possemato, S. Mavandadi, D. Lerner, H. Chang, J. Klaus, J. D. Tew, D. Barrett, E. Ingram, and D. W. Oslin. 2011. Psychiatric status and work performance of veterans of Operations Enduring Freedom and Iraqi Freedom. *Psychiatric Services* 62(1):39-46.

Al Nassir, F., R. Lipari, and K. Matos. 2012. Response to notes regarding the 2006 survey of active duty spouses. *Armed Forces and Society* [Epub].

Angrist, J. D. 1998. Estimating the labor market impact of voluntary military service using Social Security data on military applicants. *Econometrica* 66(2):39.

Angrist, J. D., S. H. Chen, and B. R. Frandsen. 2010. Did Vietnam veterans get sicker in the 1990s? The complicated effects of military service on self-reported health. *Journal of Public Economics* 94(11-12):824-837.

Blough, D. K., S. Hubbard, L. V. McFarland, D. G. Smith, J. M. Gambel, and G. E. Reiber. 2010. Prosthetic cost projections for servicemembers with major limb loss from Vietnam and OIF/OEF. *Journal of Rehabilitation Research and Development* 47(4):387-402.

BLS (Bureau of Labor Statistics). 2012a. *BLS Inflation Calculator*. http://www.bls.gov/data/inflation_calculator.htm (accessed April 24, 2012).

———. 2012b. *Employment Situation of Veterans—2011*. Washington, DC: BLS.

Burnett-Zeigler, I., M. Valenstein, M. Ilgen, A. J. Blow, L. A. Gorman, and K. Zivin. 2011. Civilian employment among recently returning Afghanistan and Iraq National Guard veterans. *Military Medicine* 176(6):639-646.

Cesur, R., J. J. Sabia, and E. Tekin. 2013. The psychological costs of war: Military combat and mental health. *Journal of Health Economics* 32(1):51-65.

Chan, D., A. D. Cheadle, G. Reiber, J. Unutzer, and E. F. Chaney. 2009. Health care utilization and its costs for depressed veterans with and without comorbid PTSD symptoms. *Psychiatric Services* 60(12):1612-1617.

Christensen, E., J. McMahon, E. Schaefer, T. Jaditz, and D. Harris. 2007. *Final Report for the Veterans' Disability Benefits Commission: Compensation, Survey Results, and Selected Topics.* Alexandria, VA: CNA.

CBO (Congressional Budget Office). 2007. *CBO Testimony: Statement of Matthew S. Goldberg, Deputy Assistant Director for National Security, Before the Committee on Veterans Affairs, U.S. House of Representatives, October 17, 2007*. Washington, DC: CBO.

———. 2010. *Potential Costs of Veterans' Health*. Washington, DC: CBO.

———. 2012. *The Veterans Health Administration's Treatment of PTSD and Traumatic Brain Injury Among Recent Combat Veterans.* Washington, DC: CBO.

DOD (Department of Defense). 2009. *Report of the 2nd Quadrennial Quality of Life Review.* Washington, DC: United States Department of Defense.

Edwards, R. D. 2012. Overseas deployment, combat exposure, and well-being in the 2010 National Survey of Veterans. *National Bureau of Economic Research Working Paper Series* No. 18227.

Egendorf, A., C. Kadushin, and R. Laufer. 1981. *Legacies of Vietnam: Comparative Adjustment of Veterans and Their Peers, Vol 1-5.* Washington, DC: Government Printing Office.

Elbogen, E. B., S. C. Johnson, R. H. Wagner, V. M. Newton, and J. C. Beckham. 2012. Financial well-being and postdeployment adjustment among Iraq and Afghanistan war veterans. *Military Medicine* 177(6).

Elman, C., and A. M. O'Rand. 2004. The race is to the swift: Socioeconomic origins, adult education, and wage attainment. *American Journal of Sociology* 110(1):123-160.

GAO (Government Accountability Office). 2009. *VA Vocational Rehabilitation and Employment: Better Incentives, Workforce Planning, and Performance Reporting Could Improve Program.* Washington, DC: GAO.

Harrell, M. C., N. Lim, L. Werber Castaneda, and D. Golinelli. 2004. *Working Around the Military: Challenges to Military Spouse Employment and Education.* Santa Monica, CA: RAND Corporation.

Hearst, N., T. B. Newman, and S. B. Hulley. 1986. Delayed effects of the military draft on mortality. A randomized natural experiment. *New England Journal of Medicine* 314(10):620-624.

Heaton, P. 2012. *The Effects of Hiring Tax Credits on Employment of Disabled Veterans.* Santa Monica, CA: RAND Corporation.

Heaton, P., and D. S. Loughran. 2010 (unpublished). *Post-Traumatic Stress Disorder and the Earnings of Military Reservists*. RAND Corporation.

Heaton, P., A. Miller, and D. S. Loughran. 2012. *Compensating Wounded Warriors: An Analysis of Injury, Labor Market Earnings, and Disability Compensation Among Veterans of the Iraq and Afghanistan Wars.* Santa Monica, CA: RAND Corporation.

Hoge, C. W., C. A. Castro, S. C. Messer, D. McGurk, D. I. Cotting, and R. L. Koffman. 2004. Combat duty in Iraq and Afghanistan, mental health problems, and barriers to care. *New England Journal of Medicine* 351(1):13-22.

Hosek, J., B. Asch, C. C. Fair, C. Martin, and M. Mattock. 2002. *Married to the Military: The Employment and Earnings of Military Wives Compared with Those of Civilian Wives.* Santa Monica, CA: RAND Corporation.

IOM (Institute of Medicine). 2010. *Returning Home from Iraq and Afghanistan: Preliminary Assessment of Readjustment Needs of Veterans, Service Members, and Their Families.* Washington, DC: The National Academies Press.

Katz, L. F. 1998. Wage subsidies for the disadvantaged. In *Generating Jobs: How to Increase Demand for Less-Skilled Workers*, edited by R. Freeman and P. Gottschalk. New York: Russell Sage Foundation. Pp. 21-53.

Kilmer, B., C. Eibner, J. S. Ringel, and R. L. Pacula. 2011. Invisible wounds, visible savings? Using microsimulation to estimate the costs and savings associated with providing evidence-based treatment for PTSD and depression to veterans of Operation Enduring Freedom and Operation Iraqi Freedom. *Psychological Trauma: Theory, Research, Practice, and Policy* 3(2):201-211.

Kleykamp, M. 2009. A great place to start?: The effect of prior military service on hiring. *Armed Forces and Society* 35(2):266-285.

———. 2012. *Employment, Earnings and Enrollment Among Post 9/11 Veterans (working paper).* College Park, MD: University of Maryland.

Leslie, D. L., J. Goulet, M. Skanderson, K. Mattocks, S. Haskell, and C. Brandt. 2011. VA health care utilization and costs among male and female veterans in the year after service in Afghanistan and Iraq. *Military Medicine* 176(3):265-269.

Losinger, W. C. 2010. Notes regarding the 2006 survey of active duty spouses. *Armed Forces and Society* 36(3).

Loughran, D. S., and J. A. Klerman. 2008. *Explaining the Increase in Unemployment Compensation for Ex-servicemembers During the Global War on Terror.* Santa Monica, CA: RAND Corporation.

———. 2010. *The Effect of Activation on the Post-activation Civilian Earnings of Reservists.* Santa Monica, CA: RAND Corporation.

Loughran, D. S., P. Martorell, T. Miller, and J. A. Klerman. 2011. *The Effect of Military Enlistment on Earnings and Education.* Santa Monica, CA: RAND Corporation.

Masini, B. D., S. M. Waterman, J. C. Wenke, B. D. Owens, J. R. Hsu, and J. R. Ficke. 2009. Resource utilization and disability outcome assessment of combat casualties from Operation Iraqi Freedom and Operation Enduring Freedom. *Journal of Orthopaedic Trauma* 23(4):261-266.

McSally, M. E. 2007. *Women in Combat: Is the Current Policy Obsolete?* Air War Coll., Maxwell Air Force Base, AL.

Neumark, D. 2011 (unpublished). *Spurring Job Creation in Response to Severe Recessions: Reconsidering Hiring Credits.* Cambridge, MA: NBER Working Paper.

Noonan, M. E., and C. J. Mumola. 2007. *Veterans in State and Federal Prison, 2004.* Washington, DC: Bureau of Justice Statistics.

Resnick, S. G., and R. A. Rosenheck. 2008. Posttraumatic stress disorder and employment in veterans participating in Veterans Health Administration Compensated Work Therapy. *Journal of Rehabilitation Research and Development* 45(3):427-435.

Riviere, L. A., A. Kendall-Robbins, D. McGurk, C. A. Castro, and C. W. Hoge. 2011. Coming home may hurt: Risk factors for mental ill health in US reservists after deployment in Iraq. *British Journal of Psychiatry* 198:136-142.

Rohlfs, C. 2010. Does combat exposure make you a more violent or criminal person? Evidence from the Vietnam draft. *Journal of Human Resources* 45(2):271-300.

Ruggles, S., J. T. Alexander, K. Genadek, R. Goeken, M. B. Schroeder, and M. Sobek. 2010. *Integrated Public Use Microdata Series: Version 5.0 [machine-readable database]*. Minneapolis, MN: University of Minnesota.

Sayer, N. A., S. Noorbaloochi, P. Frazier, K. Carlson, A. Gravely, and M. Murdoch. 2010. Reintegration problems and treatment interests among Iraq and Afghanistan combat veterans receiving VA medical care. *Psychiatric Services* 61(6):589-597.

Senate Health Education Labor and Pension Committee. 2011. *New data on post-9/11 GI Bill Benefits Show Disproportionate Share of Taxpayer Dollars Going to For-profit Colleges with Concerning Outcomes.* http://harkin.senate.gov/documents/pdf/4e7b5d0253b75.pdf (accessed July 14, 2012).

Sewall, M. 2010. Bill to expand veterans' education benefits begins moving through Congress. *Chronicle of Higher Education*, August 5.

Sheftick, G. W. 2012. New Transition Assistance Program set for November launch. *Army News Service.* http://www.defense.gov/news/newsarticle.aspx?id=117959 (accessed November 1, 2012).

Smith, M. W., P. P. Schnurr, and R. A. Rosenheck. 2005. Employment outcomes and PTSD symptom severity. *Mental Health Services Research* 7(2):89-101.

Steele, J. L., N. Salcedo, and J. Coley. 2011. *Service Members in School: Military Veterans' Experiences Using the Post-9/11 GI Bill and Pursuing Postsecondary Education.* Santa Monica, CA: RAND Corporation.

Stiglitz, J. E., and L. Bilmes. 2008. *The Three Trillion Dollar War*. New York: Norton.

Tanielian, T., and L. H. Jaycox. 2008. *Invisible Wounds of War: Psychological and Cognitive Injuries, Their Consequences, and Services to Assist Recovery*. Santa Monica: RAND Corporation.

Wang, L., J. Glen Elder, and N. J. Spence. 2012. Status configurations, military service, and higher education. *Social Forces* 91(2):397-422.

# 9

# ACCESS AND BARRIERS TO CARE

This chapter begins with a discussion of what access to health care means. It then presents a discussion of how active-duty military and veterans access their health care through the Department of Defense (DOD) and the Department of Veterans Affairs (VA) health care systems with a focus on mental-health care. Mental-health issues are highlighted because of the large numbers of returning Operation Enduring Freedom (OEF) and Operation Iraqi Freedom (OIF) that have been diagnosed with posttraumatic stress disorder (PTSD) and other mental-health disorders (see Chapter 4). The chapter then presents a discussion of issues related to fragmentation of care and disparities in care, in particular, disparities based on gender and ethnicity. The chapter highlights many of the barriers to care and examines the DOD's and VA's programmatic responses to those barriers; finally, the committee provides its recommendations. Returning OEF and OIF military and veterans have been diagnosed with a host of physical- and mental-health outcomes (as documented in earlier chapters of this report). The DOD and VA health care systems have been struggling in certain health care areas to provide timely care to the over 2 million service members who have been deployed since 2001. While the DOD and VA have excelled in providing acute care and care to patients with polytrauma, areas such as mental-health care services have fallen behind.

As documented and discussed in several chapters of this report and other sources, OEF and OIF deployed service members are returning with high rates of mental-health disorders; concerns regarding the availability and adequacy of mental-health services have been highlighted in numerous reports (e.g., Tanielian and Jaycox, 2008). That is troubling as untreated mental-health disorders are strongly linked to numerous adverse outcomes (see Chapter 4).

A 2009 report of mental-health care for OEF and OIF veterans (Burnam et al., 2009) found that the mental-health workforce had insufficient capacity to address the mental-health needs of service members returning home. The study also found that the workforce lacked sufficient training in evidence-based practices and that there were inadequate organizational systems and tools to support mental-health quality improvements. Other concerns about VA health care have been highlighted and include perceptions that programs and service options are not adequate or uniform across different locations, facilities or providers, that services are not welcoming to certain groups (e.g., women and minorities) (GAO, 2011b), and that their availability differs across regions. For example, studies indicate that VA patients in rural areas have reduced access to health services and fewer alternatives to VA care (Weeks et al., 2004; West and Weeks, 2006).

## ACCESS TO HEALTH CARE

This section begins with a definition of *access* to health care and provides information about how active-duty service members and veterans access care through the DOD's Military Health System (MHS) and the VA's Health Care System. Access to care has been defined as "the timely use of personal health services to achieve the best possible health outcomes" (IOM, 2001). A related concept is *perceived access*, defined as the individual's subjective impression of his or her personal access to services. Perceived access is influenced by personal knowledge, actual experience in obtaining preferred services, and degree of satisfaction with those services. Satisfaction in turn is influenced by utilization, quality, and patient outcomes experience, all of which are influenced by the individual's perceived need for care. Perceived access may be greater or less than actual access. For example, someone who is not attempting to obtain care may be unaware of impediments they would likely encounter; thus, their perceived access may be greater than actual access (Fortney et al., 2011).

**TABLE 9.1** Patient, Community, Health System and Provider Determinants of Access

| Dimension of Access | Actual Access | Perceived Access | Examples of Measures |
|---|---|---|---|
| Geographic | Road travel distance and travel time to nearest provider or nearest facility with telemedicine equipment; number and choice of providers | Self-report of one's travel | Distance to nearest provider or telehealth provider |
| Temporal | Time delay between when services are needed and how long it actual takes to receive the service; length of time to get an appointment or to communicate digitally with the provider; time spent waiting in the reception area, receiving the treatment, and wait time for next appointment | Self-reported time burden and temporal convenience of receiving services | Appointment wait times |
| Financial | Eligibility and cost of utilizing the services, including insurance premiums, out-of-pocket costs, and opportunity costs, cost of digital connectivity, and other computer health applications. | Influenced by perceptions of eligibility and affordability | Copayments |
| Cultural | Whether language of the patient is offered, and whether service is discriminatory free | Patients trust and understanding of their provider; trust in their treatment plan; degree to which a patient internalizes any provider discrimination or public stigma | Linguistic match between provider and patient |

| Dimension of Access | Actual Access | Perceived Access | Examples of Measures |
|---|---|---|---|
| Digital | Connectivity and adequate tools required to engage in synchronous or asynchronous digital communication with providers, caregivers, peers, and computerized health applications | Perception about the opportunity and simplicity of the digital interaction, which includes connectivity issues, user problems, provider responsiveness, and security and privacy concerns | Web-based access to health records |

SOURCE: Fortney et al., 2011 (adapted).

Successfully achieving "access" requires that there be a unique fit among the above elements, the patient, and health care system (Fortney et al., 2011). Thus, the DOD and VA health systems must be flexible enough to adapt to the individual patient's characteristics and specific needs as they relate to the domains above (see Table 9.1), both on the actual and perceived level. As noted in Fortney et al. (2011), policy makers are responsible for developing and implementing performance measures across the five dimensions as they relate to all components influencing access and barriers to care.

Below is a description of how active-duty service members, their families, and veterans access care through the DOD's Military Health Care System and the VA's Health Care System.

## MILITARY HEALTH CARE SYSTEM

The DOD's MHS provides the resources, health professionals, and direction necessary to promote the health of its beneficiary population. It is one of the largest health care organizations in the country, providing services to 9.6 million beneficiaries and employing 140,000 military, civilian, and contract personnel in the MHS setting who work with an additional 380,000 civilian providers in the United States and overseas (DOD, 2011b). The MHS provides direct care to most active-duty service members through military treatment facilities (MTFs) and clinics. The direct care is supplemented by care purchased from the civilian sector. Retirees and dependent family members of active-duty service members are also eligible to receive care at an MTF on a space-available basis; priority is given to those enrolled in TRICARE Prime (described below). Responsibility for delivering health care to garrisoned and deployed troops remains with the health departments of the individual services—Army, Navy,[1] and Air Force—which have considerable autonomy in facility and personnel management (DOD, 2011a; IOM, 2010). In addition to providing health care to its beneficiaries, the health system funds education and training in accredited medical and graduate school programs and devotes approximately $600 million per year on research and development (Merlis, 2012).

[1]The medical department of the Navy oversees health care delivery for the Marine Corps.

## TRICARE

TRICARE refers to the DOD's collective medical programs, which provide care to all active-duty military, activated members of the National Guard and reserves, retired military personal, and their dependents who are eligible for coverage. Services may be provided through managed-care providers directly in DOD facilities,[2] which includes 44 inpatient hospitals and medical centers, 291 ambulatory care clinics, 213 dental clinics in the United States, or through the purchased care system which includes 379,233 network individual providers (primary care, mental-health, and specialty care) and 3,146 TRICARE network acute care hospitals (DOD, 2011a; Merlis, 2012). There is also a fee-for-service option for care administered by civilian providers who are not part of the network (Deployment Health Clinical Center, 2012).

### Eligibility and Enrollment

The total number of eligible beneficiaries stationed or residing in the United States at the end of fiscal year (FY) 2010 was 9.09 million (0.60 million were stationed or residing abroad). Retirees and their family members under the age of 65 constitute the largest percentage of the eligible population (3.07 million, 55%); followed by retirees and their family members over the age of 65 (1.88 million, 215); active-duty family members (1.91 million, 21%); active duty (1.28 million, 14%); and National Guard and reserve family members (0.58 million, 6%) (DOD, 2011a). Figure 9.1 shows the extent to which the MHS population has geographic access to direct care by providing a visual of the US distribution of the 9.09 million beneficiaries eligible for TRICARE coverage overlaid with the DOD MTFs (medical centers, community hospitals, and medical clinics).

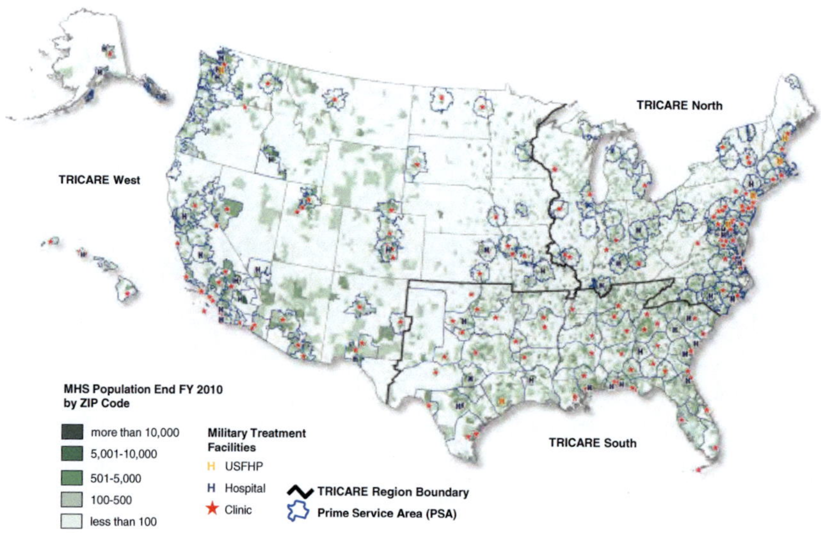


**FIGURE 9.1** Military Health System population distribution in the United States relative to military treatment facilities in FY2010.
SOURCE: DOD, 2011a.

---

[2]Direct care treatment facilities are operated under one of the three service branches: Army, Navy, and Air Force.

To enroll in any TRICARE plan, service members, their families, and retirees must first establish eligibility through the Defense Enrollment Eligibility Reporting System (DEERS). Active-duty and retired service members, including National Guard and reserve members activated for at least 30 days, are automatically registered in DEERS, but individual service members are responsible for registering their family members, updating their status, and ensuring that their information is current and correct (TRICARE Management Activity, 2009). Active-duty service members, including members of the reserve components activated for at least 30 days, automatically enroll in TRICARE Prime[3] at no cost. Eligible service members may also enroll their dependent family members in TRICARE Prime at no cost. Dependents, however, may also choose to pay extra to enroll in TRICARE Extra, an option within the TRICARE Standard program that functions similar to a preferred provider organization where participants may pay lower coinsurance if using a contracted network provider or seek coverage through a civilian health-insurance provider. There is no enrollment fee; however, an annual deductible must be met (Andrews et al., 2009; Military.com, 2012b).

In addition to active-duty members and their families, the following beneficiary groups are also eligible for coverage under TRICARE Prime: retired National Guard and reserve members (age 60 and receiving retired pay but not eligible for TRICARE for Life) and their families, survivors, Medal of Honor recipients and their families, and qualified former spouses. However, these individuals (non-active-duty members and their families) are also eligible for and may choose TRICARE Standard, a fee-for-service option that allows beneficiaries to obtain care from any TRICARE-authorized provider; there is a deductible, and coinsurance of 20–25% but no enrollment fee. About one-third of non-active-duty individuals eligible for TRICARE Prime (mostly retirees under the age of 65 and their families) live in areas without access to the Prime network and thus must choose TRICARE Standard (Military.com, 2012b).

Reserve component members and their eligible family members are covered by TRICARE up to 180 days prior to reporting to active duty (preactivation) and up to 180 days after deactivation through the Transitional Assistance Management Program (TAMP). When not in mobilized status, reservists may purchase TRICARE Select Reserve coverage, which is premium-based and offers comprehensive health care coverage similar to the TRICARE Standard and TRICARE Extra options (DOD, 2011a).

### Access to Facilities

TRICARE Prime is available in the United States in areas known as Prime Service Areas. After enrolling in TRICARE Prime, a primary care manager (PCM) is assigned to the beneficiary at either an MTF or from the TRICARE network. The PCM will provide referral to care specialists when they are unable to provide the necessary care, coordinate with the regional contractor for authorization, find a specialist in the network, and file claims on the beneficiary's behalf. Active-duty service members and their families pay no out-of-pocket costs for any type of care as long as it is received from the PCM or from another provider with a referral (DOD, 2012).

Military hospitals have historically been defined by two geographic boundaries: a 40-mile catchment area (59 catchment areas) for inpatient and referral care and a 20-mile Provider

[3]TRICARE Prime is a point-of-service health-maintenance organization that covers 100% of care at MTFs or any civilian provider that is a member of the TRICARE network.

Requirement Integrated Specialty Model (PRISM) (290 PRISM areas) for outpatient care. Stand-alone clinics or ambulatory care centers have only a PRISM area boundary.[4] From FY 2004 to FY 2010 there was a downward trend (from 51 to 46%) in the proportion of beneficiaries living in catchment areas, due mostly to Base Realignment and Closure (BRAC) actions; the percentage living in PRISM has remained relatively constant at 64%.

Most active-duty members and their families (91%) live in MTF service areas. Ninety-six percent live in Prime Service Areas, which are geographic areas that in the least include catchment areas where the TRICARE Managed Care Support Contractors offer the TRICARE Prime benefits through an established network of providers. The percentage of Reserve Component members[5] and families with access to MTF-PRIME (those living in a catchment or PRISM area) is 44.8%. TRICARE Prime is available at MTFs, in areas around most MTFs, and in some areas where an MTF was recently removed as a result of BRAC (DOD, 2011a). Note that non-active-duty beneficiaries that do not live in a catchment or a PRISM area have limited or no access to MTF-based Prime (DOD, 2011a). Figure 9.2 provides further information on beneficiaries and their geographic access to catchment and PRISM areas.

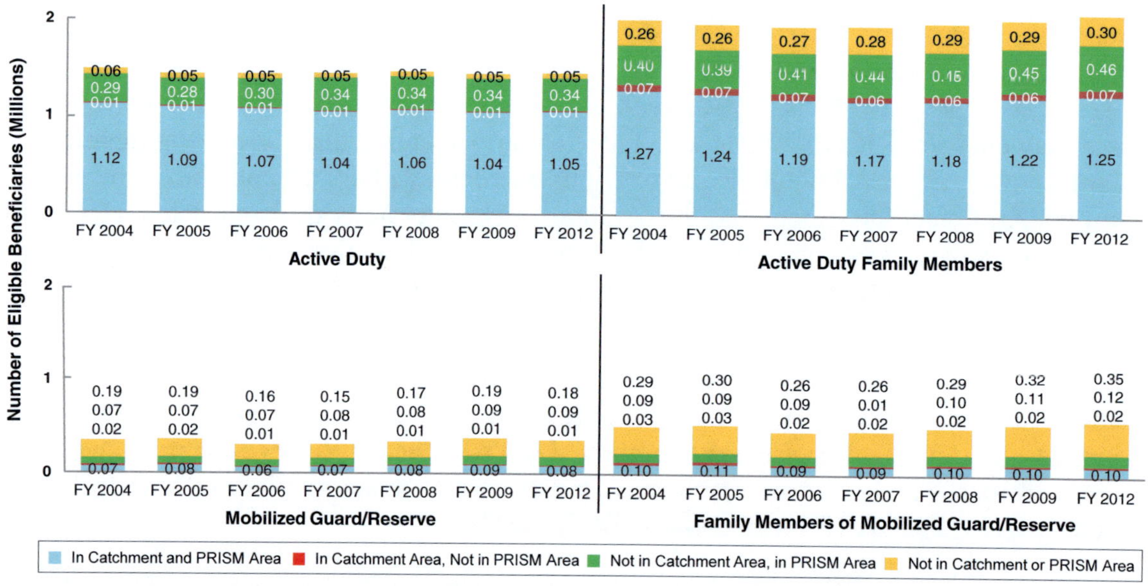


**FIGURE 9.2** Trend in the number of eligible beneficiaries living in and out of MTF catchment and PRISM areas (year-end population).
NOTE: In Catchment and PRISM Area = within 20 miles of a military hospital (proximity to both inpatient and outpatient care); In Catchment, Not in PRISM Area = beyond 20 miles but within 40 miles of a military hospital (proximity to inpatient care); Not in Catchment Area, in PRISM Area = within 20 miles of a freestanding military clinic (no military hospital nearby; proximity to outpatient care only); Not in Catchment or PRISM Area = beyond 20 miles of a freestanding military clinic (lack of proximity to either inpatient or outpatient MTF-based care).
SOURCE: DOD, 2011a.

[4]The distance-based catchment and PRISM area concepts have been superseded within MHS by a time-based geographic concept referred to as an MTF Enrollment Area. An MTF Enrollment Area is defined as the area within a 30-minute drive time of an MTF in which a commander may require TRICARE Prime beneficiaries to enroll with the MTF. However, because this is a relatively new concept, it has not yet been implemented within DEERS or in MHS administrative data and is consequently unavailable for use in this report.

[5]Reserve component includes ready, standby, and retired reserve.

Since 2007, the population of beneficiaries has grown by about 400,000. However, the direct care system has decreased—70 hospitals in 2004 to 59 in 2009. To handle the increase in eligible beneficiaries while accounting for the decrease in direct care facilities, TRICARE must rely more heavily on civilian providers. Eligible beneficiaries are also choosing TRICARE Prime with more frequency, and, consequently, purchased care workload has grown (DOD, 2011b). In addition, mobilizations of National Guard and reserve contributed disproportionately to the number of beneficiaries living outside the catchment areas. Most members live in noncatchment areas when they are called to and leave for active duty; however, their families usually remain in the same location (DOD, 2011a). That may explain the shift in MHS workload from direct care to purchase care in the 2004–2010 period.

## Mental-Health Care Within the MHS

The DOD provides mental-health services through military treatment facilities and clinics for active-duty service members and their families as well as eligible military retirees, eligible reserve-component members, and their respective families (Burnam et al., 2009). Some combat veterans have access to community-based networks of practitioners through TRICARE. TRICARE requires active-duty service members (ADSMs) to seek nonemergency mental-health care at MTFs, when available. If not available, ADSMs must obtain referrals from their MTFs or service points of contact before receiving civilian care. Non-active-duty service members do not need referrals or prior authorization for the first eight outpatient mental-health care visits per fiscal year to a network provider for a medically diagnosed and covered condition. Services provided include psychotherapy, psychoanalysis, psychologic testing, medical management, telemental-health program, acute inpatient psychiatric care, psychiatric partial hospitalization program, residential treatment center care, inpatient detoxification, rehabilitation, and outpatient substance abuse care.

## Transitional Health Care Coverage

Separating active-duty members and their dependents are eligible for transitional TRICARE coverage for 180 days through TAMP if they were involuntarily separated under honorable conditions, separated following involuntary retention (stop-loss) in support of a contingency operation, separated following a voluntary agreement to stay on active duty in support of contingency operation, received a sole survivorship discharge, or separated and agreed to become a member of Selected Reserve. Deactivated National Guard and reserve members who were called to active duty for at least 30 days in support of a contingency operation and their dependents are also usually eligible to receive health care coverage for 180 days through TAMP (Military.com, 2012a).

If not eligible for TAMP or within 60 days of terminating TAMP coverage, active-duty members leaving the military under other than adverse conditions and their dependent family members can purchase a health plan similar to TRICARE Standard for up to 18 months of coverage through the Continued Health Care Benefit Program (CHCBP) if family coverage is selected. Children and spouses who were enrolled in TRICARE and lose eligibility can purchase CHCBP coverage for up to 36 months if individual coverage is selected (Military.com, 2012a).

## VA Health Care System

VA is the second-largest cabinet-level department in the federal government, next to the DOD. Like other large government agencies, the VA administers its many programs through a number of subcabinet agencies, the primary ones being the Veterans Benefits Administration (VBA), the Veterans Health Administration (VHA), and the National Cemetery Administration (NCA). The VBA administers veteran's compensation and pension, home loan, educational, life insurance, vocational rehabilitation, and other non–health care benefits; VHA administers the Veterans Health Care System; and the NCA oversees 136 national cemeteries and other memorials.

The VA Health Care System was established in the early 1900s to care for disabled and poor veterans. Expansion of the system was catalyzed first by the 2 million veterans returning home from World War I and second by the 12 million new veterans from World War II. The VA Health Care System grew rapidly after 1945. Today, it is the nation's largest and only national direct care delivery system. Integral to its clinical services, the VA also provides transportation, housing, vocational rehabilitation, and other social support services rarely offered by private health plans (CBO, 2009; Panangala, 2010).

The VA began affiliating with academic health centers in 1947 (CBO, 2009). It operates the nation's largest health care professions training program, providing training on a yearly basis for about 110,000 aspiring health care workers in more than 40 health care disciplines through affiliations with some 1,100 universities, colleges, and other institutions of higher education. VA funds more than 9,500 graduate medical education positions, and 85% of its medical centers are teaching hospitals, and almost one-third of all postgraduate physicians receive some portion of their training at a VA facility. Thus, the VA is the nation's largest provider of training for nurses, pharmacists, optometrists, podiatrists, clinical psychologists, and other health care professions.

The VHA also conducts a broad portfolio of research on veterans. In FY2010, the VHA's research program had a total budget of $1.8 billion, including intramural funding of $575 million and an additional indeterminate amount of medical care funds to support clinical research.

Embedding a biomedical, health services delivery and quality-improvement research program in a national health care delivery system and serving a stable population with an unusually high prevalence of chronic conditions, the VA has been very productive. Because veterans often have been a sentinel population for health conditions affecting the public at large, VA research about amputations and prosthetics, organ transplants, end-stage renal disease, traumatic brain injury, diabetes, geriatrics, mental-health, and quality improvement, among other areas, have materially benefitted all Americans. A description of VHA-funded studies that are currently in progress on the OEF, OIF, and OND population are provided in Appendix D.

### Health Care Facilities

Since 1924, the VA has served as a national health care safety net for veterans (Kizer and Dudley, 2009; Koenig, 2003; Wilson and Kizer, 1997). Approximately 30% of VA enrollees have one or more mental-health conditions (Liu et al., 2005; Ralston et al., 2007; Seal et al., 2007), making VA the nation's largest provider of mental-health services.

In federal FY 2010, the VA Health Care System had an operating budget of $45.1 billion, 8.3 million enrollees, and 222,551 full-time employees, including some 14,000 staff physicians and more than 40,000 nurses (CBO, 2009; Panangala, 2010). Medical treatment facilities are located in all 50 states and essentially every major metropolitan area of the country, as well as in Puerto Rico, the US Virgin Islands, Guam, American Samoa, and the Philippines.

Health care is delivered through Veterans Affairs Medical Centers (VAMCs) that provide acute and long-term care delivery facilities through 152 hospitals; more than 800 ambulatory care clinics (CBOCs), 135 community living centers, 140 home-based primary care programs, 299 readjustment counseling centers, and 43 residential care facilities. VHA also co-funded 133 state-operated nursing facilities for elderly veterans in FY 2010 and managed 9 purchased care programs that bought more than $6 billion of services from private providers (Himmelstein et al., 2007; Koenig, 2003). The various components of the system provide a wide spectrum of medical services, including inpatient and outpatient care, mental-health care, rehabilitation, complex specialty care, and pharmaceutical benefits and distribution.

Finally, services may be provided to veterans in non-VA facilities and fall into two broad categories: contract care and noncontract care purchased on a fee-for-service basis. The use of non-VA care is justified if there is geographic inaccessibility, a lack of clinical capacity, if medical expertise or technology is not available at the local facility, or in an emergency situation.

## Eligibility

With the enactment of the National Defense Authorization Act (PL 110-181), veterans who served in a combat theater (including National Guard and reserves) after November 11, 1998, and were discharged or released for reasons other than dishonorable on or after January 28, 2003, now have 5 years from their date of discharge to enroll in and obtain health care coverage from the VA. This includes all OEF and OIF veterans. Effective January 28, 2003, OEF and OIF veterans who enroll within the first 5 years after separating from the military are eligible for enhanced enrollment placement into priority group 6 (see Table 9.2) for 5 years after discharge. Injuries or conditions related to combat service are treated by the VA health care system free of charge (IOM, 2010). After the designated 5 years, enrolled veterans are placed in the appropriate priority group (see Table 9.2) on the basis of income and disability; placement determines the extent of coverage and copayment amounts. Each year, VA determines whether appropriations are adequate to cover all priority groups; if not, those in the lowest groups may lose coverage (Panangala, 2007).

In general, VHA does not provide health care services or coverage to spouses or dependents of veterans (IOM, 2009; VA, 2009). However, in accordance with the Veterans' Mental-health and Other Care Improvements Act of 2008 (S. 2162, 110th Congress), if VA health care services for family members are necessary for the proper treatment of a veteran, then various family members also will have access. Previously, family members were only allowed to take part in such services if they were initiated during a veteran's hospitalization and continued only if necessary for hospital discharge (IOM, 2010).

**TABLE 9.2** Enrollment Priority Groups

| Priority Group | Definition |
|---|---|
| 1 | Veterans with VA service-connected disabilities 50% or more disabling.<br>Veterans assigned a total disability rating for compensation based on unemployability. |

| Priority Group | Definition |
|---|---|
| 2 | Veterans with VA service-connected disabilities rated 30% or 40%. |
| 3 | Veterans who are former Prisoners of War.<br>Veterans awarded a Purple Heart Medal.<br>Veterans awarded the Medal of Honor.<br>Veterans whose discharge was for a disability incurred or aggravated in the line of duty.<br>Veterans with VA service-connected disabilities rated 10% or 20%.<br>Veterans awarded special eligibility classification under Title 38, U.S.C. § 1151, "benefits for individuals disabled by treatment or vocational rehabilitation." |
| 4 | Veterans receiving increased compensation or pension based on their need for regular Aid and Attendance or by reason of being permanently Housebound.<br>Veterans determined by VA to be catastrophically disabled. |
| 5 | Non-service-connected Veterans and noncompensable service-connected Veterans rated 0%, whose annual income and/or net worth are not greater than the VA financial thresholds.<br>Veterans receiving VA Pension benefits.<br>Veterans eligible for Medicaid benefits. |
| 6 | Compensable 0% service-connected veterans.<br>Veterans exposed to ionizing radiation during atmospheric testing or during the occupation of Hiroshima and Nagasaki.<br>Project 112/SHAD participants.<br>Veterans who served in the Republic of Vietnam between January 9, 1962, and May 7, 1975.<br>Veterans who served in the Southwest Asia theater of operations from August 2, 1990, through November 11, 1998.<br>Veterans who served in a theater of combat operations after November 11, 1998, as follows:<br>Veterans discharged from active duty on or after January 28, 2003, for 5 years post discharge. |
| 7 | Veterans with incomes **below** the geographic means test (GMT) income thresholds and who agree to pay the applicable copayment. |
| 8 | Veterans with gross household incomes above the VA national income threshold and the geographically adjusted income threshold for their resident location and who agrees to pay copays.<br>**Veterans eligibility for enrollment:** Noncompensable 0% service-connected and:<br>• Subpriority a: Enrolled as of January 16, 2003, and who have remained enrolled since that date and/ or placed in this subpriority due to changed eligibility status.<br>• Subpriority b: Enrolled on or after June 15, 2009, whose income exceeds the current VA National Income Thresholds or VA National Geographic Income Thresholds by 10% or less<br>**Veterans eligible for enrollment:** Non-service-connected and:<br>• Subpriority c: Enrolled as January 16, 2003, and who remained enrolled since that date and/ or placed in this subpriority due to changed eligibility status<br>• Subpriority d: Enrolled on or after June 15, 2009, whose income exceeds the current VA National Income Thresholds or VA National Geographic Income Thresholds by 10% or less<br>**Veterans not eligible for enrollment**: Veterans not meeting the criteria above:<br>• Subpriority e: Noncompensable 0% service-connected<br>• Subpriority g: Non-service-connected |

SOURCE: Department of Veterans Affairs website:
http://www.va.gov/healthbenefits/resources/priority_groups.asp (accessed October 3, 2012).

## Cost of Care

All enrolled veterans are provided treatment and medications for service-connected illness of injury by the VA free of charge. Those who are in the higher-priority groups usually do not pay a copayment for services unrelated to their military service, while those veterans in the lower-priority groups usually pay $15 for a primary care visit and $50 for a specialist care visit (VA, 2012a). With the passage of the Veterans Millennium Health Care Act in 1999 (effective in FY 2002) the copayment for outpatient prescriptions increased from $2 to $7 per 30-day supply (Zeber et al., 2007). As of January 2006, the copayment for veterans in priority categories 2 through 6 increased to $8 per prescription with a maximum annual copayment of $960. Veterans with higher incomes (priority group 7 and 8) pay $9 per 30-day supply; there is no annual cap for this group (VA, 2012a). For those with very low income or a disability rating of 50% of higher, all copayments are waived (CBO, 2009; Stroupe et al., 2007). Thus, veteran's health care is provided at no cost to veterans in high-priority groups and at low cost to veterans in other priority categories. Furthermore, in its attempt to reduce or eliminate costs for some treatments, the VA no longer requires a copayment for telehealth (discussed later in this chapter) (VA, 2012b).

## VA Electronic Health Record

In an effort to improve access through communication between health care provider and patient, the website MyHealth*e*Vet was introduced by the VHA in 2003. It is a Web-based personal health record that provides information on health conditions, benefits, and VA facility locations and contains a personalized patient health record, which allows patients to perform certain functions related to their health care, such as refilling prescriptions, making appointments, and viewing the results of certain laboratory tests (Jackson et al., 2011; Turvey et al., 2012). More broadly, it is intended to improve co-managed care and empower patients to play a more active role in their health care (Nazi et al., 2010).

In 2010, a survey was conducted using the American Customer Satisfaction Index. Veterans who had viewed at least four pages of MyHealth*e*Vet were invited to participate in the survey regarding utilization of the website. The majority of the users were male (91%), between 51 and 70 years old (68%), and served during Vietnam (60%). Most rated their health in the "good" or "very good" category, one-third live 1 or more hours away from a VA facility, and 75% use the system to refill prescriptions (Nazi, 2010). Results also indicated that 40% of users printed out their information, 21% saved their information to their computers, 4% sent to other users, 18% shared their medication lists with VA providers, and 9.6% shared with non-VA providers. As of April 2011, the website had registered over 1.2 million users. While MyHealth*e*Vet has the capacity to improve access through increased coordination of care, VHA will need to determine how to increase usage among veterans.

## Mental-Health Care Within the VA

The VA offers acute inpatient care, intensive and regular outpatient care (e.g., psychotherapy, pharmacotherapy, and telemedicine), residential care, and supported work settings. Services include treatment for depression and anxiety, substance abuse, PTSD, severe mental illnesses (e.g., schizophrenia, schizoaffective disorder, and bipolar disorder), and special programs for veteran populations with special needs (e.g., suicide prevention services, sexual trauma, services for women veterans, homeless veterans, older veterans, and veterans within the criminal justice system).

In 2004, when the VA adopted a new approach to mental-health care designed to focus on recovery, it integrated mental-health care into overall health care for veteran patients. The VA also developed a 5-year action plan that includes more than 200 initiatives, including initiatives aimed at raising awareness of the importance of mental-health, eliminating disparities in the availability and quality of mental-health services for veterans, and providing comprehensive mental-health care services to veterans with mental illness (VA, 2011b).

In 2008, the VA published a handbook specifying which mental-health and substance-use treatment services VA hospitals and clinics are required to offer veterans and their families; in 2011 a simplified version to help beneficiaries navigate services was published (VA, 2011a; VA and VHA, 2008).

## FRAGMENTATION OF CARE

Fragmentation of care diminishes continuity and coordination, often resulting in higher use of emergency departments, increased hospitalization, duplication of tests, and increased costs. It has also been shown to increase the likelihood of adverse effects and medical errors. Persons with chronic conditions and mental-health diagnoses are especially vulnerable to these consequences, as are young adult males who are more likely to seek care from multiple providers (Kizer, 2011, 2012). Continuity of care is an essential element in health care service delivery and includes availability of patient information, clinician consistency and availability, coordination during transition events, and ongoing patient and provider communication (Donaldson, 2001). The transition between the DOD and the VA systems is a vulnerable period when continuity of care might be compromised.

### Transitions Within the DOD and VA

Military service men and women experience frequent changes in geographic location related to their military service. Those changes necessitate changes in primary care and mental-health care, which can delay treatment (until new providers are identified and appointments secured) and change treatment protocols. Transfer of medical records within the military health system might not capture all medical information, particularly treatment for mental-health visits. Paper records for mental-health evaluations might not be available, and repeat examinations might occur as might treatments that had previously proved ineffective (Tanielian and Jaycox, 2008).

When active-duty members leave military service and return to civilian status, their health care coverage transitions from DOD to the VA health care system. That requires successful completion of several handoffs, from MTFs and TRICARE network providers to VA facilities. Critical handoffs include enrollment in the VA system, identification of and enrollment in programs, and the successful transfer of medical records. Additionally, some reserve members might receive care from both DOD and VA, and although both use electronic health records, the two systems are not yet compatible.

In general, transition points pose risks to access and quality of care, including disruption of relationships with care providers, treatment interruption, and handoff errors. Risks are increased for service members receiving mental-health care as they make the transition. Furthermore, the VA requires consent for medical records to be transferred from DOD to VA for reserve members, creating another potentially risky transition point.

Programs have been developed by both DOD and VA to bridge gaps in care and decrease fragmentation. For example, DOD utilizes the inTransition Program, which offers specialized assistance and coaching aimed at enhancing continuity for service members receiving mental-health care as they make any of the following transitions: relocating to another assignment, returning from deployment, transitioning from active duty to reserve or vice versa, and leaving military service (Office of the Assistant Secretary of Defense, 2010). The Federal Recovery Coordination Program (FRCP) was jointly developed by DOD and VA to coordinate care for severely wounded service members and veterans. It was designed to complement existing programs such as DOD's Recovery Coordination Program, the Wounded Warrior Program operated by the individual military services,[6] Army Warrior Transition Units, VA's OEF and OIF Care Management Program, VA's Spinal Cord Injury Disorders Program, and the VA Polytrauma System of Care. FRCP coordinators are assigned to link together multiple case managers, oversee their enrollment in programs, and serve as the single point of contact for the injured service member and their families (CBO, 2011; Yano et al., 2003).

A major limitation and concern of the FRCP is the inability to share information across DOD and VA and the general incompatibility among systems used by different programs. Service members are typically enrolled in multiple programs—in September 2010, 84% of FRCP enrollees were also enrolled in a military service wounded warrior program. That limits coordination of services, increases duplications of services, and may result in enrollee confusion. Accordingly, FRCP is making efforts to address those limitations and improve information sharing; however, as noted by the GAO (2011a), it appears that increased efforts to improve data exchange between the two systems and interdepartmental coordination are needed.

### Electronic Health Records

Successful transfer of medical records is a necessary component of the DOD-to-VA transition and, more broadly, a way in which to decrease fragmentation of care resulting from movements between health systems and providers. Electronic health records have the potential to facilitate communication between patients and providers, especially from differing health care systems, to improve coordination and reduce redundant care, medication errors, and costs (Kaelber and Pan, 2008; Ralston et al., 2007; Ross et al., 2004; Schnipper et al., 2009; Zhou et al., 2007). Additionally, electronic health records should allow patients the ability to transfer their records to providers who are not in the system; for example, rural veterans who often receive both VA and non-VA care.

The DOD and the VA health systems currently employ electronic health records and the Federal Health Information Exchange (HIE) supports the transfer of electronic health information from the DOD to VA at time of separation. That one-way exchange of information

[6]The Wounded Warrior Program includes the Army Wounded Warrior Program, the Marine Wounded Warrior Regiment, Navy Safe Harbor, the Air Force Warrior and Survivors Care Program, and the Special Operations Command's Care Coalition.

allows VA providers to view the clinical data record, and the deployment and postdeployment health assessments (DOD, 2011a). Additionally, there is a Bidirectional Health Information Exchange that provides bidirectional health care data transfers between VA and DOD health care facilities for shared patients. For example, the Clinical Health Data Repository (CHDR) provides, at a minimum, outpatient pharmacy and drug allergy records; and the Laboratory Data Sharing and Interoperability supports the sharing of secure encrypted laboratory orders and results between the two agencies. Despite those technologies, service members have indicated poor management throughout medical record transfer.

In an effort to address those problems, the DOD and the VA have announced that they are working to integrate their health records; currently the goal is to reach that milestone by 2017. The goal of the new system is to provide a seamless transition of care between the DOD and the VA. The development of the Integrated Electronic Health Record (iEHR) is to be tested in two sites by 2014 that offer DOD and VA care: San Antonio, Texas, and Hamptons Roads, Virginia (Pellerin and Marshall, 2012).

## DISPARITIES IN HEALTH CARE

Providing uniform services within the DOD and VA health care systems across geographic locations, facilities, and providers should be a priority; as should providing quality care to women and ethnic minorities (GAO, 2011b). There is a paucity of information regarding disparities in health care in the OEF and OIF active duty and veteran populations. This section, however, highlights issues regarding health care in women, racial and ethnic minorities, and rural veterans. As discussed below, disparities in health might manifest in subtle ways; for example, the type of diagnoses received by women or different ethnic groups.

### Women in the Military

As noted in Chapter 4, women comprise about 14% of all active-duty military, and 17.6% of National Guard and reserves; about 12% of women veterans served in OEF, OIF, or OND.[7] Historically, the research on the health of veterans has focused on the health consequences of combat service in men with little scientific research or longitudinal study of the health consequences of military service for women. Research that has examined gender differences is generally mixed, and a recent review (Street et al., 2009) highlighted the need to conduct studies with larger samples of women to understand issues relevant specifically for women. Women in the military cope with some unique stressors that might amplify their risk for mental-health problems, such as military sexual trauma (MST); histories of premilitary trauma, pregnancy, and the multiple family roles (e.g., mother, spouse, caregiver).

Recent studies of OEF and OIF female veterans suggest that they exhibit higher need for mental-health care than that evidenced in previous conflicts, with reports that 17% are diagnosed with PTSD (compared to other eras, in which 8–9% of women veterans were diagnosed with current PTSD) and 23% are diagnosed with depression (Litz et al., 1997; Maguen et al., 2009; Schlenger et al., 1992). Recent data suggest that between half to a third of women veterans indicated that they needed counseling for depression (48%), relationship issues (38%), anxiety

[7]See http://www.womenshealth.va.gov/WOMENSHEALTH/facts.asp.

(36%), and anger management (30%) (Shekelle et al., 2011). In addition, a greater number of deployments seem to be associated with screening positive for mental-health problems (Bean-Mayberry et al., 2011).

MST appears to be an important risk factor for PTSD. Suris and Lind (2008) reviewed research on health consequences of MST and found higher rates of PTSD, depression, and substance abuse in female veterans with a history of sexual assault. In fact, female veterans with a history of MST were nine times more likely to develop PTSD than female veterans with no history of sexual trauma. Recent research on OEF and OIF veterans supports those findings. Kimerling et al. (2010) reviewed medical records of OEF and OIF veterans (17,580 women and 108,149 men) for diagnoses of mental-health disorders and found that those with a history of MST were significantly more likely to receive a diagnosis of PTSD, other anxiety disorders, depression, or substance-use disorders than those with no history of abuse. Odds ratios remained significant after adjusting for other significant associations, and effect sizes for women were substantially stronger than those for men.

Estimates of MST have been reported based on a universal screening program implemented by the VA. In 2003, shortly after implementation of VA screening, 21.5% of women and 1.1% of men reported experiencing MST (Kimerling et al., 2007). It has been noted that those estimates have remained fairly consistent, and as of 2008 those percentages translate into 48,106 women and 43,693 men screening positive for MST (Hyun et al., 2009). DOD estimates of MST report that the annual prevalence of sexual assault for women was 6.8% and 1.8% for men (Lipari et al., 2008). A study of reservists examined sexual harassment and assault during military service and found that sexual assault was reported by 13.1% of the women and 1.6% of the men (Street et al., 2008).

There are mixed findings regarding the relationship between women's health care use and sexual assault. Kelly et al. (2008) found MST to be associated with greater use of VHA care but less satisfaction with VHA services. Other studies found that women with a positive history of any form of sexual assault were more likely to meet the criteria for PTSD but accessed fewer health care services (Suris et al., 2004). Women veterans who have experienced MST and access health care report significant anxiety if treated by a male provider, particularly if subjected to any invasive exam, a concern with regard to aggravating mental-health symptoms and accessing future health care (Bean-Mayberry et al., 2010).

**Utilization**

Utilization of mental-health services provides an interesting comparison between men and women serving in OEF and OIF. Differences in gender use of DOD or VA mental-health services might be linked to type of psychiatric condition, since some data seem to suggest that there are no disparities across gender groups when adjusting for differences in need. For example, Maguen et al. (2012) conducted a retrospective study to examine gender differences in VA health care use among a national sample of newly returning OEF and OIF veterans with PTSD seeking care from 2001–2010. The study population consisted of 159,705 OEF and OIF veterans (15,303 women, 144,402 men) who had at least one clinical VA facility visit from 2001 through 2010 and were diagnosed with PTSD. Mean number of visits for each type of use were similar for men and women with PTSD; both had a median of about 3 mental-health outpatient visits per year. Other research has shown, however, that 9 or more sessions of evidence-based treatment is needed to reduce PTSD severity (Foa et al., 2005).

There were a few small, statistically significant differences in the incidence rate ratio for those initiating care. Women with PTSD initiating care were more likely than male veterans with PTSD to have lower use of inpatient mental-health hospitalization, higher rates of outpatient mental-health service use, higher use of primary care visits, and higher use of emergency care visits. These findings are consistent with research of women in the general (nonmilitary) population that shows that women use primary care and emergency services at higher rates than men (Bertakis et al., 2000).

Men and women with comorbid PTSD and depression (respectively 57% and 72%) were more likely to use all categories of services more frequently than those with PTSD alone. For example, the rate of mental-health inpatient use by women with PTSD and depression was 12.5 times greater than for those without depression, while that figure for men was only 6.7 times greater. Comorbid alcohol use disorders and PTSD was present in 8.2% of women and 29% of men. Again, both women and men in the comorbid group were more likely to have used all categories of VA services (Maguen et al., 2012).

Washington et al. (2006) conducted a study to determine why women do or do not use VA health care services. A telephone survey was conducted in 2004 among women veterans eligible for VA health care; the women lived in southern California and southern Nevada. The most often cited reasons for VA use included the following: affordability (67.9%), availability of a women's health clinic (58.8%), quality of care (54.8%), and convenience (47.9%). Findings also indicated reasons for choosing non-VA care, such as having health insurance (71.0%), greater convenience of non-VA care (66.9%), lack of knowledge about VA eligibility and services (48.5%), and perceived better non-VA quality of care (34.5%). Thus, lack of information about VA health care, poor perceptions about quality, and inconvenience reduce utilization of VA health care.

The National Survey of Women Veterans, a national population-based telephone survey, was conducted in 2008–2009 to examine health care needs of women veterans. Of the 10,638 contacted households, 3,611 (33.9%) participants were eligible for and consented to enroll in the survey. Overall, 18.9% of the population delayed or went without needed health care in the prior 12 months, including 14.3% of insured and 54.6% of uninsured. Younger age was associated with a higher prevalence of delayed care or unmet need (35% of 18–34-year-olds). Women veterans with delayed care were more likely to be OEF and OIF veterans, a high-priority group for VA enrollment, and to have experienced MST. In the study, 4.8% (n = 173) of the overall population sampled were OEF and OIF veterans, of which more than a third (37.2%) experienced an unmet need for care. The most commonly cited reason for unmet need was not being able to afford medical care. The independent predictors of delayed or unmet need for OEF and OIF women veterans health care were the following: being uninsured (OR = 6.5; 95% CI: 3.0–14.0) followed by being in the under-35 age group (OR = 4.5; 95% CI 1.8–11.3). After controlling for potential confounders, other predictors of delayed care were the perception that VA providers are not gender sensitive (Shekelle et al., 2011) and having a history of MST.

## Racial and Ethnic Minorities

There is a paucity of literature on disparities in health care in racial and ethnic minorities in the OEF and OIF populations. Therefore, the committee includes studies in this section on all minority veterans, in particular African American, Latino, American Indian, and Alaskan Native veterans.

In 2007, the VA conducted a systematic review of racial and ethnic disparities in its health care system. Findings from several studies indicate that black and Hispanic patients were more frequently diagnosed and treated for psychotic disorders (e.g., schizophrenia), while white veterans were more frequently diagnosed and treated for affective disorders (e.g., bipolar disorder and depression). The difference in patterns of diagnosis and treatment are unclear. The review notes, however, that black veterans might benefit from having black clinicians (Saha et al., 2007).

A small study of Puerto Rican OEF and OIF veterans and family members following deployment examined unmet health needs. Hannold et al. (2011) found that Puerto Rican veterans tend to deny symptoms of stress and do not seek psychologic examinations. The authors also found that the families of these veterans experience emotional problems and expressed the need for family support groups. The veterans also indicated that they had physical problems and needed pain treatment. The authors concluded that there is a need for "veteran-centric" and family-focused health care.

The Native American Indian, Pacific Islander, native Hawaiian, and Alaska Native (AIAN) populations serve at the highest rate per capita in the Armed Forces (Holiday et al., 2006; Kramer et al., 2009). Nearly half of all Native veterans reside in rural locations on tribal or Alaska Native lands. According to the American Indian Vietnam Veterans Project, a community-based epidemiological study, Native veterans have high rates of combat-related mental-health disorders, 31% current and 59% lifetime, and alcohol abuse and dependence, 72% current, 84% lifetime. These figures are significantly higher than any other ethnic group (Beals et al., 2002). AIAN veterans have 1.9 higher odds of being uninsured compared with non-Latino white veterans (Johnson et al., 2010). They have a disproportionate amount of service-related military conditions, and they are more likely to use the Indian Health Service as opposed to the VA system (Johnson et al., 2010). The Indian Health Service, similar to the VA, struggles to find and retain physicians, especially those who have the necessary cultural awareness (Brod et al., 1982; Fannin and Barnes, 2007; Hostetter and Felsen, 1975; Johnson and Cameron, 2001).

The AIAN population, similar to other rural veterans as described below, experiences significant barriers in accessing care, such as underfunded resources (i.e., time, money, and transportation), lack of culturally appropriate care, inability to recruit and retain health care professionals, and geographic access issues (Kaufman et al., 2010). AIAN veterans are more likely than their white counterparts to report delays in care because of not getting a timely appointment, not being able to reach a contact by phone, or because of transportation problems. Despite the growing evidence on telehealth effectiveness, acceptance and implementation in the rural areas where these veterans reside remain a challenge (Barton et al., 2007; Grigsby et al., 2007; Spaulding et al., 2005). For example, one study examined the differences in administering a mental-health assessment, the SCID, by teleconference versus in person to AIAN veterans. Attitudes did not differ significantly between the groups; however, participants expressed lower ratings of satisfaction and comfort in the telehealth interviews (Shore et al., 2008).

**Utilization**

There is a dearth of knowledge on disparities in mental-health care in the OEF and OIF veterans, and available studies show mixed findings on whether disparities exist. For example, one study found racial disparities in the granting of service connection for PTSD by the VA for black patients compared to non-Latino white patients. In the study of 20,284 veterans, black veterans were significantly less likely to have received services connected for PTSD (Murdoch et al., 2003) compared to their non-Latino white counterparts. Service-connected veterans receive priority for VA enrollment due to documented, compensative conditions related to or aggravated by military service. For many, service connection represents the difference between access to VA health care facilities and no access. Although black and Hawaiian/Pacific Islander veterans were as likely as non-Latino whites to receive psychotropic medications, they were less likely to receive at least four 1-month supplies of the medication (Murdoch et al., 2003). Similarly, the authors discuss that even among poor, homeless veterans who are eligible for VA care because of their low income, lack of service connection decreased their odds of using VA services. However, another study found no disparities in the use of intensive VA treatment programs for PTSD among black and Hispanic patients compared to white patients (Rosenheck and Fontana, 2002).

There are also mixed findings among the few studies conducted in OEF and OIF veterans on racial and ethnic disparities in mental-health care. One recent study found that ethnicity (i.e., Latino) was not a contributing factor to mental-health service use among veterans with a new diagnosis of PTSD, and that once engaged in mental-health services, all veterans were more likely to use counseling and complete at least eight counseling sessions of treatment (Spoont et al., 2009). However, veteran race (i.e., African American and Hawaiian/Pacific Islander) contributed to lower use (Spoont et al., 2009). Another recent study found that black veterans were less likely than white veterans to receive guideline concordant depression care at the VA and less likely to receive or adhere to pharmacotherapy (Chermack et al., 2008).

Black and Hispanic veterans are most significantly affected by racial and ethnic disparities in the VA (Saha et al., 2007). Race and ethnicity was related to the number of VA outpatient visits among veterans, with black and Latino veterans having more visits (reverse disparity) and Asian and Pacific Islanders having fewer visits (greater disparity) than non-Latino white veterans (Harada et al., 2002). Black, Latino, and Asian/Pacific Islander veterans were less likely than non-Latino white veterans to persist with health care services over a 12-month period, with ambulatory care varying by race/ethnicity (Washington et al., 2005). Black and Latino veterans were less likely to indicate having a primary care physician than whites. Despite these disparities, black and Latino veterans are more likely to use VA-only health services, with Asian/Pacific Islanders and non-Latino white veterans more likely to seek help outside the VA system (Washington et al., 2002).

## Rural Veterans

Health disparities between rural and urban communities have been well documented (IOM, 2005). Health care in rural populations poses challenges such as limited specialized providers, limited options for assessment and treatment referrals, and the lack of providers' cultural awareness of the community (Richardson et al., 2009). Rural veterans are less likely to access mental-health services because they are hindered by challenges such as greater distance and travel time than their urban counterparts. According to VA's Office of Rural Health, as of FY 2010, veterans living in rural areas make up 41% of those enrolled in the VA system (GAO, 2011b); 39% of enrolled OEF and OIF veterans are from rural areas (VA, 2012d). Although 11.8% of 18–24-year-old military recruits are from rural areas, that number decreases to 7.6% of 18–24-year-olds in the general population (Kane, 2006).

Studies have shown that VA patients in rural areas have more physical comorbidities and worse health-related quality of life than those residing in suburban or urban settings. In addition, they have reduced access to health services and fewer alternatives to VA care (Weeks et al., 2004; West and Weeks, 2006). Compared to urban and suburban veterans, rural veterans live further from private-sector and VA hospitals, have access to fewer mental-health and specialty services, and visit their providers less frequently, but they have more physical- and mental-health problems (Weeks et al., 2004). Among veterans seeking treatment for serious mental illness, travel distance was found to be the strongest predictor of poor service (McCarthy et al., 2006). Increasing travel distance also predicts poor retention for alcohol abuse treatment, especially among older and younger veterans (but less so among the middle-aged) (Fortney et al., 1995).

Outpatient service utilization trends were examined for rural veterans with PTSD compared to their urban counterparts. Data were obtained for 415,617 veterans with PTSD who received outpatient care at a VA facility. Results indicate that veterans from rural and highly rural areas had 19% (CI = 0.80–0.82) and 25% (CI = 0.72–0.79), respectively, fewer outpatient visits than those who lived in an urban setting. Results are similar for visits to specialized PTSD clinics with 22% (CI = 0.87–0.89) fewer visits for those in rural and 33% (CI = 0.64–0.71) fewer visits for those in highly rural areas compared to their counterparts in urban areas. Service use was contingent on proximity to services, with a larger effect seen for those requiring specialized mental-health care. There is concern that those living further distances from a facility might not receive optimal care (Brooks et al., 2012).

The effect of distance on access to care for rural veterans was assessed through surveys (n = 96 patients, 88 providers/staff), interviews (42 patient, 64 providers/staff), and focus groups (n = 7 consisting of providers and staff) at 15 VHA primary care clinics in the Midwest (VISN 23). "Distance to drive" was the most frequently selected barrier by patient and provider; other barriers included travel related challenges such as time, limited transportation, and cost or expense. Veterans indicated that the same travel distance was more burdensome when seeking care for routine services (e.g., laboratory, podiatry) as compared to specialty care (e.g., cardiology, neurology) (Buzza et al., 2011).

Numerous studies have noted an increased risk of suicide for those living in rural areas (Kapusta et al., 2008; Levin and Leyland, 2005; Middleton et al., 2003; Razvodovsky and Stickley, 2009; Singh and Siahpush, 2002). McCarthy et al. (2012) examined rural–urban differences in suicide rates in a population of veterans receiving services in the VA health system. Suicide mortality was assessed in two periods: FY 2004–FY 2005 and FY 2007–FY 2008; and suicide risks were assessed for two cohorts—those that had VA inpatient or outpatient encounters in those time periods. Median distance to the nearest VA mental-health provider was greater for patients in rural areas. In the two cohorts, residence in rural areas was associated with increased rates of suicide and increased suicide risk. Although previous studies have documented decreased service utilization and continuity of care with greater distances to health system providers, the McCarthy et al. (2012) study noted that distance measures were not necessarily related to suicide risk. That finding suggested that elevated suicide risks observed among rural populations might have less to do with health system accessibility barriers and more to do with socioeconomic or sociocultural factors.

## BARRIERS TO CARE

Barriers to care imply impediments that make it difficult for a service member or veteran to receive treatment. Numerous studies have detailed barriers to care. For example, Britt et al. (2008) and Hoge et al. (2008) highlight issues such as veterans not knowing where to go for treatment, not having enough leave time, long distances to travel to a facility, lengthy wait times, workforce shortages, and stigma. Furthermore, among military personnel who screened positive for a mental disorder, 55% stated it would be difficult to obtain time off from work, and 45% stated it would be difficult to schedule an appointment (Hoge et al., 2008). Similarly, a recent GAO report (2011b) notes logistical challenges for veterans in accessing mental-health care, including difficulty in scheduling and coordinating appointments, long distances to facilities and other transportation challenges, cost of services, challenges in arranging child care or spousal support, and other time constraints.

The section below begins with a discussion of stigma, a barrier that has been well documented in the military population as it relates to mental-health; additional barriers discussed include wait times, workforce capacity, and geographic accessibility.

### Stigma, the Military Environment, and Attitudes About Treatment

In the military, stigma refers to the belief that treatment seeking might cause harm to one's career, diminish the trust and confidence of fellow service members, or affect how a soldier will be perceived by his colleagues and superiors (Britt, 2000; Christensen et al., 2009; Greene-Shortridge et al., 2007; Hoge et al., 2008; Link and Phelan, 2001). Furthermore, stigma in military populations, as in the general population, has been found to have a negative impact on treatment seeking, treatment initiation, and adherence to treatment (Kim et al., 2011).

Research indicates that stigma deters individuals in the military from seeking help for mental illness because service members might interpret seeking such care as a weakness and that it is possible to "tough it out" (Dickstein et al., 2010). Stecker et al. (2007) notes that the most frequently reported barrier to mental-health care by soldiers and Marines deployed to Iraq was the belief that one "ought to handle it on my own." Hoge et al. (2004) found that service members with mental-health disorders felt they "would be seen as weak" if they engaged in treatment.

Rae Olmsted et al. (2011) examined the differences in perceived stigma among soldiers in treatment for substance abuse (n = 12), for mental-health treatment (n = 388), for both substance use and mental-health (n = 70), and those not in treatment (n = 966). Soldiers were recruited from two Army installations between October 2009 and February 2010. Those reporting any treatment within the past 12 months indicated more stigma with regard to both substance abuse and mental-health treatment than those without treatment. Results of the study demonstrate that while all military personnel reported stigma related to treatment of mental-health and substance use, those in treatment reported increased perceptions of stigma regarding mental-health treatment. The authors note that stigma may be a barrier to care and that it might result in treatment failure or dropout from treatment.

Seeking treatment is often at odds with several aspects of military culture. It has been noted that military culture promotes individual strength and selfless devotion to the nation and to one's comrades. Soldiers fear loss of support from their unit as well as fear of career repercussions, as mental-health treatment will appear on medical records (Tanielian and Jaycox, 2008). Gorman et al. (2011) conducted a study of 332 National Guard troops who had been deployed to OEF and OIF, and their partners. Findings indicate that 49% of National Guard members and 34% of their partners met screening criteria for one or more mental-health symptoms. Although 53% of the National Guard soldiers who met screening criteria reported getting some type of care, concerns about treatment influencing career advancement among service members was a barrier for those not seeking care.

Gibbs et al. (2011) reported on results from 48 focus-group interviews conducted at six Army installations regarding the perception of treatment for substance abuse and mental-health in the military environment. Study participants varied in that some were currently in the Army Substance Abuse Program (n = 80), others in treatment for mental-health (n = 56), and others were not in any treatment program (n = 134). Those in treatment for alcohol abuse or mental-health issues were more likely to describe negative attitudes from command and peers. The negative perceptions of treatment for alcohol abuse were based on potential infractions, in addition to "social distancing" from peers that was felt by those in treatment. Ironically, high alcohol use prior to treatment was associated with bonding with peers and as a way to respond to stressors (similar results were reported by Ames et al., 2007).

Another frequent reason reported by service members for not seeking treatment was negative perceptions from leadership (Kim et al., 2011). Britt et al. (2012) studied perceived stigma and barriers to care for mental-health treatment. The authors examined leadership behaviors (in noncommissioned officers[8] [NCOs] and officers) and the effect on stigma and practical barriers to seeking mental-health treatment in 1,455 soldiers following a 15-month deployment to Afghanistan. Positive and negative leadership by NCOs were more strongly correlated with stigma and practical barriers than officers. Only NCO behaviors were uniquely predictive of stigma over time, with higher ratings of negative behaviors and lower ratings of positive behaviors being associated with higher reports of stigma.

Wright et al. (2009) studied soldiers in combat support units (n = 680) 3 months postreturn from combat in Iraq. A relatively small but statistically significant relationship was found between factors such as officer leadership and unit cohesion as predictors of stigma and subsequent treatment seeking. Not only were both factors related independently to reduced stigma and greater use, but positive leader behavior in conjunction with unit cohesion enhanced access to care (Wright et al., 2009). This study supports other work indicating that leadership behaviors, along with unit cohesion, override the relationship between high symptom levels of mental-health issues and higher perceptions of stigma in terms of seeking treatment (Britt et al., 2012; Hoge et al., 2008; Kessler et al., 2001). In addition, a study of OEF and OIF National Guard and reservists found that lower unit support was related to higher perception of barriers in accessing care as well as perceived stigma (Pietrzak et al., 2009).

[8]Noncommissioned officers (NCOs) are the front-line supervisors of most military personnel and have a more direct daily impact on service members than commissioned officers.

Hoerster et al. (2012) examined the effect of perceived barriers on prospective mental-health care use among a sample 305 OEF and OIF veterans who sought care and presented with symptoms of depression (n = 273), PTSD (n = 231), or alcohol misuse (n = 91) at a VA postdeployment health clinic. Barriers related to stigma such as "it would harm my career, members of my unit might have less confidence in me, my unit leadership might treat me differently, and I would be seen as weak" were most commonly cited among the sample (n = 111; 37% endorsed at least one stigma-related barrier). Despite those stated barriers, they did not interfere with receipt of adequate treatment in this population of care-seeking veterans. The results may not accurately reflect those who have not sought or initiated care (Hoerster et al., 2012).

Finally, negative attitudes toward treatment, including perceived effectiveness of treatment and prior experiences with providers can also be barriers to seeking care. Positive experiences with mental-health providers improve the likelihood of seeking additional treatment. For example, studies have found that the use of mental-health services in National Guard troops was associated with previous mental-health care satisfaction and belief in treatment efficacy (Kehle et al., 2010; Pietrzak et al., 2009).

Kim et al. (2011) analyzed data from self-reported questionnaires on barriers to care, treatment utilization, and mental-health risk in 2,623 soldiers approximately 6 months postdeployment to OEF or OIF. Results indicate that those reporting a mental-health issue were significantly more likely to report barriers to accessing care and more likely to endorse negative attitudes toward treatment than those not reporting mental-health concerns. Negative perceptions from peers and leadership were a frequently reported concern with utilizing mental-health care. Controlling for age, gender, and education, negative attitudes toward treatment were also negatively associated with use of mental-health professionals and military facilities; those reporting negative attitudes were 42% less likely to utilize care in a military facility. Negative attitudes were identified as the only unique predictor of utilization and treatment seeking. It is, however, unclear whether those negative attitudes stem from the soldier's belief that they could address their own problems or because of their negative perceptions on efficacy of the treatment itself.

Britt et al. (2011) conducted a cross-sectional survey in a sample of National Guard and reserve members from the Army, Marine Corps, and Air Force (n = 760) and members of the Pennsylvania National Guard (n = 334) who had been deployed in support of a military operation since 2003. Survey results indicated that 27.5% reported a "mild problem," 11.7% reported a "moderate problem," and 2.6% reported a "severe problem" when asked about current experience with a psychologic problem. Thirty-four percent of veterans (n = 120) reporting a mental-health problem had no interest in obtaining care. The most frequently cited reason for not obtaining care was that "the problem was not severe enough" (26.6%), followed by a lack of resources in being able to seek treatment, such as cost, time, and transportation (16.5%), followed by negative beliefs about the treatment itself (12%). Overall attitude and beliefs about psychologic problems was a unique predictor of whether one reported treatment seeking for mental-health. Those who had a positive attitude toward treatment and those not believing they could handle the problem on their own were more likely to seek care.

## Wait Times

Excessive wait times are a frequent complaint expressed by both active-duty and veteran service members. The DOD's MHS is supposed to meet statutory access standards[9] for its TRICARE beneficiaries. For example, the wait time for an appointment must be less than 4 weeks for a well-patient visit or a specialty care referral, less than 1 week for a routine visit, and less than 24 hours for an urgent care visit. MTF enrollees see their assigned primary care manager about 40% of the time; if beneficiaries call for an acute care appointment, they should be offered at least three options within 24 hours about 50% of the time; that figure increases to 70% for routine appointments (DOD, 2011a, 2011b).

Evaluations of TRICARE reveal that active-duty service members and their families complain about delays in receiving TRICARE mental-health services primarily because of long wait times for appointments and difficulty in locating providers accepting TRICARE (Avery and MacDermid Wadsworth, 2011; Bagchi et al., 2007; National Council on Disability, 2009).

Problems with access to mental-health services have been highlighted (Tanielian and Jaycox, 2008) and include shortages of uniformed mental-health specialty providers, long wait times, and unfilled training slots. Numerous studies have shown such organizational barriers to seeking care (Britt et al., 2008; Wright et al., 2009). An earlier example is the study by Hoge et al. (2004). The authors examined mental-health problems and barriers to care in three Army units and one Marine unit before deployment to OEF or OIF and 3–4 months after deployment. Among military personnel who screened positive for a mental-health disorder, nearly half reported difficulty in scheduling an appointment (45%); other barriers included being seen as weak (65%), problems with leadership such as being blamed (51%) and being treated differently (63%), and harming ones career (50%).

Kim et al. (2011) collected data from 3,380 soldiers approximately 6 months postdeployment from OEF or OIF (with 2,623 reported being deployed at least once). Numerous barriers to care were examined. Specific to wait times, among respondents with mental-health problems, 32.5% of those receiving care indicated it was difficult to get an appointment vs 16.8% of those not receiving care.

VHA policy requires that first-time patients requesting mental-health care be seen within 24 hours for an initial evaluation with followup for a comprehensive exam within 14 days. However, a recent review of access to mental-health care in the VHA has been conducted and findings indicate that the VHA does not have a "reliable and accurate method" of determining whether they are meeting that standard (VA Office of the Inspector General, 2012). In addition to the finding above, the VA Office of the Inspector General (OIG) found that the VHA does not provide first-time patients with timely mental-health exams as patients often waited more than 14 days; VHA schedulers did not consistently follow procedures outlined in VHA directives; and vacancies in mental-health staffing might affect VHA's timeliness goals.

Prior to the VA OIG report (noted above) in July 2011, the US Senate Committee on Veterans Affairs requested that the VA conduct a survey among mental-health professionals regarding whether their medical center had adequate staff to meet the veterans' demands for treatment. Seventy-one percent indicated that their medical centers did not have adequate staffing to meet the needs. The VA OIG interviewed clinicians at four of the sites participating in

---

[9]CFR § 199.17(p)(5)(ii).

the survey and found that three of the four sites had vacant positions in psychiatry. It was determined that a patient in need of a mental-health visit at one of those sites[10] had to wait, on average, 86 days to see a psychiatrist (VHA, 2011).

In general, long wait times can compromise health due to delayed utilization, lead to poorer health outcomes, and decrease patient satisfaction (Pizer and Prentice, 2011). Several studies have examined the effects of wait times on health outcomes in the VA (Pizer and Prentice, 2011; Prentice and Pizer, 2007; Prentice et al., 2011) and found that there are statistically significant decreases in utilization particularly in the elderly and vulnerable veteran populations. In addition, long-term outcomes such as mortality and preventable hospitalizations are worse for veterans who seek care at facilities with longer waits compared to veterans at facilities with shorter wait periods.

### Workforce Capacity

Poor availability and distribution of mental-health specialists in many parts of the United States presents a significant barrier for OEF and OIF veterans to access mental-health care. Many specialists are in urban areas, and even in those areas there are disparities in concentrations of psychiatrists. For example, according to Burnam et al. (2009) in the mid-Atlantic region there are 8.2 psychiatrists per 100,000 people. However, in New England, there are 53 psychiatrists per 100,000 people. In some rural areas, psychiatrists are entirely absent.

For active-duty service members, limited participating provider networks is a primary barrier for accessing mental-health care. In Indiana, for example, providers in markets with higher populations are more likely to accept the TRICARE plan than providers in rural, less populated areas (Avery and MacDermid Wadsworth, 2011). Additionally, provider lists for TRICARE consumers may be confusing and inaccurate; certain providers are listed in the TRICARE directory of providers but are no longer providing services to TRICARE.

A study by Avery and MacDermid Wadsworth (2011) examined access to mental-health services for active-duty service members and National Guard in Indiana. The authors found several discrepancies in the TRICARE outpatient network—of the 907 providers in the list, only 404 were distinct providers in 551 office locations. Of those, only 339 were nonredundant, listed with correct contact information, and answered telephones during office hours. Furthermore, only 235 (25%) of the listed providers were accepting TRICARE, and only 200 of these were accepting new patients. It was also noted that providers in areas with the greatest density of National Guard troops were more likely to report that they were no longer accepting TRICARE coverage.

With regard to veterans' access to mental-health services, some states have established public–private collaborative programs so veterans can seek care in areas of poor availability of VHA mental-health services. The VA also has recently hired more than 3,500 mental-health professionals, increasing the mental-health staff to more than 21,000 (VHA, 2011). However, even with the increase in personnel, concerns remain with regard to maldistribution of providers.

Finally, the literature documents a lack of training in combat-related mental-health treatments in the civilian workforce, despite the need for such programs (Burnam et al., 2009). For example, self-reports of mental-health problems and barriers to care in 200 active-duty Air

[10]The Salisbury VA Medical Center.

Force members indicated that some service members expressed hesitation to seek care from civilian providers due mainly to the inability to relate to the deployment experience (Visco, 2009).

### Geographic Accessibility

Most active-duty service members and families live within 20 miles of a medical treatment facility and within 40 miles of inpatient services; however, less than 50% of National Guard and reserve members live within those described areas (DOD, 2011b). Time to travel to a treatment facility has been highlighted as a barrier to seeking care (see discussion above), although, as noted in Fortney et al. (2011), long distance to travel to a treatment facility has less impact on those with high levels of perceived need for care (e.g., cardiac issues) as opposed to those with lower levels of perceived need (e.g., substance use disorders).

Veterans enrolled in a low-priority group (as described in Table 9.1) with long distances to travel to VHA facilities will likely be deterred from seeking treatment (Burnam et al., 2009). Seal et al. (2010) conducted a study examining VA mental-health service utilization in nearly 85,000 OEF and OIF veterans who had received a new mental-health diagnosis. The veterans had at least one followup mental-health visit during the first year of the diagnosis. One finding was that veterans living more than 25 miles from a VA facility were less likely to receive the recommended PTSD treatment compared to veterans living within 25 miles of their treatment.

## RESPONSE TO BARRIERS

Earlier in the chapter, the committee noted that important barriers to care included stigma, the military environment, and attitudes about treatment; wait times; clinical capacity; and geographic accessibility. Telemedicine is one response to most of those barriers in accessing care.

### Telemedicine

Telemedicine has been defined as "the use of electronic information and communication technologies to provide support in health care when distance separates the participants (IOM, 1996). Historically, that definition included a variety of modalities such as e-mail, the Internet, phone, Fax, still imaging, and video-conferencing (Antonacci et al., 2008). A more recent and broader interpretation defines "virtual health care" as the use of communication and information technologies to bridge geographic distance and to facilitate the interactions and relationships necessary for providing accessible, coordinated, and high-quality care (Kizer, 2011).

Telemedicine provides a mechanism by which many access barriers might be overcome, particularly with regard to wait time, cost of care, travel distance to a treatment facility, and stigma (Pietrzak et al., 2009; Wong et al., 2007). The VHA has been in the forefront of information technology, and telemedicine has been a focus for recent VHA funding (Hill et al., 2010). Initiatives have been employed to expand services into a national telemental-health clinical and technical infrastructure. In FY 2011, 55,000 patients and 140,000 telemental-health visits were provided from 146 VA hospitals to 531 CBOCs (Darkins, 2012). The VHA currently provides various types of telehealth services, including services linking clinical settings with each other and in-home telehealth delivered directly to the patient's home, which eliminates the need for travel (VA, 2012b). Resulting from those VA initiatives, there is a growing body of literature describing and evaluating telemedicine, including telemental-health services in the veteran population, with the majority of studies focused on the treatment of PTSD and depression.

Two studies by Detweiler et al. (2011, 2012) describe the clinical experience of a collaborative telepsychiatry clinic between the VA and the US Army Warrior Transition Clinic (WTC). There are 38 WTCs on US military bases nationally and internationally that were developed to treat soldiers with the most severe health problems. Telepsychiatry offers a mechanism for VA mental-health professionals to treat returning OEF and OIF veterans with one or more mental-health diagnosis, and other medical comorbidities, in areas where there is limited access to timely evaluation and treatment. The authors examined data from telepsychiatry encounters at the Womack WTC (North Carolina Womack Army Medical Center) between September 2008 and August 2009. During those 12 months, 120 active-duty soldiers were seen for a total of 394 clinic visits. Prior to the implementation of the telepsychiatry team, soldiers on average waited more than 30 days to see a psychiatrist; after, the wait decreased to 22 days with a range of 1–79 days. At the start, 10% of the WTC psychiatry caseload was managed by the VA team; at the end of the 12-month period, that figure increased to 47%. The two most frequent diagnoses at psychiatry intake and at the last psychiatry visit were anxiety and mood disorders. Findings indicate that there was an increase in the incidence of anxiety and mood disorders from the VA psychiatric intake (anxiety, 59.2%, and mood disorders, 45.8%) to the final 12-month VA psychiatry visit (anxiety, 65.0%, and mood disorders, 46.7%). The authors acknowledge that the mental-health profile of this group is not representative of the entire OEF and OIF population, as the WTC typically treats the most traumatized soldiers. This innovative approach demonstrates an opportunity for collaboration between the DOD and VA in addressing the potential shortage of US Army psychiatrists. However, considering that the VA is also experiencing issues related to capacity, understaffing, and delivery of timely care, this approach may not be feasibly deployed as a systematic nationwide effort, but rather implementation on a site-by-site basis might be further explored (Detweiler et al., 2011, 2012).

Godleski et al. (2012) reports on outcomes in 98,609 veterans newly enrolled in telemental-health services between 2006 and 2010. Findings indicate that the total number of hospital admissions among the telemental-health patients dropped from 3,948 before enrollment in the program to 2,994 after enrollment; the total days for hospitalization fell from 35,532 before enrollment to 26,080 after enrollment. Several smaller studies, for example, also found positive outcomes using telemental-health. Morland et al. (2010) conducted a randomized controlled study to compare the effectiveness of cognitive behavioral anger management treatment delivered via televideoconferencing vs traditional in-person service delivery for rural combat veterans with PTSD. The study included 125 male veterans: one group received televideoconferencing treatment (n = 61), and the other received in-person treatment (n = 64). There was a significant reduction of PTSD symptoms posttreatment for both videoconferencing and in-person treatment, and both groups reported positive outcomes with no statistically significant differences; there was, however, high group therapy alliance observed in the in-person treatment group. Mohr et al. (2011) conducted a randomized controlled trial in a group of veterans meeting the *DSM-IV* diagnosis of depression to compare the effectiveness of telephone-administered cognitive behavioral therapy (T-CBT) vs treatment as usual (TAU). Results indicated no significant treatment effects for the 16-session course of T-CBT and no statistically significant difference between the T-CBT and TAU group.

Ruskin et al. (2004) conducted a study comparing treatment outcomes and satisfaction of patients receiving treatment for depression remotely vs in person. Veterans suffering from depression who were referred to VA mental-health clinics (n = 119) were randomized to receive treatment through telepsychiatry (n = 59) or in person (n = 60). Results indicate scores on the Hamilton Depression Rating Scale and the Beck Depression Inventory improved significantly over the study period, however, with no significant differences between the two treatment modalities. There was also no difference in dropout rates or medication adherence between the two groups. General patient satisfaction also did not differ; however, psychiatrist satisfaction was greater for patients who received in-person treatment.

Hill et al. (2010) conducted a systematic review of 19 VHA-sponsored telemedicine interventions published between 2000 and 2009. The studies included populations over the age of 60 with issues of chronic disease management for multiple morbidities. Studies with a mean population age under 60 targeted mental-health, including PTSD and clinical depression. Conclusions indicate that telehealth interventions had distinct advantages, such as enhanced patient access to treatments, a medium for patient–provider communication, access to electronic medical record information, and the facilitation of collaborative care. The studies demonstrated that frequent contact between patient and provider fostered a therapeutic alliance and may increase patient satisfaction and willingness to participate in collaborative care. The authors concluded that telemedicine was one method of addressing issues for veterans struggling with access to care or living in areas without adequate facilities.

Remote health services such as diagnosis, assessment, case management, and treatment are provided by a VA-credentialed psychiatric practitioner at a main facility in Denver to patients located at a CBOC or tribal facility in a rural reservation. From April 2002 through February 2011, there have been 3,845 total sessions (3,220 individual followups and 44 group sessions) and 4,610 patient contacts. Clinical feasibility of services was established (Shore and Manson, 2004a, 2004b, 2005), and a high degree of patient and provider satisfaction was documented (Shore et al., 2008). Diagnostic reliability of videoconferencing was supported by evidence from a randomized controlled trial (Shore et al., 2007). Longitudinal clinical data showed a significant increase in medical service utilization associated with the subset of the clinics (Shore et al., 2012).

Wilson et al. (2008) conducted a study in 352 active-duty soldiers regarding their attitudes on the use of technology such as computerized therapy, video teleconferencing, and virtual reality in mental-health care. The majority were willing to use technology-based approaches to treatment (84%). Notably, 33% of soldiers who were not willing to speak to a counselor in person were willing to use at least one type of technology for mental-health treatment.

The VA is in a unique position to conduct national studies on the outcomes of telehealth because of the size of the telemental-health network and because of access to patient data from the electronic medical record (Godleski et al., 2012). The VA also has the opportunity to transform itself into an exemplary model of continuous and coordinated health care wherein patients can exchange secure messages through MyHealth*e*Vet, and have automated transmission of patient data from in-home devices (i.e., videoconferencing) (Hogan et al., 2011; IOM, 2001). Also, many returning OEF and OIF service members and veterans are comfortable with the use of technology.

Thus, telemedicine offers an alternative to traditional health care delivery. It addresses most of the issues related to barriers to care identified in this report. Although its acceptance among active-duty service members and veterans is mixed, it appears to be more positive than negative. Telemedicine offers rural veterans the opportunity to access health care that they might not otherwise obtain and reduces wait time and addresses workforce capacity issues. Continued study on the efficacy of telemedicine will be needed to determine the value of this approach.

### VHA Strategies to Improve Geographic Accessibility

In the early 1990s, the VHA implemented a system of CBOCs, which were designed to provide primary care, mental-health services, pharmacy benefits, and the management of acute and chronic conditions for veterans (Panangala and Mendez, 2010). CBOCs are separate entities from their parent medical facility; they can be either VA-owned and staffed or contracted to an HMO. The VA currently has more than 812 CBOCs throughout the United States and its territories, with plans to open 13 new facilities in nine states; it is expected that they will be operational over the next 3 years (VA, 2012c).

In a recent review, Kehle and Greer (2011) describe four studies that examined the impact of CBOCs on access to care (Fortney et al., 2002, 2005a, 2005b; Rosenheck, 2000). Findings from that review indicate a positive impact on geographic accessibility for veterans: CBOCs attracted more new users to the VA than did VAMCs; there was a decrease in travel distance to the closest VA facility for those in the CBOC catchment areas; and there was a higher rate of accessing VA medical services in counties with a CBOC. It was also noted that decreases in travel distance significantly predicted an increase in number of primary care encounters; however, improvements in health outcomes were small and not clinically significant.

The Government Accountability Office (GAO) highlighted other efforts to remove barriers and improve access for veterans (GAO, 2011b). These include VA integration of mental-health care into primary care, increasing the number of Vet Centers to provide confidential and free mental-health counseling; increasing the use of VA call centers; increasing VA mental-health staff; and expanded use of VA telemental-health services (discussed above). Additionally, the GAO notes that more than 2 million unique veterans received mental-health care at the VA between FY 2006 and FY 2010, with each year seeing an increase in veterans. The OEF and OIF veteran population accounts for that increase. VA began requiring its primary care clinics to conduct mental-health screenings for PTSD, depression, substance-use disorders, and history of MST. Since 2008, the VA requires mental-health providers to be on-site in mental-health clinics that treat more than 1,500 veterans annually. Those measures have been associated with a doubling of the number of unique patients receiving mental-health care in primary care clinics from 2008 through 2010.

The VA has continued to increase the number of Vet Centers as a mechanism to overcome barriers such as stigma and geographic accessibility. These centers provide confidential and free mental-health counseling services. VA increased the number of its Vet Centers from 232 to 292, from FY 2008 through August 2011. The VA has also increased the availability Vet Centers through the use of about 70 mobile Vet Centers to provide counseling services, especially to rural veterans.

VA call centers connect veterans with telephone-based counseling services. The VA has expanded the use of such centers, which, like Vet Centers, are free and confidential. One of the call centers is a Veterans Crisis Line that allows not only veterans, but their family members to call and receive counseling. According to the VA, since 2007 it has received more than 400,000 calls and has referred more than 55,000 veterans to suicide-prevention coordinators for same-day or next-day services. The VA has also implemented programs to assist veterans and their family members with mental-health care. The VA now needs to study the effectiveness of those efforts in improving veterans' access to mental-health care and determine how well they eliminate barriers. This will enable the VA to expand policies and programs that are effective and eliminate those that are not attaining their stated goals.

## DOD MENTAL-HEALTH PREVENTION PROGRAMS

In response to recommendations from the DOD Mental-health Task Force, DOD has taken steps to reduce stigma while building psychologic fitness and resilience in service members. Prevention programs aim to foster more robust mental-health, involve leadership, and increase cohesion among service members. There are numerous prevention programs for mental-health issues within the DOD, almost all of which are aimed at promoting resilience. Resilience in these programs is rarely and inconsistently defined, according to RAND, which catalogued 23 resilience programs (Meredith et al., 2011). Moreover, there are few studies of program effectiveness. Here the committee focuses on the most prominent prevention programs for which there is evidence of efficacy in alleviating the occurrence of psychiatric symptoms or disorders.[11] Both the RAND report and a recent IOM report (IOM, 2012) comprehensively describe the wide-ranging prevention programs. Two of these programs are highlighted below.

### Battlemind

Battlemind—now referred to as Resilience Training—is a training program originally developed by Army researchers to ease returning troops' transition from combat to civilian life. Its explicit purpose is to promote resilience and prevent postcombat psychosocial problems. Battlemind is a group training intervention that draws on positive psychology and cognitive behavioral techniques to reframe combat experience into adaptive experiences at home, away from the front lines (Castro et al., 2006; Orsingher et al., 2008). The Army mandated Battlemind in 2007, and since then some of its components have been extended to different stages of deployment (Williams, 2008).

The term "Battlemind" is an acronym, each letter of which stands for a strength or skill to adapt from the combat mindset to that in civilian life. The "B" in Battlemind stands for "buddies," and the intervention strives to teach that reliance on buddies, while essential to unit cohesiveness, can be detrimental at home, where service members need to make the shift from buddies to reliance on family and friends. A pervasive problem is that service members, upon return, tend to withdraw from family and friends because they feel that only their buddies can understand what they have experienced. Battlemind seeks to prevent withdrawal from families and friends through skill training. Similarly, the program teaches that hypervigilance, which is crucial during combat, is maladaptive at home; in fact, hypervigilance in civilian life is one of the hallmarks of PTSD.

---

[11]Programs for family members are discussed in Chapter 6.

The concepts behind Battlemind have also been incorporated into a new variant of psychologic debriefing known as "Battlemind debriefing" (Adler et al., 2009a, 2009b). It is a group-level intervention run by a specially trained professional facilitator to resemble the more familiar critical incident debriefing or a military after-action review (Adler et al., 2009a). The goal is for the group to arrive at lessons learned after a traumatic event and to focus on reintegration through resilience. Participants are encouraged to recall traumatic events, but in a limited way to prevent their own retraumatization or prevent exposing others to trauma. Standard psychologic debriefing has been criticized for its heavy emphasis on the traumatic experience, which risks retraumatization and worsening of mental-health (McNally et al., 2003).

The efficacy of Battlemind has been measured in a few studies. Adler and colleagues compared Battlemind training and Battlemind debriefing in 2,297 Army active-duty service members returning from a 12-month deployment to Iraq (Adler et al., 2009a). Platoons were randomly assigned to Battlemind training, Battlemind debriefing, or the Army's standard postdeployment stress education. A cluster randomization was conducted at the level of the platoon (rather than the individual). The study assessed symptoms of PTSD, depression, and sleep problems, once at the beginning of the 7-day reintegration period and then 4 months later (n = 1,060). Compared with stress education, the Battlemind debriefing was associated with fewer symptoms of PTSD, depression, and sleep problems, but only among those with high combat exposure. Battlemind training that was delivered in a small group (18–45 individuals), as compared to stress education, was associated with fewer PTSD and depression symptoms, again only among those highly exposed to combat. Battlemind training that was delivered in a large group setting (126–225 individuals) reported fewer symptoms of PTSD, fewer stigmatizing beliefs about mental-health, and, irrespective of combat exposure, fewer depression symptoms. The researchers concluded that both types of Battlemind programs were efficacious for service members with high combat exposure.

The findings propelled UK researchers to test an anglicized version of Battlemind in a cluster randomized controlled trial similar in design to that of Adler and colleagues. Mulligan et al. (2012) compared Battlemind to "standard care" by the UK military, i.e., a postdeployment standardized lecture on stress and homecoming. The most prominent change to Battlemind was an increased emphasis on alcohol, as alcohol problems are more prevalent in the United Kingdom than in the US military. Researchers assessed outcomes on the PTSD Checklist, the General Health Questionnaire, the Patient Health Questionnaire, and the Alcohol Use Disorders Identification Test (AUDIT). Six months after the program, the investigators found no improvement in mental-health or the overall AUDIT score, but those who received Battlemind were less likely to report binge drinking. The effect size, however, was small.

## Comprehensive Soldier Fitness

Comprehensive Soldier Fitness (CSF) is an Army-wide resilience program introduced in 2009. Its broad goal is to prevent adverse consequences of combat through resilience and mental fitness. More specifically, the goals are to enhance soldiers' ability to handle adversity, prevent depression and anxiety, prevent PTSD, and enhance overall well-being and performance (Reivich et al., 2011). The program was derived from an evidence-based civilian program, the Penn Resiliency Program (Brunwasser et al., 2009), which draws on cognitive-behavioral theories of depression. The CSF program has four components (Cornum et al., 2011):

1. *Assessment*. Psychologic fitness is assessed through a comprehensive questionnaire known as the Global Assessment Tool (GAT), which was expressly developed for the CSF. The GAT measures psychologic fitness in four domains: emotional, social, family, and spiritual fitness. Service members are expected to take the GAT at recruitment and then on an annual basis thereafter to monitor their own growth. The results are confidential, with the Army only monitoring aggregate data. The key point about the GAT is that measuring psychologic fitness is seen as important as measuring physical fitness (Peterson et al., 2011). A special GAT is available for family members.
2. *Universal resilience training*. This is accomplished by online training modules that focus on teaching specific resilience skills. Thus far there are 20 such modules focusing on each of the dimensions measured by the GAT (emotional, social, family, and spiritual fitness).
3. *Individualized training*. This component of the program tailors resilience training to domains that are needed according to performance on the GAT. It is not a one-size-fits-all approach, unlike universal resilience training (above).
4. *Master Resilience Trainer Course* (*MRT*). This is a train-the-trainer approach via a 10-day resilience training course for noncommissioned officers, primarily Staff Sergeants or Sergeants First Class. The MRT course is designed to train resilience skills to noncommissioned officers in a way that they in turn can teach these skills to their soldiers. The Army's goal is to have MRT experts in every company for the purpose of monitoring CSF and its component domains (Reivich et al., 2011).

The efficacy of Comprehensive Soldier Fitness has not yet been formally evaluated, but its predecessor program, the Penn Resiliency Program, has been evaluated by at least 17 controlled studies. A meta-analysis of those studies found a modest effect of the Penn program in reducing depression symptoms 12 months after the program's introduction (Brunwasser et al., 2009). The meta-analysis found no significant effect of the program in preventing diagnoses of depression.

Several research projects are planned or are currently in progress regarding the CSF program. One assessment will focus on whether the CSF program influences the rate of suicide, divorce, PTSD, crime, reenlistment, and promotion of rank (Lester et al., 2011). A longitudinal study is currently under way to determine if the Master Resilience Training program and the computer modules foster longstanding resilience. Another evaluation effort is designed to measure the empirical validity of the GAT (Peterson et al., 2011). A final study will be examining physiological and neurobiological correlates of psychologic resilience.

## CONCLUSIONS

Access to heath care is defined as the timely use of service to achieve the best possible health care outcome. Active-duty military and veterans access their health care through the DOD's military health system, TRICARE, and the VA's health care system, respectively. Fragmentation of care in both those systems does occur. Electronic health records offer the promise of minimizing fragmentation of care, but the DOD and VA have not yet integrated their health records.

There are disparities in health care in the DOD and VA health care systems. In particular, women face some unique stressors, and more study is needed to understand issues relevant to them. Military sexual assault needs to be addressed both in the DOD and the VA. There are limited studies in racial and ethnic minorities; however, studies show patterns of diagnostic inconsistencies between different racial groups. Those variations might be due to provider insensitivity toward cultural behaviors regarding mental-health. Rural veterans face many challenges in gaining access to care, and those veterans typically have more physical comorbidities and worse health-related quality of life than veterans in more urban areas.

Barriers to health care access include stigma, the military culture, and attitudes about treatment; long wait times for care; limited workforce capacity; and geographic accessibility. There is a continued high prevalence of stigma associated with mental-health problems and their treatment. Many active-duty service members are concerned about possible adverse effects of mental-health diagnoses and treatment on career advancement. Service members are reluctant to seek care for mental-health problems due to concerns about the privacy of their health information. The DOD and the VA have initiated policies and procedures to address those barriers, but clearly more needs to be done. Telemedicine offers promise as a mechanism to address those barriers; however, continued evaluation should occur to determine its acceptance and efficacy. Finally, the DOD has implemented programs for prevention of mental-health and resiliency training; those programs should be evaluated.

## RECOMMENDATIONS

Transitioning from the DOD health care system to the VA health care system presents challenges for OEF and OIF service men and women. There are numerous difficulties in navigating services because of the complexities of both systems. Although DOD and VA are making administrative changes to alleviate some of the problems, information sharing between the two agencies remains a problem.

**The committee recommends improved coordination of care and services between the Department of Defense and the Department of Veterans Affairs medical treatment facilities, including the completion of an interoperable or single combined electronic health record for all care that begins with entry into military service and continues throughout care in the Department of Veterans Affairs system after transition.**

Stigma is still a problem for military personnel in care or seeking care for mental-health or substance-abuse problems. Active-duty military fear that visits to a mental-health provider will jeopardize their careers because of the military's long-standing policy of reporting mental-health and substance-abuse problems to the chain of command. Mixed messages about seeking treatment and concerns about health-information privacy remain disincentives to seeking care.

**The committee recommends that the Department of Defense continue to promote an environment that reduces stigma and encourages treatment for mental-health and substance-use disorders. The committee recommends that the department undertake a systematic review of its policies regarding mental-health and substance-abuse treatment with regard to issues of confidentiality and the relation**

**between treatment-seeking and military advancement. The committee recommends that the department regularly issue reports describing actions taken with regard to its policies and procedures to determine progress in this area.**

Excessive wait time is a complaint often expressed by both active-duty and veteran service members. Long wait times can compromise health because of delayed use and decreased patient satisfaction. In addition, adverse long-term outcomes, such as death and preventable hospitalizations, are more common for veterans who seek care at facilities that have longer wait times than for veterans at facilities that have shorter wait times.

Poor availability and misdistribution of mental-health specialists in many parts of the United States, especially in rural areas, present substantial barriers to OEF and OIF veterans' access to mental-health care. For active-duty service members, inadequate participating provider networks present a challenge for accessing mental-health care.

**The committee recommends that the Department of Defense and the Department of Veterans Affairs conduct a needs assessment to determine the numbers and types of providers needed to address the long-term health needs of Operation Enduring Freedom, Operation Iraqi Freedom, and Operation New Dawn active-duty service members and veterans. The Department of Defense and the Department of Veterans Affairs should determine the optimal team composition—for example, MDs, PhDs, RNs, master's-trained professionals, and peer counselors—needed to ensure that providers function efficiently and perform at the upper level of their credentials and privileges.**

There is evidence of cultural insensitivity to nonwhite service members, who might have different or more severe physical-health and mental-health problems than their white counterparts. For example, black personnel are less likely than white personnel to use mental-health services and quicker to drop out of treatment. Issues related to types of diagnoses and potential misdiagnoses have also been raised. Whether clinicians who have ethnic characteristics similar to those of their patients would alleviate those problems is unknown.

**The committee recommends that the Department of Defense, the Department of Veterans Affairs, and other federal agencies fund research to determine whether culturally sensitive clinicians and treatment approaches improve retention in care and improve clinical outcomes.**

Women now constitute 14% of deployed forces in the US military, and an unprecedented number of female soldiers are deployed to combat areas. Although all service members are exposed to high levels of workplace stress, women in the military face some unique stressors, such as MST, which may affect their mental-health and emotional well-being. Female veterans report a higher burden of medical illness and worse quality-of-life outcomes than do men who are exposed to the same levels of trauma. MST appears to be an important risk factor for the development of PTSD.

**The committee recommends that the Department of Defense and the Department of Veterans Affairs consider ways to remove barriers and improve women's access to and use of health care in their systems. The two departments should examine**

**issues related to women's circumstances and stressors—such as military workplace stress, sexual harassment and assault, posttraumatic stress disorder, and premilitary trauma—in an effort to reduce disparities and to provide health care that is sensitive to their needs and preferences.**

## REFERENCES

Adler, A. B., P. D. Bliese, D. McGurk, C. W. Hoge, and C. A. Castro. 2009a. Battlemind debriefing and battlemind training as early interventions with soldiers returning from Iraq: Randomization by platoon. *Journal of Consulting and Clinical Psychology* 77(5):928-940.

Adler, A. B., C. A. Castro, and D. McGurk. 2009b. Time-driven battlemind psychological debriefing: A group-level early intervention in combat. *Military Medicine* 174(1):21-28.

Ames, G. M., C. B. Cunradi, R. S. Moore, and P. Stern. 2007. Military culture and drinking behavior among US Navy careerists. *Journal of Studies on Alcohol and Drugs* 68(3):336-344.

Andrews, K., K. Bencio, J. Brown, L. Conwell, C. Fahlman, and E. Schone. 2009. *Health Care Survey of DOD Beneficiaries 2008 Annual Report.* Washington, DC: Mathematica Policy Research, Inc.

Antonacci, D. J., R. M. Bloch, S. A. Saeed, Y. Yildirim, and J. Talley. 2008. Empirical evidence on the use and effectiveness of telepsychiatry via videoconferencing: Implications for forensic and correctional psychiatry. *Behavioral Sciences and the Law* 26(3):253-269.

Avery, G. H., and S. MacDermid Wadsworth. 2011. Access to mental-health services for active duty and National Guard TRICARE enrollees in Indiana. *Military Medicine* 176(3):261-264.

Bagchi, A., K. Bencio, J. Kim, M. Lee, and E. Schone. 2007. *Health Care Survey of DOD Beneficiaries 2007 Annual Report.* Washington, DC: Mathmatica Policy Research, Inc.

Barton, P. L., A. G. Brega, P. A. Devore, K. Mueller, M. J. Paulich, N. R. Floersch, G. K. Goodrich, S. G. Talkington, J. Bontrager, B. Grigsby, C. Hrincevich, S. Neal, J. L. Loker, T. M. Araya, R. E. Bennett, N. Krohn, and J. Grigsby. 2007. Specialist physicians' knowledge and beliefs about telemedicine: A comparison of users and nonusers of the technology. *Telemedicine Journal and E-Health* 13(5):487-499.

Beals, J., S. M. Manson, J. H. Shore, M. Friedman, M. Ashcraft, J. A. Fairbank, and W. E. Schlenger. 2002. The prevalence of posttraumatic stress disorder among American Indian Vietnam veterans: Disparities and context. *Journal of Traumatic Stress* 15(2):89-97.

Bean-Mayberry, B., C. Huang, F. Batuman, C. Goldzweig, D. L. Washington, E. M. Yano, and I. M. Miake-Lye. 2010. *Systematic Review of Women Veterans Health Research 2004-2008.* Los Angeles, CA: Evidence-based Synthesis Program (ESP) Center.

Bean-Mayberry, B., E. M. Yano, D. L. Washington, C. Goldzweig, F. Batuman, C. Huang, I. Miake-Lye, and P. G. Shekelle. 2011. Systematic review of women veterans' health: Update on successes and gaps. *Womens Health Issues* 21(4 Suppl):S84-S97.

Bertakis, K. D., R. Azari, L. J. Helms, E. J. Callahan, and J. A. Robbins. 2000. Gender differences in the utilization of health care services. *Journal of Family Practice* 49(2):147-152.

Britt, T. W. 2000. The stigma of psychological problems in a work environment: Evidence from the screening of service members returning from Bosnia. *Journal of Applied Social Psychology* 30(8):1599-1618.

Britt, T. W., T. M. Greene-Shortridge, S. Brink, Q. B. Nguyen, J. Rath, A. L. Cox, C. W. Hoge, and C. A. Castro. 2008. Perceived stigma and barriers to care for psychological treatment: Implications for reactions to stressors in different contexts. *Journal of Social and Clinical Psychology* 27:19.

Britt, T. W., E. A. Bennett, M. Crabtree, C. Haugh, K. Oliver, A. McFadden, and C. L. S. Pury. 2011. The theory of planned behavior and reserve component veteran treatment seeking. *Military Psychology* 23(1):82-96.

Britt, T. W., K. M. Wright, and D. Moore. 2012. Leadership as a predictor of stigma and practical barriers toward receiving mental-health treatment: A multilevel approach. *Psychological Services* 9(1):26-37.

Brod, R. L., P. A. May, and T. J. Stewart. 1982. Recruitment and retention of federal physicians on the Navajo reservation. *Social Science Journal* 19(4):47-66.

Brooks, E., D. K. Novins, D. Thomas, L. Jiang, H. T. Nagamoto, N. Dailey, B. Bair, and J. H. Shore. 2012. Personal characteristics affecting veterans' use of services for posttraumatic stress disorder. *Psychiatric Services* 63(9):862-867.

Brunwasser, S. M., J. E. Gillham, and E. S. Kim. 2009. A meta-analytic review of the Penn Resiliency program's effect on depressive symptoms. *Journal of Consulting and Clinical Psychology* 77(6):1042-1054.

Burnam, M. A., L. S. Meredith, T. Tanielian, and L. H. Jaycox. 2009. Mental-health care for Iraq and Afghanistan war veterans. *Health Affairs* 28(3):771-782.

Buzza, C., S. S. Ono, C. Turvey, S. Wittrock, M. Noble, G. Reddy, P. J. Kaboli, and H. S. Reisinger. 2011. Distance is relative: Unpacking a principal barrier in rural healthcare. *Journal of General Internal Medicine* 26(2 Suppl):648-654.

Castro, C. A., C. W. Hoge, C. W. Milliken, D. McGurk, and A. B. Adler. 2006. *Battlemind Training: Transitioning Home from Combat.* Silver Spring, MD: Walter Reed Army Institute of Research.

CBO (Congressional Budge Office). 2009. *Quality Initiatives Undertaken by the Veterans Health Administration.* Washington, DC: Congressional Budget Office.

———. 2011. CBO Testimony: Statement of Randall B. Williamson, Director, Health Care Federal Recovery Coordination Program: Enrollment, Staffing, and Care Coordination Pose Significant Challenges before Subcommittee on Health, Committee on Veterans' Affairs, House of Representatives, May 13, 2011.

Chermack, S. T., K. Zivin, M. Valenstein, M. Ilgen, K. L. Austin, J. Wryobeck, and F. C. Blow. 2008. The prevalence and predictors of mental-health treatment services in a national sample of depressed veterans. *Medical Care* 46(8):813-820.

Christensen, E., P. Netzer, E. Schaefer, C. Hill, D. Farr, and J. McMahon. 2009. *Economic Impact on Caregivers of the Seriously Wounded, Ill, and Injured.* Alexandria, VA: Center for Naval Analyses.

Cornum, R., M. D. Matthews, and M. E. P. Seligman. 2011. Comprehensive soldier fitness building resilience in a challenging institutional context. *American Psychologist* 66(1):4-9.

Darkins, A. 2012. Experiences of the Department of Veterans Affairs and the Indian Health Services. Paper read at *Workshop on the Role of Telehealth in an Evolving Health Care Environment*, August 9, Washington, DC.

Deployment Health Clinical Center. 2012. *DOD/VA/Federal Healthcare Services.* http://www.pdhealth.mil/hss/healthcare_services.asp#mhs (accessed September 25, 2012).

Detweiler, M. B., S. Arif, J. Candelario, J. Altman, P. F. Murphy, M. H. Hailing, J. G. Detweiler, and S. Vasudeva. 2011. A telepsychiatry transition clinic: The first 12 months experience. *Journal of Telemedicine and Telecare* 17(6):293-297.

Detweiler, M. B., S. Arif, J. Candelario, J. Altman, P. F. Murphy, M. H. Halling, S. Vasudeva, and J. G. Detweiler. 2012. Salem VAMC-US Army Fort Bragg warrior transition clinic telepsychiatry collaboration: 12-month operation clinical perspective. *Telemedicine Journal and E-Health* 18(2):81-86

Dickstein, B. D., D. S. Vogt, S. Handa, and B. T. Litz. 2010. Targeting self-stigma in returning military personnel and veterans: A review of intervention strategies. *Military Psychology* 22(2):224-236.

DOD (Department of Defense). 2011a. *Evaluation of the TRICARE Program.* Washington, DC: DOD.

———. 2011b. *MHS Stakeholder's Report.* Washington, DC: DOD.

———. 2012. *TRICARE (webpage).* http://www.tricare.mil/mybenefit/ProfileFilter.do;jsessionid=PQ2hM96Jx9ybGG8xnbhCwqnvK331Lxql3d5vQgcLjC1pNv21J2ND!349025571?puri=%2Fhome (accessed March 2, 2012).

Donaldson, M. S. 2001. Continuity of care: A reconceptualization. *Medical Care Research and Review* 58(3):255-290.

Fannin, J. M., and J. N. Barnes. 2007. Recruitment of physicians to rural America: A view through the lens of transaction cost theory. *Journal of Rural Health* 23(2):141-149.

Foa, E. B., E. A. Hembree, S. P. Cahill, S. A. Rauch, D. S. Riggs, N. C. Feeny, and E. Yadin. 2005. Randomized trial of prolonged exposure for posttraumatic stress disorder with and without cognitive restructuring: Outcome at academic and community clinics. *Journal of Consulting and Clinical Psychology* 73(5):953-964.

Fortney, J. C., B. M. Booth, F. C. Blow, and J. Y. Bunn. 1995. The effects of travel barriers and age on the utilization of alcoholism treatment aftercare. *American Journal of Drug and Alcohol Abuse* 21(3):391-406.

Fortney, J. C., S. J. Borowsky, A. N Hedeen, M. L. Maciejewski, and M. K. Chapko. 2002. VA community-based outpatient clinics: Access and utilization performance measures. *Medical Care* 40(7):561-569.

Fortney, J. C., M. L. Maciejewski, J. J. Warren, and J. F. Burgess, Jr. 2005a. Does improving geographic access to VA primary care services impact patients' patterns of utilization and costs? *Inquiry* 42(1):29-42.

Fortney, J. C., D. E. Steffick, J. F. Burgess, Jr., M. L. Maciejewski, and L. A. Petersen. 2005b. Are primary care services a substitute or complement for specialty and inpatient services? *Health Services Research* 40(5 Pt 1):1422-1442.

Fortney, J. C., J. F. Burgess, Jr., H. B. Bosworth, B. M. Booth, and P. J. Kaboli. 2011. A re-conceptualization of access for 21st century healthcare. *Journal of General Internal Medicine* 26(2 Suppl):639-647.

GAO (Government Accountability Office). 2011a. *DOD and VA Health Care: Federal Recovery Coordination Program Continues to Expand but Faces Significant Challenges.* Washington, DC: GAO.

———. 2011b. *VA Mental-health: Number of Veterans Receiving Care, Barriers Faced, and Efforts to Increase Access.* Washington, DC: GAO.

Gibbs, D. A., K. L. Rae Olmsted, J. M. Brown, and A. Clinton-Sherrod. 2011. Dynamics of stigma for alcohol and mental-health treatment among army soldiers. *Military Psychology* 23(1):36-51.

Godleski, L., A. Darkins, and J. Peters. 2012. Outcomes of 98,609 US Department of Veterans Affairs patients enrolled in telemental-health services, 2006-2010. *Psychiatric Services* 63(4):383-385.

Gorman, L. A., A. J. Blow, B. D. Ames, and P. L. Reed. 2011. National Guard families after combat: Mental-health, use of mental-health services, and perceived treatment barriers. *Psychiatric Services* 62(1):28-34.

Greene-Shortridge, T. M., T. W. Britt, and C. A. Castro. 2007. The stigma of mental-health problems in the military. *Military Medicine* 172(2):157-161.

Grigsby, B., A. G. Brega, R. E. Bennett, P. A. Devore, M. J. Paulich, S. G. Talkington, N. R. Floersch, P. L. Barton, S. Neal, T. M. Araya, J. L. Loker, N. Krohn, and J. Grigsby. 2007. The slow pace of interactive video telemedicine adoption: The perspective of telemedicine program administrators on physician participation. *Telemedicine Journal and E-Health* 13(6):645-656.

Hannold, E. M., I. M. Freytes, and C. R. Uphold. 2011. Unmet health services needs experienced by Puerto Rican OEF/OIF veterans and families post deployment. *Military Medicine* 176(4):381-388.

Harada, N. D., J. Damron-Rodriguez, V. M. Villa, D. L. Washington, S. Dhanani, H. Shon, M. Chattopadhyay, H. Fishbein, M. Lee, T. Makinodan, and R. Andersen. 2002. Veteran identity and race/ethnicity: Influences on VA outpatient care utilization. *Medical Care* 40(1 Suppl):I117-I128.

Hill, R. D., M. K. Luptak, R. W. Rupper, B. Bair, C. Peterson, N. Dailey, and B. L. Hicken. 2010. Review of Veterans Health Administration telemedicine interventions. *American Journal of Managed Care* 16(12 Suppl):e302-e310.

Himmelstein, D. U., K. E. Lasser, D. McCormick, D. H. Bor, J. W. Boyd, and S. Woolhandler. 2007. Lack of health coverage among US veterans from 1987 to 2004. *American Journal of Public Health* 97(12):2199-2203.

Hoerster, K. D., C. A. Malte, Z. E. Imel, Z. Ahmad, S. C. Hunt, and M. Jakupcak. 2012. Association of perceived barriers with prospective use of VA mental-health care among Iraq and Afghanistan veterans. *Psychiatric Services* 63(4):380-382.

Hogan, T. P., B. Wakefield, K. M. Nazi, T. K. Houston, and F. M. Weaver. 2011. Promoting access through complementary ehealth technologies: Recommendations for VA's home telehealth and personal health record programs. *Journal of General Internal Medicine* 26(2 Suppl):628-635.

Hoge, C. W., K. Wright, P. Bliese, A. Adler, and J. Thomas. 2004. *Prevalence and Screening of Mental-health Problems Among US Combat Soldiers Pre- and Post- Deployment.* Silver Spring, MD: Walter Reed Army Institute of Research.

Hoge, C. W., C. A. Castro, S. C. Messer, D. McGurk, D. I. Cotting, and R. L. Koffman. 2008. Combat duty in Iraq and Afghanistan, mental-health problems and barriers to care. *US Army Medical Department Journal*:7-17.

Holiday, L. F., G. Bell, R. E. Klein, and M. R. Wells. 2006. *American Indian and Alaska Native Veterans: Lasting Contributions*. Washington, DC: Assistant Secretary for Policy, Planning, and Preparedness, Department of Veterans Affairs.

Hostetter, C. L., and J. D. Felsen. 1975. Multiple variable motivators involved in the recruitment of physicians for the Indian Health Service. *Public Health Reports* 90(4):319-324.

Hyun, J. K., J. Pavao, and R. Kimerling. 2009. Military sexual trauma. *PTSD Research Quarterly* 20(2).

IOM (Institute of Medicine). 1996. *Telemedicine: A Guide to Assessing Telecommunications for Health Care*. Washinton, DC: National Academy Press.

———. 2001. *Crossing the Quality Chasm: A New Health System for the 21st Century.* Washington, DC: National Academy Press.

———. 2005. *Quality Through Collaboration: The Future of Rural Health Care*. Washington, DC: The National Academies Press.

———. 2009. *Combating Tobacco Use in Military and Veteran Populations*. Washington, DC: The National Academies Press.

———. 2010. *Returning Home from Iraq and Afghanistan: Preliminary Assessment of Readjustment Needs of Veterans, Service Members, and Their Families.* Washington, DC: The National Academies Press.

———. 2012. *Treatment for Posttraumatic Stress Disorder in Military and Veteran Populations: Initial Assessment*. Washington, DC: The National Academies Press.

Jackson, G. L., S. L. Krein, D. C. Alverson, A. W. Darkins, W. Gunnar, N. D. Harada, C. D. Helfrich, T. K. Houston, T. F. Klobucar, K. M. Nazi, R. K. Poropatich, J. D. Ralston, and H. B. Bosworth. 2011. Defining core issues in utilizing information technology to improve access: Evaluation and research agenda. *Journal of General Internal Medicine* 26(2 Suppl):623-627.

Johnson, J. L., and M. C. Cameron. 2001. Barriers to providing effective mental-health services to American Indians. *Mental-health Services Research* 3(4):215-223.

Johnson, P. J., K. F. Carlson, and M. O. Hearst. 2010. Healthcare disparities for American Indian veterans in the United States: A population-based study. *Medical Care* 48(6):563-569.

Kaelber, D., and E. C. Pan. 2008. The value of personal health record (PHR) systems. *AMIA Annual Symposium proceedings*:343-347.

Kane, T. 2006. *Who Are the Recruits? The Demographic Characteristics of US Military Enlistment, 2003-2005.* Washington, DC: The Heritage Foundation.

Kapusta, N. D., A. Zorman, E. Etzersdorfer, E. Ponocny-Seliger, E. Jandl-Jager, and G. Sonneck. 2008. Rural-urban differences in austrian suicides. *Social Psychiatry and Psychiatric Epidemiology* 43(4):311-318.

Kaufman, C., E. Brooks, T. Noe, B. Bair, N. Dailey, and J. Shore. 2010. *How Rural are American Indian and Alaska Native Veterans?* Salt Lake City, UT: Veterans Rural Health Resource Center, Western Region Native Domain.

Kehle, S., and N. Greer. 2011. *Interventions to Improve Veterans' Access to Care: A Systematic Review of the Literature.* Washington, DC: Department of Veterans Affairs, Evidence-Based Synthesis Program Center.

Kehle, S. M., M. A. Polusny, M. Murdoch, C. R. Erbes, P. A. Arbisi, P. Thuras, and L. A. Meis. 2010. Early mental-health treatment-seeking among US National Guard soldiers deployed to Iraq. *Journal of Traumatic Stress* 23(1):33-40.

Kelly, M. M., D. S. Vogt, E. M. Scheiderer, P. Ouimette, J. Daley, and J. Wolfe. 2008. Effects of military trauma exposure on women veterans' use and perceptions of Veterans Health Administration care. *Journal of General Internal Medicine* 23(6):741-747.

Kessler, R. C., P. A. Berglund, M. L. Bruce, J. R. Koch, E. M. Laska, P. J. Leaf, R. W. Manderscheid, R. A. Rosenheck, E. E. Walters, and P. S. Wang. 2001. The prevalence and correlates of untreated serious mental illness. *Health Services Research* 36(6 Pt 1):987-1007.

Kim, P. Y., T. W. Britt, R. P. Klocko, L. A. Riviere, and A. B. Adler. 2011. Stigma, negative attitudes about treatment, and utilization of mental-health care among soldiers. *Military Psychology* 23(1):65-81.

Kimerling, R., K. Gima, M. W. Smith, A. Street, and S. Frayne. 2007. The Veterans Health Administration and military sexual trauma. *American Journal of Public Health* 97(12):2160-2166.

Kimerling, R., A. E. Street, J. Pavao, M. W. Smith, R. C. Cronkite, T. H. Holmes, and S. M. Frayne. 2010. Military-related sexual trauma among Veterans Health Administration patients returning from Afghanistan and Iraq. *American Journal of Public Health* 100(8):1409-1412.

Kizer, K. W. 2011. The emerging era of virtual healthcare. Paper read at *VHA Visioning Summit on Virtual Health Care Delivery*, October 13, 2010, Arlington, VA.

———. 2012. Veterans and the Affordable Care Act. *Journal of the American Medical Association* 307(8):789-790.

Kizer, K. W., and R. A. Dudley. 2009. Extreme makeover: Transformation of the veterans health care system. *Annual Review of Public Health* 30:313-339.

Koenig, K. L. 2003. Homeland security and public health: Role of the Department of Veterans Affairs, the US Department of Homeland Security, and implications for the public health community. *Prehospital and Disaster Medicine* 18(4):327-333.

Kramer, B. J., M. Wang, S. Jouldjian, M. L. Lee, B. Finke, and D. Saliba. 2009. Veterans Health Administration and Indian Health Service: Healthcare utilization by Indian Health Service enrollees. *Medical Care* 47(6):670-676.

Lester, P. B., S. McBride, P. D. Bliese, and A. B. Adler. 2011. Bringing science to bear an empirical assessment of the Comprehensive Soldier Fitness program. *American Psychologist* 66(1):77-81.

Levin, K. A., and A. H. Leyland. 2005. Urban/rural inequalities in suicide in Scotland, 1981–1999. *Social Sciences and Medicine* 60(12):2877-2890.

Link, B. G., and J. C. Phelan. 2001. Conceptualizing stigma. *Annual Review of Sociology* 27:363-385.

Lipari, R. N., P. J. Cook, L. M. Rock, and K. Matos. 2008. *2006 Gender Relations Survey of Active Duty Members.* Arlington, VA: Defense Manpower Data Center.

Litz, B. T., S. M. Orsillo, M. Friedman, P. Ehlich, and A. Batres. 1997. Posttraumatic stress disorder associated with peacekeeping duty in Somalia for US military personnel. *American Journal of Psychiatry* 154(2):178-184.

Liu, C. F., M. L. Maciejewski, and A. E. Sales. 2005. Changes in characteristics of veterans using the VHA health care system between 1996 and 1999. *Health Research Policy and Systems* 3(1):5.

Maguen, S., T. J. Metzler, B. T. Litz, K. H. Seal, S. J. Knight, and C. R. Marmar. 2009. The impact of killing in war on mental-health symptoms and related functioning. *Journal of Traumatic Stress* 22(5):435-443.

Maguen, S., B. Cohen, G. Cohen, E. Madden, D. Bertenthal, and K. Seal. 2012. Gender differences in health service utilization among Iraq and Afghanistan veterans with posttraumatic stress disorder. *Journal of Women's Health* 21(6):666-673.

McCarthy, J. F., J. D. Piette, J. C. Fortney, M. Valenstein, and F. C. Blow. 2006. Outpatient visit chaining among patients with serious mental illness. *Medical Care* 44(3):257-264.

McCarthy, J. F., F. C. Blow, R. V. Ignacio, M. A. Ilgen, K. L. Austin, and M. Valenstein. 2012. Suicide among patients in the Veterans Affairs health system: Rural–urban differences in rates, risks, and methods. *American Journal of Public Health* 102(S1):S111-S117.

McNally, R. J., R. A. Bryant, and A. Ehlers. 2003. Does early psychological intervention promote recovery from posttraumatic stress? *Psychological Science in the Public Interest* 4(2):45-79.

Meredith, M., C. D. Sherbourne, S. Gailot, L. Hansell, H. V. Ritschard, A. M. Parker, and G. Wrenn. 2011. *Promoting Psychological Resilience in the US Military.* Santa Monica, CA: RAND Corporation.

Merlis, M. 2012. *The Future of Health Care for Military Personnel and Veterans.* Washington, DC: Academy Health.

Middleton, N., D. Gunnell, S. Frankel, E. Whitley, and D. Dorling. 2003. Urban-rural differences in suicide trends in young adults: England and Wales, 1981-1998. *Social Science and Medicine* 57(7):1183-1194.

Military.com. 2012a. *Transition Assistance Management Program.* http://www.military.com/benefits/tricare/transition-assistance-management-program.html (accessed November 8, 2012).

———. 2012b. *TRICARE: Benefits*. http://www.military.com/benefits/tricare (accessed September 25, 2012).

Mohr, D. C., T. Carmody, L. Erickson, L. Jin, and J. Leader. 2011. Telephone-administered cognitive behavioral therapy for veterans served by community-based outpatient clinics. *Journal of Consulting and Clinical Psychology* 79(2):261-265.

Morland, L. A., C. J. Greene, C. S. Rosen, D. Foy, P. Reilly, J. Shore, Q. He, and B. C. Frueh. 2010. Telemedicine for anger management therapy in a rural population of combat veterans with posttraumatic stress disorder: A randomized noninferiority trial. *Journal of Clinical Psychiatry* 71(7):855-863.

Mulligan, K., N. T. Fear, N. Jones, H. Alvarez, L. Hull, U. Naumann, S. Wessely, and N. Greenberg. 2012. Postdeployment Battlemind training for the U.K. Armed Forces: A cluster randomized controlled trial. *Journal of Consulting and Clinical Psychology* 80(3):331-341.

Murdoch, M., J. Hodges, D. Cowper, L. Fortier, and M. van Ryn. 2003. Racial disparities in VA service connection for posttraumatic stress disorder disability. *Medical Care* 41(4):536-549.

National Council on Disability. 2009. *Invisible Wounds: Serving Service Members and Veterans with PTSD and TBI.* Washington, DC: National Council on Disability.

Nazi, K. M. 2010. Veterans' voices: Use of the American Customer Satisfaction Index (ACSI) survey to identify *My Healthevet* personal health record users' characteristics, needs, and preferences. *Journal of the American Medical Informatics Association* 17(2):203-211.

Nazi, K. M., T. P. Hogan, T. H. Wagner, D. K. McInnes, B. M. Smith, D. Haggstrom, N. R. Chumbler, A. L. Gifford, K. G. Charters, J. J. Saleem, K. R. Weingardt, L. F. Fischetti, and F. M. Weaver. 2010. Embracing a health services research perspective on personal health records: Lessons learned from the VA *My Healthevet* system. *Journal of General Internal Medicine* 25(1 Suppl):62-67.

Office of the Assistant Secretary of Defense. 2010. *Department of Defense 'In Transition' Program.* Washington, DC: Department of Defense.

Orsingher, J. M., A. T. Lopez, and M. E. Rinehart. 2008. Battlemind training system: Armor for your mind. *US Army Medical Department Journal* Jul-Sep:66-71.

Panangala, S. V. 2007. *Veterans Health Care Issues.* Washington, DC: Congressional Research Service.

———. 2010. *Veterans Medical Care: FY2011 Appropriations.* Washington, DC: Congressional Research Service.

Panangala, S. V., and B. H. P. Mendez. 2010. *Veterans Health Administration: Community Based Outpatient Clinics.* Washington, DC: Congressional Research Service.

Pellerin, C., and T. C. Marshall. 2012. *DOD, VA Announce Joint Health Record Milestone.* http://www.defense.gov/news/newsarticle.aspx?id=116437 (accessed October 6, 2012).

Peterson, C., N. Park, and C. A. Castro. 2011. Assessment for the US Army Comprehensive Soldier Fitness program the Global Assessment Tool. *American Psychologist* 66(1):10-18.

Pietrzak, R. H., D. C. Johnson, M. B. Goldstein, J. C. Malley, and S. M. Southwick. 2009. Perceived stigma and barriers to mental-health care utilization among OEF-OIF veterans. *Psychiatric Services* 60(8):1118-1122.

Pizer, S. D., and J. C. Prentice. 2011. What are the consequences of waiting for health care in the veteran population? *Journal of General Internal Medicine* 26 (2 Suppl):676-682.

Prentice, J. C., and S. D. Pizer. 2007. Delayed access to health care and mortality. *Health Services Research* 42(2):644-662.

Prentice, J. C., B. G. Fincke, D. R. Miller, and S. D. Pizer. 2011. Outpatient wait time and diabetes care quality improvement. *American Journal of Managed Care* 17(2):e43-e54.

Rae Olmsted, K. L., J. M. Brown, J. Vandermaas-Peeler, S. J. Tueller, R. E. Johnson, and D. A. Gibbs. 2011. Mental-health and substance abuse treatment stigma among soldiers. *Military Psychology* 23(1):52-64.

Ralston, J. D., D. Carrell, R. Reid, M. Anderson, M. Moran, and J. Hereford. 2007. Patient web services integrated with a shared medical record: Patient use and satisfaction. *Journal of the American Medical Informatics Association* 14(6):798-806.

Razvodovsky, Y., and A. Stickley. 2009. Suicide in urban and rural regions of Belarus, 1990-2005. *Public Health* 123(1):27-31.

Reivich, K. J., M. E. P. Seligman, and S. McBride. 2011. Master resilience training in the US Army. *American Psychologist* 66(1):25-34.

Richardson, L. K., B. C. Frueh, A. L. Grubaugh, L. Egede, and J. D. Elhai. 2009. Current directions in videoconferencing tele-mental-health research. *Clinical Psychology* 16(3):323-338.

Rosenheck, R. 2000. Primary care satellite clinics and improved access to general and mental-health services. *Health Services Research* 35(4):777-790.

Rosenheck, R., and A. Fontana. 2002. Black and hispanic veterans in intensive VA treatment programs for posttraumatic stress disorder. *Medical Care* 40(1 Suppl):I52-I61.

Ross, S. E., L. A. Moore, M. A. Earnest, L. Wittevrongel, and C. T. Lin. 2004. Providing a web-based online medical record with electronic communication capabilities to patients with congestive heart failure: Randomized trial. *Journal of Medical Internet Research* 6(2):e12.

Ruskin, P. E., M. Silver-Aylaian, M. A. Kling, S. A. Reed, D. D. Bradham, J. R. Hebel, D. Barrett, F. Knowles 3rd, and P. Hauser. 2004. Treatment outcomes in depression: Comparison of remote treatment through telepsychiatry to in-person treatment. *American Journal of Psychiatry.* 161(8):1471-1476.

Saha, S., M. Freeman, J. Toure, K. M. Tippens, C. Weeks, and S. Ibrahim. 2007. *Racial and Ethnic Disparities in the VA Healthcare System: A Systematic Review.* Washington, DC: Department of Veterans Affairs.

Schlenger, W. E., R. A. Kulka, J. A. Fairbank, R. L. Hough, B. Kathleen Jordan, C. R. Marmar, and D. S. Weiss. 1992. The prevalence of post-traumatic stress disorder in the Vietnam generation: A multimethod, multisource assessment of psychiatric disorder. *Journal of Traumatic Stress* 5(3):333-363.

Schnipper, J. L., C. Hamann, C. D. Ndumele, C. L. Liang, M. G. Carty, A. S. Karson, I. Bhan, C. M. Coley, E. Poon, A. Turchin, S. A. Labonville, E. K. Diedrichsen, S. Lipsitz, C. A. Broverman, P. McCarthy, and T. K. Gandhi. 2009. Effect of an electronic medication reconciliation application and process redesign on potential adverse drug events: A cluster-randomized trial. *Archives of Internal Medicine* 169(8):771-780.

Seal, K. H., D. Bertenthal, C. R. Miner, S. Sen, and C. Marmar. 2007. Bringing the war back home: Mental-health disorders among 103,788 US veterans returning from Iraq and Afghanistan seen at Department of Veterans Affairs facilities. *Archives of Internal Medicine* 167(5):476-482.

Seal, K. H., S. Maguen, B. Cohen, K. S. Gima, T. J. Metzler, L. Ren, D. Bertenthal, and C. R. Marmar. 2010. VA mental-health services utilization in Iraq and Afghanistan veterans in the first year of receiving new mental-health diagnoses. *Journal of Traumatic Stress* 23(1):5-16.

Shekelle, P. G., F. Batuman, B. Bean-Mayberry, C. Goldzweig, C. Huang, I. M. Miake-Lye, D. L. Washington, E. M. Yano, and L. C. Zephyrin. 2011. *Health Effects of Military Service on Women Veterans*. Washington, DC: VA Evidence-based Synthesis Program, Department of Veterans Affairs.

Shore, J. H., and S. M. Manson. 2004a. The American Indian veteran and posttraumatic stress disorder: A telehealth assessment and formulation. *Culture, Medicine and Psychiatry* 28(2):231-243.

———. 2004b. Telepsychiatric care of American Indian veterans with post-traumatic stress disorder: Bridging gaps in geography, organizations, and culture. *Telemedicine Journal and E-Health* 10(1 Suppl):S64-S69.

———. 2005. A developmental model for rural telepsychiatry. *Psychiatric Services* 56(8):976-980.

Shore, J. H., D. Savin, H. Orton, J. Beals, and S. M. Manson. 2007. Diagnostic reliability of telepsychiatry in American Indian veterans. *American Journal of Psychiatry* 164(1):115-118.

Shore, J. H., E. Brooks, D. Savin, H. Orton, J. Grigsby, and S. M. Manson. 2008. Acceptability of telepsychiatry in American Indians. *Telemedicine and eHealth* 14(5):461-466.

Shore, J. H., E. Brooks, H. Anderson, B. Bair, N. Dailey, L. J. Kaufmann, and S. Manson. 2012. Characteristics of telemental-health service use by American Indian veterans. *Psychiatric Services* 63(2):179-181.

Singh, G. K., and M. Siahpush. 2002. Increasing rural-urban gradients in US suicide mortality, 1970-1997. *American Journal of Public Health* 92(7):1161-1167.

Spaulding, R. J., T. Russo, D. J. Cook, and G. C. Doolittle. 2005. Diffusion theory and telemedicine adoption by Kansas health care providers: Critical factors in telemedicine adoption for improved patient access. *Journal of Telemedicine and Telecare* 11(1 Suppl):107-109.

Spoont, M. R., J. Hodges, M. Murdoch, and S. Nugent. 2009. Race and ethnicity as factors in mental-health service use among veterans with PTSD. *Journal of Traumatic Stress* 22(6):648-653.

Stecker, T., J. C. Fortney, F. Hamilton, and I. Ajzen. 2007. An assessment of beliefs about mental-health care among veterans who served in Iraq. *Psychiatric Services* 58(10):1358-1361.

Street, A. E., J. Stafford, C. M. Mahan, and A. Hendricks. 2008. Sexual harassment and assault experienced by reservists during military service: Prevalence and health correlates. *Journal of Rehabilitation Research and Development* 45(3):409-419.

Street, A. E., D. Vogt, and L. Dutra. 2009. A new generation of women veterans: Stressors faced by women deployed to Iraq and Afghanistan. *Clinical Psychology Review* 29(8):685-694.

Stroupe, K. T., B. M. Smith, T. A. Lee, E. Tarlov, R. Durazo-Arvizu, Z. Huo, T. Barnett, L. Cao, M. Burk, F. Cunningham, D. M. Hynes, and K. B. Weiss. 2007. Effect of increased copayments on pharmacy use in the Department of Veterans Affairs. *Medical Care* 45(11):1090-1097.

Suris, A., and L. Lind. 2008. Military sexual trauma: A review of prevalence and associated health consequences in veterans. *Trauma, Violence, and Abuse* 9(4):250-269.

Suris, A., L. Lind, T. M. Kashner, P. D. Borman, and F. Petty. 2004. Sexual assault in women veterans: An examination of PTSD risk, health care utilization, and cost of care. *Psychosomatic Medicine* 66(5):749-756.

Tanielian, T., and L. H. Jaycox. 2008. *Invisible Wounds of War: Psychological and Cognitive Injuries, Their Consequences, and Services to Assist Recovery*. Santa Monica, CA: RAND Corporation.

TRICARE Management Activity. 2009. *DEERS.* http://tricare.mil/mybenefit/home/overview/Eligibility/DEERS (accessed July 6, 2009).

Turvey, C. L., D. M. Zulman, K. M. Nazi, B. J. Wakefield, S. S. Woods, T. P. Hogan, F. M. Weaver, and K. McInnes. 2012. Transfer of information from personal health records: A survey of veterans using *My Healthevet*. *Telemedicine Journal and E-Health* 18(2):109-114.

VA (Department of Veterans Affairs). 2009. *Stats at a Glance: VA Benefits and Health Care Utilization, April 2009*. http://www1.va.gov/vetdata (accessed July 9, 2009).

———. 2011a. *Guide to VA Mental-health Services for Veterans and Families*. Washington, DC: VA.

———. 2011b. *Strategic Plan Refresh: Fiscal Year (FY) 2011-2015*. Washington, DC: Office of the Secretary.

———. 2012a. *Copays*. http://www.va.gov/healthbenefits/cost/copay_rates.asp (accessed August 14, 2012).

———. 2012b. Exempting in-home video telehealth from copayments: Direct final rule. *Federal Register* 77(44):13195-13198.

———. 2012c. *VA to Expand Health Care Service by Opening 13 New Community-based Outpatient Clinics*. http://www.va.gov/opa/pressrel/pressrelease.cfm?id=2358 (accessed September 25, 2012).

———. 2012d. *VHS Office of Rural Health*. http://www.ruralhealth.va.gov (accessed March 1, 2012).

VA and VHA (Veterans Health Administration). 2008. *VHA Handbook 1160.01: Uniform Mental-health Services in VA Medical Centers and Clinics*. Washington, DC: Department of Veterans Affairs.

VA Office of the Inspector General. 2012. *Veterans Health Administration: Review of Veterans' Access to Mental-health Care*. Washington, DC VA Office of Inspector General.

VHA (Veterans Health Administration). 2011. *A Query of VA Mental-health Professionals: Executive Summary and Preliminary Analysis.* Washington, DC: Veterans Health Administration.

Visco, R. 2009. Postdeployment, self-reporting of mental-health problems, and barriers to care. *Perspectives in Psychiatric Care* 45(4):240-253.

Washington, D. L., N. D. Harada, V. M. Villa, J. Damron-Rodriguez, S. Dhanani, H. Shon, and T. Makinodan. 2002. Racial variations in Department of Veterans Affairs ambulatory care use and unmet health care needs. *Military Medicine* 167(3):235-241.

Washington, D. L., V. Villa, A. Brown, J. Damron-Rodriguez, and N. Harada. 2005. Racial/ethnic variations in veterans' ambulatory care use. *American Journal of Public Health* 95(12):2231-2237.

Washington, D. L., E. M. Yano, B. Simon, and S. Sun. 2006. To use or not to use. What influences why women veterans choose VA health care. *Journal of General Internal Medicine* 21(3 Suppl):S11-S18.

Weeks, W. B., L. E. Kazis, Y. Shen, Z. Cong, X. S. Ren, D. Miller, A. Lee, and J. B. Perlin. 2004. Differences in health-related quality of life in rural and urban veterans. *American Journal of Public Health* 94(10):1762-1767.

West, A., and W. B. Weeks. 2006. Physical and mental-health and access to care among nonmetropolitan Veterans Health Administration patients younger than 65 years. *Journal of Rural Health* 22(1):9-16.

Williams, J. 3rd. 2008. *Army Expands Battlemind Training*. http://www.army.mil/article/9548/army-expands-battlemind-training (accessed September 30, 2012).

Wilson, J. A., K. Onorati, M. Mishkind, M. A. Reger, and G. A. Gahm. 2008. Soldier attitudes about technology-based approaches to mental-health care. *Cyberpsychology and Behavior* 11(6):767-769.

Wilson, N. J., and K. W. Kizer. 1997. The VA health care system: An unrecognized national safety net. *Health Affairs* 16(4):200-204.

Wong, E. C., G. N. Marshall, V. Shetty, A. Zhou, H. Belzberg, and D. D. Yamashita. 2007. Survivors of violence-related facial injury: Psychiatric needs and barriers to mental-health care. *General Hospital Psychiatry* 29(2):117-122.

Wright, K. M., O. A. Cabrera, P. D. Bliese, A. B. Adler, C. W. Hoge, and C. A. Castro. 2009. Stigma and barriers to care in soldiers postcombat. *Psychological Services* 6(2):108-116.

Yano, E. M., D. L. Washington, C. Goldzweig, C. Caffrey, and C. Turner. 2003. The organization and delivery of women's health care in Department of Veterans Affairs Medical Center. *Womens Health Issues* 13(2):55-61.

Zeber, J. E., K. L. Grazier, M. Valenstein, F. C. Blow, and P. M. Lantz. 2007. Effect of a medication copayment increase in veterans with schizophrenia. *American Journal of Managed Care* 13(6 Pt 2):335-346.

Zhou, Y. Y., T. Garrido, H. L. Chin, A. M. Wiesenthal, and L. L. Liang. 2007. Patient access to an electronic health record with secure messaging: Impact on primary care utilization. *American Journal of Managed Care* 13(7):418-424.

# 10

# PROPOSED DATA ANALYSES

As the committee members read the legislation that directed their charge and reviewed the literature, they recognized that not all areas of concern were addressed by available information. Thus, they conceived a detailed data-analysis plan that they believed would provide clarity on many of the issues of concern. Initially, the committee thought it might carry out the proposed analyses and researched sources of potential data, developed data-analysis plans, data use agreements, and provided the institutional review boards of the National Academies, Department of Defense (DOD), and Department of Veterans Affairs (VA) with the appropriate documents. The committee abandoned its plans because of time and funding constraints, however, this chapter describes the committee's efforts for exploring and gathering data for the development of a database that would provide the foundation for linking data from multiple data sources (e.g., linking basic demographic data with data on diagnoses, types of treatments received, and employment and earnings records before and after deployment). The chapter details the committee's vision for the database, the questions the committee hoped to address with the data, the data sources the committee believed would provide answers to its questions, and the committee's overall process for approaching this task.

Through that process, the committee identified a variety of data and databases available from the DOD, VA, and other federal agencies that could be used to address many of the questions posed by the legislation that motivated its work. Appendix F describes a small sample of the databases explored by the committee as the list of potentially useful data sources continued to increase with additional queries and searches.

On the basis of its investigations, the committee determined that it should expand its initial approach in responding to its task by proposing data analyses that could be conducted by using existing government databases. Very limited quantitative characterization of the issues described in the legislation existed in the published literature, so the committee proposed using available government data and linking them. There are no databases or files that fully integrate basic deployment and demographic data with health outcomes, treatment or transition of care, access to care, employment and earnings records before and after deployment, family records, and other processes and outcomes. Thus, the committee decided to develop an analytic database for that purpose and attempted to begin linking the data. As noted, the committee ultimately abandoned its approach, however, it details its efforts so that others might carry out its vision.

## COMMITTEE'S APPROACH

First, the committee reviewed the legislation to determine which sections could be addressed with data and which could not; it then divided each section into discrete tasks that would be overseen by the committee's work groups. Second, each work group developed an analytic plan that highlighted the questions to be answered and the data sources that could potentially provide the necessary information; thus, the issues and questions posed were aligned with available data sources. Third, the committee prepared its analytic plans for the institutional review board (IRB) at the National Academy of Sciences and for data-use agreements (DUAs) with various government agencies. Fourth, the work groups attempted to secure the necessary data; but they were often faced with impediments that prevented accessing them. Finally, the committee recognized that not all the questions that it would like to have answered would have a data source and that some questions would remain unanswered.

## COMMITTEE PROCESS

The need and request for each specific file and variable within a file from various data sets would be supported by different sections of the legislation (see Appendix A). Because the legislation was broad and covered so many aspects of deployment—not only in active duty but in veterans, family members, and communities—the committee members reviewed the legislation carefully and developed questions that would need to be answered in an effort to respond to each section of it. The committee members also had to determine which agencies collected the information that might enable them to answer the questions and which datasets would provide the data that they needed. Data dictionaries were secured and reviewed so that the committee members were able to identify the files that they needed and to determine whether the information was held in a particular database. On the basis of the legislation, several data groups were organized according to the need for similar data (rather than according to the committee's work groups). For example, the outcomes, treatment, family, and economic work groups wished to understand how the number of deployments affected outcomes of the conditions of interest, such as posttraumatic stress disorder (PTSD) and traumatic brain injury (TBI). The committee members planned to send the Defense Manpower Data Center (DMDC) file of all deployed persons to the VA and DOD health systems to identify those who had the *International Classification of Diseases* (*ICD*) diagnoses of interest. Those persons would then be followed through the DOD and VA health system to determine the types of treatment provided and the numbers of visits to treatment facilities, they would then be linked to employment records and earnings so that the committee could determine the impact of deployment. The committee secured the demographic files of all those deployed (see Chapters 2 and 3), but linking them with the additional files needed became too time-consuming and the committee would not be able to complete its work before the termination of its contract with the DOD.

## DATA-COLLECTION PLAN AND ANALYSIS QUESTIONS

The following is a breakdown of the legislation according to the types of data needed, samples of the types of questions developed by each group (to be answered by the data), and the data sources that the committee believed would provide answers to the questions. In some cases, more than one work group examined the same section of the legislation, but each group had its own focus.

**Public Law 110-181. Section 1661.** Study on physical and mental health and other readjustment needs of members and former members of the armed forces who deployed in Operation Iraqi Freedom and Operation Enduring Freedom and their Families.

(2) A second phase, to be completed not later than three years after the date of the enactment of this Act, to carry out a comprehensive assessment, in accordance with the parameters identified under the preliminary report required by paragraph (1), of the physical and mental health and other readjustment needs of members and former members of the Armed Forces who deployed in Operation Iraqi Freedom or Operation Enduring Freedom and their families as a result of such deployment, including, at a minimum—

(c) POPULATIONS TO BE STUDIED.—the study required under subsection (a) shall consider the readjustment needs of each population of individuals as follows:

(1) Members of the regular components of the Armed Forces who are returning, or have returned, to the United States from deployment in Operation Iraqi Freedom or Operation Enduring Freedom.
(2) Members of the National Guard and Reserve who are returning, or have returned, to the United States from deployment in Operation Iraqi Freedom or Operation Enduring Freedom.
(3) Veterans of Operation Iraqi Freedom or Operation Enduring Freedom.
(4) Family members of the members and veterans described in paragraphs (1) through (3).

## Data Group 1

**Relevant Sections of the Law**
(B) an assessment of the particular impacts of multiple deployments in Operation Iraqi Freedom or Operation Enduring Freedom on such members and former members and their families;

(C) an assessment of the full scope of the neurological, psychiatric, and psychological effects of traumatic brain injury on members and former members of the Armed Forces, including the effects of such effects on the family members of such members and former members, and an assessment of the efficacy of current treatment approaches for traumatic brain injury in the United States and the efficacy of screenings and treatment approaches for traumatic brain injury within the Department of Defense and the Department of Veterans Affairs;

(D) an assessment of the effects of undiagnosed injuries such as post-traumatic stress disorder and traumatic brain injury.

**Data Files Required**

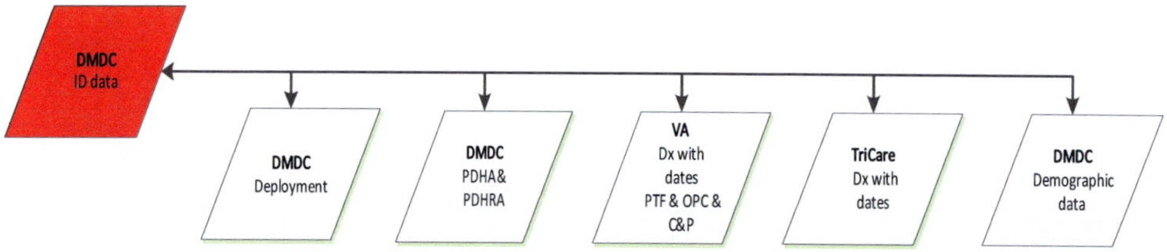


**Sample Questions to Be Answered by the Data**

- How many people who were deployed screen positive for TBI, PTSD, or both? How many people who were deployed receive a diagnosis of TBI, PTSD, or both (in theater vs posttheater)? How long after deployment do service members and veterans receive a diagnosis of PTSD, TBI, or both?
- What are the major comorbidities associated with TBI, PTSD, depression, substance use, and suicidal ideation?
- What is the impact of multiple deployments, length of deployment, and site of deployment on TBI, PTSD, or both?
- How do the above questions vary by sex, ethnicity, marital status, age, service, rank, education attained, criminal record, home of record on service entry, aptitude, occupational category, branch of service, reserve, guard, or active duty?
- Does higher education affect TBI or PTSD outcomes? Does alcohol use before deployment increase or decrease the risk of TBI or PTSD?
- In a longitudinal cohort of deployed service members, what are the frequency, course (timing), and co-occurrence of screening for, diagnosis of, and treatment for TBI, PTSD, substance-use disorder, depression, and suicide risk?
- When treatment is provided for one of the five conditions (as indicated by *ICD-9* code), what approach is used? That is, if pharmacologic, what medication? If behavioral, what method, by whom, and were sessions individual or group?
- What is the person's current functioning: What diagnoses is the person still being treated for? What is the person's current employment status? Quality of life?
- Does the course of screening, diagnosis, and treatment vary by branch of military, where processed through the immediate postdeployment period, ZIP code of postdeployment residence, urban vs rural setting, rank, race or ethnicity, sex, marital status, waivers granted to allow enlistment, Armed Forces Qualification Test (AFQT) or General Classiification Test, pre-enlistment disorders, or predeployment disorders?
- What are the number of deployments and the length of deployments of each person? What are the number and pattern of medical visits? What proportion of people who have a particular diagnosis are using services in DOD or in VA?

**Data Group 2**

**Relevant Sections of the Law**

(A) an assessment of the psychological, social, and economic impacts of such deployment on such members and former members and their families;

(B) an assessment of the particular impacts of multiple deployments in Operation Iraqi Freedom or Operation Enduring Freedom on such members and former members and their families;

(C) an assessment of the full scope of the neurological, psychiatric, and psychological effects of traumatic brain injury on members and former members of the Armed Forces, including the effects of such effects on the family members of such members and former members, and an assessment of the efficacy of current treatment approaches for traumatic brain injury in the United States and the efficacy of screenings and treatment approaches for traumatic brain injury within the Department of Defense and the Department of Veterans Affairs;

(I) an assessment of the impacts of increasing numbers of older and married members of the Armed Forces on readjustment requirements.

**Data Files Required**

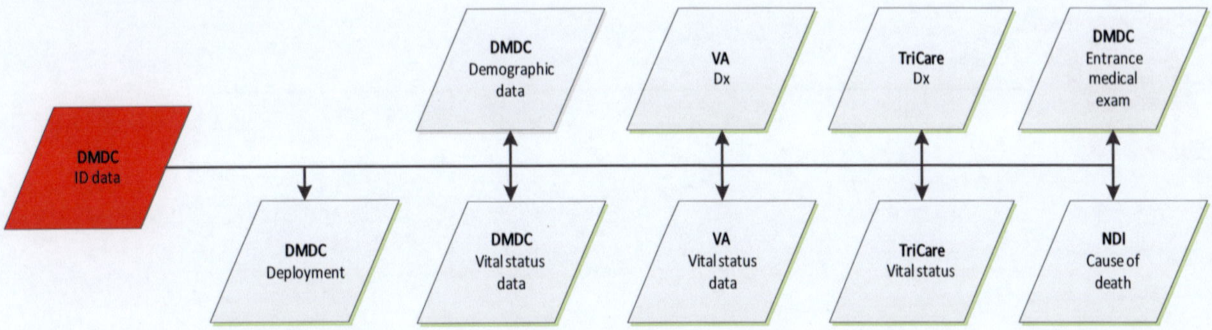


**Sample Questions to Be Answered by the Data**

- Is mortality higher on return from deployment than among the nondeployed?
- What are the effects of multiple deployments, length of deployment, and location of deployment?
- Does TBI or PTSD increase mortality? Is a person more likely to be in a motor-vehicle accident within 2 years after a TBI or PTSD diagnosis than a person who does not have a TBI or PTSD diagnosis?
- How do answers to the above questions vary by sex, ethnicity, marital status, age, service, rank, educational attainment, criminal record, home of record on service entry, aptitude, occupational category, or branch of service?
- Do people who have TBI or PTSD who are deployed have a higher risk of being killed or injured in action than others who are deployed? How many people who have TBI or PTSD complete their deployment?

## Data Group 3

**Relevant Sections of the Law**

(A) an assessment of the psychological, social, and economic impacts of such deployment on such members and former members and their families;

(B) an assessment of the particular impacts of multiple deployments in Operation Iraqi Freedom or Operation Enduring Freedom on such members and former members and their families;

(C) an assessment of the full scope of the neurological, psychiatric, and psychological effects of traumatic brain injury on members and former members of the Armed Forces, including the effects of such effects on the family members of such members and former members, and an assessment of the efficacy of current treatment approaches for traumatic brain injury in the United States and the efficacy of screenings and treatment approaches for traumatic brain injury within the Department of Defense and the Department of Veterans Affairs;

(E) an assessment of the gender- and ethnic group-specific needs and concerns of members of the Armed Forces and veterans.

**Data Files Required**

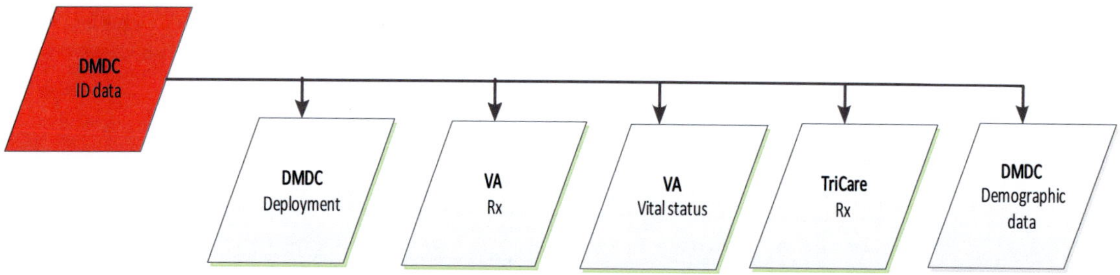


**Sample Questions to Be Answered by the Data**

- How many people are deployed or redeployed while on antidepressants, antianxiety agents, or narcotic pain medications?
- How does the answer to the above question vary by sex, ethnicity, marital status, age, service, rank, education attained, criminal record, home of record on service entry, aptitude, occupational category, or branch of service? For example, the outcomes, treatment, family, and economic groups wished to understand how the number of deployments affected positive screens and subsequent diagnoses with the conditions of interest (e.g., PTSD or TBI)?
- Are people who report antidepressant or antianxiety medication use before deployment at increased or decreased risk for TBI and PTSD?
- Are deployed people who are using antianxiety or antidepressant medication at higher or lower risk for injury or death than those not taking the drugs?
- When treatment was provided for one of the five conditions (as indicated by *ICD-9* code), what approach was used? That is, if pharmacologic, what medication? If behavioral, what method, by whom, and were sessions individual or group?

**Data Group 4**

**Relevant Sections of the Law**
(A) an assessment of the psychological, social, and economic impacts of such deployment on such members and former members and their families;

(B) an assessment of the particular impacts of multiple deployments in Operation Iraqi Freedom or Operation Enduring Freedom on such members and former members and their families;

(D) an assessment of the effects of undiagnosed injuries such as post-traumatic stress disorder and traumatic brain injury, an estimate of the long-term costs associated with such injuries, and an assessment of the efficacy of screenings and treatment approaches for post-traumatic stress disorder and other mental health conditions within the Department of Defense and Department of Veterans Affairs;

(E) an assessment of the gender- and ethnic group-specific needs and concerns of members of the Armed Forces and veterans.

**Data Files Required**

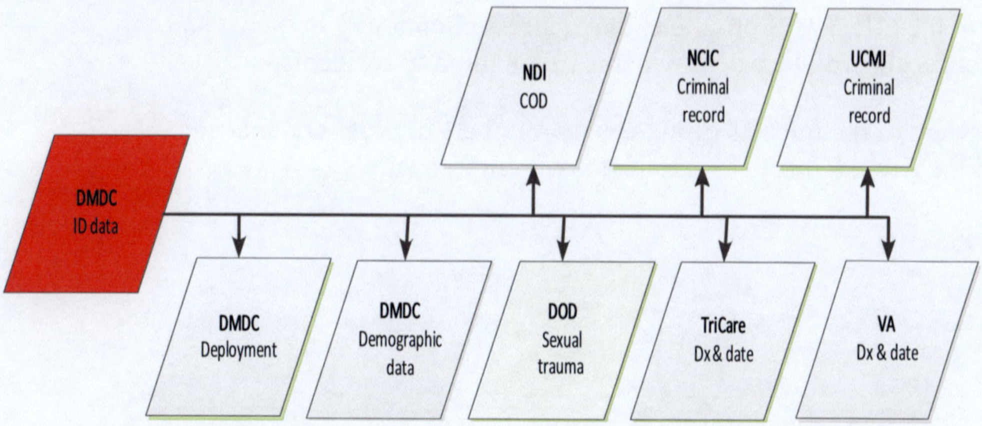


**Sample Questions to Be Answered by the Data**

- How many people report sexual trauma or harassment during deployment?
- What are long-term outcomes of sexual trauma (in men and women) during deployment?
- Does sexual trauma increase the risk of PTSD, TBI, or both?
- Does TBI or PTSD increase the risk of sexual trauma among women and men?
- Does TBI or PTSD diagnosis increase the risk of becoming a victim of domestic abuse or of committing domestic abuse?
- Do education, age, sex, race, ethnicity, service branch and component, residence of origin, number and length of deployments, and marital status increase the risk of domestic abuse in people diagnosed with TBI, PTSD, or both?

**Data Group 5**

**Relevant Sections of the Law**
(A) an assessment of the psychological, social, and economic impacts of such deployment on such members and former members and their families;

(B) an assessment of the particular impacts of multiple deployments in Operation Iraqi Freedom or Operation Enduring Freedom on such members and former members and their families;

(D) an assessment of the effects of undiagnosed injuries such as post-traumatic stress disorder and traumatic brain injury, an estimate of the long-term costs associated with such injuries, and an assessment of the efficacy of screenings and treatment approaches for post-traumatic stress disorder and other mental health conditions within the Department of Defense and Department of Veterans Affairs;

(H) an assessment of the impacts on communities with high populations of military families, including military housing communities and townships with deployed members of the National Guard and Reserve, of deployments associated with Operation Iraqi Freedom and Operation Enduring Freedom, and an assessment of the efficacy of programs that address community outreach and education concerning military deployments of community residents;

(I) an assessment of the impacts of increasing numbers of older and married members of the Armed Forces on readjustment requirements.

**Data Files Required**

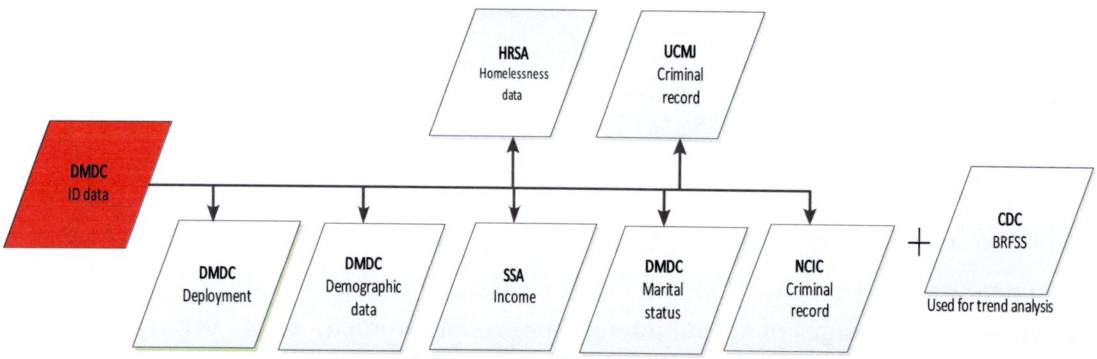


**Sample Questions to Be Answered by the Data**

- How is quality of life affected by PTSD or TBI? Professionally? Personally? Domestically?
- How many of those who have TBI or PTSD are unemployed? Incarcerated? Divorced?
- Does TBI or PTSD diagnosis affect income, employment, or vocational needs (such as the need to change profession)?
- Do such factors as education, age, sex, race, ethnicity, service branch and component, residence of origin, number and length of deployments and marital status increase the risk of homelessness in people who have TBI, PTSD, or both?
- What is the person's current functioning? What diagnoses are still being treated for? What is the current employment status? What is the current quality of life?
- What are the longitudinal effects of deployment to OEF and OIF on active-duty personnel and recent veterans with respect to earnings? Military earning? Employment? Homelessness? Arrest?

- How have changes in the benefits provided under the GI Bill affected educational attainment? How might they affect earnings (as a consequence of increased educational attainment)? How are the effects this moderated by deployment?
- What are the economic effects of deployment on spouses in particular and families in general?

## Data Group 6

**Relevant Section of the Law**

(C) an assessment of the full scope of the neurological, psychiatric, and psychological effects of traumatic brain injury on members and former members of the Armed Forces, including the effects of such effects on the family members of such members and former members, and an assessment of the efficacy of current treatment approaches for traumatic brain injury in the United States and the efficacy of screenings and treatment approaches for traumatic brain injury within the Department of Defense and the Department of Veterans Affairs.

**Data Files Required**

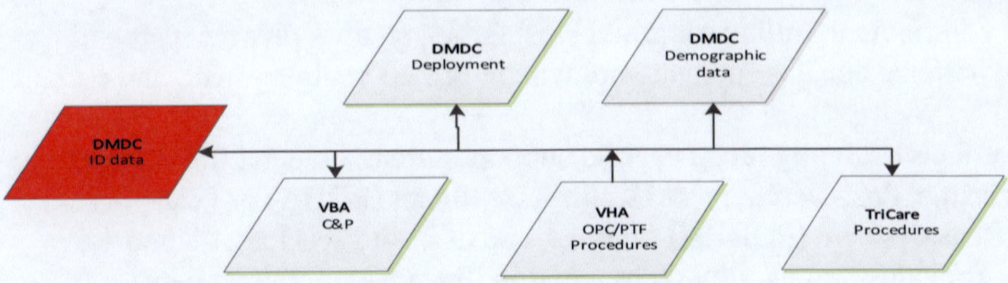


**Sample Questions to Be Answered by the Data**

- How many people who receive diagnoses of TBI, PTSD, or both receive military or VA disability compensation? How many receive vocational rehabilitation services?
- How frequently was imaging used to assist in diagnosis of TBI?

## Data Group 7

**Relevant Sections of the Law**

(A) an assessment of the psychological, social, and economic impacts of such deployment on such members and former members and their families;

(B) an assessment of the particular impacts of multiple deployments in Operation Iraqi Freedom or Operation Enduring Freedom on such members and former members and their families;

(F) an assessment of the particular needs and concerns of children of members of the Armed Forces, taking into account differing age groups, impacts on development and education, and the mental and emotional well-being of children.

**Data Files Required**

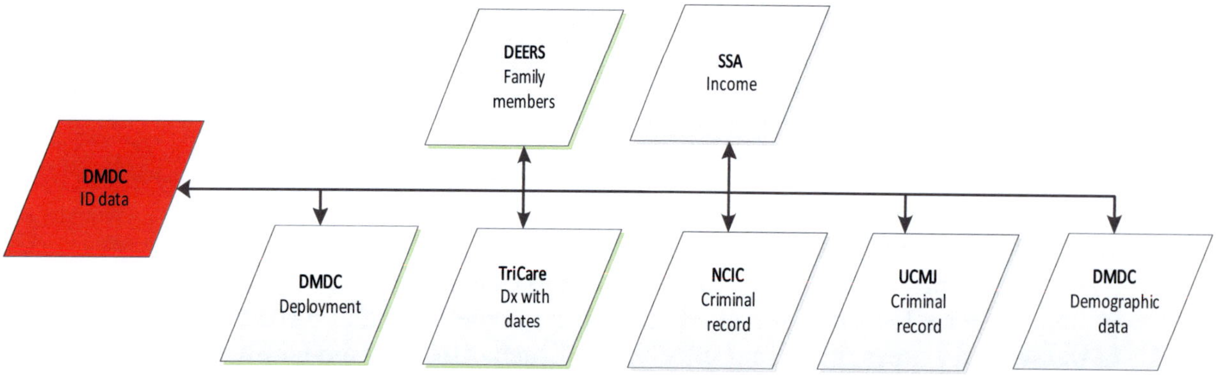


**Sample Questions to Be Answered by the Data**

- What are the implications for children's (and other family members') well-being and functioning of each of the following characteristics: deployment frequency and duration, dwell time, location, type of mission, parental injury or death and the aftermath, and perinatal stressors (such as low birth weight and maternal smoking and drinking)?
- What characteristics contribute to military families' instability, such as divorce, parental estrangement, young parental age, parental unemployment or underemployment, and parental educational level?
- What are the family effects of family income, child support, parental mental illness, parental drug abuse, parental crime, Post-Deployment Health Assessment (PDHA) or Post-Deployment Health Reassessment (PDHRA) findings, use of health services, diagnosed injury or illnesses, or previous trauma, illness, psychiatric diagnoses, and treatment?
- How should military families be defined—such as by using deployment data, demographic data, rank, grade, income, military occupational specialty, AFQT score, or education level?

Thus, the committee read the legislation, decided on questions that needed to be answered, and identified data sources. After reviewing the questions, which were organized by data groups, and examining potential data sources, the committee planned to link the data into a central database that was developed specifically for it. Figures 10.1 and 10.2 illustrate the committee's vision for data-gathering and data inputs. The committee expected to conduct analyses to answer its questions and to shed light on the issues posed by the legislation. Other groups undertaking such analyses will likely develop their own view of database development and data inputs.

The committee proposed to incorporate the details on all those (including active-duty, reserve, and National Guard personnel) deployed to OEF, OIF, and OND during 2001–2010 and to compare them with a matched cohort of personnel who were not deployed during that period. The database would include files provided by DOD, for example, by the DMDC (demographic data), TRICARE, the Defense Enrollment Eligibility Reporting System, the PDHA, and the PDHRA; by VA, specifically, by the Veterans Benefit Administration and Veterans Health Administration, such as Patient Treatment Files, Outpatient Clinic Visits, and Compensation and Pension; by the Centers for Disease Control and Prevention, such as the National Death Index and the Behavioral Risk Factor Surveillance System; by the Health Resources and Services Administration (data on homelessness); by the Department of Health and Human Services

(Medicare and Medicaid data); by the Social Security Administration; by the Internal Revenue Service; and by the Federal Bureau of Investigation (crime data) (see Appendix F for database descriptions).

Initially, the committee requested the DMDC demographic database on all service members (regular, reserve, and National Guard Components) who were deployed to OEF and OIF during the period September 11, 2001–December 31, 2010, and those who were not deployed during the same period. In addition, the committee requested the available PDHA and PDHRA data files on deployed personnel. The DMDC files constituted the sampling frame from which multiple cohorts would be selected—initially with deidentified files that contained no names and no Social Security numbers and then, after selection, with unique person identifiers that permitted linkage to records from the different DMDC databases.

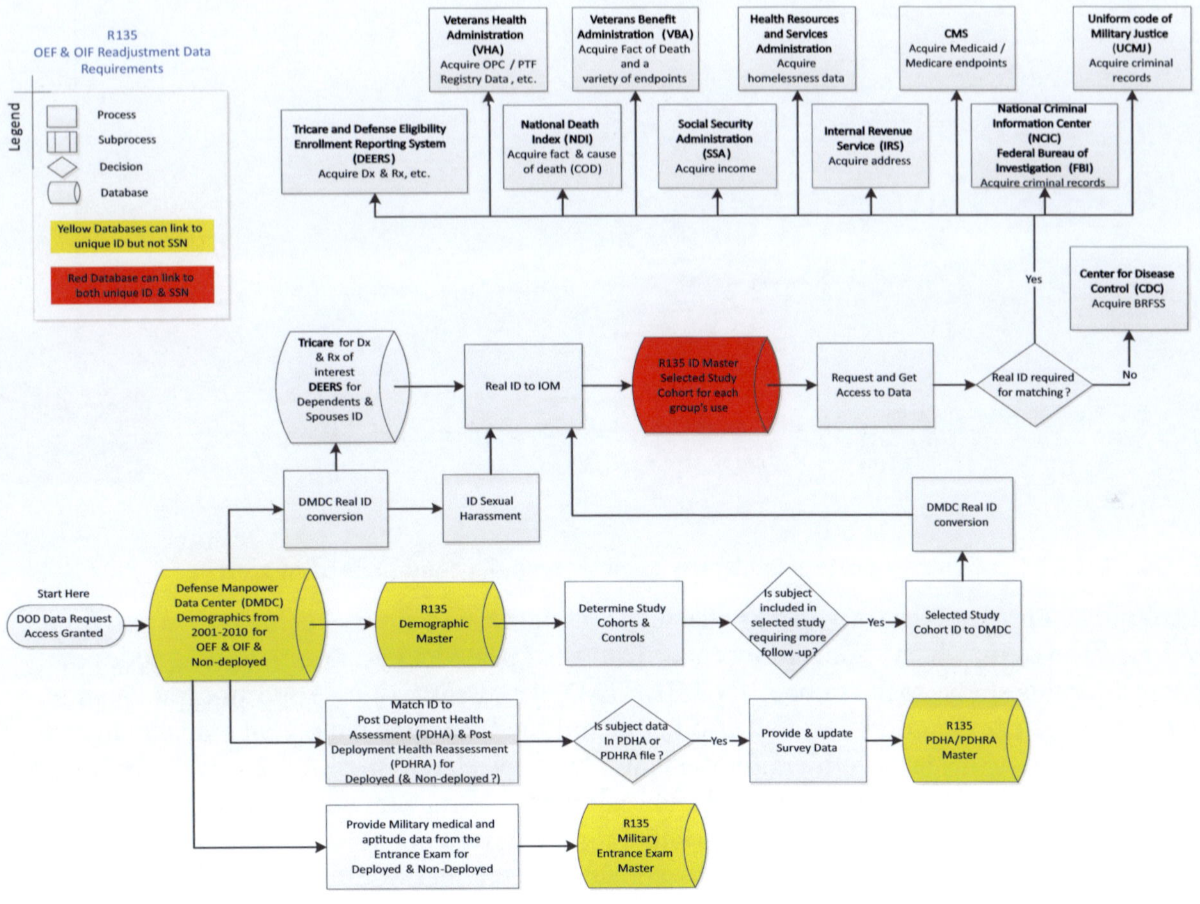


**FIGURE 10.1** Committee's database and data requirements.

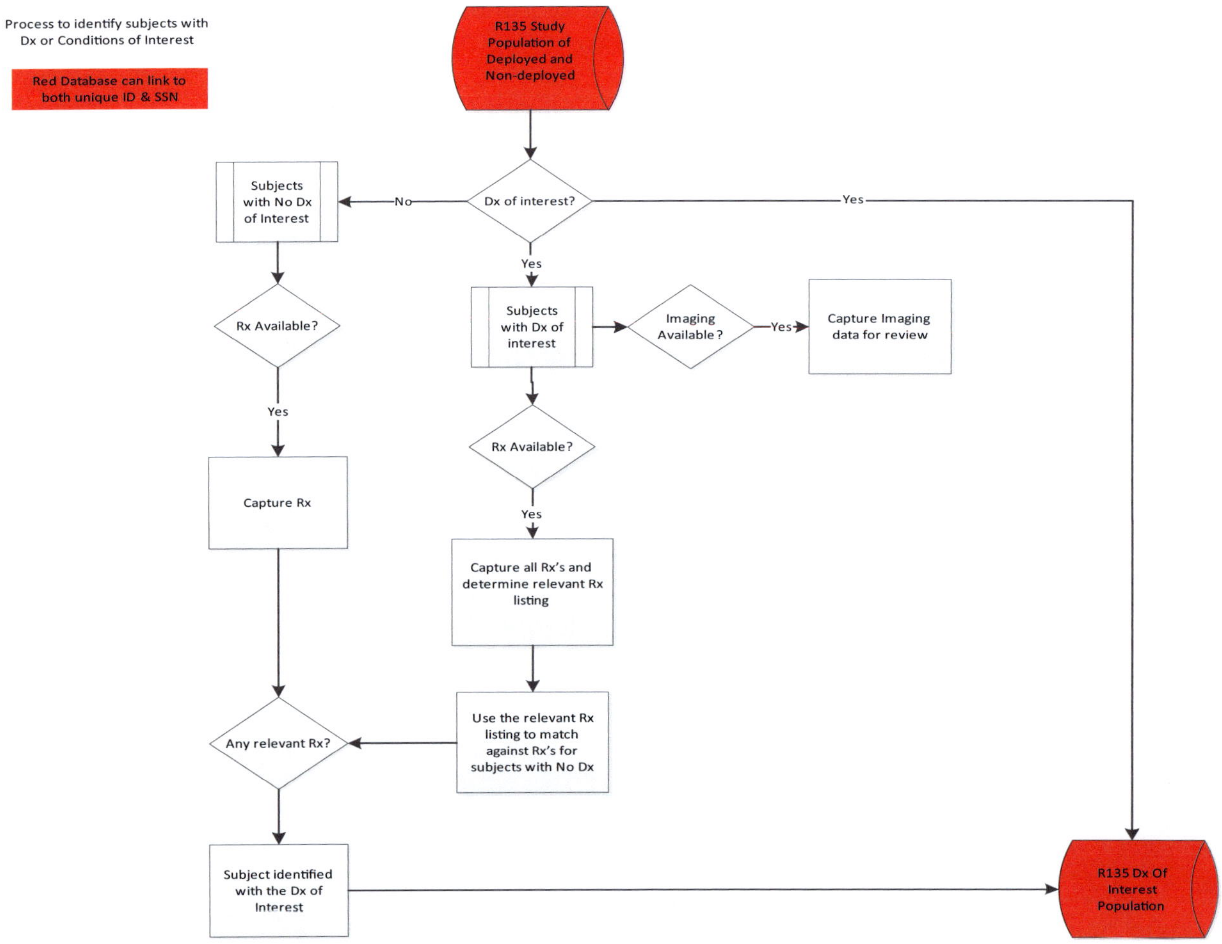


**FIGURE 10.2** Committee's process to identify subjects with the conditions of interest.

Through that process, data would be collected from the DOD military health system and from the VA health system, which would allow classification of personnel according to ICD codes of interest for this study (such as codes for TBI, PTSD, depression, suicide and suicidal ideation, and substance-use disorders), as well as other records and outcome data. That plan would have required access to actual identifiers for the individuals selected as part of the sample for further study. In effect, the ability to link the selected sampled cohorts with other databases and back to the DMDC database would have been essential for the development of the committee's analytic database. However, all committee analyses and later report data would have used only deidentified or aggregated information.

## SUMMARY

The US government collects numerous useful datasets. Understanding how to gain access, the requirements for receiving data, what information is in the databases, and the terminology used can be difficult, expensive, and time-consuming. Time became an issue for the committee, and it abandoned most of its data-collection efforts; the committee considers that an important missed opportunity. In the end, the committee relied primarily on the published literature to respond to the legislation; however, with respect to many issues of concern, there was a paucity of published data. Limited analyses, that is, descriptive analyses of those deployed to OEF and OIF were completed.

## RECOMMENDATIONS

There has been little quantitative characterization of the issues described in the legislation, but the committee identified a wide array of data and databases available in DOD, VA, and other federal agencies that could be used to address many of the questions posed by the legislation that motivated its work. On the basis of available data, the committee developed a comprehensive data-analysis plan. The committee notes that in addition to its recommendation for comprehensive data analyses, privacy experts will need to be involved with data owners before data are linked and made accessible to researchers. The committee believes that privacy and confidentiality are essential alongside issues of coordination and synchronization of data sources.

**The committee recommends that the Department of Defense and the Department of Veterans Affairs support comprehensive analyses of relevant data that reside in the two departments and other agencies of the federal government. Their databases should be linked and integrated so that they can be used effectively to address questions regarding readjustment that are not answered in the peer-reviewed literature.**

The committee's preliminary work in this area has provided a clear rationale, justification, and roadmap for comprehensive data analyses. Comprehensive data analyses will require establishment of systematic, timely processes for using available government data and linking them in such a way as to improve the characterization of issues of interest. No databases or files fully integrate basic deployment and demographic data with data on health outcomes, treatment or transition-of-care files, data on access to care, records of employment before and after deployment, and data on other processes and outcomes. A comprehensive analytic database will have to be created and maintained.

**The committee recommends that the secretary of defense and the secretary of veterans affairs establish an interagency work group to identify and examine the feasibility of linking data that exist in Executive Branch departments and agencies throughout the federal government. The work group should be tasked to explore issues related to coordination among agencies, for example, defining common goals, establishing common policies and procedures, creating mechanisms for data-sharing, establishing records systems, and overcoming legal impediments and meeting legal requirements. The work group should provide the secretaries with options and recommendations for establishment of a sustainable program for long-term cooperation and data-sharing to improve understanding of the outcomes of military service and readjustment after combat deployment.**

The committee believes that many of the issues examined in this study can be addressed through analyses of data already maintained by numerous federal agencies. The committee tried to gain access to the data files so that it could begin such analyses, but it faced numerous obstacles in its attempts to access them. In light of those difficulties, the committee recommends the following actions to address many of the problems that it faced.

**The committee recommends that clear procedures be developed for accessing data held by the Department of Defense, the Department of Veterans Affairs, and other federal agencies. The procedures should appear on each agency's website with access to its data dictionaries. That would enable researchers and others wishing to access data to understand all the requirements before they begin their data-gathering efforts and would provide information about the types of data that are available and how to access them.**

The questions posed to the committee are complex and critical to the well-being of US veterans, their families, and the communities in which they live. A major finding of the committee is that there is no way to provide data-based answers to those questions. All agencies that collect, store, and manage information relevant to veterans and their families should give high priority to coordination of those efforts throughout the federal statistical system so that informed decisions about veterans' readjustment needs can be made in the near future.

The committee believes that such coordination will greatly enhance the ability of researchers and the government to link data held by multiple agencies to allow the types of analyses recommended above.

# 11

# RECOMMENDATIONS

The committee was tasked with examining a wide array of issues as presented in PL 110-181, Section 1661, including the effects of deployment on physical and mental health; community, family, and economic issues; treatment for physical-health and mental-health problems; and issues related to access and barriers to care of active-duty personnel and veterans who were deployed to Operation Enduring Freedom (OEF) and Operation Iraqi Freedom (OIF). The committee examined those issues and conducted its study amid an evolving landscape. The wars in Iraq and Afghanistan have continued throughout the committee's deliberations. New research that will probably shed light on issues that the committee is addressing has been published. What might have been important 2 or 3 years ago might now be overshadowed by new information and concerns, such as the current wave of suicides in the military. Different priorities for readjustment concerns and needs are emerging. Thus, the committee's conclusions and recommendations have been formed against a backdrop of constantly changing conditions.

## KEY FINDINGS

The readjustment needs of service members, veterans, and families that have experienced deployment to OEF or OIF encompass a complex set of health, economic, and social issues. Below are the committee's key findings, which to a large extent are the focus of its recommendations.

- Many veterans return from deployment relatively unscathed by their experience, but others return from deployment with a multitude of complex health outcomes that present life-long challenges and hinder readjustment.
- Not all veterans who need treatment receive it despite the offering of evidence-based treatments by the Department of Veterans Affairs (VA) and the Department of Defense (DOD) health systems, because systemwide challenges exist.
- Military families often endure the adverse consequences of deployments, for example, health effects, family violence, and economic burdens.
- Numerous programs exist to respond to the needs of returning OEF and OIF active-duty personnel, veterans, and family members, but there is little evidence regarding their effectiveness.
- Unemployment and underemployment are acute problems for military veterans.
- Published data on the effects of deployment on military communities are sparse.

- DOD, VA, and other federal agencies have data that can answer many of the questions posed in the legislation; however, numerous barriers must be overcome to facilitate sharing and linking of data.

The federal government, in particular DOD and VA, is actively seeking to understand the scope of readjustment challenges, implement appropriate policies, and provide programs and services. In many cases, however, the response does not match the magnitude of the problems, and many readjustment needs are unmet or unknown. The urgency of addressing those issues is heightened by the sheer number of people affected, the rapid drawdown of personnel from Afghanistan and Iraq, and the long-term effects that many of the issues might have not only on military personnel and veterans and their families but on the country as a whole. Previous wars have demonstrated that veterans' needs peak several decades after the war in which they served, and that highlights the need for managing current problems and planning future resources.

The legislation that directed the study advised that it be conducted in two phases. In the Phase 1 report, published in March 2010, the committee raised an issue that remains important: research conducted on OEF and OIF military and veterans has many limitations that might hinder informed policy making and resource planning. The committee found that those limitations remain. They include the following:

- Reliance on samples of convenience, which limits the external validity (generalizability) of research.
- Reliance on brief screening instruments to identify key outcomes and to estimate prevalence, which limits the internal validity of research.
- Use of cross-sectional designs, which limits the ability to support causal inference and to elucidate the course of disorders.
- Assessment of narrow sets of risk and protective factors, which results in underspecified models that have a high risk of bias.
- Conduct of many studies by the VA or the DOD, rather than by independent third parties, which raises important questions about the accuracy of respondents' self-reports, particularly with regard to sensitive issues.

All those limitations are understandable, given the fiscal and practical challenges involved in conducting long-term outcome studies (for example, longitudinal epidemiologic studies are expensive and difficult to implement). However, the committee emphasizes again that future research should adhere to the criteria described in the Phase 1 report, as expressed in this Phase 1 recommendation:

**The committee recommends that the Department of Defense, the Department of Veterans Affairs, and other federal agencies fund research on readjustment needs of returning OEF and OIF veterans, their families, and their communities that explicitly addresses methodologic and substantive gaps in completed and ongoing research. For example, the support of large-scale, independent studies with longitudinal designs, probability sampling, comprehensive clinical assessment of key outcomes, and more fully specified models that include objective biologic measures should be considered.**

To inform its work during the second phase of its study, the committee read the literature, collected data and attempted data analyses, oversaw ethnographic research, and tabulated current research in the OEF and OIF populations. The remainder of this chapter summarizes the committee's Phase 2 recommendations.

## OUTCOMES

The literature on the outcomes of military deployment has grown dramatically over the last two decades. Although discrepant findings do emerge, there is a clear consensus in the literature that the stressors of deployment, from exposure to combat to multiple deployments away from home and family, can lead to a number of adverse conditions. The committee concentrated on deployment-related outcomes—such as traumatic brain injury (TBI), posttraumatic stress disorder (PTSD), depression, substance use, and suicidal ideation—but the list could be expanded to many additional psychiatric conditions and a host of physical conditions. The data on short-term outcomes (outcomes in 6 months or less) is extensive, but data on long-term outcomes (over years) less extensive and both can be challenged on methodologic grounds. To capture the true long-term outcomes of deployment to war zones and plan services to address them, more data will be essential.

**The committee recommends that the Department of Defense and the Department of Veterans Affairs sponsor longitudinal studies to answer many of the questions regarding long-term effects of traumatic brain injury, posttraumatic stress disorder, and other mental-health disorders. Such studies should strive to improve the validity of exposure measurements, identification and use of biomarkers, and recruitment and retention of subjects. Attention should be paid to whether the outcomes of traumatic brain injuries depend on the severity and number of such injuries, on the presence of comorbid conditions, and on sex and ethnicity.**

Current studies might be the most appropriate platform for developing a strategy for long-term followup, such as the Millennium Cohort Study and the Longitudinal Health Study of Gulf War Era Veterans. Those studies can be augmented with supplementary samples of OEF, OIF, and Operation New Dawn (OND) veterans. Other factors that should define such studies include the ability to collect biologic specimens, oversampling of OEF, OIF, and OND female and minority-group populations, and planning for add-on studies to address new needs as they are identified.

Many health consequences of service in OEF, OIF, and OND are related to the inherently dangerous nature of the wartime environment or resulting trauma. However, one major exposure, military sexual trauma (MST), is unrelated to war but rather is due to noncombat violent assault. Studies show that MST has been occurring at high rates in the US military, including during OEF, OIF, and OND. Research demonstrates that MST is associated with poor readjustment and adverse mental-health and physical outcomes. The burden of physical and mental-health consequences for the victims and their family members is high. Increased efforts by DOD are necessary, and a zero-tolerance approach should be implemented.

**The committee recommends that the Department of Defense develop policies to eliminate military sexual trauma as research demonstrates that it is associated with poor readjustment and mental-health and physical-health outcomes. The committee further recommends that the department reinforce existing policies on**

**military sexual trauma by adding specific mandatory evaluation criteria regarding how well military leaders address the issue, for example, in the formal performance-appraisal and promotion systems.**

The breadth and depth of the challenges faced by military service members and veterans who served in Iraq and Afghanistan result from the complex interaction of issues that must be addressed by primary prevention, diagnostics, treatment, rehabilitation, education and outreach, and community support programs if readjustment after combat service is to be successful.

## TREATMENT

Screening, assessment, and treatment approaches for brain injuries and psychologic health problems are not always implemented between and within DOD and VA in a consistent manner or aligned with the evidence base. DOD and VA use different thresholds for some of the same mental-health screening and assessment instruments, such as the Primary-Care PTSD screen and the PTSD Checklist for PTSD and the Patient Health Questionnaire for depression. Parts of VA and DOD clinical guidance lack recommendations for a specific assessment instrument and leave the selection of instrument to the clinician, for example, for suicide-risk assessments and TBI neurocognitive assessments.

The committee identified topics on which VA and DOD policies are out of step with the evidence base. There is a lack of clear scientific evidence supporting the effectiveness of the neurocognitive assessment tool (Automated Neuropsychological Assessment Metrics) used by DOD to assess cognitive function after a head injury. With respect to suicide prevention, DOD policy prohibits restricting access to privately owned weapons for those who might be at risk for of suicide, but research shows that restricting access to lethal means prevents suicides. VA has included Acceptance and Commitment Therapy for depression in its national rollout of evidence based treatments, however, there is not sufficient evidence to support its use as a first-line intervention. Moreover, the limited data that are available suggest that patients in need of evidence-based care might not be receiving it. The committee has serious concerns about inadequate and untimely clinical followup and low rates of delivery of evidence-based treatments, particularly psychotherapies to treat PTSD and depression and approved pharmacotherapies for substance use disorder.

**The committee recommends that the Department of Defense and the Department of Veterans Affairs select instruments and their thresholds for mental health screening and assessment in a standardized way on the basis of the best available evidence. The committee also recommends that the two departments ensure that treatment offerings are aligned with the evidence base, particularly before national rollouts, and that all patients consistently receive first-line treatments as indicated.**

Unwarranted variability in clinical practices and deviations from the evidence base presents threats to high-quality patient care. Such variability also hampers opportunities to make research comparisons that can inform and improve the effectiveness of screening, assessment, and treatment practices. The committee notes that the emphasis on promoting evidence-based practices should not discourage the use of new or experimental interventions where there is reason to believe that they might lead to better outcomes than standard interventions.

In many ways, DOD and VA clinicians are at the forefront of providing evidence-based care for service members and veterans who have brain injuries and psychologic-health problems. But there are opportunities to improve processes of training and evaluating clinicians. DOD does not have a standardized process for assessing clinicians' competence to administer the Military Acute Concussion Evaluation for TBI. VA is implementing a robust clinician-training program to disseminate evidence-based psychotherapies, but the program appears to lack periodic clinician assessments beyond the 6-month training period to ensure that continued treatment fidelity is maintained. Current approaches for training clinicians on the management of comorbid conditions (by disseminating clinician resources, for example) are not adequate.

**The committee recommends that the Department of Defense and the Department of Veterans Affairs incorporate continuing supervision and education into programs that train clinicians in the use of selected assessment instruments and evidence-based treatments. Once clinicians are trained, the two departments should systematically and periodically evaluate them to assess the degree to which therapeutic interventions are accurately implemented according to a manual, protocol, or model as supported by evidence. The committee also recommends that the two departments place greater focus on coordinated, interdisciplinary care to ensure optimal treatment for service members and veterans.**

The committee determined that there are few data on whether screening, assessment, and treatment interventions in DOD and VA are being implemented according to clinical guidelines and VA and DOD policy. Minimal data is readily available on the numbers of people who have been screened and the extent to which followup is appropriate and timely for those who screen positive. There is a dearth of data on which treatments patients receive and whether the treatments were appropriate, timely, and delivered at the recommended intensity level (for example, individual vs group format and frequency and duration of sessions).

**The committee recommends that the Department of Defense and the Department of Veterans Affairs conduct systematic assessments to determine whether screening and treatment interventions are being implemented according to clinical guidelines and department policy. Data systems should be developed to assess treatment outcomes, variations among treatment facilities, and barriers to the use of evidence-based treatment.**

## MILITARY FAMILIES

The committee found that DOD has many programs and policies to support families. However, DOD policies, programs, and practices typically do not take into consideration the full spectrum of military families. By focusing almost exclusively on traditional families (married heterosexual spouses and their children), DOD is missing critical opportunities to support the readjustment needs of many service members' nontraditional families. To be able to support all families, DOD will need data on the full constellation of service members' family.

**The committee recommends that the Department of Defense ensure that policies, programs, and practices aim to support and strengthen all military families, including nontraditional ones.**

Healthy families help service members to do their jobs effectively and readjust after deployment. The demands placed on military family members call for support in the areas of relationship-building, family and individual function, and reduction of risk of psychologic and physical-health problems. The committee found that little information is available on the potential effectiveness of broad-based, universal prevention efforts aimed at military children and their families. In addition, most treatment interventions for family members have been developed and tested in civilian communities and lack evidence of their effectiveness for military families. The committee concludes that military families would benefit from increased efforts to identify, develop, and test new prevention and treatment interventions targeted toward military families, including interventions directed at children and adolescents.

**The committee recommends that the Department of Defense use evidence-based primary prevention programs and treatments that have been specifically evaluated in service members and their families and that are focused on preventing and treating mental-health and relationship problems.**

The committee concludes that there are substantial gaps in knowledge about the effects of deployment on military families that hinder DOD's ability to meet the needs of military service members and their families effectively. The committee found that—although some important large-scale, well-designed studies are under way—much of the research heretofore has been methodologically flawed, suffering, for example, from the use of small convenience samples, use of cross-sectional designs, and the like. The committee concludes that well-designed studies that use rigorous and diverse methods (both qualitative and quantitative) are needed to increase understanding of the challenges faced by military service members and their families.

**The committee recommends that the Department of Defense and other relevant federal agencies fund methodologically rigorous research on the social, psychologic, and economic effects of deployments on families, including nontraditional families.**

Studies of families of service members deployed to OEF and OIF have documented a rise in domestic violence (typically including abuse of spouses or neglect of children). In the FY 2000 National Defense Authorization Act (PL 106-65, Section 591), Congress directed the secretary of defense to establish a Defense Task Force on Domestic Violence to make recommendations for reducing the prevalence of domestic violence in military families. The task force submitted a report in 2003 report that identified multiple shortcomings in the current systems and recommended many improvements. The Government Accountability Office, in 2006 and 2010, issued reports concerning progress in implementing the nearly 200 recommendations made by the task force. Both reports described progress on some recommendations but little on others, including a recommendation for reliable documentation of violent events.

**The committee recommends that the Department of Defense place high priority on reducing domestic violence because it degrades force readiness and the well-being of military family members.**

## COMMUNITY

There has been too little research on community effects of deployments to OEF and OIF. To supplement the published research, the committee completed ethnographic assessments in six communities that are near large military installations or that have recently deployed National Guard populations. Those efforts provided some insight, but the lack of community-wide assessments of the effects of OEF and OIF deployments on communities made it difficult to respond to this aspect of the committee's charge.

**The committee recommends that the Department of Defense, the Department of Veterans Affairs, and other relevant federal agencies fund research on the effects of Operation Enduring Freedom and Operation Iraqi Freedom deployments on communities. Such research should include current indicators of community well-being, such as measures of economic performance, availability of social and support services, law-enforcement activity, and school and educational functioning.**

Relevant data are available, but data linkages are needed to allow specific analyses that can more clearly illuminate opportunities to mitigate potential adverse community consequences after service members deploy, return, and separate.

## SOCIOECONOMIC IMPACTS

Problems of unemployment and underemployment, which are broadly felt by the US civilian population today, appear to be more acute for veterans of the post-9/11 era, particularly young veterans. In 2011, the unemployment rate among all post-9/11 veterans 18 years old and older was more than one-third higher than that among equivalent nonveterans—12.1% compared with 8.7%. Among veterans 18–24 years old, the rate was almost twice as high—30.2% compared with 16.1%. The sources of those disparities remain unclear and could include skills mismatch, impeded ability to maintain or obtain employment because of physical or mental-health trauma, stigma or discrimination, or some combination of those factors or other elements. Successful readjustment depends on reentry into the civilian workforce, and the available evidence suggests that this is an important gap for policy to address. The committee found that the literature assessing the effectiveness of DOD's and VA's transition-assistance programs is relatively thin, even though reentry into the labor force is one of the most important readjustment challenges. One study suggests that recent expansions of hiring tax credits might have been effective in raising rates of employment of older veterans who have disabilities. But OEF, OIF, and OND veterans did not appear to benefit from the expansions.

**The committee recommends that the Department of Defense and the Department of Veterans Affairs evaluate the effectiveness of transition-assistance programs to ensure that they are effective in reducing unemployment among returning**

**veterans of Operation Enduring Freedom, Operation Iraqi Freedom, and Operation New Dawn.**

Evaluation of the effectiveness of transition-assistance programs, with research that examines employment patterns after separation from the military over time, will provide data to ensure that scarce resources can be allocated to effective programs. Further study might focus on whether employment tax credits are a cost-effective means of expanding employment for Operation Enduring Freedom and Operation Iraqi Freedom veterans and whether programs to counsel and prepare service members for long-term postservice careers are effectively implemented.

The Post-9/11 GI Bill is one of the largest expansions of educational subsidies to veterans and their families on record, but its effectiveness is difficult to gauge. The committee is aware of no studies that have explicitly evaluated the effects of deployment to OEF and OIF on the use of the Post-9/11 GI Bill or the effects of the Post-9/11 GI Bill.

**The committee recommends a comprehensive evaluation of the effects of the Post-9/11 GI Bill on the educational attainment of veterans and eligible family members.**

The committee views the current evidence on the costs of caring for injured veterans as an overwhelming challenge. There is a need to assess the costs of caring for injured veterans systematically and publicly. The Congressional Budget Office publicly assesses short-term and medium-term costs, and, as the VA stated in response to the committee's Phase 1 report, it already produces some forecasts of health and disability spending. But the committee continues to believe that long-term planning for veterans' care requires public long-term cost forecasts in the same way that Social Security and Medicare require them, and these forecasts should take a similar form to be internally and externally useful.

**The committee reiterates its call for comprehensive long-term forecasts of the costs of the Veterans Health Administration's medical care and the Veterans Benefits Administration's disability benefits associated with combat deployments; these forecasts should be conducted annually and should be released publicly by the Department of Veterans Affairs and confirmed by an independent external authority.**

## ACCESS AND BARRIERS TO CARE

Transitioning from the DOD health care system to the VA health care system presents challenges for OEF and OIF service men and women. There are numerous difficulties in navigating services because of the complexities of both systems. Although DOD and VA are making administrative changes to alleviate some of the problems, information sharing between the two agencies remains a problem.

**The committee recommends improved coordination of care and services between the Department of Defense and the Department of Veterans Affairs medical treatment facilities, including the completion of an interoperable or single**

**combined electronic health record for all care that begins with entry into military service and continues throughout care in the Department of Veterans Affairs system after transition.**

Stigma is still a problem for military personnel in care or seeking care for mental-health or substance-abuse problems. Active-duty military fear that visits to a mental-health provider will jeopardize their careers because of the military's long-standing policy of reporting mental-health and substance-abuse problems to the chain of command. Mixed messages about seeking treatment and concerns about health-information privacy remain disincentives to seeking care.

**The committee recommends that the Department of Defense continue to promote an environment that reduces stigma and encourages treatment for mental-health and substance-use disorders. The committee recommends that the department undertake a systematic review of its policies regarding mental-health and substance-abuse treatment with regard to issues of confidentiality and the relation between treatment-seeking and military advancement. The committee recommends that the department regularly issue reports describing actions taken with regard to its policies and procedures to determine progress in this area.**

Excessive wait time is a complaint often expressed by both active-duty and veteran service members. Long wait times can compromise health because of delayed use and decreased patient satisfaction. In addition, adverse long-term outcomes, such as death and preventable hospitalizations, are more common for veterans who seek care at facilities that have longer wait times than for veterans at facilities that have shorter wait times.

Poor availability and misdistribution of mental-health specialists in many parts of the United States, especially in rural areas, present substantial barriers to OEF and OIF veterans access to mental-health care. For active-duty service members, inadequate participating provider networks present a challenge for accessing mental-health care.

**The committee recommends that the Department of Defense and the Department of Veterans Affairs conduct a needs assessment to determine the numbers and types of providers needed to address the long-term health needs of Operation Enduring Freedom, Operation Iraqi Freedom, and Operation New Dawn active-duty service members and veterans. The Department of Defense and the Department of Veterans Affairs should determine the optimal team composition—for example, MDs, PhDs, RNs, master's-trained professionals, and peer counselors—needed to ensure that providers function efficiently and perform at the upper level of their credentials and privileges.**

There is evidence of cultural insensitivity to nonwhite service members, who might have different or more severe physical-health and mental-health problems from their white counterparts. For example, black personnel are less likely than white personnel to use mental-health services and quicker to drop out of treatment. Issues related to types of diagnoses and potential misdiagnoses have also been raised. Whether clinicians who have ethnic characteristics similar to those of their patients would alleviate those problems is unknown.

**The committee recommends that the Department of Defense, the Department of Veterans Affairs, and other federal agencies fund research to determine whether culturally sensitive clinicians and treatment approaches improve retention in care and improve clinical outcomes.**

Women now constitute 14% of deployed forces in the US military, and an unprecedented number of female soldiers are deployed to combat areas. Although all service members are exposed to high levels of workplace stress, women in the military face some unique stressors, such as MST, which may affect their mental health and emotional well-being. Female veterans report a higher burden of medical illness and worse quality-of-life outcomes than do men who are exposed to the same levels of trauma. MST appears to be an important risk factor for the development of PTSD.

**The committee recommends that the Department of Defense and the Department of Veterans Affairs consider ways to remove barriers and improve women's access to and use of healthcare in their systems. The two departments should examine issues related to women's circumstances and stressors—such as military workplace stress, sexual harassment and assault, posttraumatic stress disorder, and premilitary trauma—in an effort to reduce disparities and to provide health care that is sensitive to their needs and preferences.**

## PROPOSED DATA ANALYSES

There has been little quantitative characterization of the issues described in the legislation, but the committee identified a wide array of data and databases available in DOD, VA, and other federal agencies that could be used to address many of the questions posed by the legislation that motivated its work. On the basis of available data, the committee developed a comprehensive data-analysis plan. The committee notes that in addition to its recommendation for comprehensive data analyses, privacy experts will need to be involved with data owners before data are linked and made accessible to researchers. The committee believes that privacy and confidentiality are essential alongside issues of coordination and synchronization of data sources.

**The committee recommends that the Department of Defense and the Department of Veterans Affairs support comprehensive analyses of relevant data that reside in the two departments and other agencies of the federal government. Their databases should be linked and integrated so that they can be used effectively to address questions regarding readjustment that are not answered in the peer-reviewed literature.**

The committee's preliminary work in this area has provided a clear rationale, justification, and roadmap for comprehensive data analyses. Comprehensive data analyses will require establishment of systematic, timely processes for using available government data and linking them in such a way as to improve the characterization of issues of interest. No databases or files fully integrate basic deployment and demographic data with data on health outcomes, treatment or transition-of-care files, data on access to care, records of employment before and after deployment, and data on other processes and outcomes. A comprehensive analytic database will have to be created and maintained.

**The committee recommends that the secretary of defense and the secretary of veterans affairs establish an interagency work group to identify and examine the feasibility of linking data that exist in Executive Branch departments and agencies throughout the federal government. The work group should be tasked to explore issues related to coordination among agencies, for example, defining common goals, establishing common policies and procedures, creating mechanisms for data-sharing, establishing records systems, and overcoming legal impediments and meeting legal requirements. The work group should provide the secretaries with options and recommendations for establishment of a sustainable program for long-term cooperation and data-sharing to improve understanding of the outcomes of military service and readjustment after combat deployment.**

The committee believes that many of the issues examined in this study can be addressed through analyses of data already maintained by numerous federal agencies. The committee tried to gain access to the data files so that it could begin such analyses, but it faced numerous obstacles in its attempts to access them. In light of those difficulties, the committee recommends the following actions to address many of the problems that it faced.

**The committee recommends that clear procedures be developed for accessing data held by the Department of Defense, the Department of Veterans Affairs, and other federal agencies. The procedures should appear on each agency's website with access to its data dictionaries. That would enable researchers and others wishing to access data to understand all the requirements before they begin their data-gathering efforts and would provide information about the types of data that are available and how to access them.**

The questions posed to the committee are complex and critical to the well-being of US veterans, their families, and the communities in which they live. A major finding of the committee is that there is no way to provide data-based answers to those questions. All agencies that collect, store, and manage information relevant to veterans and their families should give high priority to coordination of those efforts throughout the federal statistical system so that informed decisions about veterans' readjustment needs can be made in the near future.

The committee believes that such coordination will greatly enhance the ability of researchers and the government to link data held by multiple agencies to allow the types of analyses recommended above.

# A

# LEGISLATION FRAMING THE COMMITTEE'S TASK

PUBLIC LAW 110–181—JAN. 28, 2008 122 STAT. 477

**Subtitle E—Studies and Reports**

**SEC. 1661. STUDY ON PHYSICAL AND MENTAL HEALTH AND OTHER READJUSTMENT NEEDS OF MEMBERS AND FORMER MEMBERS OF THE ARMED FORCES WHO DEPLOYED IN OPERATION IRAQI FREEDOM AND OPERATION ENDURING FREEDOM AND THEIR FAMILIES.**

(a) STUDY REQUIRED.—The Secretary of Defense shall, in consultation with the Secretary of Veterans Affairs, enter into an agreement with the National Academy of Sciences for a study on the physical and mental health and other readjustment needs of members and former members of the Armed Forces who deployed in Operation Iraqi Freedom or Operation Enduring Freedom and their families as a result of such deployment.

(b) PHASES.—The study required under subsection (a) shall consist of two phases:

(1) A preliminary phase, to be completed not later than one year after the date of the enactment of this Act—

(A) to identify preliminary findings on the physical and mental health and other readjustment needs described in subsection (a) and on gaps in care for the members, former members, and families described in that subsection; and (B) to determine the parameters of the second phase of the study under paragraph (2).

(2) A second phase, to be completed not later than three years after the date of the enactment of this Act, to carry out a comprehensive assessment, in accordance with the parameters identified under the preliminary report required by paragraph (1), of the physical and mental health and other readjustment needs of members and former members of the Armed Forces who deployed in Operation Iraqi Freedom or Operation Enduring Freedom and their families as a result of such deployment, including, at a minimum—

(A) an assessment of the psychological, social, and economic impacts of such deployment on such members and former members and their families;

(B) an assessment of the particular impacts of multiple deployments in Operation Iraqi Freedom or Operation Enduring Freedom on such members and former members and their families;

(C) an assessment of the full scope of the neurological, psychiatric, and psychological effects of traumatic brain injury on members and former members of the Armed Forces, including the effects of such effects on the family members of such members and former members, and an assessment of the efficacy of current treatment approaches for traumatic brain injury in the

United States and the efficacy of screenings and treatment approaches for traumatic brain injury within the Department of Defense and the Department of Veterans Affairs;

(D) an assessment of the effects of undiagnosed injuries such as post-traumatic stress disorder and traumatic brain injury, an estimate of the long-term costs associated with such injuries, and an assessment of the efficacy of screenings and treatment approaches for post-traumatic stress disorder and other mental health conditions within the Department of Defense and Department of Veterans Affairs;

(E) an assessment of the gender- and ethnic group specific needs and concerns of members of the Armed Forces and veterans;

(F) an assessment of the particular needs and concerns of children of members of the Armed Forces, taking into account differing age groups, impacts on development and education, and the mental and emotional well being of children;

(G) an assessment of the particular educational and vocational needs of such members and former members and their families, and an assessment of the efficacy of existing educational and vocational programs to address such needs;

(H) an assessment of the impacts on communities with high populations of military families, including military housing communities and townships with deployed members of the National Guard and Reserve, of deployments associated with Operation Iraqi Freedom and Operation Enduring Freedom, and an assessment of the efficacy of programs that address community outreach and education concerning military deployments of community residents;

(I) an assessment of the impacts of increasing numbers of older and married members of the Armed Forces on readjustment requirements;

(J) the development, based on such assessments, of recommendations for programs, treatments, or policy remedies targeted at preventing, minimizing, or addressing the impacts, gaps, and needs identified; and

(K) the development, based on such assessments, of recommendations for additional research on such needs.

(c) POPULATIONS TO BE STUDIED.—The study required under subsection (a) shall consider the readjustment needs of each population of individuals as follows:

(1) Members of the regular components of the Armed Forces who are returning, or have returned, to the United States from deployment in Operation Iraqi Freedom or Operation Enduring Freedom.

(2) Members of the National Guard and Reserve who are returning, or have returned, to the United States from deployment in Operation Iraqi Freedom or Operation Enduring Freedom.

(3) Veterans of Operation Iraqi Freedom or Operation Enduring Freedom.

(4) Family members of the members and veterans described in paragraphs (1) through (3).

(d) ACCESS TO INFORMATION.—The National Academy of Sciences shall have access to such personnel, information, records, and systems of the Department of Defense and the Department of Veterans Affairs as the National Academy of Sciences requires in order to carry out the study required under subsection (a).

(e) PRIVACY OF INFORMATION.—The National Academy of Sciences shall maintain any personally identifiable information accessed by the Academy in carrying out the study required under subsection (a) in accordance with all applicable laws, protections, and best practices regarding the privacy of such information, and may not permit access to such information by any persons or entities not engaged in work under the study.

(f) REPORTS BY NATIONAL ACADEMY OF SCIENCES.—Upon the completion of each phase of the study required under subsection (a), the National Academy of Sciences shall submit to the Secretary of Defense, the Secretary of Veterans Affairs, and the congressional defense committees a report on such phase of the study.

(g) DOD AND VA RESPONSE TO NAS REPORTS.—Not later than 90 days after the receipt of a report under subsection (f) on each phase of the study required under subsection (a), the Secretary of Defense and the Secretary of Veterans Affairs shall develop a final joint Department of Defense-Department of Veterans Affairs response to the findings and recommendations of the National Academy of Sciences contained in such report.

# B

# PHASE 1 SUMMARY

The United States began combat operations in Afghanistan on October 7, 2001, in response to the September 11, 2001, terrorist attacks. That war is officially referred to as Operation Enduring Freedom (OEF), and the war in Iraq, which began in March 2003, is referred to as Operation Iraqi Freedom (OIF). Since October 2001, about 1.9 million US troops have been deployed to Afghanistan and Iraq. OEF and OIF have many unique features with regard to the military force being sent to fight those wars. The all-volunteer military has experienced multiple redeployments to the war zone, great use of the reserve components of the military and National Guard, deployment of high numbers of women and of parents of young children, and a high number of military personnel who survive severe injuries that in previous wars would have resulted in death.

Many men and women return from the war zone successfully and adjust to their lives out of theater, but others have had difficulty in readjusting or transitioning to family life, to their jobs, and to living in their communities after deployment. Numerous reports and articles in the popular press have drawn attention to those readjustment issues and have suggested that onset or exacerbation of mental disorders—particularly posttraumatic stress disorder (PTSD), anxiety disorders, and depression—might hinder readjustment. In addition, traumatic brain injury (TBI), often called the signature wound of OEF and OIF, is associated with a host of long-term adverse health outcomes, such as unprovoked seizures, decline in neurocognitive function, dementia, and adverse social-function outcomes, including unemployment and diminished social relationships, depression, and aggressive behaviors.

## BACKGROUND

In response to the growing needs of OEF and OIF active-duty service members, veterans, and families, Congress passed Section 1661 of the National Defense Authorization Act for FY 2008. That section required that the secretary of defense, in consultation with the secretary of veterans affairs, enter into an agreement with the National Academies for a study of the physical and mental health and other readjustment needs of members and former members of the armed forces who were deployed to OIF or OEF and their families as a result of such deployment. The study was assigned to the Institute of Medicine (IOM) and is to be conducted in two phases. This report is a response to the congressional legislation for phase 1 of the study.

## STATEMENT OF TASK

The statement of task for this study evolved out of discussions among the Department of Defense (DOD), the Department of Veterans Affairs (VA), and IOM. Specifically, it was determined that in phase 1, the IOM committee would identify preliminary findings regarding the physical and mental health and other readjustment needs for members and former members of the armed forces who were deployed to OEF or OIF and their families as a result of such deployment.

The committee would also determine how it would approach phase 2 of the study, which is meant to be a comprehensive assessment of the physical, mental, social, and economic effects and to identify gaps in care for members and former members of the armed forces who were deployed to OIF or OEF, their families, and their communities.

## COMMITTEE'S APPROACH TO ITS CHARGE

IOM appointed a committee of 16 experts to carry out this study. The committee members have expertise in sociology, psychiatry, rehabilitation, neurology, economics, epidemiology, survey research, and health policy and management. The Committee on Readjustment Needs of Military Personnel, Veterans, and Their Families decided, at its first meeting, that its approach to gathering information would include consideration of data in the peer-reviewed literature; gathering of data directly from DOD and VA; review of government articles, reports, and testimony presented before Congress; and review of recent IOM reports on PTSD, TBI, and physiologic, psychologic, and psychosocial effects of deployment-related stress. The committee would also seek input from the affected groups and communities.

The committee conducted extensive searches of the peer-reviewed literature in its attempts to understand readjustment needs, and it considered about 1,000 articles that were identified through those searches. Many of the articles, however, focused on outcomes primarily of service in the Vietnam War rather than OEF and OIF. There was a paucity of information in the literature about the current wars; thus, the articles reviewed, although instructive about the numerous outcomes and long-term effects of deployment and redeployment, were in effect a substitute for the information that the committee would like to have had. The committee also requested data from DOD and VA.

The committee examined the basic demographic data on the active-duty forces, the reserve components of the military, and the National Guard that DOD and VA provided, such as number of troops deployed and redeployed, dwell time, marital status, numbers of women deployed, types of injuries reported, and health-care use by OEF and OIF veterans. DOD data were provided by the Defense Manpower Center and the Armed Forces Health Surveillance Center. Committee members reviewed numerous reports that informed it about DOD and VA programs developed for those who have served in OEF and OIF and the costs of such programs. They reviewed reports from the Government Accountability Office, the Congressional Budget Office, and the Congressional Research Service; inspector general reports for VA and DOD; and congressional testimony relevant to the committee's task. And they reviewed several IOM reports on PTSD diagnosis, PTSD treatment, the effects of deployment-related stress, and long-term outcomes related to TBI.

Members of the committee understood that to carry out their task it would be important to talk to people who had first-hand knowledge of readjustment needs—active-duty personnel, veterans, family members, health-care providers, and community leaders. Therefore, in addition to its six meetings and literature reviews, the committee held several town hall meetings. The committee tried different venues and approaches for meeting with active-duty military personnel, veterans, and family members; some of the approaches were more successful than others.

Ultimately, the committee met with active-duty personnel, National Guard members, family members, veterans, and community leaders in cities, towns, and rural areas where there are large military bases and that were home to troops deployed to Iraq and Afghanistan. The committee held those meetings in Killeen, Texas (near Fort Hood); in Austin, Texas (at Camp Mabry); in Jacksonville and Fayetteville, North Carolina (near Camp Lejeune and Fort Bragg, respectively); and in Oceanside, California (near Camp Pendleton). Several committee members also met with the Marine and Family Services Division of Marine Corps Community Services at Camp Pendleton to gain a better understanding of the needs of marines and their family members and to become aware of the services offered. Those meetings were invaluable in providing the committee with an understanding of the challenges faced, not only by active-duty military with regard to accessing services but by providers who were trying to meet all the needs of service members and their families. Groups of committee members and staff went to Toledo, Ohio, to meet with National Guard members and representatives of the Ohio, Michigan, and Indiana Guard and to Watertown, New York, to meet with community leaders who serve those stationed at Fort Drum. The information-gathering sessions were open to the public. The committee also solicited comments from military-service and veteran-service organizations.

As a result of its approach to gathering information and its meetings and discussions, the committee decided to focus its findings on readjustment needs and gaps related to the conditions most frequently diagnosed in returning OEF and OIF active-duty personnel and veterans, such as PTSD and other mental health conditions, TBI, and social outcomes.

## FINDINGS AND RECOMMENDATIONS

The committee is aware that it is addressing a dynamic set of issues in that the conflicts in Iraq and Afghanistan are going on now and issues and needs will continue to change. The committee also recognizes that VA, DOD, and other government agencies are actively responding to changing needs of active-duty service members, veterans, and their family members, and that many of the committee's recommendations consequently might already be in the process of being addressed. Overall, the committee has found

- Relevant data on previous conflicts that are useful in addressing issues in the OEF and OIF populations.
- A relative paucity of data on OEF and OIF populations that are adequate to support evidence-based policy on most issues of concern.
- Information on a multitude of programs that have been developed to address the needs of the OEF and OIF populations.
- A scarcity of systematic or independent evaluation of such programs.

As the committee notes in Chapter 3, every war is unique in important respects. Empirical evidence collected from multiple wars documents that exposure to combat, other war-zone stressors, or even deployment itself can have immediate and long-term physical, psychologic, and other adverse consequences. Some of the consequences have been generally constant throughout the history of warfare, even though the context and nature of warfare have changed dramatically. However, throughout history, society and culture have played a powerful role in how the effects of war on soldiers have been viewed, in the perceived nature and causes of the effects, and in how soldiers were treated for them. Although the experiences of those deployed to Iraq or Afghanistan bear similarities to the experiences of those deployed in previous conflicts, there are a number of distinctive and important differences in who is serving, how they are deployed, and how the conflicts are being fought. The differences have important consequences for the types and severity of challenges and readjustment problems likely to be experienced by the men and women serving in OEF and OIF and for the types of support that they and their families need both in theater and on their return home. Most of the differences are notable in that our armed forces and our country as a whole have not had relevant experience with the key features of organization and warfare that make these conflicts most distinctive. Furthermore, the research that has been conducted shares a set of limitations with studies of the experiences in prior conflicts. Those limitations include

- Reliance on samples of convenience, which limits their external validity (generalizability).
- Reliance on brief screening instruments to identify key outcomes and to estimate prevalence, which limits internal validity.
- Use of cross-sectional designs, which limits the ability to support causal inference and to elucidate the course of disorders.
- Assessment of narrow sets of risk and protective factors, which results in under-specified models with a high risk of bias.
- Conduct of many studies by VA or DOD, rather than by independent third parties, which raises important questions about the accuracy of respondents' self-reports, particularly with regard to sensitive issues.

All those limitations are understandable given the fiscal and practical challenges involved in conducting long-term outcome studies (for example, longitudinal epidemiologic studies are expensive and difficult to implement). To be useful in the formulation of policy, however, studies need to be both scientifically sound and comprehensive. The committee is aware of the Millennium Cohort Study, several studies being conducted by RAND, and other studies that are in progress. Additional studies that address some of the methodologic challenges identified above—for instance, using probability sampling, diagnostic interviewing, and longitudinal designs—will be needed to move the field forward.

**The committee recommends that the Department of Defense, the Department of Veterans Affairs, and other federal agencies fund research on readjustment needs of returning OEF and OIF veterans, their families, and their communities that explicitly addresses methodologic and substantive gaps in completed and ongoing research. For example, the support of large-scale, independent studies with longitudinal designs, probability sampling, comprehensive clinical assessment of key outcomes, and more fully specified models that include objective biologic measures should be considered.**

In Chapter 4, the committee presents many of its preliminary findings and notes that research and program development are needed to substantiate the potential efficacy and cost effectiveness of developing protocols for the long-term management of TBI and polytrauma. The array of potential health outcomes associated with TBI suggests that injured service members will have long-term psychosocial and medical needs from both persistent deficits and problems that develop in later life. Access to rehabilitation therapies—including psychologic, social, and vocational—is required initially with the onset of deficits and will persist over time as personal and environmental factors change leading to loss of functional abilities.

VA has put into place a comprehensive system of rehabilitation services for polytrauma, including TBI (see Chapter 5), that addresses acute and chronic needs that arise in the initial months and years after injury. However, protocols to manage the lifetime effects of TBI are not in place and have not been studied for either military or civilian populations. As in other chronic health conditions, long-term management for TBI may be effective in reducing mortality, morbidity, and associated costs.

**The committee recommends that the Department of Veterans Affairs conduct research to determine the potential efficacy and cost effectiveness of developing protocols for the long-term management of service members who have polytrauma and traumatic brain injury. The approaches considered should include**

- **Prospective clinical surveillance to allow early detection and intervention for health complications.**
- **Protocols for preventive interventions that target high-incidence or high-risk complications.**
- **Protocols for training in self-management aimed at improving health and well-being.**
- **Access to medical care to treat complications.**
- **Access to rehabilitation services to optimize functional abilities.**

Another issue of concern, discussed in Chapter 4, is the critical shortage of health-care professionals—especially those specializing in mental health—to meet the demands of those returning from theater in Iraq and Afghanistan and their family members. Psychologists, psychiatrists, social workers, and other mental health professionals who do serve the military and veteran communities have large caseloads, especially in some locations that result in underserving of patients, high rates of burnout, and turnover. The committee heard of those problems repeatedly in its town hall meetings both from mental health professionals and from those who were waiting for appointments for treatment. Many of the people who spoke at the committee's meetings, from Fort Hood to Camp Pendleton, emphasized that those who are in need of mental health treatment have to wait too long for initial appointments or between appointments.

**The committee recommends that the Department of Defense and the Department of Veterans Affairs quantify the number and distribution of mental health professionals needed to provide treatment to the full population of returning service members, veterans, and their families who suffer from mental health disorders, such as PTSD, major depression, and substance abuse, so that they can**

**readjust to life outside of theater. The committee also recommends that the Department of Defense and the Department of Veterans Affairs continue to implement programs for the recruitment and retention of mental health professionals, particularly to serve those in hard-to-reach areas.**

Stigma, real or imagined, is perceived by military personnel who are (or are considering) seeking care for mental health or substance-abuse problems. And active-duty military and veterans fear that visits to a mental health provider will jeopardize their careers because of the military's long-standing and understandable policy of reporting mental health and substance-abuse problems to the chain of command. Such a policy is a disincentive to seeking care, underestimates the extent of the problem or the disease burden, and may ultimately compromise readiness.

**The committee recommends that the Department of Defense actively promote an environment to reduce stigma and encourage treatment for mental health and substance-use disorders in an effort to improve military readiness and ability to serve. The committee also recommends that the Department of Defense undertake a systematic review of its policies regarding mental health and substance-abuse treatment with regard to issues of confidentiality and the relation between treatment-seeking and military advancement.**

As noted in Chapter 4, the demands of the current conflicts have made compliance with DOD's rotational policies (for example, length of deployments and length of time between deployments) difficult. The implications and potential consequences of shorter dwell time and more frequent deployments are of obvious importance for understanding the readjustment needs of service members and their families; policies that help to ease reintegration are paramount. Little research has been conducted to evaluate whether service members who undergo third-location decompression (that is, for service members to have time with their comrades and peers in a restful situation and prepare themselves for going back to their families and communities) have better outcomes than those who do not, but anecdotal reports from foreign troops have been favorable. For example, Canadian forces have returned home from Afghanistan via Guam or Cyprus by spending 5 days of structured time with their units, which allows some time for decompression; they are also required to work about three half-days at their home base, and this provides additional time to adjust to life back in Canada and to ease the transition back into family life.

**The committee recommends that the Department of Defense formally assess whether a "third-location decompression" program would be beneficial for US combat troops. Third-location decompression has the potential to allow troops to have time to begin to readjust before returning home and to family responsibilities.**

Primarily on the basis of studies of previous conflicts, Chapter 4 highlights many issues related to families, spouses, children, women, and racial and ethnic minority-group members. It also discusses preliminary findings related to social issues related to deployment, such as employment, education, income, debt, wages, and earnings, also on the basis of data on previous wars. The committee found that active-duty service members, reservists, and veterans face hardships resulting from service in Iraq and Afghanistan that extend beyond physical and mental health problems. They also face numerous readjustment needs that affect their ability to adjust to life outside theater. Those needs, in turn, create hardships for their families.

**The committee recommends that the Department of Defense, the Department of Veterans Affairs, and other federal agencies fund research on the social and economic effects of deployment and multiple deployments on families. For example, research should examine the effects of multiple deployments on domestic violence and maltreatment of children, as well as on financial well-being.**

Women now constitute 14% of deployed forces in the US military, and, although technically they are barred from serving in combat, a growing and unprecedented number of female soldiers are deployed to combat areas where their lives are at risk. Although all service members are exposed to high levels of workplace stress, women in the military face some unique stressors, such as sexual harassment and trauma exposure that may affect their mental health and emotional well-being. Female veterans report a higher burden of medical illness, worse quality-of-life outcomes, and earlier psychologic morbidity than do men who are exposed to the same levels of trauma. Both the military and family life require commitment and loyalty, and servicewomen who have families may experience intense conflict between the demands of their military roles and their family roles. Some of the specific issues for women are military-related sexual harassment and assault and the resulting mental health problems, histories of premilitary trauma, specific health-care needs, pregnancy and the postpartum period, and the configuration of family roles (such as mother, spouse, and caregiver of aging parents).

**The committee recommends that the Department of Defense, the Department of Veterans Affairs, and other federal agencies fund studies to evaluate the effectiveness of mental health treatments currently being provided to women and to identify potential new treatments designed specifically to address women's unique circumstances and stressors, such as sexual harassment and assault, PTSD, and premilitary trauma.**

Although the military has a tradition of being one of the most desegregated institutions in US society, there is evidence that minority-group members have greater health and mental health needs than their white counterparts. For example, some minority groups may be at greater risk for PTSD and other adverse outcomes than nonminority groups exposed to comparable traumatic events. In addition, minority groups are less likely than nonminority groups to use mental health services and quicker to drop out of treatment. Therefore, health-care needs and other needs of minorities might be different from those of whites and are not yet well understood. All those issues raise a number of research questions that should be addressed.

**The committee recommends that the Department of Defense, the Department of Veterans Affairs, and other federal agencies fund research on culturally sensitive treatment approaches targeted toward minorities. Research is also needed on utilization patterns of currently available services by minority populations and the efficacy of such services to improve health outcomes.**

The burden borne by wounded warriors and their families, and thus the public responsibility to treat or compensate them, will persist for many years. Historically, the peak demand for compensation has lagged behind the end of hostilities by 30 years or more, so the maximum stress on support systems for OEF and OIF veterans and their families might not be felt until 2040 or later. To produce timely, accurate, and transparent forecasts of veterans' needs and demands on the system, it will be important to put into place mechanisms for anticipating the needs of veterans and their families so that the needs can begin to be addressed. Although long-term costs are less predictable and potentially are the subject of much controversy, because the costs are certain to be substantial and will be acutely felt by veterans and their families, high-quality cost forecasts are needed so that resources can be allocated better.

**The committee recommends that Congress appropriate funds and direct the Department of Veterans Affairs to expand the role of its actuary to produce annual long-term forecasts of costs associated with all health and disability benefits that are consistent with the practices of Social Security and Medicare.**

As the committee notes in Chapter 5, numerous programs exist or have been developed to meet the readjustment needs of OEF and OIF service members, veterans, and their families. There appears to be little coordination between programs and a lack of communication about the programs to those who need the services (there are notable exceptions, such as Military OneSource), especially those living in remote areas. Furthermore, the efficacy of the programs is unknown inasmuch as most programs have not been evaluated and there is no clear chain of accountability. No specific organization is providing stewardship of the available programs to assist those in need.

**The committee recommends that the Department of Defense and the Department of Veterans Affairs oversee coordination and communication of the multitude of programs that have been created in response to the needs of Operation Enduring Freedom and Operation Iraqi Freedom service members, veterans, and their family members in an effort to maximize their reach and effectiveness. The committee also recommends that there be independent evaluation of these programs with standardized evaluation designs and assessment of outcomes.**

## PHASE 2

As previously noted, the legislation (see Appendix A) that mandated this study directed that it be conducted in two phases. The specific aims of the second phase are to carry out a comprehensive assessment of the physical and mental health and other readjustment needs of members and former members of the armed forces who were deployed to OEF or OIF and their families as a result of such deployment and to assess the psychologic, social, and economic effects of such deployment on members, former members, and their families, including

- Effects of multiple deployments to OEF and OIF on members, former members, and their families.
- The scope of the neurologic, psychiatric, and psychologic effects of TBI on members and former members of the armed forces and their family members, including the efficacy of

current approaches to treatment for TBI in the United States and the efficacy of approaches to screening and treatment for TBI in DOD and VA.

- Effects of undiagnosed injuries, such as PTSD and TBI, an estimate of the long-term costs associated with such injuries, and the efficacy of approaches to screening and treatment for PTSD and other mental health conditions in DOD and VA.
- Sex-specific and ethnic-group–specific needs and concerns of members of the armed forces and veterans.
- Particular needs and concerns of children of members of the armed forces, taking into account different age groups, effects on development and education, and the mental and emotional well-being of children.
- An assessment of the particular educational and vocational needs of members and former members and their families and the efficacy of existing educational and vocational programs to address such needs.
- Effects of deployments associated with OEF and OIF on communities that have high populations of military families, including military housing communities and townships that are home to deployed members of the National Guard and reserves, and an assessment of the efficacy of programs that address community outreach and education concerning military deployments of community residents.
- Effects of increases in numbers of older and married members of the armed forces on readjustment requirements.
- The development, based on such assessments, of recommendations for programs, treatments, or policy remedies targeted at preventing, minimizing, or addressing the identified effects, gaps, and needs.
- The development, based on such assessments, of recommendations for additional research on identified needs.

The committee has given considerable thought to a framework to advance its task. The remainder of this chapter will describe the committee's approach to the formidable task given to it by Congress.

Inasmuch as the situations in Afghanistan and Iraq continue to evolve—as do the needs of OEF and OIF active-duty service members, veterans, family members, and communities—the committee suggests a flexible approach that can respond to the dynamic circumstances. The committee will expand its ranks by adding experts to assist in data collection and analysis, and it expects to have the input of its new members in the final approach for phase 2 before making its plan final. Phase 2 will probably involve collecting both qualitative and quantitative data. Possible approaches to address the statement of task that will be considered by the committee are described below.

**1. Review of funded research and gap analysis**

In phase 2, the committee expects to conduct a comprehensive assessment of newly completed and current research on OEF and OIF populations to determine what additional research is needed to identify and assess the magnitude of readjustment needs. The committee will perform a gap analysis based on the concerns outlined in the legislation (see Appendix A) and the funded research; the committee members will recommend topics for additional studies and provide the details for the approach to the research. The committee will require the cooperation of DOD and VA to compile a comprehensive list of newly completed and currently funded research.

**2. Systematic reviews of interventions**

The committee will conduct systematic literature reviews on interventions to address readjustment problems for social services and physical and mental health services and will recommend evidence-based interventions. There is a need to define optimal standards of care to restore and maintain health for OEF and OIF active-duty service members and veterans. The committee will review the literature on treatment modalities for TBI and PTSD and make recommendations for the best treatment approaches and for culturally sensitive treatments.

**3. Identify access-to-care issues**

The committee intends to examine issues related to access to care, specifically the extent to which DOD and VA treatment facilities are in areas where the need is greatest. The committee will gather data on demographics and on the number and types of services and programs that are available on the installations and in the surrounding communities (such as local hospitals, social services, and VA medical centers) to map actual resource allocation. The committee will also gather data on the numbers and types of health and mental health diagnoses being made by DOD and VA and examine the numbers of health and mental health professionals in an effort to determine workforce needs. The committee will need the cooperation of DOD and VA as it attempts to gather information to complete this task. DOD has already been helpful in providing detailed demographic information to the committee.

**4. Generate opportunities for research to fill identified knowledge gaps**

Informed by knowledge gaps identified in paragraphs 1 and 2 above, the committee plans to develop a request for proposals for a large-scale independent study or a suite of studies that would aim to improve understanding of the scope of the consequences of OEF and OIF and that would offer solutions to remediate those needs. Such a study should not duplicate current efforts but rather should be complementary and reflect the state of the science. In general, we anticipate that the study should have longitudinal designs inasmuch as not all consequences of deployment are immediately obvious (or even immediately measurable). It should use probability sampling so that all who served have a nonzero probability of being in the sample (that is, sampling cannot be complete until the war ends, or the sample would be drawn from all those who had served as of a specified date). That will be critical for external validity (generalizability) and to capture the varying nature of exposure by time and place of service. In addition, incorporation of clinical assessment, moving beyond screening instruments, will be required. We expect that some research started in phase 2 might not be completed by the time phase 2 concludes. However, our intention is that this work will lay a comprehensive base for future implementation science that deals directly with the readjustment needs of OEF and OIF active-duty service members, veterans, their families, and their communities. We also note that the committee will lay the foundation for qualitative research if a need for it becomes apparent in the reviews being discussed in paragraphs 1 and 2 above.

**5. Identify policy remedies**

Implicit in much of what the committee has found and has written is that dealing with the population-level consequences of OEF and OIF will require policy changes. The scope of potential policy remedies will be targeted at preventing, minimizing, or addressing the impacts, gaps, and needs identified during the committee's work. It is anticipated that this work will generate specific recommendations that may require statutory changes to implement.

# APPENDIX C

# THE DOD AND VA RESPONSE TO THE PHASE 1 REPORT

# Report to Congress Section 1661 of the National Defense Authorization Act for Fiscal Year 2008 Phase 1 Supporting Adjustment and Readjustment of Active Military, Veterans, and Family Members:

IOM's March 31, 2010

*Returning Home from Iraq and Afghanistan: Preliminary Assessment of Readjustment Needs of Veterans, Service Members, and Their Families*

**September 2010**

# Table of Contents

## I. Introduction

To address a 2008 Congressional mandate to study the physical and mental health and other readjustment needs of members and former members of the Armed Forces who deployed in Operation Enduring Freedom (OEF) or Operation Iraqi Freedom (OIF) and their families as a result of such deployment (Public Law 110-181), the Institute of Medicine (IOM) of the National Academy of Sciences published *Returning Home from Iraq and Afghanistan: Preliminary Assessment of Readjustment Needs of Veterans, Service Members and Their Families* on March 31, 2010. This document presents a joint response from the Secretary of Defense and the Secretary of Veterans Affairs in response to the IOM report. This report on the first phase of a two-part study describes data collection methodology, summarizes preliminary findings, and proffers ten recommendations for future research. In general, the Department of Defense (DoD ) and the Department of Veterans Affairs (VA) support the majority of IOM's recommendations, and are pleased to report that many of the recommended actions are already well underway, with particular emphasis on OEF and OIF Service members and Veterans.

In the sections that follow, comments are provided for each recommendation that include descriptions of the ongoing and completed studies and programs that address the suggested actions. Lists and brief descriptions of studies and publications are included in appendices A through H.

IOM considered data from numerous sources to include:

- searches of peer-reviewed literature;
- data from DoD and VA;
- reports from the Government Accountability Office;
- reports from the Congressional Budget Office;
- reports from the Congressional Research Service;
- reports in the popular press;
- relevant Congressional testimony;
- IOM reports on PTSD, PTSD treatment, the effects of deployment-related stress, and the long-term outcomes related to TBI: and
- six town hall meetings with active duty personnel, Veterans, family members, health-care providers, and community leaders.

Because information on specific readjustment needs of OEF/OIF Service members, Veterans, and their families is limited, IOM included in its review reports and studies on the Service members and Veterans of the Second World War, Korea, Vietnam, and the Gulf War. The authors make it clear that direct comparisons may not be appropriate because many more Service members now survive wounds they would not have survived in earlier conflicts.

Not surprisingly, much of the data included in IOM's chapter on preliminary findings has been reported elsewhere and complete citations are provided in the text. We have culled IOM's preliminary findings for those that are specific to the OEF/OIF conflicts and have included them as appendix I. As they do in the text, the OEF/OIF-specific findings address six areas of interest to include:

- TBI and related blast injuries;
- polytrauma;
- mental health disorders;
- deployment;
- women and minorities; and
- projecting the lifelong burden of war.

We look forward to Phase 2 of the study, "a comprehensive assessment... of the physical and mental health and other readjustment needs of members and former members of the Armed Forces who deployed in OEF or OIF and their families as a result of such deployment" (P.L. 110-181). Among the minimum requirements for Phase 2 outlined in the legislation, DoD and VA are particularly interested in new information on:

- An assessment of the particular impacts of multiple deployments
- An assessment of the full scope of effects of TBI and the efficacy of current treatment approaches
- An estimate of the long-term costs associated with "undiagnosed" injuries such as PTSD and
- "Recommendations for programs, treatments, or policy remedies targeted at preventing, minimizing, or addressing the impacts, gaps, and needs identified."

## II. Response to IOM's Recommendations

In general, the Department of Defense (DoD ) and the Department of Veterans Affairs (VA) support the majority of IOM's recommendations, and are pleased to report that many of the recommended actions are already underway, with particular emphasis on OEF and OIF Service members. Comments are provided for each recommendation that include descriptions of the ongoing and completed studies and programs that address the suggested actions.

### *A. IOM Recommendation 1*

**The committee recommends that the Department of Defense, the Department of Veterans Affairs, and other federal agencies fund research on readjustment needs of returning OEF and OIF [V]eterans, their families, and their communities that explicitly addresses methodologic and substantive gaps in completed and ongoing research. For example, the support of large-scale, independent studies with longitudinal designs, probability sampling, comprehensive clinical assessment of key outcomes, and more fully specified models that include objective biologic measures should be considered.**

#### 1. DoD Response to IOM Recommendation 1

DoD and VA agree with this recommendation and have worked steadily to develop and implement the most rigorous scientific investigations possible. In 2007, representatives from DoD, VA, various NIH (National Institutes of Health) institutes (e.g., National Institute of Mental Health [NIMH], National Institute of Neurological Disorders and Stroke [NINDS]), other federal agencies, and subject matter experts, primarily from academia, met as a working group to identify and prioritize research gaps in post-deployment military readjustment literature. This major effort directly informed the planning and development of the largest targeted research funding opportunity for deployment-related mental health and brain injury conditions in U.S. history. Supplemental Fiscal Year 2007 (FY07) DoD funding provided $150 million for Posttraumatic Stress Disorder (PTSD) research and an additional $150 million for traumatic brain injury (TBI) research. In FY09, Congress provided an additional appropriation of $55 million for psychological health (PH) and TBI research. Currently, DoD is investing more than $20.1 million in longitudinal studies on readjustment needs of Warriors and their families. One such study is described below.

**Study to Assess Risk and Resilience in Service Members (Army STARRS)**

Funded by the U.S. Army, and conducted by NIMH and an interdisciplinary team from four leading academic research institutions, this is the largest study of suicide and mental health among military personnel ever undertaken. The research team, from the Uniformed Services University of the Health Sciences (USUHS), Harvard University, the University of Michigan, and Columbia University, is internationally known for its expertise and experience in research on military health, health and behavior surveys, epidemiology, and suicide, including genetic and neurobiological factors involved in suicidal behavior. The study will have both a retrospective and a prospective component.

Investigators will undertake a retrospective case-control study, comparing Soldiers with suicidal behavior (cases) to similar Soldiers without suicidal behavior (controls) in order to identify characteristics, events, experiences, and exposures that may be predictive of Soldiers' suicides. This study design will make it possible to begin generating information on risk and protective factors—and how to determine who is at high risk—very rapidly. Study investigators will produce actionable information that the Army can use to develop and refine interventions to prevent future suicides and address related PH issues.

For the prospective study, investigators will follow a representative sample of approximately 90,000 active duty Soldiers (including mobilized Reserve Component and National Guard Soldiers), from whom they will collect detailed information on psychological and physical health, exposure to adverse events, attitudes, social supports, leadership and unit climate, training and knowledge, employment and economic status, family history, and other potentially relevant domains over the life of the study. Biological specimens (e.g., saliva and/or blood) will be collected for genetic and neurobiological studies. This will provide rich longitudinal information relating Soldiers' characteristics and experiences to subsequent psychological health, suicidal behavior, and other relevant outcomes and will identify high-risk periods in a military career.

**Other Ongoing Studies**

In its report, the IOM comments that the "committee is aware of the Millennium Cohort study [and] several studies being conducted by RAND" (p. 156). Two of these studies are summarized briefly below.

**The Millennium Cohort Study (MCS)**

Launched in the summer of 2001, this study follows a random sample of over 150,000 U.S. military personnel from all Services, including both active duty and Reserve/National Guard members, for up to 21 years. Approximately 50 percent of the cohort has been deployed in OEF and OIF. The MCS study is designed to investigate exposures and health outcomes temporally, to detect outcomes with longer latency, and to ascertain symptom and illness duration, resolution, and chronicity. The unique aspect of this study is its ability to link this data to a wealth of DoD and VA electronic data that includes personnel files, birth and infant health, inpatient and outpatient health care use, pharmaceutical use, vaccination history, deployment experience, exposures, and mortality. Links with other federal databases (e.g., Centers for Disease Control and Prevention [CDC], National Death Index [NDI], and Social Security Administration [SSA]) are being utilized in this ongoing study.

The study is in its eighth year and current areas of research include investigations differentiated by deployment focusing on diabetes; weight change; hearing loss; migraine headaches; unit cohesion; complementary and alternative medicine and health care use; physical activity and PTSD symptoms; professional care provider occupations; PTSD and depressive symptoms; chronic multi-symptom illnesses and associated co-morbidities; motor vehicle accidents; head trauma; back pain; tendonopathies and other injuries; and cause-specific mortality including suicide.

The impact of military service and deployment health on families will be evaluated through a spousal assessment component in the 2010-11 survey cycle. This study will be the first of its kind to use a large cohort to assess the impacts on spouses and co-resident children, and to evaluate the quality of family relationships.[1]

Funded by DoD through the Military Operational Medicine Research Program (MOMRP) and conducted at the Navy Health Research Center (NHRC) with co-investigators from all Services and VA, this large study will assess career-span health outcomes beyond military service and serve as a showcase for DoD and VA cooperation.

**RAND Corporation's Deployment Life Study (DLS)**

The DLS is a 3-year longitudinal study that began in March 2009 to examine the impact of deployment on the health and well-being of military families. This study will recruit approximately 9,600 Army, Navy, Marine and Air Force families, following them across an OEF/OIF deployment cycle, and assessing a number of outcomes over time. These outcomes include: (i) the emotional and physical health of each family member, (ii) family relationship quality and longevity, (iii) financial well-being and role performance, and (iv) for children, school performance, and social development.

The project will collect longitudinal data from approximately 5,000 (anticipated at follow-up) military families, including the Service member, his or her spouse, and, if one exists, one child 11 years of age or older (with parental consent). The baseline interview will be conducted by phone. Every 4 months after baseline, the respondent will log into a Website to complete an on-line survey. The project will take place over 36 months for nine waves of data collection, spanning a period of 6-12 months pre-deployment, throughout deployment, and post-

---

[1] The study team estimates that 10,000 spouses will be enrolled in this component, and that about half of these will be the spouses of individuals deployed at least once to OEF and OIF.

deployment. The project will examine specific behaviors as mediators of the deployment effects, such as: accessing health care or social support services, shifts in the division of labor within the family, changes in communication patterns and style, etc. Investigators will also be able to examine how changes in some outcomes (e.g., the marital relationship) account for changes in other outcomes (e.g., child school performance).

The DLS is being conducted within the RAND Center for Military Health Policy Research, a joint research initiative between RAND Health and the RAND Arroyo Center. This project is funded by the offices of the U.S. Army Surgeon General and the Assistant Secretary of Defense for Health Affairs.

Appendix A lists active DoD-funded longitudinal studies on PH and TBI.[2] The list includes studies from the Congressionally Directed Medical Research Programs (CDMRP) FY07 and FY09 rounds as well as other DoD funding entities and mechanisms (e.g., US Army Medical Research and Materiel Command's (USAMRMC), MOMRP, and Telemedicine and Advanced Technology Research Center [TATRC]).

### 2. VA Response to IOM Recommendation 1

VA notes the following points regarding research-related limitations the Committee highlighted in the Phase I assessment:

- The question of sampling is critical to validity, as the Committee noted. While samples of convenience may limit generalizability, it is more likely the case that this issue could relate to some smaller, single-site studies, although scientific peer review committees also consider generalizability carefully. Larger studies, especially those being conducted by VA's Cooperative Studies Program (CSP), address the ability to generalize as a working principle. In VA's large-scale cohort studies, national samples considered to be representative of the population are the norm (e.g., CSP 575, a study of genetic factors related to PTSD in OEF/OIF, randomly assesses from the entire DoD manpower roster [see Appendix B).

- Brief screening instruments have some utility in clinical assessments as well as in overall surveillance of a population. According to VA Office of Mental Health Services, OEF/OIF Veterans coming to VA for the first time are screened for the presence of symptoms of PTSD, depression, and alcohol abuse. The same screening for these conditions is repeated on an annual basis for new or existing Veterans of any service era. Should the Veteran screen positive for any of these conditions, further evaluation and appropriate treatment are provided. Veterans who screen positive for PTSD or

[2] Some studies may appear in more than one appendix.

depression are also assessed for risk of suicidal behavior. This is important information for clinical purposes and may be legitimately reported at the level of surveillance.

- In VA's research portfolio, a small number of studies have examined the validity of the screening instruments directly. However, in the more definitive large cohort studies and clinical trials, the battery of assessments is quite extensive as a rule and they are not dependent upon brief screening measures. In working group recommendations on PTSD methodology, consideration of reliability, validity, including cultural appropriateness and practicality are recommended for outcome measures. (See "Advancing Research Standards for PTSD Interventions," 2008.)

- Knowledge of VA's research portfolio will be key to further assessment by the Committee and will inform the stated limitations regarding cross sectional vs. longitudinal studies as well as focus in risk/protective factor studies. VA portfolio addresses these concerns by supporting a wide range of efforts. In some cases, specific hypotheses are being tested on a limited set of factors by design; however, in other cases, extensive batteries are used to study risk and protective factors (e.g., CSP 575). See Appendix B.

- VA research program does support cross-sectional approaches in certain cases, but it is also informed by large-scale longitudinal studies. An example of this is CSP 566 (see Appendix B) with multiple post-deployment follow up assessments of an Army cohort with pre-deployment baseline performance prior to service in Iraq.

- VA conducts an appreciable number of studies in the population of Veterans who have served in Iraq and Afghanistan. While some studies may rely on self-report, our Human Subjects Protection Program allows extensive oversight to ensure confidentiality and appreciation of sensitive issues. Examples include: (a) VA's consent process that includes information provided to participants stating that their participation in the research will not affect VA benefits or VA health care, (b) VA clinical researchers are encouraged to obtain a Certificate of Confidentiality, and this information is also conveyed to research participants. VA believes that scientific results from Veterans participating in VA research are not *a priori* tainted by this limitation.

As a general operating principle, VA closely coordinates post-deployment readjustment research efforts with other federal agencies. The coordination ranges from informal phone calls between offices to co-sponsored meetings and joint solicitations. Notably, VA initially led in convening expert work groups to identify research priorities for the Veterans of Iraq and Afghanistan (see "Mapping the Landscape of Deployment Related Adjustment and Mental Disorders," 2006). The recommendations from these work groups led to publication of multiple research solicitations focused on identified gaps.

VA and NIMH have issued a series of joint solicitations on readjustment disorders in OEF/OIF Veterans, including: "Intervention and Practice Research for Combat Related Mental Disorders and Stress Reactions," "Network(s) for Developing PTSD Risk Assessment Tools," and, "Clinical Pharmacotherapy for PTSD: Single and Collaborative Studies." Both VA and NIMH committed funds for these efforts.

Probably the largest interagency effort in the area of substance use/abuse co-morbidities among active duty Service members and Veterans followed discussions with multiple federal funding agencies in 2008. At a co-sponsored meeting in January 2009, VA and its federal partners set the stage for a Request for Applications (RFA) issued by VA together with the National Institute on Drug Abuse (NIDA), the National Institute of Alcohol Abuse and Alcoholism (NIAAA), and the National Cancer Institute (NCI), with a total of up to $7 million committed by all agencies. Proposals in response to this RFA will be evaluated and approved in FY 2010.

A notable gap identified by the federal research funding agencies was the use of common measures and terminology for studies focused on TBI and PH. One major recent effort has therefore been collaborative work toward defining common data elements for PH and TBI. VA research with NIH's NINDS, the National Institute on Disability and Rehabilitation Research (NIDRR), and the Defense Centers of Excellence for Psychological Health and Traumatic Brain Injury (DCoE), co-sponsored an initiative to adopt common data elements (CDEs). Scientific experts participated in working groups for specific topic-driven CDEs, which were discussed in a workshop, "Advancing Integrated Research in Psychological Health and Traumatic Brain Injury: Common Data Elements," held on March 23-24, 2009, with 137 national and international PH and TBI experts.

The process leading to the workshop and the subsequent recommendations by the working groups led to a series of manuscripts (Overview, Agency Background, TBI Definition, TBI Demographics and Clinical Assessment, Biomarkers, TBI Neuroimaging, TBI Outcomes, PTSD, and Operational Anxiety) expected to be published in the Archives of Physical Medicine and Rehabilitation in 2010. The CDEs themselves appear on a Web site launched April 1, 2010, and hosted by NINDS (http://www.nindscommondataelements.org/). The site contains a mechanism to capture feedback and suggestions for the CDEs from the community of users. Four new working groups met in March 2010 to review and adapt the TBI CDEs for pediatric relevance. Manuscripts with recommendations are in progress.

**Other Methodology-Directed Activities**

VA has long been considered a leader in the area of PTSD research, and in 2006 co-sponsored a work group with NIMH on the topic of clinical treatment research methodology for PTSD studies ("Advancing Research Standards for PTSD Interventions," 2008; Leon and Davis, 2009). This meeting resulted in recommendations that were disseminated widely to the scientific community and have been incorporated in the joint solicitations (see above) issued by VA and NIMH.

One notable VA program that has advanced the methodological rigor in clinical research is the CSP. With five coordinating centers and other multiple resource centers, the methodological rigor in CSP studies is developed through a cooperative planning process and scientific peer review in which proponents and methodological/statistical experts meet face-to-face with a review panel to defend the proposal and answer questions about concerns. When a CSP study is approved for funding, it is overseen by multiple bodies including an Executive Committee, Data Monitoring Committee (for safety and data reviews), as well as an Institutional Review Board (IRB). Appendix B lists and briefly describes some of the CSP programs related to the OEF/OIF population.

The CCTA program has made strides to incorporate the methodological rigor of the CSP studies into all clinical trials, irrespective of size. One strong example of this is the CCTA funding mechanism, which pairs the methodological expertise from a CSP coordinating center with a principal investigator to conduct small, early phase interventional work. Although this is a relatively new program, two of the initially approved studies are focused on novel TBI and PTSD treatments for the OEF/OIF population. The goal of the program is to identify treatments that appear to warrant testing at the multi-site CSP level.

**VA Deployment Health Research Related to OEF/OIF Veterans**

VA has an open solicitation for Deployment Health Services Research to support studies focused on deployment health care needs and services. The solicitation targets three major areas: 1) health delivery system resources, structures, and processes of utilization; 2) population characteristics; and 3) health and satisfaction outcomes. This research also has direct relevance for other Veterans, as well as for civilians experiencing disability due to injury or disease.

### *B. IOM Recommendation 2*

**The committee recommends that the Department of Veterans Affairs conduct research to determine the potential efficacy and cost effectiveness of developing protocols for the long-term management of Service members who have polytrauma and traumatic brain injury. The approaches considered should include:**

- **Prospective clinical surveillance to allow early detection and intervention for health complications,**
- **Protocols for preventive interventions that target high-incidence or high-risk complications,**

- **Protocols for training in self-management aimed at improving health and well-being,**
- **Access to medical care to treat complications, and**
- **Access to rehabilitation services to optimize functional abilities.**

### 1. VA Response to IOM Recommendation 2

VA has been and will continue to address the long-term management of Service members and Veterans who require it. VA has an established research program on polytrauma and TBI, and translates research outcomes into improved clinical care and management. For example, the Polytrauma and Blast-Related Injury Quality Enhancement Research Initiative (PT/BRI (QUERI) Coordinating Center works closely with Polytrauma Rehabilitation Centers (PRCs) to identify needs and gaps in care, as well as best practices for TBI with polytrauma and traumatic amputation with polytrauma. In addition, the four PRCs and Defense Veterans Brain Injury Center (DVBIC) have established a joint VA/DoD initiative for ongoing clinical care, research, and service delivery for Veterans and active duty Service members with brain injury.

In June 2009, VA and DVBIC developed a 5-year pilot program to assess the effectiveness of providing Assisted Living (AL) services to Veterans with functional disabilities due to TBI. Veterans placed in private facilities that specialize in rehabilitation services for TBI continue to be monitored by VA care managers, and outcome data are being collected (e.g., demographic and health information, functional status, satisfaction with care, and quality of life). A report of this pilot will be provided to Congress upon the program's conclusion in 2013.

VA is also presently collaborating with NIDRR on the national TBI Model Systems (TBIMS) project to benchmark rehabilitation and longitudinal functional outcomes with those of other TBIMS Centers, and to collaborate on research initiatives. Lastly, VA's Office of Research and Development (ORD) has numerous priorities for TBI/polytrauma-related research, including investigating long-term care and management of Veterans with polytrauma, blast-related injuries, or TBI.

Appendix C summarizes a sampling of the studies in polytrauma and TBI from VA research portfolio. Appendix D provides key associated bibliographic references.

## *C. IOM Recommendation 3*

**The committee recommends that the Department of Defense and the Department of Veterans Affairs quantify the number and distribution of mental health**

**professionals needed to provide treatment to the full population of returning Service members, Veterans, and their families who suffer from mental health disorders, such as PTSD, major depression, and substance abuse, [so] that they can readjust to life outside of theater. The committee also recommends that the Department of Defense and the Department of Veterans Affairs continue to implement programs for the recruitment and retention of mental health professionals, particularly to serve those in hard-to-reach areas.**

### 1. DoD Response to IOM Recommendation 3

Significant progress has been made to recruit additional mental health personnel in order to meet the growing demand for services in DoD and VA. Between 2007 and the second quarter of 2009, the number of DoD mental health specialists grew 47 percent from 4,129 to 6,061 in military medical treatment facilities (MTFs) and the number of TRICARE Network providers increased 26 percent from 39,587 to 49,807. A gap analysis performed at the end of the third quarter of 2009 revealed that 93 percent of current Service-determined mental health provider "requirements" or "needs" at MTFs were filled. The substantial increase in the numbers of mental health providers is attributable largely to recruitment efforts.

DoD established a mental health recruiting and retention strategy to help develop new programs to attract and retain uniformed and civilian mental health professionals. A Directive-Type Memorandum (DTM) established the Health Profession Incentive Working Group to adjust incentives and pay annually to maximize recruitment and retention of those with high-needs skill sets. DoD developed another DTM (09-009) for the "Implementation of Special Pay for Health Professions Officers (HPOs)" on July 23, 2009, allowing DoD to offer mental health professionals within DoD special pay and bonuses.

This action is expected to enhance significantly DoD's ability to recruit and retain mental health professionals, particularly psychologists and social workers, through direct accession recruitment. As an additional effort to boost provider availability, DoD entered into a Memorandum of Agreement with the Department of Health and Human Services (HHS) to use uniformed Public Health Service (PHS) mental health providers. More than 70 PHS officers have been hired as a result of this agreement.

Another potential effort on the horizon is the Civilian Health Professions Scholarship Program (CHPS), a recruitment program that would provide health care scholarship funds and related educational expenses to prospective health care professionals in return for a DoD service commitment when the providers have completed their training.

DoD has initiated several joint efforts to improve access to mental health care. These include the following.

- DCoE's National Center for Telehealth and Technology (T2) has embarked on a program to develop and deliver Web-based telehealth care that will extend the reach of services to underserved military beneficiaries, particularly the Reserve Component and those in historically underserved areas, by leveraging the Services, TRICARE, VA, and civilian provider partnerships;
- DoD provides training to, coordination for, and oversight of a national network of systems delivering psychological health care via technology;
- DoD collaborated with VA's National Center for PTSD in three states–Massachusetts, California, and Hawaii–to create Afterdeployment.org, a Web-based portal focused on post-deployment issues and the PH needs of Service members and their families;
- In coordination with other stakeholders, DoD developed and published common access standards for mental health services;
- To further assist telehealth treatment, a telemental health standard of care was created through the Office of the Chief Medical Officer; and.
- T2 is evaluating a program to deliver PH care through mobile platforms. This program has promise as an effective way to provide needed psychological care to Service members and their families who might not otherwise have access to care. The benefits of the Mobile TeleHealth Unit project include the ability to reach all DoD and VA beneficiaries.

To teach best clinical practices to community-based mental health staff who are addressing the behavioral health needs of military personnel, Veterans, and their families, the Center for Deployment Psychology at the USUHS has established the Military and Veteran Behavioral Health Post-Master's Certificate Program. The program takes from 6 months to 1 year to complete and includes the following required workshops:

- Military Culture, Terminology, and the Deployment Cycle;
- Etiology and Assessment of PTSD and Co-morbid Problems;
- Assessment and Treatment of Sleep Disturbance Associated with Deployment,
- Traumatic Brain Injury Sustained in Combat;
- Assessment and Treatment of Deployment-Related Depression;
- Identification, Prevention, and Treatment of Suicidal Behavior; and
- Evidence-Based Treatment of PTSD: Prolonged Exposure Therapy.

In addition, DoD is developing the Psychological Health Risk-Adjusted Model for Staffing (PHRAMS) for use by medical department personnel within Army, Air Force, Navy, and staff within the Office of Health Affairs to model predicted psychological health staffing requirements. Each Service's medical department and Office of the Assistant Secretary of Defense (Health Affairs) staff provided input for this project.

Using deployment history data from the Defense Manpower Data Center (DMDC) and eligibility, demographic, and medical data from the Military Health System Data Repository (MDR), PHRAMS is able to provide a forecast for the total staffing requirements to meet the annual need for psychological health services by beneficiaries over a 5-year period for each type of specialty provider (e.g., psychiatrists, psychologists, psychiatric nurse practitioners, and clinical social workers) and for others who provide PH services as part of the care they offer (e.g., primary care providers and chaplains).

DoD Health Affairs is working with the Services to determine how Service staffing aligns with the PHRAMS predictions of mental health providers needed for beneficiary psychological services. Currently, a projection of requirements for each mental health specialty has been made for the Services from 2009 through 2014, including mental health specialty providers embedded into operational units and integrated into primary care clinics. The Services will determine the gaps between these requirements and existing providers in order to establish specific hiring and recruitment goals.

## 2. VA Response to IOM Recommendation 3

VA has increased mental health staff 36 percent in the last 3 years (from 14,208 in FY 2006 to 19,283 in FY 2009) through Mental Health Expansion Initiative (MHEI) funds and has increased the number of Veterans treated for mental health problems by 21 percent in the same time period (from 1,183,819 to 1,428,858). VA is tracking total Core Mental Health Staffing full-time equivalent employee (FTEE) positions funded under annual budget processes and those funded by special purpose and MHEI funds.

Veterans Integrated Service Network (VISN) and facilities are required to maintain a staffing level of greater than 90 percent of the filled and approved mental health staff positions that existed at the end of FY 2009. As of the end of the first quarter of 2010, all VISNs have surpassed this minimum standard, and 20 out of the 21 VISNs have produced a net gain in mental health staffing over that time period.

The Uniform Mental Health Services Handbook delineates the essential components of the mental health program to ensure that all Veterans, wherever they obtain care in the Veteran's Health Administration (VHA), have access to needed services. The Handbook specifies those services that must be provided at each VA Medical Center and Community Based Outpatient Clinic (CBOC). VA actively employs the use of remote clinical videoconferencing technology to improve access, fill gaps in mental health services, and provide remote national expert consultation to Veterans at any VA facility in the country.

A National Telemental Health Center will be operational by the end of FY10. The Office of Telehealth Services (OTS) and Office of Mental Health Services (OMHS) are currently staffing the center and planning delivery of remote expert consultation services. OTS and OMHS have identified opportunities for the delivery of telemental health services into the home for the care of Veterans with substance abuse problems and for the management of depression using interactive voice response (IVR) technology. VA continues to explore opportunities for using telemental health to fill any gaps identified in mental health services.

VA has a number of initiatives in place to ensure that access and continuity of care is facilitated as close to home as possible. Three VISNs are in the process of negotiating contracts with community providers as part of a 3-year pilot program. Results from this effort will provide valuable information on how VA can develop partnerships with community providers to expand access to mental health services for rural-residing Veterans.

An expansion of the Mental Health Intensive Case Management – Rural Access Network for Growth Enhancement (MHICM-RANGE) initiative has been supported by VA's Office of Rural Health. This initiative adds mental health staff to CBOCs, enhances telemental health services, and uses referrals to community mental health services and other providers to increase access to mental health care in rural areas. The expansion of MHICM-RANGE has also led to four research studies on clinical policies or programs that improve access, quality, and outcomes of mental health and substance abuse treatment services for rural and underserved Veterans.

OMHS has partnered with the My Health*e*Vet program office and the Office of Information and Technology (OI&T) to develop online resources designed to complement traditional mental health services, and to expand access to these services to Veterans in rural areas. OMHS is working closely with the Office of Health Information (OHI) and OI&T to develop My Recovery Plan – an online, interactive application designed to support Veteran-centered, evidence-based mental health practices. Sections of My Recovery Plan will be available for self-paced independent work, while other areas will be made available to Veterans in conjunction with work with a provider. Both approaches are expected to facilitate treatment for Veterans in rural areas.

Among the OMHS initiatives in place to assist community and rural health care providers is an Internet Website (www.mentalhealth.va.gov/College/index.asp) with basic information on assessment and treatment of PTSD. The site is designed for college mental health counselors who, like many community providers, may not have knowledge about military service or experience treating combat-related PTSD and other disorders associated with war. Access to services is supported increasingly by Internet-based resources such as VA OEF/OIF Web site (www.oefoif.va.gov) and the National Center for PTSD's Web site (www.ptsd.va.gov), as well as a VA presence on social media sites such as Facebook and Twitter.

A two-part VHA Productivity and Staffing study conducted by OMHS in collaboration with the Office of Productivity, Efficiency, and Staffing (OPES) used electronic workload and provider data from psychiatrists and associated mental health providers (psychologists, social workers, nurse practitioners (NPs), clinical nurse specialists (CNSs), and physician assistants (PAs) working in mental health. The results of the study are being used to establish reasonable productivity and staffing standards, to be completed this year.

To ensure adequate inpatient minimum staffing standards, OMHS established a workgroup to review current utilization of inpatient mental health services across VISNs and Medical Centers, determining the sources of geographic variability in individuals with extended lengths of stay, and evaluating the extent of variability when these individuals are excluded from analyses. Administrative data on utilization and staffing are expected to be translated into staffing guidelines this year.

Vet Centers are community-based counseling centers, within Readjustment Counseling Service (RCS), that provide a wide range of social and psychological services including professional readjustment counseling to Veterans and families, military sexual trauma counseling, and bereavement counseling for families who experience an active duty death. This program also facilitates community outreach and the brokering of services with community agencies that link Veterans with other needed VA and non-VA services. A core value of the Vet Center program is to promote access to care by helping Veterans and families overcome barriers that impede them from using those services.

The Vet Center program has provided services to more than 40 percent (450,162) of all separated OEF/OIF Veterans since the beginning of the wars in Afghanistan and Iraq (cumulative through March 31, 2010). Furthermore, 40 percent of all Vet Center clients do not receive services at any other VA facility. To meet this growing need, the Vet Center program has increased its counseling staff by 103 percent since 2003. In addition, more than 34 percent of Vet Center staff has served in either the Afghanistan or Iraq combat theaters. (See Appendix E for a list of Vet Centers.)

To extend the geographical reach of Vet Center services, RCS has implemented initiatives to ensure that Veterans have access to care. Following the onset of the current hostilities in Afghanistan and Iraq, the Vet Center program hired 100 OEF/OIF Veteran Outreach Specialists to contact their fellow returning Veterans at military demobilization sites, including National Guard and Reserve locations, and in the community. Further, to facilitate access to services for Veterans in hard-to-reach outlying areas, RCS has deployed 50 Mobile Vet Centers (MVCs) across the country. A full time driver/outreach specialist and counselor are attached to each of these vehicles. The placement of the vehicles is designed to cover a national network of designated Veterans Service Areas (VSAs) that collectively cover every county in the continental

United States. The 50 MVCs are used to provide early access to returning combat Veterans via outreach to a variety of military and community events. The vehicles are also extending Vet Center outreach to more rural communities that are isolated from existing VA services.

In FY 2010, the Vet Center program is authorized to employ a total of 1,391 counseling staff in 300 Vet Centers and 50 Mobile Vet Centers. Further, by the end of 2010, RCS will have a qualified family and marriage counselor at every Vet Center. To meet this goal, RCS has partnered with the VHA Healthcare Retention and Recruitment Office to initiate a national recruitment and targeted marketing campaign to find qualified professionals to meet the diverse needs of Veterans, their families, and the community in which they live.

In recent years, RCS and the Vet Center programs have been the subject of program evaluations by several different agencies and organizations. According to the President's Advisory Committee on Gulf War Veterans' Illnesses[3]:

> The Department of Defense and VA should follow the model of field-based outreach demonstrated in the Vet Centers when developing health education and risk communication campaigns for active duty service members, Reserve and Guard personnel, and other Veterans. The prompt response by the Vet Centers to the acute PTSD and other post-war readjustment difficulties, such as family and employment problems, illustrate VA's commitment to early intervention and outreach (p. 1).

Further, the U.S. Medicine Institute for Health Studies, with participants from DoD, Substance Abuse and Mental Health Services Administration (SAMHSHA) and VA, reported "VHA's Vet Centers have proven a 'best practice' model in fostering peer-to-peer relationships for those with combat stress disorders. The best way to overcome concerns about stigmatization is through person-to-person contact with someone who has recovered."[4] The Vet Center program is also the gold standard in both internal and external VA surveys measuring Veteran and employee satisfaction.

### *D. IOM Recommendation 4*

**The committee recommends that the Department of Defense actively promote an environment to reduce stigma and encourage treatment for mental health and substance-use disorders in an effort to improve military readiness and ability to serve. The committee**

---

3 Persian Gulf Veterans Coordinating Board. (1997, March). *The Final Report of The Presidential Advisory Committee on Gulf War Veterans' Illnesses (PAC).*

4 U.S. Medicine Institute for Health Studies. (2004, October). *Executive Summary- USMI Roundtable Discussion: The Changing Face of Mental Health Services in the Veteran Health Administration.*

**also recommends that the Department of Defense undertake a systematic review of its policies regarding mental health and substance-abuse treatment with regard to issues of confidentiality and the relation between treatment-seeking and military advancement.**

1. **DoD and VA Response to IOM Recommendation 4**

Both DoD and VA are working actively to reduce stigma and encourage treatment for mental health and substance use disorders (SUDs). Some of the efforts are outlined below.

**Real Warriors Campaign**

DCoE launched the "Real Warriors, Real Battles, Real Strength" national public awareness campaign in May 2009, emphasizing that seeking help for psychological concerns is a sign of strength. Supporting initiatives have been implemented across the Services to target their individual cultures. To date, the campaign has produced eight Public Service Announcements (PSAs) that aired more than 4,000 times to 1.3 million Service members in 177 countries on the Armed Forces Radio and Television Service (AFRTS). PSAs have also aired domestically on 144 civilian national, regional, and local television networks and stations. Posters for the campaign have been displayed 254 military installations worldwide, and more than 90 organizations have collaborated with the campaign to further its reach. The campaign has been featured on CNN, NBC's Today Show, USA Today, Associated Press, and LA Times.

The Real Warriors Campaign Website (www.realwarriors.net) includes several unique features that help educate and connect Service members, Veterans, and their families to the resources they need to build resilience and access appropriate care for invisible wounds, including: 40 articles on a wide array of topics related to PH, handling deployments, and TBI; a live online chat feature; and online message boards where individuals can connect with others who have shared similar experiences.

**Screening, Brief Intervention, Referral and Treatment**

Another strategy to reduce stigma is the utilization of the Screening, Brief Intervention, Referral and Treatment (SBIRT) model to identify depression and PTSD in primary care clinics. If the Service member who is seeking care from his or her primary care clinic is identified via this mechanism, the treating physician would present the Service member to a care coordinator for screening and evaluation within the confines of the primary care venue. Substance use and abuse also may be addressed using the same methodology. The SBIRT model targets those with nondependent substance use and provides effective strategies for intervention prior to the need for more extensive or specialized treatment.

The model involves a system within community and/or medical settings, including physicians' offices, hospitals, educational institutions, and mental health centers. Screening determines the severity of substance use and identifies the appropriate level of intervention. The system provides for brief intervention or brief treatment within the community setting or motivates and refers those identified as needing more extensive services to a specialist for assessment, diagnosis, and appropriate treatment. Currently, the U.S. Army has 42 primary care clinics assessing and treating depression and PTSD and is in the process of expanding this primary care model. The Air Force and Navy have already integrated mental and primary health care.

**Education through Conferences**

Recently, the Center for the Study of Traumatic Stress (CSTS) hosted a conference on stigma, bringing together more than 100 national subject matter experts (SMEs) to discuss the current state of knowledge on stigma. SMEs from DoD, VA, and the civilian sector presented on current programs and research, and identified gaps. The conference highlighted stigma because of institutional, external, and internal cultural factors, all of which must be addressed to reduce stigma.

**Policy Review**

The Office of the Assistant Secretary of Defense (Health Affairs) is currently undertaking a systematic review of policies related to substance use treatment and confidentiality issues mandated by National Defense Authorization Act (NDAA) FY10 Section 596, "Comprehensive Plan on Prevention, Diagnosis, and Treatment of Substance Use Disorders and Disposition of Substance Abuse Offenders in the Armed Forces." Some extant policies have already been reviewed and endorsed by the Services.

There have been some relevant policy memoranda issued over the past several years. For example, a policy memorandum co-issued by the Under Secretaries of Defense for Intelligence and Personnel and Readiness and endorsed by DoD leadership including the Secretary of Defense resulted in the immediate revision of Question 21 of SF 86, "Questionnaire for National Security Positions," regarding prior mental health treatment. The revision explicitly excludes the reporting of counseling that was "strictly marital, family, grief not related to violence by you; or strictly related to adjustments from service in a military combat environment." These two reasons for seeking services address a substantial percentage of the reasons why a Service member might seek deployment-related counseling in the first place.

Perhaps more important than the specific questionnaire revisions was the language in the memorandum that indicated seeking care to mitigate adjustment difficulties was the responsible thing to do, and not doing so was less responsible. Similarly, "Policy Guidance for Deployment-Limiting Psychiatric Conditions and Medication," issued by the Assistant Secretary of Defense for Health Affairs in November 2006, indicates that seeking care is the appropriate/responsible action for a Service member to take. While recognizing that psychological fitness for duty in the context of deployment is very important and may entail higher levels of mental health status in general, the guidance indicates that deployment and psychiatric treatment (to include treatment with psychotropic medications) are not automatically and mutually exclusive

There have been policy enactments and actions that make available models of counseling that do not entail medical record keeping and are inherently more confidential (e.g., the Military OneSource program). A July 2009 DTM entitled "Command Notification Requirements to Dispel Stigma in Providing Mental Health Care to Military Personnel" (DTM 09-006) specifies those situations for which Command notification is not required. A DoDI will replace this DTM and provide additional guidance.

**Leadership Training**

The relationship between treatment seeking and military advancement is now an integral aspect of the Services' leadership training developed and implemented over the past several years. This training has a strong anti-stigma objective and theme. Again, an essential message is that seeking care for psychological difficulties is the responsible and courageous thing for Service members to do and should be strongly encouraged by all levels of leadership.

See Appendix F for a sample of VA research that is exploring the effects of stigma in the veteran population.

## *E. IOM Recommendation 5*

**The committee recommends that the Department of Defense formally assess whether a "third-location decompression" program would be beneficial for US combat troops. Third-location decompression has the potential to allow troops to have time to begin to readjust before returning home and to family responsibilities.**

### 1. DoD Response to IOM Recommendation 5

Third-Location Decompression (TLD) "refers to a process that is designed to allow Service personnel returning from deployment to adapt to the home environment in a graduated way, with the aim of reducing the potential for maladaptive psychological adjustment."[5] It has been used in multiple settings with varying results and, as noted in the IOM report, no published evidence exists that indicates the TLD process is effective. However, DoD and VA agree that TLD

---

[5] Hughes, J., Hacker, G.H., Earnshaw, N.M., Greenberg, N., Eldridge, R, Fear, N.T., French, C., Deahl, M.P., & Wessley, S. (June, 2008). Use of Psychological Decompression in Military Operational Environments, Military Medicine, p. 1. Downloaded 4/8/10 from http://findarticles.com/p/articles/mi_qa3912/is_200806/ai_n27995836/

programs are worthy of further study, to determine whether they do result in benefits for stress-exposed troops (e.g., improved social support, lower rates of PTSD). To this end, DoD will work to ensure analyses of TLD programs and potential benefits are included in research investment strategic plans and future funding opportunities in a way that leverages prior investments and ongoing studies.

### *F. IOM Recommendations 6, 7, and 8*

**Recommendation 6: The committee recommends that the Department of Defense, the Department of Veterans Affairs, and other federal agencies fund research on the social and economic effects of deployment and multiple deployments on families. For example, research should examine the effects of multiple deployments on domestic violence and maltreatment of children, as well as on financial well-being.**

**Recommendation 7: The committee recommends that the Department of Defense, the Department of Veterans Affairs, and other federal agencies fund studies to evaluate the effectiveness of mental health treatments currently being provided to women and to identify potential new treatments designed specifically to address women's unique circumstances and stressors, such as sexual harassment and assault, PTSD, and premilitary trauma.**

**Recommendation 8: The committee recommends that the Department of Defense, the Department of Veterans Affairs, and other federal agencies fund research on culturally sensitive treatment approaches targeted toward minorities. Research is also needed on utilization patterns of currently available services by minority populations and the efficacy of such services to improve health outcomes.**

#### 1. DoD Response to IOM Recommendations 6, 7, and 8

As discussed above, DoD has dedicated substantial resources to PH and TBI research, and recognizes that studies on families, women, and minorities are important components of its research program. Broad Agency Announcements (BAAs) (i.e., requests for proposals) reflect the explicit requirements of legislation and input from not only DoD SMEs, but also SMEs from the NIH, VA, and other federal agencies. Funded studies explore novel areas of research or build upon work done by other researchers.

These published BAAs include the following language, which is intended to ensure adequate consideration of families, women, and minorities in all appropriate research.

> "Priorities include interventions across the deployment lifecycle for warriors, Veterans, families, caregivers, and communities, particularly those at risk for mental disorders and psychosocial problems. Investigators are encouraged to take into account considerations for special populations, such as gender-specific or racial/ethnic groups as a focus. Consideration of Active Duty, Reserve Component, National Guard, and/or Veteran populations is also encouraged."[6]

Currently, more than $48.2 million in DoD funding is invested in 42 active studies focused on families, women, and/or minorities. Specifically

- More than $40.1 million is invested in research on families,
- More than $3.6 million is invested in research on the particular needs of women, and
- More than $2.4 million is invested in research on the needs of minority populations.

The DoD repeatedly re-evaluates the priority focus areas of its research portfolio in light of emerging knowledge, preliminary data from studies in progress, and previous investments, but studies of the specific needs of families, and female and/or minority Service members will remain a priority in future research investments.

A complete list of the studies reviewed appears in Appendix G. Note that some studies are included in more than one appendix.

### 2. VA Response to IOM Recommendations 6, 7, and 8

VA health care is provided only to Veterans and their families as it relates to the care of the Veteran. By advancing treatment and improving care for the individual Veteran, VA attempts to mitigate the issues faced by spouses and children. The health and well-being of the Veteran's family is, however, of vital concern to VA.

The overall research agenda is richly described in Conference Proceedings from the Trauma Spectrum Disorders Conference, 2009. The conference focused on the impact of military service on families and caregivers, with sponsorship by DCoE, NIH Office of Research on Women's Health, and VA Research.

Over 11 percent of OEF/OIF Veterans are women. VA Research supports a robust portfolio of studies related to women Veteran's health, including studies on diseases prevalent solely or predominantly in women, research focusing on women Veterans, and research addressing the goals of the Women Veterans Health Strategic Health Care Group's (WVHSHG) to develop a

---

6 FY09 PH/TBI Concept Award BAA, pg 2-3; W81XWH-09-PH/TBIRP-CA

comprehensive practice redesign to enhance primary care delivery for women, and redesign of primary care delivery to integrate gender-specific care (Yano, 2009).

The focus of VA-supported research on women Veterans, including those who served in the National Guard and Reserves as well as the regular military in past conflicts and OEF/OIF ranges widely, and includes

- Research aimed at improving the organization and quality of health care for women Veterans;
- Women-specific prevalence and treatment of PTSD;
- The impacts of deployment and military service on physical and mental health of women Veterans;
- Comorbid conditions such as substance use and PTSD among women Veterans;
- Access to mental health care and predictors of mental health care use by women Veterans;
- Special concerns of reintegration for women Veterans;
- Intimate partner violence among women Veterans; and
- The implementation and sustainability of VA's women's mental health clinics.

A brief description of many of these studies appears in Appendix H.

VA Research has been laying the groundwork for improved health care services to women Veterans and the development of effective programs and treatments to address the mental health needs and readjustment and reintegration issues related to service in Iraq and Afghanistan. Armed with a growing and comprehensive body of research, VA is prepared to take the next steps in transforming VA health care to women Veterans through a research program focused on intervention, implementation, and dissemination of best practices, especially regarding mental health care. Some of these studies have already been implemented and some completed. The current initiative includes

- An update of the systematic review of women Veterans' health literature, initially conducted in 2004, with a focus on post-deployment health and mental health issues (expected to be available in summer 2010);
- Another systematic review that focuses solely on mental health issues and treatments, including gender differences. This accumulated evidence will facilitate design of a treatment and outcome pilot and multi-center trial studies;;
- A Long Term Health Outcomes of Women's Service during the Vietnam Era, a comprehensive 3-year study of an anticipated 10,000 women to assess the prevalence of PTSD and other mental and physical health conditions for women Vietnam Veterans, and explore the relationships between PTSD and other conditions and the Vietnam

deployment experience. The study will include both VA users and women Vietnam Veterans who do not use VA for their health care, and will include both self-report, extensive survey, and medical record data. This large-scale study will help to explain relationships between stressful and traumatic experiences and mental and physical health outcomes in women Vietnam Veterans, and older women in general. It will also look at the relationship of these outcomes to disability and functioning. Knowledge from this study will help VA organize and offer its services, not only for these aging women Veterans, but for future generations of women Veterans as well;

- The first national survey of women Veterans since 1985, already fielded, is now providing VA with comprehensive data on health care needs and VA experiences, differences among cohorts of women Veterans by military era, and women Veterans' preferences and perceptions about access and quality. Approximately a third of the almost 3,500 survey respondents are OEF/OIF Veterans and their survey data indicates a higher need for mental health services, as well as higher utilization of services. The survey will provide important information to guide future efforts to improve outreach, access, and care of women Veteran;
- A field-based conference planned for July 2010 on "Building the Evidence Base to Improve Health Care and Outcomes for Women Veterans." One of the goals of the meeting is to foster methodological and other research advances in support of improving the quality and quantity of VA women's health research in high priority areas, with special emphasis on accelerating movement to interventions and implementation research. Post-deployment mental health is one of the areas of emphasis;
- A women Veterans' practice-based research network (PBRN) will provide a laboratory for examining new treatments, quality performance and quality improvements, models of care (e.g., integrated mental health and primary care), and provider education and training innovations. One of the initial planned studies will survey a representative sample of women Veterans, including OEF/OIF Veterans, to identify socioeconomic and health status and determine preferences for mental health interventions in primary care settings; and
- VA continues to work with DCoE, as well as various NIH offices (including the Office of Research on Women's Health) to explore and document the impact of trauma in the military on those who have served, as well as their families and caregivers, by sponsoring annual conferences addressing various issues related to trauma, evaluating the current evidence, and determining research gaps.

VA has devoted significant resources toward the reduction and elimination of health disparities in quality of care and health outcomes in VA, sponsoring special equity research solicitations since the late 1990s. As the largest national health care system, VA offers a unique opportunity to understand and analyze the complex reasons for disparities among different racial, ethnic, and minority populations. VA also offers the ideal setting in which to evaluate and implement patient-centered and culturally sensitive approaches to care that will meet the needs of diverse populations of Veterans and provide equitable access to quality health care.

VA has an extensive portfolio of research on disparities, and devotes significant resources and infrastructure to this area. VA funds a Center of Excellence for Health Equity Research and Promotion, which has a mission to reduce disparities and promote equity in health and health care among vulnerable groups of Veterans and other populations. VA also funds a Targeted Research Enhancement Program to understand racial and ethnic variations in health outcomes for chronic diseases (e.g., diabetes and hypertension), focusing on patient trust, patient preferences for care, and the incremental effect of patient-level factors on disparities in health outcomes.

A recent solicitation calls for the development and evaluation of interventional studies to reduce ethnic minority health care disparities, including interventions that address provider and patient beliefs and attitudes, patient preferences and knowledge that impact medical decision-making and access to or use of health services, patient-provider relationships, and system-wide or facility-specific policies and characteristics that can reduce variations in treatment or outcomes. VA also supports implementation research through VA QUERI, which works collaboratively with VA's Office of Quality and Performance (OQP), to translate the findings of disparities research into changes in clinical practice in VA's health care system.

In order to guide future VA research, deliver high-quality care in an equitable manner, and eliminate racial and ethnic disparities in health care, VA directed an Evidence-Based Synthesis Project (ESP) on racial and ethnic disparities in health care within VA to determine 1) the clinical areas in which racial and ethnic disparities are prevalent; 2) what is known about the sources of those disparities; and 3) synthesize that knowledge to determine the most promising areas for future research aimed at improving quality in VA health care.

The synthesis suggests that the reasons for disparities are complex and that variability in study settings and populations, clinical topics and services, data collection methods, and measures sometimes makes it difficult to generate unifying theories that are generalizable across settings and services. However, the review suggested a number of promising areas for future research, including: decision aids and information tools; patient activation interventions; patient-centered communication training; determining sources of variation in clinician judgment by patient race; interventions to promote evidence-based decision-making by providers; and adherence-support interventions (Saha, Freeman, Toure et al., 2008). VA continues to work with other federal agencies to advance research on disparities and minority health, including through the Federal Collaboration on Health Disparities Research, and also as part of ongoing efforts with the DCoE and NIH to improve treatment to OEF/OIF Service members, Veterans, and their families and caregivers.

## *G. IOM Recommendation 9*

**The committee recommends that Congress appropriate funds and direct the Department of Veterans Affairs to expand the role of its actuary to produce annual long-term forecasts of costs associated with all health and disability benefits that are consistent with the practices of Social Security and Medicare.**

### 1. VA Response to IOM Recommendation 9

VA's Office of the Actuary (OACT) provides long term projections of veteran population. The veteran population projection is used for VA's strategic planning (e.g., healthcare) and benefits valuations (e.g., disability). OACT is expanding its projections and advanced modeling activities to support VA strategic planning and policy improvement. All the actuarial projections follow actuarial standards of practice and are consistent with SSA, HHS and other government agency practices.

OACT maintains a model of future benefits for the compensation, pension and burial programs administered by the Veterans Benefits Administration (VBA). The model projects future cash flows, including the effect of Cost of Living Adjustments (COLA), for any future period up to a hundred years. The model covers current VA beneficiaries, as well as Veterans who will become beneficiaries in the future and those who have yet to separate from the military. The model is currently used for financial reporting. The model and the data inputs used for that purpose were audited in 2009 by the external accounting firm of Deloitte and Touche.

Since 1999, VHA has partnered with Milliman, Inc., a premier global actuarial and consulting firm, to develop and support a health care actuarial model to project demand for VA health care. VA's Enrollee Health Care Projection Model (Model) produces annual, 20-year projections of the number of Veterans expected to be enrolled in VA health care, their utilization of VA's health care services, and the expenditures associated with those services. The model methodology is consistent with actuarial principles and practices and accounts for the unique demographics of the Veteran enrollee population and VA health care delivery system.

Each year, VA assesses the expected demand for inpatient and ambulatory medical services based on its most recent experience for both VA and fee-based care provided to enrolled Veterans. Projections are updated to reflect the changing demographics of the enrolled Veteran population including factors such as aging, priority transition, and geographic migration. The methodology and assumptions used in the Model also are reviewed to ensure that the Model is projecting Veteran demand as accurately as possible. In addition, VA conducts a rigorous review to understand health care trends in VA, which may also affect the number of services and the expected cost of providing these services to enrolled Veterans. Some services, such as long-term care, are not included in the Model, which currently projects approximately 84 percent of VA medical care budget. Actions are underway to include non-modeled services, including long-term care.

VA has successfully collaborated with internal and external stakeholders to enhance the Model. For example, the annual Model update is done in active collaboration with myriad program offices to ensure the Model reflects VA's current health care delivery system, specific program initiatives to improve service delivery and access, and reflects VA's vision for its health care system in the future. VA currently has approximately 9.2 FTEE working on the Model and VA's consulting health actuary, Milliman, dedicates an estimated 8 FTEE to support the Model.

Since 2007, VHA's model estimates that portion of the Veteran population that represents the number of new OEF/OIF Veterans each year. Through discussion and collaboration with the Congressional Budget Office (CBO) and monitoring recent policy decisions by the administration, VA has revised its model to reflect the current deployment levels and strategy in support of OEF and OIF. This year's Model uses the same methodology to project OEF/OIF enrollment as the previous Model but reflects an updated OEF/OIF Veteran separation model. Experience supports an increase in the assumed number of Service members required to support a given deployment level. As a result, a given deployment level causes more Service members to be given OEF/OIF status than in the previous model and this leads to more unique OEF/OIF Veterans. In comparison with the 2009 model, the updated model projects more OEF/OIF Veterans.

VA's Enrollee Health Care Projection Model projects OEF/OIF Veteran enrollment and utilization apart from non-OEF/OIF Veterans and the Model is updated annually to reflect VA's most recent experience in terms of enrollment and utilization.

### *H. IOM Recommendation 10*

**The committee recommends that the Department of Defense and the Department of Veterans Affairs oversee coordination and communication of the multitude of programs that have been created in response to the needs of Operation Enduring Freedom and Operation Iraqi Freedom Service members, [V]eterans, and their family members in an effort to maximize their reach and effectiveness. The committee also recommends that there be independent evaluation of these programs with standardized evaluation designs and assessment of outcomes.**

#### 1. DoD Response to IOM Recommendation 10

DoD and VA continue to work together and with other federal, state, local, academic, and not-for-profit institutions to oversee the coordination and communication of the multitude of programs that have been created in response to OEF and OIF.

One ongoing effort is participation in the Federal Partners Priority Working Groups led by SAMHSA to leverage a wide range of professionals from federal partners in building an optimal model of programs and best practices dissemination strategy.

In a second effort, the agencies are harnessing technology and social media tools. The use of technology provides Service members and their families access to resources even in the most extreme and remote circumstances while maximizing reach and effectiveness.

The National Leadership Summit on Military Families provides a third example of collaboration, coordination, and communication. A partnership between the Military Community and Family Policy within the Office of the Secretary of Defense (OSD), the Department of Agriculture (USDA),[7] and the University of Maryland, the summit took place on November 9-10, 2009. Summit participants included senior military family policymakers, family program leaders and their staff, military family researchers, representatives from DoD, VA, all military Service components, and other non-governmental partners. Summit participants identified the following priorities

- Categorize and evaluate programs to enhance effectiveness, consistency, and return on investment,
- Develop and implement a strategic communications strategy that reaches Service members, Veterans, and their families with what they need to know, and connects them with those who have the capacity and resources to provide support, and
- Strengthen the ability of DoD and VA to provide for the psychological well-being of military personnel and their families.

DoD is addressing the coordinated outreach of programs through several other mechanisms. The Army and Marine Corps have established outreach and case management programs as well as Warrior Transition Units. The Office of the Assistant Secretary of Defense (Health Affairs) monitors and evaluates these programs to assess their applicability to other services and to ensure the continuum of care for Service members, Veterans, and their families as they navigate the system of care. In a similar effort, VA hired the Federal Recovery Coordinators to work in MTFs and other selected sites in the United States. The goal is to assist in the recovery, rehabilitation, and reintegration into the community of severely injured Service members who are unlikely to return to active duty.

---

[7] USDA's Cooperative Extension Service is a key education partner for military families.

Recovery care coordinators are part of the Services' wounded Warrior programs and also assist the Service members and their families as they navigate the continuum of care. The overall goal of transition and coordination of care is to improve quality of care, including rapid and effective information sharing to support the continuity of care. In order to synchronize department-wide transition efforts for our Service members, DoD stood up the Office of Transition Policy and Care Coordination (now called Wounded Warrior Care and Transition Policy) in October 2008. The goals for this office include ensuring equitable, consistent, and high-quality care coordination and transition support for members of the Armed Forces, including wounded Warriors and their families through appropriate interagency collaboration, responsive policy, and effective program oversight.

Clearly, there is a need for collaborative program evaluations that capture PH and TBI project and program effectiveness information and provide practical evidence to support collaboration and knowledge-sharing across the Services, DoD, and VA. Such evaluation will enable the Military Health System (MHS) to leverage project performance information to enhance care delivery for our Service members, Veterans, and their families. However, the challenge to date has been determining how to take advantage of the Services', DoD's, and VA's respective PH-TBI program portfolio evaluations in order to leverage existing data and reduce duplication. A second challenge is how to pursue a strategic analysis of the full DoD/VA portfolio in order to identify gaps in programs and services, and to collect and disseminate information on evidence-based practices and lessons learned.

As program evaluations can be initiated at different points in a project's lifecycle, it is important to gather additional information from stakeholders to identify what may drive an evaluation. For example, while still in its formative stages, DCoE proposed the development of an annual plan that systematically identifies innovative and necessary programs. This plan prioritizes how best to obligate finite staff and other resources, further evaluating those programs, and identifying important lessons learned across the Services. Furthermore, planning requires gathering sufficient information in order to gain an initial understanding of the projects, their current and planned focus, how they are organized, and where they are located. Finally, there may be specific stakeholder considerations that will further define the information gathering activities.

As these relevant programs are identified and begin to be evaluated, common metrics must be created. Desirable measures have three attributes: 1) importance (i.e., relevance to stakeholders, health importance, applicable to measuring equitable distribution of care, and potential for improvement), 2) scientific soundness (i.e., explicitness and strength of the evidence, reliability, and validity), and 3) feasibility (i.e., explicit definitions and count specifications for its components, and the availability of the data).

## 2. VA Response to IOM Recommendation 10

Over the past 3 years, DoD and VA have made a significant investment to improve the level of coordination and collaboration between the departments to meet the needs of OEF/OIF Service members, Veterans, and their families. The Departments established the Senior Oversight Committee (SOC), co-chaired by the Deputy Secretaries of both departments, to provide oversight of the many programs and policies established to assist wounded, ill, and injured Service members and Veterans. The SOC meets monthly to address issues related to improving the delivery of benefits and services. As an example, the SOC is currently providing oversight for the expansion of the DoD/VA Disability Evaluation System (DES) Pilot that was established to create a seamless, transparent, and joint disability evaluation system.

To support the efforts of the SOC within VA, the department created the Collaboration Service in October 2008. The mission of the Collaboration Service is to facilitate the development and oversight of joint policies and programs. DoD has created its own organizational structure as well through the Office of Wounded Warrior Care and Transition Policy and the Executive Secretariat under the Under Secretary of Defense (Personnel and Readiness). The level of oversight provided by this new infrastructure has improved the level of coordination between the departments and consequently improved the reach and effectiveness of programs and services created in response to the needs of returning Service members.

VA meets its statutory mandate to evaluate its programs using standardized evaluation designs to collect and analyze data in the assessment of outcomes. VA program evaluations are conducted by independent third parties and follow systematic research designs to ensure that final outcome data are valid and reliable.

VA is currently conducting a 4-year multi-million dollar program evaluation study on mental health services and outcomes in the VHA for Veterans with PTSD, schizophrenia, major depression, bipolar disorder, and substance use disorder, with a particular emphasis on OEF/OIF Veterans. This program evaluation specifically addresses the number and distribution of mental health professionals needed to provide treatment to Veterans returning with PTSD, major depression and substance use disorder through a survey of all VA facilities conducted in May 2007 and again in late 2009. The use of evidence-based treatments, particularly for PTSD, is a focus of the Mental Health study. The evaluation has identified 114,000 OEF/OIF Veterans who received care for the five study diagnoses during FY 04-08. Their utilization of care, outcomes, and costs are being evaluated.

Coordination of care and communication between DoD and VA is essential when transitioning severely ill and injured Service members from DoD to VA's system of care. VA Liaisons for Health Care, strategically placed in MTFs with concentrations of recovering Service members returning from Afghanistan and Iraq, are critical to this process. VA has 33 social worker or nurse VA Liaisons stationed at 18 MTFs to facilitate the transfer of Service members and Veterans from the MTF to a VA health care facility closest to the Veteran's home or most appropriate for the specialized services required. These Liaisons have greatly improved the communication between VA and DoD and enhanced the coordination of care as Service members transition from active duty to Veteran status.

VA Liaisons are co-located with DoD Case Managers at MTFs for onsite consultation and collaboration regarding VA resources and treatment options. VA Liaisons educate Service members and their families about VA's system of care, coordinate the Service member's initial registration with VA, and secure outpatient appointments or inpatient transfer to a VA health care facility as appropriate. VA Liaisons make early connections with Service members and families to promote a positive relationship with VA.

In addition, each VA Medical Center has an OEF/OIF Care Management team in place to coordinate patient care activities and ensure that Service members and Veterans are receiving patient-centered, integrated care and benefits. Members of the OEF/OIF Care Management Program team include: a program manager, clinical case managers, a VBA Veterans service representative, and a transition patient advocate. The program manager, who is either a nurse or social worker, has overall administrative and clinical responsibility for the team and ensures that Service members and Veterans receive case management services if needed. Clinical case managers, also either nurses or social workers, coordinate patient care activities and ensure that all clinicians providing care to the patient are doing so in a cohesive and integrated manner. VBA team members assist Veterans by educating them about VA benefits and assisting with the benefit application process. The transition patient advocate assists the Veteran and family in navigating VA's system of care.

All severely ill and injured OEF/OIF Service members and Veterans receiving care at VA are provided a case manager. All others are screened for case management needs and, based upon the assessment; a case manager is assigned as indicated. The patient and family serve as integral partners in the assessment and treatment care plan. Since many of the returning OEF/OIF Veterans connect to more than one specialty care system, VA introduced a new concept of a "lead" case manager. The lead case manager now serves as a central communication point for the patient and family. Case managers maintain regular contact with Veterans and their families to provide support and assistance to address any health care and psychosocial needs that may arise. To improve communication and coordination internally, a multi-disciplinary Care Management Review Team oversees coordination of patient care activities and integration of services.

## III. Conclusion

The Secretary of Defense and the Secretary of Veterans Affairs agree with most of the recommendations of the IOM report and, as noted, have many projects underway to address the issues raised. We look forward to the phase 2 study, a comprehensive assessment of the physical and mental health and other adjustment needs of Service members and former members who deployed in OEF/OIF and the families of these Service members as a result of such deployment (P.L. 110-181). Among the minimum requirements for the Phase 2 requirement outlined in the legislation, DoD and VA are particularly interested in new information on

- An assessment of the particular impacts of multiple deployments;
- An assessment of the full scope of effects of TBI and the efficacy of current treatment approaches;
- An estimate of the long-term costs associated with "undiagnosed" injuries such as PTSD and mild traumatic brain injury (mTBI); and
- "Recommendations for programs, treatments, or policy remedies targeted at preventing, minimizing, or addressing the impacts, gaps, and needs identified."

# IV. Appendices

## *Appendix A (IOM Recommendation 1): Rigorous DoD Studies on Readjustment Needs*

| Title | Amount | Synopsis |
|---|---|---|
| Understanding Resilience in Wounded Warriors and Their Families | $264,778 | Examine the natural course of wounded Warrior family functioning. Determine major stressors, family resiliency factors, risk factors related to decreased family functioning, and the impact of clinical intervention to improve family functioning of wounded Warriors. Develop and validate a needs assessment screening tool for supportive services referral. |
| Addressing the Needs of Children and Families of Combat Injured | $497,584 | Identify immediate and progressive impact of parental combat injury on child, parent and family functioning. Evaluate post-traumatic combat injury impact in five major clinical categories of child and family function: 1) acute child and parent traumatic stress symptoms; 2) levels of parental efficacy (e.g., emotional availability, disciplinary style); 3) parent-child communication; 4) alterations to family schedule and structure; and 5) long-term impact of injury on child, parent, and family function. |
| National Warfighter Health and Sustainment Study: Implement Family Member Assessment Component in the Millennium Cohort Study (Family Cohort Study) | $10,000,000 | Examine association between deployment stressors and adverse behavioral and related health outcomes for spouses and children of deployed service members. Add a 2010 family impact component to the Millennium Cohort Study. Assess spouse perceptions of deployment stressors, current mental health status, spouse's perception of mental health and related symptoms of their children and quality of family relationships. |
| Family Maltreatment, Substance Problems, and Suicidality: Prevalence Surveillance and Ecological Risk/Protective Factors Models | $952,491 | Derive and validate an innovative public health surveillance Air Force (AF) wide system for family maltreatment, suicidality, and problematic alcohol/drug use. A biennial survey of individual, family, workplace, and community functioning along with a supplement specifically designed to assess secretive problems will be given to AF members and spouses worldwide. Develop complex statistical algorithms to estimate secretive problems from data sets. |
| A Longitudinal Study of the Impact of Combat Deployments on Military Personnel and Their Families | $900,189 | Examine the role of family adjustment and support in promoting resilience among military personnel following combat deployments; model the longitudinal course of adjustment over the course of the deployment cycle using state-of-the-art data analytic techniques. Evaluations will begin about 1 month prior to deployment and continue approximately every 4 months following. Approximately 500 deploying military service members and their spouses will participate. |

*Appendix A (IOM Recommendation 1): Rigorous DoD Studies on Readjustment Needs CONTINUED*

| Title | Amount | Synopsis |
|---|---|---|
| Case for Support: Children of Military Fathers with PTSD | $1,700,000 | Compare the wellbeing of military children who have fathers with PTSD with children whose fathers do not have PTSD to examine the relationship between parental PTSD and anxiety disorders and depression in children. A two-group comparison study, nested within a large randomly selected United Kingdom (UK) military cohort of the children's wellbeing as measured by the Strengths and Difficulties Questionnaire (SDQ). The two groups are children with fathers with PTSD and children with fathers without PTSD. |
| Land Combat Study | $1,015,000 | Determine the effects of combat operations in Iraq and Afghanistan on mental health and physical functioning of Soldiers and families. Continue work to 1) determine the risk factors for mental health problems (e.g., combat, deployment length and frequency, and operational stressors) and determine predictors of resetting; 2) identify factors that improve mental health and well-being (e.g., good leadership, unit cohesion, social support, and individual background); 3) identify ways to reduce mental health stigma and barriers which hinder access to care; and 4) identify relationship between mild TBI, PTSD, and physical health problems post-deployment. Survey active and reserve component Soldiers from Brigade Combat Teams (BCTs) in a repeated cross-sectional and longitudinal design. |
| Family-Based Intervention with Traumatized Service Members and Their Young Children | $1,583,843 | Describe the interplay between returning service member PTSD symptoms and reintegration, including the parent-child relationship and parenting role. Develop and pilot an evidence-based family intervention addressing trauma impact on the parent-child relationship for families in which the returning member parent has PTSD and a child less than 5 years. Conduct an RCT with pre-, post-, and 6-month follow up assessments. |

*Appendix A (IOM Recommendation 1): Rigorous DoD Studies on Readjustment Needs CONTINUED*

| Title | Amount | Synopsis |
|---|---|---|
| Parental Stress, PTSD, and Infant Health Outcomes in U.S. Military Families | $202,990 | Study to 1) Identify the prevalence of adverse reproductive health outcomes among infants born to parents who are participants in the Millennium Cohort Study (MCS); 2) evaluate the occurrence of these adverse reproductive health outcomes in relation to parental PTSD symptoms and diagnosis; and 3) identify how temporal differences in parental stress, in particular PTSD, and pregnancy onset impact reproductive health outcomes. The primary study population will include all infants born to service members who are participants in the MCS. Self-reported data from the MCS, including occupational exposures, and demographic and behavioral characteristics are supplemented with objective data on occupation, deployments, and healthcare utilization. These data will be linked to birth and infant health information obtained from the DoD Birth and Infant Health Registry, a database that captures all inpatient and outpatient healthcare data on all infants born to military families, and has been validated to define birth defects and preterm births. A complementary analysis will evaluate infant health among women exposed to the acute stress of 11 September 2001 during pregnancy. |
| Development of a PTSD Population Registry | $954,935 | Develop and implement registry of combat-exposed men and women with PTSD to identify clinical characteristics, risk factors, and co-morbidities of PTSD, including disparities by gender, race/ethnicity, and socioeconomic status; evaluate neuropsychological and psychosocial outcomes; and evaluate treatment trajectories and outcomes in a sample of combat-exposed Veterans |
| Understanding Psychological Recovery through Resilience Army National Guard Veterans | $429,114 | Investigate psychosocial resiliency and recovery processes in Army National Guard Soldiers returning from OEF and OIF. The study aims to reduce the occurrence of combat-related PTSD and other psychological disorders, such as depression and substance abuse. The study will examine psychologically well-adjusted soldiers to identify psychosocial factors that contribute to successful redeployment adjustment and reintegration into their communities. Through both qualitative and quantitative methods, the study will attempt to identify factors in soldiers' individual positive coping strategies, military leadership, and family and community support systems. |

*Appendix A (IOM Recommendation 1): Rigorous DoD Studies on Readjustment Needs CONTINUED*

| Title | Amount | Synopsis |
|---|---|---|
| Epidemiological Study of Mild Traumatic Brain Injury Sequelae Caused by Blast Exposure During Operations Iraqi Freedom and Enduring Freedom | $1,604,313 | Identify proportion of service members experiencing blast events that develop persisting symptoms. Identify multiple predictive factors for developing post-concussion syndrome (PCS) after blast-related mTBI (presence of retrograde and/or anterograde amnesia). Describe blast-induced mTBI objective cognitive and neurophysical impairments on various measures. Examine whether Service members with PCS after blast-induced mTBI show symptom improvement over time with current standard of care treatment, but have significant long-term disability. |
| Reintegrating Troops with Mild Traumatic Brain Injury (mTBI) into Their Communities: Understanding the Scope and Timeline of Post-Deployment Driving Problems | $208,463 | Determine extent to which combat driving behaviors are carried over into post-deployment driving on American roads by Troops with and without mTBI; separate driving behaviors associated with military service from those associated with mTBI or deployment to OEF/OIF; and establish military respondents' self-recognition of driving behaviors relative to an informed third party report. |
| Longitudinal Risk and Resilience Factors Predicting Psychiatric Disruption, Mental Health Service Utilization, and Military Retention in OIF National Guard | $787,176 | Identify prospective psychosocial predictors of military retention and attrition by assessing pre-deployment, deployment, and post-deployment levels of mental health disruptions, mental health service utilization, and important individual and organizational risk and resiliency factors. |

*Appendix B (IOM Recommendation 1): Rigorous VA Studies on Readjustment Needs*

| Title | Synopsis |
|---|---|
| CSP #256, "Contribution of Emotionally Traumatic Events and Inheritance to the Report of Current Physical Health Problems in 4042 Vietnam Era Veteran Twin Pairs" | The Vietnam Era Twin Registry consists of over 7,000 male twin pairs born between 1939 and 1957 with both brothers having served in the United States military during the Vietnam War. This study was designed to determine the contributions of psychological trauma (exposure to combat during the Vietnam War), genetic factors, childhood experiences shared by twin siblings, and unmeasured experiences not shared by twin siblings to the reporting of current physical health problems a mean of 19 years after military service |
| CSP #470, "A Randomized, Multi-Center, Controlled Trial of Multi-Modal Therapy in Veterans With Gulf War Illnesses" | Determine if multi-modal therapy will significantly improve clinical outcomes in Veterans with Gulf War illnesses. The primary endpoint is the proportion of patients improved at one year relative to baseline on the Physical Component Summary (PCS) scale of the Veterans Short Form 36 (SF-36V) questionnaire. |
| CSP #475, "Persian Gulf - Antibiotic Treatment Trial of Gulf War Veterans' Illnesses" | Randomized placebo-controlled trial to determine whether a 1-year course of doxycycline treatment in deployed Gulf War Veterans with illnesses (GWVI) and testing as Mycoplasma species positive will improve their overall functional status as measured by the PCS of the SF-36V questionnaire. |
| CSP #494, "A Randomized Clinical Trial of Cognitive-Behavioral Treatment for PTSD in Women" | This completed study found a psychotherapeutic approach to be advantageous in women Veterans suffering from PTSD, and was specifically cited by the IOM as fulfilling the requirement for methodological rigor in trials (IOM Report on PTSD Treatment Effectiveness). |
| CSP #500, "An Epidemiological Investigation Into the Occurrence of Amyotrophic Lateral Sclerosis (ALS) Among Gulf War Veterans" | Epidemiologic investigation into the occurrence of ALS among Veterans of the Gulf War This study will further define the epidemiology of this neurological disease among younger individuals while determining whether there is a higher than expected occurrence. |
| CSP #500A, "National Registry of Veterans With Amyotrophic Lateral Sclerosis" | In response to concern about the development of ALS among Veterans of the U.S. armed forces, particularly Gulf War Veterans, the Department of Veterans Affairs established a national registry of Veterans with ALS. This Registry will identify living Veterans with ALS, track the progression of their disease, and serve as a vehicle to facilitate study of epidemiological risk factors for ALS in a military context. |
| CSP #504, "Risperidone Treatment for Military Service Related Chronic Post-Traumatic Stress Disorder" | Examine the effects of antipsychotics on PTSD, after other treatments for PTSD have failed. This study is large, with multi-site trials |

*Appendix B (IOM Recommendation 1): Rigorous VA Studies on Readjustment Needs CONTINUED*

| Title | Synopsis |
|---|---|
| CSP #519, "Integrating Practice Guidelines for Smoking Cessation Into Mental Health Care for PTSD" | Study the complexities of integrated care for smoking cessation and PTSD. Subject follow-up has been completed and the study is now in the data analysis phase. The primary study objective is to conduct a prospective, randomized controlled clinical trial that compares the effectiveness of two approaches for delivering smoking cessation treatment for Veterans with PTSD. An approach in which smoking cessation treatment is integrated into mental health care for PTSD and delivered by mental health providers (experimental condition) will be compared to specialized smoking cessation clinic referrals (VA's usual standard of care). Results are anticipated late in 2010. |
| CSP #535, "Anabolic Steroid Therapy on Pressure Ulcer Healing in Persons With Spinal Cord Injury" | Test whether the use of oxandralone, an anabolic steroid, can heal pressure ulcers in persons with spinal cord injury. Following a feasibility study, all sites will participate in a blind randomized treatment study. A total of 400 patients will be enrolled over a 4-year period. |
| CSP #556, "[Repetitive transcranial magnetic stimulation (rTMS)] in Depression" | Evaluate the efficacy, safety, durability of benefits and cost-effectiveness of repetitive transcranial magnetic stimulation in the resolution of treatment-resistant major depression (TRMD) with emphasis on the unique VA population of depressed patients that are commonly co-morbid for substance abuse and/or PTSD. |
| CSP #563, "Prazosin and Combat Trauma PTSD (PACT)" | Currently enrolling participants, the primary objective is to demonstrate in a large multi-site placebo-controlled trial in Veterans with war zone trauma-induced PTSD that prazosin is efficacious for PTSD trauma nightmares, sleep disturbance, and global clinical status. A secondary objective is to demonstrate prazosin's effectiveness for these outcome measures during clinically meaningful long-term (26-week) maintenance treatment of PTSD. |
| CSP #566, "Neuropsychological and Mental Outcomes of Operation Iraqi Freedom (OIF): A Longitudinal Cohort Study" | Considered a landmark longitudinal effort, this study is directed to the population of OIF Veterans. This study was the first to use a prospective longitudinal design for assessing neurocognitive performance prior to deployment to Iraq. The incorporation of a prospective pre-, post-deployment design provides a powerful tool that will help explicate changes related to military service. This study has just initiated another long-term follow up phase. Since the successful launch of CSP #566, other non-CSP studies have also begun to use the repeated assessment approach in different cohorts. One of these, VA's Marine Resiliency Study, adds the unique contribution of including physiological measures, which may define some objective biological markers. |

*Appendix B (IOM Recommendation 1): Rigorous VA Studies on Readjustment Needs CONTINUED*

| Title | Synopsis |
|---|---|
| CSP #569, "Twin Study of the Course and Consequences of PTSD in Vietnam Era Veterans" | Study to: 1) estimate the longitudinal course and current prevalence of PTSD; 2) identify the relationships between the longitudinal course of PTSD and Veterans' current mental and physical health conditions e.g., cardiovascular disease, diabetes, depression, and substance use disorders); and 3) identify the relationships between PTSD and Veterans' current functional status and disability. |
| CSP #575, "PTSD [Genome-wide Association Studies (GWAS)] of OEF/OIF Deployed Military Personnel: Phase 1" | Study genetic factors related to PTSD in OEF/OIF Veterans randomly selected from the entire DoD manpower roster. |
| CSP #579, "Long Term Health Outcomes of Women's Service During the Vietnam Era" | Determine the current physical and mental health status of Vietnam women Veterans. Information gleaned from this effort is expected to inform our understanding of contemporary generations. |
| CSP #585, "Gulf War Illness GWAS" - Planned | Study genetic factors related to Gulf War Illness. |
| CSP #717B, "Prospective Cohort Study of Respiratory Function and Illness in Chronic [Spinal Cord Injury (SCI)]" | Prospective cohort study of respiratory function and illness in spinal cord injury. |
| CSP #723D, "Olfactory Functioning in Gulf War Veterans" | Assess possible neurotoxic sequelae of Gulf War participation, olfactory identification performance, neurocognitive functioning, health perceptions, and emotional distress in 72 Veterans. |

## *Appendix C (IOM Recommendation 2): VA Long-term Management Studies*

| Title | Synopsis |
|---|---|
| TBI Screening and Evaluation | All eligible OEF/OIF Veterans who receive medical care within the Veterans Health Administration (VHA) are screened for possible TBI. Those whose screening suggests they may have sustained a TBI are offered further evaluation and treatment by clinicians with expertise in TBI. This study will determine the clinical validity and reliability of VA's TBI Clinical Reminder and Comprehensive TBI Evaluation. |
| Clinical Tracking Form (CTF) Study | VA is collaborating with the DVBIC on this study of individuals who have been diagnosed with TBI while in the military service. The study evaluates enrolled subjects at both DoD and VA sites at 6 months, 12 months, and annually, up to 10 years after enrollment. VA and DVBIC will also collaborate on a more extensive 15-year follow-up study. |
| Neurorehabilitation: Neurons to Networks" Center of Excellence at the Houston VA Medical Center (VAMC) | Study to: 1) improve the diagnosis of mild to moderate TBI using structural and functional neuroimaging; and 2) measure the process and outcome of state-of-the art rehabilitation techniques with validated assessment tools. |
| Translational Research Center for TBI and Stress Disorders" at the Boston VAMC | Center focused on research leading to innovations in the diagnosis and treatment of Veterans with mTBI and stress-related emotional disorders such as PTSD. This includes systematic study of the impact of TBI on the efficacy of exposure-based cognitive therapies for PTSD. |
| VA Rehabilitation Research and Development Service (VA RR&D) studies using advanced technology | Innovative studies using advanced technology aimed at improving the diagnosis and treatment of TBI-related deficits. This includes the development and application of improved methods for both structural and functional imaging of the brain using magnetic resonance imaging (MRI) and diffusion tensor imaging (DTI). This research to better "map" the brain changes associated with TBI is leading to a better understanding of the biology of long-term TBI-related deficits and development of more effective evidence-based rehabilitation strategies. VA researchers in San Francisco have developed a computer-assisted intervention to improve selective attention among Veterans with TBI. They are using Functional MRI to track actual improvements in brain function associated with the intervention. |
| Blast-Related Health Problem Identification and Polytrauma Taxonomy at the Polytrauma Center at the Tampa VAMC | Investigate the epidemiology of the less visible complications of polytrauma blast injury (e.g., ear trauma and resultant hearing loss, concussion and resultant cognitive and vestibular deficits, and PTSD). |

| Title | Synopsis |
|---|---|
| Five service-directed projects for research projects examining the quality, usefulness, and potential improvement of VA's screening for TBI | Inform policy and practice involving the instrument used to screen all OEF/OIF Veterans, the processes used for clinical follow-up, clinical co-morbidity (particularly psychiatric), clinical outcomes, health care utilization, and costs. VA's Health Services Research and Development Service PT/BRI QUERI initiative focuses on filling gaps and implementing research to improve health outcomes for two high priority and prevalent blast-related injuries that occur in the context of other combat injuries: TBI and traumatic amputation. |
| Co-morbidity studies for possible links to TBI. | High-risk/high incidence complications include TBI-induced visual dysfunction and psychological health related to TBI. This study seeks to determine if visual dysfunctions are associated with mTBI, PTSD, or both. |
| Prevalence of psychological health issues and mTBI in the National Guard population. | Investigate the effects mTBI and PTSD co-morbidities on post-deployment outcomes. The primary objectives of this study were to describe the scope of mTBI/PTSD co-morbidity among returning National Guard OIF Veterans and to identify the extent to which these problems affected Veterans' psychosocial functioning, physical health, and quality of life over time. |
| Studies to determine the effectiveness of goal management training (GMT) in Veterans who have been diagnosed with mTBI. | Those with mTBI typically are employed and need the freedom in their therapy sessions that GMT offers. To meet the current needs of VA's treatment team and the mTBI population, these interventions could be administered via telemedicine and/or group sessions. |
| Developing a program of tinnitus management for Veterans | Components include: 1) online tinnitus training for VA audiologists; 2) a patient education book that provides detailed instructions for Veterans on self-managing tinnitus; 3) specialized presentations for group education sessions; 4) a patient counseling guide for use by clinicians; and 5) all supporting materials to conduct this program. A randomized clinical trial will evaluate the efficacy of this program compared to "usual care." |
| Health Care Use and Costs of Veterans with Neurotrauma | Determine the proportion of Veterans with neurotrauma who utilize VA health care services who are Medicare users, Medicaid users, and VA-only users; to describe characteristics of VA-only users and users of two or more systems; and to describe health care utilization, setting, and cost of VA, Medicare, and Medicaid services for eligible VA users. The secondary objective is to compare the patterns of health care use and costs of Veterans with neurotrauma who obtained their injuries during OEF/OIF with those of other Veterans with neurotrauma. |

*Appendix C (IOM Recommendation 2): VA Long-term Management Studies CONTINUED*

| Title | Synopsis |
|---|---|
| Gainesville VAMC study of access to rehabilitation services for returning OEF/OIF Veterans with traumatic injury. | Explore access to rehabilitation in the VHA Polytrauma System of Care and identified areas in which returning Veterans with traumatic injury were outside of reasonable drive time. |
| James Haley VAMC Telerehabilitiation study | Assess the utility of services provided to Veterans discharged from the Level 1 Polytrauma/Blast Related Injury Center at the Tampa VAMC with a diagnosis of mild and moderate TBI incurred in combat theaters. The program is rendered with assistive technology and home environmental modifications, together with providing needed medical care via telehealth. |
| Assisted Living Project | A 5-year pilot program to assess the effectiveness of providing assisted living (AL) services to eligible Veterans with moderate to severe functional disabilities due to TBI Outcome data on Veteran health status, quality of life, patient and family satisfaction with care, and the related impact and cost of providing AL services to eligible Veterans with TBI will be collected over the period of the pilot which is scheduled to run through June 30, 2013 |
| Neurobiology of Suicide Risk in Traumatic Brain Injury and Substance Abuse | Building on existing neurobiologic models of frontal function, study will extend our understanding of TBI related brain changes by applying functional MRI and diffusion tensor imaging techniques. Accordingly, we will examine blood oxygen level dependent signal changes within the cingulate and dorsolateral prefrontal cortices as well as the amygdala in TBI subjects, with and without a history of substance abuse, to characterize the nature of these patterns of signal change (higher/lower) in relation to healthy control subjects. |
| Rehabilitation Strategies to Reduce Violence and Anger in TBI and PTSD | Protocol to: 1) identify risk and protective factors empirically related to violent behavior among Veterans who have returned from Iraq and Afghanistan; 2) examine the link between specific factors related to violence among Veterans from previous conflicts and post-deployment violence risk among Iraq and Afghanistan Veterans, especially work status, PTSD, substance use disorder, and TBI; and 3) develop an evidence-based risk assessment instrument to administer to Iraq and Afghanistan Veterans in order to identify those most in need of services. |
| Understanding and Meeting the Needs of Informal Caregivers to Improve Outcomes for Traumatic Brain Injury Patients with Polytrauma | Pilot to inform participant recruitment strategies and aid in questionnaire development for the main survey study. |

## *Appendix D (IOM Recommendation 2): VA Conference Presentations and Publications*

| Reference |
|---|
| Goodrich, G.L., Arditi, A., Rubin, G., Keeffe, J., & Legge, G. The low vision timeline: An interactive history. Paper presented at: International Society for Low Vision Research and Rehabilitation Annual Conference; 2008 Jul 9; Montréal, Canada. |
| Brahm, K., Shen, M., Goodrich, G., Katsaros, J., Kirby, J., & Wilgenburg, H. Low vision eccentric viewing training: Computer vs. CCTV model. Paper presented at: International Society for Low Vision Research and Rehabilitation Annual Conference; 2008 Jul 7; Montréal, Canada. |
| Goodrich, G.L. Blasts, Brain Injury, and Vision. Paper presented at: International Society for Low Vision Research and Rehabilitation Annual Conference; 2008 Jul 7; Montréal, Canada. |
| Goodrich, G.L. Low vision services: Evolution in a time of revolution? Paper presented at: International Society for Low Vision Research and Rehabilitation Annual Conference; 2008 Jul 7; Montréal, Canada. |
| Wilgenburg, H.M., Goodrich, G., Brahm, K., Kirby, J., & Ingalla, S. Visual findings associated with traumatic brain injury in military personnel. Paper presented at: International Society for Low Vision Research and Rehabilitation Annual Conference; 2008 Jul 7; Montréal, Canada. |
| Polusny, M.A., Erbes, C.R., Arbisi, P.A., Thuras, P., Kehle, S.M., Rath, M., Courage, C., Reddy, M.K., & Duffy, C. Impact of prior Operation Enduring Freedom/Operation Iraqi Freedom combat duty on mental health in a predeployment cohort of National Guard soldiers. Mil Med. 2009 Apr; 174 (4):353-7. PubMed PMID: 19485103. |
| Ferrier-Auerbach, A.G., Kehle, S.M., Erbes, C.R., Arbisi, P.A., Thuras, P, & Polusny, M.A. Predictors of alcohol use prior to deployment in National Guard Soldiers. Addict Behav. 2009 Aug; 34 (8):625-31. Epub 2009 Apr 1. PubMed PMID: 19375239. |
| Ferrier-Auerbach, A.G., Erbes, C.R., Polusny, M.A., Rath, C.M., & Sponheim, S.R. Predictors of emotional distress reported by soldiers in the combat zone. J Psychiatr Res. 2009 Nov 25. [Epub ahead of print] PubMed PMID: 19939409. |
| Kehle, S.M., Polusny, M.A., Murdoch, M., Erbes, C.R., Arbisi, P.A., Thuras, P., & Meis, L.A. Early mental health treatment-seeking among U.S. National Guard soldiers deployed to Iraq. J Trauma Stress. 2010 Feb; 23 (1):33-40. PubMed PMID: 20104591. |
| Carter-Visscher, R., Polusny, M.A., Murdoch, M., Thuras, P., Erbes, C.R., & Kehle, S.M. Predeployment gender differences in stressors and mental health among U.S. National Guard troops poised for OIF deployment. J Trauma Stress. 2010 Feb; 23 (1):78-85. PubMed PMID: 20135681. |
| Cowper Ripley, D.C., Reker, D.M., Vogel, W.B., Hayes, J.M., Beyth, R.J., Litt, E., Dewald, L., Wang, X., & Wu, S.S. Geographic Access to VHA Rehabilitation Services by OEF/OIF Veterans. Paper presented at: VA HSR&D National Meeting; 2008 Feb 15; Baltimore, MD. |

## *Appendix E (IOM Recommendation 3): Vet Center and Mobile Vet Center Locations*

| State/Territory | Location |
|---|---|
| Alaska | Anchorage; Fairbanks; Kenai; Wasilla |
| Alabama | Birmingham; Huntsville; Mobile; Montgomery |
| American Samoa | Pago Pago |
| Arkansas | Fayetteville*; Little Rock |
| Arizona | Chinle**; Mesa; Mohave County; Phoenix; Prescott*; Tucson; Yuma; |
| California | Antelope Valley; Bakersfield; Chico; Chula Vista; Citrus Heights; Concord; Corona*; East Los Angeles; Eureka; Fresno*; High Desert; Los Angeles; Modesto; North Orange County; Northbay; Oakland; Peninsula; Redwoods**; Sacramento; San Bernardino; San Diego; San Francisco; San Jose; San Luis Obispo; San Marcos; Santa Cruz County*; Sepulveda; South Orange County; Temecula; Ventura; West Los Angeles |
| Colorado | Boulder; Colorado Springs*; Denver; Grand Junction; Pueblo |
| Connecticut | Fairfield; Hartford; New Haven; Norwich |
| District of Columbia | Washington |
| Delaware | Sussex County; Wilmington |
| Florida | Bay County; Broward County; Clearwater; Collier; Daytona Beach; Fort Lauderdale; Fort Myers; Gainesville; Jacksonville; Jupiter; Lake County; Marion County; Melbourne; Miami; Okaloosa; Orlando*; Palm Beach; Pasco County; Pensacola*; Polk County; Sarasota; St. Petersburg; Tallahassee*; Tampa |
| Georgia | Atlanta; Lawrenceville; Macon*; Marietta; Muskogee County; Richmond County; Savannah |
| Guam | Hagatna |
| Hawaii | Hilo; Honolulu; Kailua-Kona; Kauai; Maui; Western Oahu; **Iowa;** Cedar Rapids; Des Moines; Sioux City |
| Idaho | Boise*; Pocatello |
| Illinois | Aurora; Chicago; Chicago Heights; East St. Louis; Evanston; Oak Park; Orland Park; Peoria; Quad Cities; Springfield* |
| Indiana | Evansville; Fort Wayne; Gary Area; Indianapolis; St. Joseph County |
| Kansas | Manhattan; Wichita* |
| *** = Vet Center and Mobile Vet Center site; ** = Mobile Vet Center site** | |

## *Appendix E (IOM Recommendation 3): Vet Center and Mobile Vet Center Locations CONTINUED*

| State/Territory | Location |
|---|---|
| Kentucky | Lexington*; Louisville |
| Louisiana | Baton Rouge; New Orleans*; Rapides; Shreveport |
| Massachusetts | Boston; Brockton; Hyannis; Lowell; New Bedford; Springfield*; Worcester |
| Maryland | Annapolis; Baltimore; Baltimore County; Cambridge; Elkton; Prince Georges County; Silver Spring |
| Maine | Bangor; Caribou*; Lewiston*; Portland; Sanford |
| Michigan | Dearborn; Detroit; Escanaba*; Grand Rapids; Macomb County; Pontiac; Saginaw; Traverse County |
| Minnesota | Minneapolis/ Brooklyn Park**; Brooklyn Park; Duluth; St. Paul Vet Center |
| Missouri | Boone County; Kansas City; Springfield; St. Louis |
| Mississippi | Biloxi; Jackson |
| Montana | Billings*; Cascade County; Flathead County; Missoula* |
| North Carolina | Charlotte; Fayetteville; Greensboro; Greenville*; Onslow County; Raleigh |
| North Dakota | Fargo*; Minot* |
| Nebraska | Lincoln*; Omaha |
| New Hampshire | Berlin; Manchester |
| New Jersey | Bloomfield; Toms River; Secaucus; Trenton; Ventnor |
| New Mexico | Albuquerque; Farmington; Las Cruces*; Santa Fe* |
| New York | Albany; Babylon; Binghamton; Bronx; Brooklyn; Buffalo; Harlem; Hicksville; Manhattan; Middletown; Queens; Rochester; Staten Island; Syracuse; Watertown*; White Plains |
| Nevada | Henderson; Las Vegas; Reno |
| Ohio | Cincinnati; Cleveland; Columbus; Dayton*; Parma; Starks County; Toledo |
| Oklahoma | Lawton Red River; Oklahoma City; Tulsa |
| Oregon | Eugene; Deshutes County; Grants Pass; Portland; Salem* |
| Pennsylvania | Bucks County; DuBois; Erie*; Harrisburg; Lancaster; McKeesport; Montgomery County; Philadelphia; Philadelphia (NE); Pittsburgh; Scranton*; Williamsport |
| *** = Vet Center and Mobile Vet Center site; ** = Mobile Vet Center site** | |

*Appendix E (IOM Recommendation 3): Vet Center and Mobile Vet Center Locations CONTINUED*

| State/Territory | Location |
|---|---|
| Puerto Rico | Arecibo; Ponce; San Juan |
| Rhode Island | Providence |
| South Carolina | Charleston; Columbia*; Greenville; Horry County |
| South Dakota | Rapid City*; Sioux Falls |
| Tennessee | Chattanooga; Johnson City*; Knoxville; Memphis*; Nashville |
| Texas | Amarillo*; Arlington; Austin; Corpus Christi; Dallas; El Paso; Ft. Worth; Harris County; Houston; Jefferson County; Killeen Heights; Laredo; Lubbock; McAllen; Mesquite; Midland; Midland/ Abilene**; San Antonio**; San Antonio NE; San Antonio NW; Taylor County; |
| U.S. Virgin Islands | St. Croix; St. Thomas |
| Utah | Provo; Salt Lake*; Washington County |
| Virginia | Alexandria; Norfolk; Richmond*; Roanoke; Virginia Beach |
| Vermont | South Burlington; White River Junction* |
| Washington | Bellingham; Everett; King County; Seattle; Spokane*; Tacoma*; Walla Walla County; Yakima Valley |
| Wisconsin | Green Bay; Madison; Milwaukee |
| West Virginia | Beckley*; Charleston; Huntington; Lacrosse County; Martinsburg; Morgantown*; Princeton; Wheeling |
| Wyoming | Casper*; Cheyenne |
| *** = Vet Center and Mobile Vet Center site; ** = Mobile Vet Center site** | |

## *Appendix F (IOM Recommendation 4): VA Studies - Stigmatization*

| Title | Amount | Synopsis |
|---|---|---|
| Stigma, Gender, and Other Barriers to VHA Use for OEF/OIF Veterans | $520,900 | Examine individual, institutional, and, most importantly, stigma-related barriers to VA health care. Focus groups with OEF/OIF Veterans will explore the relevance of proposed stigma-related barrier categories, uncover any additional factors that are not addressed within the proposed framework, and use this information to inform the measurement of barriers to care. The study will administer measures of barriers to care and assess health-care use within a national sample of OEF/OIF Veterans and use these data to address study hypotheses. |
| Barriers and Facilitators to PTSD Treatment Seeking | $362,117 | Compare barriers and facilitators to treatment initiation for PTSD among OEF/OIF Veterans to those among Veterans from the Vietnam era. Study will develop a conceptual framework for future research and interventions on PTSD treatment initiation. |
| Telemedicine Outreach for Post Traumatic Stress (TOP) in CBOCs | $1,948,399 | Evaluate a telemedicine intervention to improve PTSD outcomes in CBOCs without on-site psychiatrists. The specific aims are to estimate diect costs and compare processes and outcomes of care delivered to CBOC patients with PTSD symptoms randomized to either the TOP intervention or to usual care. |

*Appendix F (IOM Recommendation 4): VA Research – Stigmatization CONTINUED)*

| Title | Amount | Synopsis |
|---|---|---|
| Web Intervention for OEF/OIF Veterans with Mental Health Problems | $755,298 | Project to a) develop an innovative, Web-based intervention for OEF/OIF Veterans that addresses mental health, barriers-to-care, and treatment participation issues to facilitate healthy recovery; b) develop video illustrations to facilitate learning of educational material; c) develop thorough evaluation mechanisms to assess knowledge change relevant to common symptoms, healthy coping strategies, and access-to-care issues; d) conduct a series of focus groups to guide development and refinement of intervention content; and e) conduct a preliminary evaluation of the intervention using thematic semi-structured interviews with a small sample of OEF/OIF Veterans recruited via mental health specialty clinics within the Ralph H. Johnson VA Medical Center and affiliated CBOCs. |
| Online Family Education to Promote Treatment Compliance in Schizophrenia | $627,500 | Evaluate the benefits of using the internet, accessed from participants' homes, to provide education and support to caregivers of persons with schizophrenia and schizoaffective disorder. Participation in family psychoeducational programs for schizophrenia has been found to reduce patient relapse rates and decrease relative stress. Nevertheless, participation rates are often low, reflecting both family impediments to attendance (e.g., transportation difficulties, time constraints, sensitivity to stigma) and limited availability. This study will investigate whether using newer technologies can improve accessibility to family educational programs. |
| Understanding Providers' Stigmatization of Serious Mental Illness (SMI) Among Veterans | $561,757 | This study examines the effect of provider specialty (primary care or psychiatry) and type (physician or nurse) on stigmatizing perceptions, beliefs, attitudes and practice behaviors towards persons with SMI. Explores the relationship of provider characteristics (demographics and personality traits) and the amount and nature of contact with SMI to provider stigmatizing attitudes and referral behaviors. |

| Title | Amount | Synopsis |
|---|---|---|
| Case for Support: Children of Military Fathers with PTSD | $1,700,000 | Compare the wellbeing of military children who have fathers with PTSD with children whose fathers do not have PTSD to examine the relationship between parental PTSD and anxiety disorders and depression in children. A two-group comparison study, nested within a large randomly selected UK military cohort of children, will use the SDQ to measure wellbeing. |
| Land Combat Study | $1,015,000 | Determine the effects of combat operations in Iraq and Afghanistan on mental health and physical functioning of Soldiers and families. Continue work to 1) determine the risk factors for mental health problems, such as combat, deployment length and frequency, and operational stressors and determine predictors of resetting, 2) identify factors that improve mental health and well-being, such as good leadership, unit cohesion, social support, and individual background, 3) identify ways to reduce mental health stigma and barriers which hinder access to care, and 4) identify relationship between mild TBI, PTSD, and physical health problems post-deployment. Survey active and reserve component Soldiers from BCTs in a repeated cross-sectional and longitudinal design. |
| Family-Based Intervention with Traumatized Service Members and Their Young Children | $1,583,843 | Describe the interplay between returning service member PTSD symptoms and reintegration, including the parent-child relationship and parenting role. Develop and pilot an evidence-based family intervention addressing trauma impact on the parent-child relationship for families in which the returning member parent has PTSD and a child less than 5 years. Randomized control trial with pre-, post- and 6-month follow up assessments. |

*Appendix G (IOM Recommendations 6, 7, and 8): Related DoD Studies CONTINUED*

| Title | Amount | Synopsis |
|---|---|---|
| Parental Stress, PTSD, and Infant Health Outcomes in U.S. Military Families | $202,990 | Study to: 1) identify the prevalence of adverse reproductive health outcomes among infants born to parents who are participants in the Millennium Cohort Study, 2) evaluate the occurrence of these adverse reproductive health outcomes in relation to parental PTSD symptoms and diagnosis, and 3) identify how temporal differences in parental stress, in particular PTSD, and pregnancy onset impact reproductive health outcomes.<br><br>Study Design: The primary study population will include all infants born to service members who are participants in the Millennium Cohort Study (MCS). Self-reported data from the MCS, including occupational exposures, and demographic and behavioral characteristics are supplemented with objective data on occupation, deployments, and healthcare utilization. These data will be linked to birth and infant health information obtained from the DoD Birth and Infant Health Registry, a database that captures all inpatient and outpatient healthcare data on all infants born to military families, and has been validated to define birth defects and preterm births. A complementary analysis will evaluate infant health among women exposed to the acute stress of 11 September 2001 during pregnancy. |
| Deployment Family Stress: Child Neglect and Maltreatment in U.S. Army Families | $680,937 | Study and describe the phenomenology of Army child neglect using a 3-pronged methodology. Identify child, parent, and family risk and protective factors that contribute to child neglect, to include deployment. Identify military and civilian community contributions to child neglect as well as protective factors in the current military context of frequent multiple combat deployments. |
| Child Adjustment to Parental Combat Deployment: Risk and Resilience Models | $215,141 | Examine the role of caregiver behavior in risk associated with parental deployment in the prediction of child adaptation. 400 parents (of children between 3-7 years) with a spouse/partner deployed will complete anonymous questionnaires at a single time point about parent responses to child stress and child achievement of stage-salient tasks. 8 groups of parents will be recruited to compare adaptation (toddlers vs. school aged, boy vs. girl, and mother vs. father deployed). |

| Title | Amount | Synopsis |
|---|---|---|
| FOCUS-CI: A Preventative Intervention with Children and Families | $6,475,828 | Study implementation and acute and long-term efficacy of a new preventive evidence based intervention strategy to address parent and child distress, individual and family functioning and injury communication in military families as they face significant transitions and recovery adaptations resulting from combat injury. Families Overcoming Under Stress-Combat Injury (FOCUS-CI) will be FOCUS adapted for combat injured Families and combined with the Early Combined Collaborative Care (ECCC) model. |
| Deployment-related Family Psychological Resilience | $416,000 | Determine the effects of combat deployment on spouse well-being; Develop and assess spouse Resilience Training; Assess efficacy of cognitive disclosure through emotionally expressive writing as a military couple early intervention technique. Using repeated cross-sectional methods, compare similar units in different phases of the deployment cycle. Couples will be randomly assigned to a writing condition (neither, one, or both members of the couple write about either readjusting to post-deployment or about a neutral topic). |
| The Role of Spouse Telephone Resilience Training | $760,462 | Develop therapeutic components of Spouse Telephone Resilience Training and a manual for later clinical translation. Evaluate intervention effectiveness and user-acceptability. Over 1 year, 60 OEF/OIF spouses will complete 15, 1-hr structured telephone groups focused on education, Cognitive Behavioral Therapy, and support. Telephone data will be collected at baseline, 6-, and 12-months. Primary outcome variables will include depression, general well-being, and family functioning. |
| Reintegration: The Role of Spouse Telephone Resilience Training, a RCT | $1,073,000 | A RCT to compare Spouse Telephone BATTLEMIND training to usual care in terms of participant satisfaction, participant adherence to therapeutic recommendations, and changes in spouse mental health. Half of 180 OEF/OIF spouses will be randomly assigned to one each intervention (15 groups of 6 participants and one group leader). Groups will meet 14 times over 7 months. Depression, anxiety, family functioning, and participant satisfaction will be collected at baseline, 7, and 12 months post training. |

*Appendix G (IOM Recommendations 6, 7, and 8): Related DoD Studies CONTINUED*

| Title | Amount | Synopsis |
|---|---|---|
| Combat Stress Intervention Program | $3,291,630 | Identify and remove barriers to mental health services for Guard and Reservists returning from OEF/OIF; increase level of awareness and capability of mental health and primary care providers, family and community members in southwestern PA via surveys, evaluations, and educational interventions. |
| Improving Work Outcomes for Veterans with Traumatic Brain Injury | $415,500 | Investigate efficacy of a supported employment cognitive training augmentation to improve cognitive performance and work outcomes in OEF/OIF Veterans with mild to moderate TBI. Compared to those receiving enhanced supported employment, participants receiving supported employment plus cognitive symptom management and rehabilitation therapy will demonstrate significant improvement in cognition, PCS, work outcomes, and quality of life. |
| Identification of At-Risk Interventions for Predeployment Psychophysiologic Predictors of Postdeployment Mental Health Outcomes | $2,095,025 | Develop and test early post-deployment objective predictors (physiologic reactivity and cognitive bias at 3-months post-deployment) of 12-month post-deployment PTSD outcomes. Adapt and test two pre-deployment combat resiliency training interventions: a) VR-SIT with biofeedback and b) cognitive bias modification training compared to a no intervention control group in a randomized trial. The longitudinal study design involves 500 National Guard members and includes a pre-deployment objective risk factor component and a randomized primary prevention intervention component. Physiologic reactivity, cognitive bias, and mental health outcome data will be collected 3- and 12-months post-deployment. |
| Soldier to Civilian: RCT of an intervention to promote postdeployment reintegration | $1,163,567 | Determine whether internet based-expressive writing (IB-EW), a brief, low-cost, easily disseminated, and resource-efficient intervention, can reduce psychological symptoms, including PTSD, and improve functioning among Veterans returning from hazardous deployments. |

| Title | Amount | Synopsis |
|---|---|---|
| Enhanced Resilience Training (formerly BATTLEMIND) through cognitive disclosure | $325,000 | A randomized controlled trial to assess the efficacy of cognitive disclosure through emotionally expressive writing as an early intervention technique with Soldiers recently returned from combat. The goal is to enhance the demonstrated impact of Post-Deployment Health Re-Assessment Resilience Training on psychological symptoms associated with exposure to combat events. Soldiers returning from combat will be assigned to one of three conditions: expressive writing, neutral writing, and survey only. Efficacy will be assessed using a follow-up survey at three months post-intervention and health care utilization data 12 months post-intervention. |
| Mortuary affairs Soldiers: Early intervention and altering barriers to care for traumatic stress and PTSD | $425,852 | Implement and assess the feasibility of TEAM: Troop Education for Army Morale: Units and Individuals Working Together, a unique intervention designed to meet the specific needs of Mortuary Affairs (MA) Soldiers for early and follow-up intervention to speed recovery, return to work, and limit barriers to care through individual training, active engagement in problem-solving and accessing care, enhanced buddy care, and spouse support. Assess short and longer-term outcome of TEAM effectiveness in MA Soldiers on barriers to care, disorder, health risk behaviors, work function, and marital conflict. |
| The Impact of Supported Employment Versus Standard Vocational Rehabilitation in Veterans With PTSD | $1,680,208 | Determine if: 1) participants assigned to supported employment group have a higher maintained employment rate for the 12-month observation period than standard vocational rehabilitation program (VRP) counterparts (obtained + maintained employment); 2) those who obtain competitive employment have significantly reduced symptoms of PTSD from baseline to endpoint compared to those who do not obtain competitive employment; and 3) compared to VRP participants, those assigned to individual placement and support (IPS) will have greater work intensity (number of weeks, days, and hours), higher total earnings, and greater improvement in quality of life outcomes. Exploratory outcomes include PTSD symptoms, other psychiatric symptoms, substance use, risk factors for early treatment drop-out, quality of life, and health care costs (follow up 12 months). |

| Title | Amount | Synopsis |
|---|---|---|
| Behavioral Health Family Readiness System Research Study | $849,732 | Develop and test an interactive website that will provide educational content directed expressly toward military Families. Three geographically diverse focus groups with 8-12 military family members to assess current knowledge and perceived needs. Modify web and survey content based on focus group feedback. Pilot study of 100 family member site users, web and survey content will be modified. Conduct a study up to 1000 family members who use the website to evaluate effectiveness of the website to improve PTSD knowledge and related disorders and seek care. |
| Development and Pilot of an Intervention for Military Personnel and Their Families | $248,250 | Project to: 1) better understand the mental health needs of young adult Reservists and National Guard personnel and their families of origin throughout deployment cycles, 2) understand the relationship between family criticism and PTSD, and 3) help develop a mental health treatment for young adult military personnel. The mental health treatment will be based on Project FOCUS, a family counseling program for returning military personnel and their families. Project FOCUS helps individuals and families cope with difficult emotions, learn problem solving, and improve communication between family members so they can support each other. Project staff will meet with groups of young soldiers and their families so that we may better understand their stresses and modify Project FOCUS to help them. Military personnel and families will then experience the new counseling program and give feedback on their satisfaction with it, and we will try to understand how the program may have helped them. It is expected that this project will provide useful information for future research on counseling programs that help families re-unite after deployment. |

| Title | Amount | Synopsis |
|---|---|---|
| PTSD-Focused Cognitive Behavioral Therapy for Partner Violent OIF/OEF Veterans | $1,536,334 | Proposed project to further develop, standardize, and test an intervention for recently separated combat Veterans with PTSD who engage in intimate partner violence (IPV). This intervention will incorporate components of interventions for PTSD and IPV and will target mechanisms implicated in the PTSD-IPV association. The development of this type of integrated treatment is critical because of high rates of PTSD-IPV co-occurrence and the pressing need to efficiently address both problems among military Veterans.<br><br>Objectives: 1) to develop and standardize PFCBT for recently separated male combat Veterans with PTSD. The outcome of this phase will involve the development of a clinician-friendly treatment manual detailing PFCBT and treatment adherence measures; 2) to test the efficacy of PFCBT for partner violent Veterans by conducting a randomized controlled trial (RCT) comparing those who receive 16 sessions of PFCBT with those placed on a waiting list to receive the treatment; and. 3) to empirically examine mechanisms of change involved in the PFCBT. |
| Development of a PTSD Population Registry | $954,935 | Develop and implement registry of combat-exposed men and women with PTSD to identify clinical characteristics, risk factors and comorbidities of PTSD, including disparities by gender, race/ethnicity, and socioeconomic status; evaluate neuropsychological and psychosocial outcomes, and evaluate treatment trajectories and outcomes in a sample of combat-exposed Veterans |

*Appendix G (IOM Recommendations 6, 7, and 8): Related DoD Studies CONTINUED*

| Title | Amount | Synopsis |
|---|---|---|
| Innovative Service Delivery for Secondary Prevention of PTSD in At-Risk OIF-OEF Service Men and Women | $1,445,214 | The study's two primary objectives are to: 1)develop, implement, and evaluate the Behavioral Activation and Therapeutic Exposure (BATE) treatment program for OEF/OIF Veterans with subclinical PTSD; and 2) determine whether this program delivered via telephone will be as effective as in-person treatment. Secondary objectives include determining: 1) which treatment modality is more effective in terms of process variables (e.g., treatment satisfaction, session attendance); 2) which treatment modality is more cost-effective; and 3) whether treatment effects differ across race and gender. Study participants will be randomized to two treatment conditions, BATE delivered via telephone (BATE-T) and BATE delivered in-person (BATE-IP). |
| Effectiveness of cognitive exposure and skills group manualized treatments in OIF/OEF female Veterans | $884,466 | Effectiveness study using manualized exposure, cognitive, and skills (assertiveness /relaxation) group therapy across 16-sessions in a sample of OEF/OIF female Veterans with PTSD. |
| Using Propranolol to Block Memory Reconsolidation in Female Veterans with PTSD | $388,461 | Investigate a novel method of reducing the hyper-arousal associated with combat memories in female OEF and OIF Veterans with PTSD. Based on a reconsolidation model of memory, we believe that a beta-adrenergic receptor blocker (propranolol) can drastically diminish the association between a combat memory and the physical reactions it generates. The model requires that two doses of propranolol be administered immediately following a strong recollection of the combat memory. Our proposal would compare female Veterans who take propranolol after a combat memory to both female Veterans who take a non-active placebo pill after a combat memory and those who take propranolol after a non-combat memory (to make sure that propranolol does not have a general effect on physical reactions). All participants in our study would be tested during the early follicular phase of the menstrual cycle, a time in which levels of estrogen are low. |

| Title | Amount | Synopsis |
|---|---|---|
| Evaluating PTSD on Reproductive Outcomes: Women Deployed in Iraq and Afghanistan | $214,357 | Retrospective study examining the relationship between PTSD and adverse reproductive outcomes and AFHS data on Iraq and Afghanistan deployment between 2001 and 2006; study will occur over 18 months; Study will compare women diagnosed with PTSD to those nondeployed and those deployed to the same region with a different mental disorder and without a mental disorder |
| PTSD, Comorbid Disorders, and Service Utilization in Women Veterans | $232,500 | Using existing data, the study will determine prevalence and annual incidence of PTSD and MST in female Veterans, as compared to male Veterans; Determine prevalence rates of depression, alcohol/drug use disorders, adjustment disorders, and other anxiety disorders in women with and without PTSD, with and without MST; will also determine prevalence of visits to VA primary care and emergency clinics in women and men with and without PTSD |
| Post-Traumatic Stress Disorder and Pain Comorbidity in Veterans | $198,959 | Analyze existing data to determine whether the presence of pain affects diagnosis and treatment of PTSD among female OEF/OIF VA patients with PTSD and pain comorbidity on use of mental health, primary care, and pain-related health services. |
| Hormonal Regulation of Extinction: Implications for Gender Differences in the Mechanisms of PTSD | $223,419 | Examine whether estrogen "predisposes" females to increased fear learning and/or an inability to extinguish that fear |
| Combat, Sexual Assault, and Post-Traumatic Stress in OIF/OEF Military Women | $519,608 | Identify and describe organizational, situational, and individual risk factors for physical and sexual assault in women who served or are currently serving in the Regular Military in OEF/OIF by deployment status |

| Title | Amount | Synopsis |
|---|---|---|
| Using Propranolol to Block Memory Reconsolidation in Female Veterans with PTSD | $388,461 | Investigate a novel method of reducing the hyper-arousal associated with combat memories in female OEF/OIF Veterans with PTSD. Based on a reconsolidation model of memory, we believe that a beta-adrenergic receptor blocker (propranolol) can drastically diminish the association between a combat memory and the physical reactions it generates. The model requires that two doses of propranolol be administered immediately following a strong recollection of the combat memory. Our proposal would compare female Veterans who take propranolol after a combat memory to both female Veterans who take a non-active placebo pill after a combat memory and those who take propranolol after a non-combat memory (to make sure that propranolol does not have a general effect on physical reactions). All participants in our study would be tested during the early follicular phase of the menstrual cycle, a time in which levels of estrogen are low. |

| Title | Amount | Synopsis |
|---|---|---|
| Predicting Post-Deployment Mental Health Substance Abuse and Services Needs | $758,021 | Identify risk and resilience factors that predict development of a psychiatric or substance abuse disorder and associated mental health and/or substance abuse service use within and outside the VHA. Specific objectives are: 1) examine the mental health and substance abuse status, functioning, and service use of post-deployed OEF/OIF military personnel in the two years' post-deployment, 2) identify risk and resilience factors that predict mental health status, functioning, and service use two years after their initial assessment, and 3) identify targets for interventions to promote readjustment and reintegration of post-deployed Veterans. |
| Re-Engineering Systems for the Primary Care Treatment of PTSD | $1,223,812 | Proposed randomized clinical trial of collaborative care for PTSD in Veterans who are treated in primary care settings to facilitate the management of PTSD and evaluate the effects of the intervention on patient outcomes, provider behavior, and costs. The long-term objectives are to generate information to support implementation research collaborative care for PTSD, and ultimately, implement the collaborative care for PTSD across VHA. |
| Relationships and PTSD Study: Detection of Intimate Partner Violence (IPV) | $897,799 | Research to provide foundational knowledge about the detection of IPV in a PTSD treatment-seeking sample by examining the documentation of the existence or non-existence of IPV in the clinical record; and to provide additional knowledge about what distinguishes IPV perpetrators common perpetrators in a cohort of men with military related PTSD. |

| Title | Amount | Synopsis |
|---|---|---|
| Evaluating VA's Assessment of Military Sexual Trauma in Veterans | $367,584 | Study of Veterans' understanding of the two unstudied MST screening questions, their understanding of Congressional and VA definitions of sexual harassment and assault, and how being provided these definitions change their understanding of the screening questions (or not), and their understanding of other sexual harassment/assault assessment approaches that are more comprehensive and whether they find these approaches improve their ability to describe their own definitions of MST. |
| Physical and Sexual Assault in Deployed Women: Risks, Outcomes and Services | $783,607 | Proposed cross-sectional study of Reserve and National Guard [R/NG]) women (both active duty and Veterans) serving in OEF/OIF. The health outcomes of interest include current physical and emotional health, health behaviors, and health services use. These outcomes will be studied in relation to deployment status, organizational, situational, and individual risk factors, as well as victimization during Reserve and National Guard (R/NG) service (which is our primary independent variable). |
| Combat, Sexual Assault, and Post-Traumatic Stress in OIF/OEF Military Women | $298,800 | Proposed study addresses the radically changing DoD and DVA health care delivery needs of two priority populations: women exposed to combat, and women sexually assaulted during military service. The objectives are to: 1) identify and describe organizational, situational, and individual risk factors for physical and sexual assault (i.e., victimization) in women who have served or are currently serving in OEF/OIF by deployment status; 2) determine associations between PTSD, TBI, and physical and sexual assault during OEF/OIF with current physical and mental health status and health risk behaviors by deployment status; 3) identify current internal and external barriers to DoD, DVA, and civilian health services in relationship to women's deployment and victimization status and the association between PTSD and TBI; and 4) identify and describe differences between Regular Military (RM) and R/NG populations for each of these objectives. |

| Title | Amount | Synopsis |
|---|---|---|
| Military Sexual Trauma (MST) Effects on PTSD and Health Behavior: A Longitudinal Study of Marines | $ 762,065 | Building on a previously conducted prospective longitudinal study of Marine recruits, we will examine the relationship between MST and respondents' functioning approximately 8 years after they joined the Marines. We will focus on health behaviors, with an understanding that there are risk and resilience factors that may influence trajectories following MST. This study has three main objectives: 1) determine what behaviors and areas of functioning are adversely affected by MST; 2) uncover the risk and resilience factors for poor outcomes following MST; and 3) determine if there are gender differences in the effects of MST and its moderators of poor outcomes. |
| Evaluation of Family Outreach Mental Health Programs for OEF/OIF Veterans | $210,640 | The primary objectives are to: 1) examine facilitators and barriers to participation in family-outreach programs among family members of returning OEF/OIF service members; 2) characterize the ways that Reserve and National Guard (R/NG) Veterans learn about and decide whether to use VHA services; and 3) formatively evaluate how the Iowa City VAMC mental health family-outreach efforts meet the mental health and readjustment needs of Veterans. |
| Perspectives on Enhancing Family Involvement in Treatment for PTSD | $329,503 | The proposed research will address gaps in the evidence-base for family involvement in PTSD treatment for the OEF/OIF population. Specific aims are to: 1) identify and describe the elements of the family-psychoeducation model that effectively meet the needs, and are consistent with the preferences of Veterans with PTSD and their families.;2) describe the needs and preferences of OEF/OIF service-era Veterans with PTSD and their families relevant to family involvement in care, and compare them to those of other Veterans with PTSD and their families; and 3) identify and describe major facilitators and barriers to the implementation and sustainability of a REACH-model program in VA settings. |
| Family-Supported Smoking Cessation for Chronically Ill Veterans | $1,034,362 | Randomized trial of a family-supported intervention compared to a standard Veteran-focused intervention to promote smoking cessation among cancer and heart disease patients. |

| Title | Amount | Synopsis |
|---|---|---|
| Neuroimaging in the Oklahoma Family Health Patterns Project | $600,000 | At present there are no functional neuroimaging studies of persons having standard risk factors for alcoholism. This study is a hypothesis-based approach to functional and structural neuroimaging in such persons that may provide new information on the neural mechanisms associated with risk for this disorder. |
| Understanding Race and Culture in Living Donor Kidney Transplantation | $939,800 | Examines factors related to the fact that African Americans are four times as likely as whites to have end stage renal disease, but only half as likely to receive kidney transplants. |
| Presence and Correlates of Racial Disparities in Pain Management | $383,349 | Examines whether patient verbal and nonverbal behaviors that are likely to co-vary with race/ethnicity in the clinical encounter mediate and/or moderate the expected effect of race/ethnicity on provider decision-making about pain treatment. |
| Identifying Mechanisms Linking Perceived Discrimination and Health | $640,591 | Study to examine the association between perceived discrimination in health care and utilization of preventive health services. |
| Comparing Quality and Equity of Care in VA's and Medicare Managed Care | $969,445 | Project to assess clinical performance trends in the areas of diabetes, cardiovascular, depression and cancer screening care in the Veterans Affairs Health Care System and Medicare managed care program from 1997-2005. The study will compare both overall performance and the magnitude of racial disparity in quality measures within these two systems of care. |
| VA Facility Determinants of Racial-Ethnic Variations in Quality of Care | $411,100 | Proposed research to: 1) Identify modifiable VA facility-level characteristics associated with quality of care for specific racial-ethnic minority groups, and do so within the context in which VA facilities deliver care; and 2) Identify modifiable VA facility-level characteristics associated with racial-ethnic disparities in VA quality of care, also doing so within the local area and fixed facility contexts, and describe the characteristics of high disparity facilities. |

| Title | Amount | Synopsis |
|---|---|---|
| Telemental Health and Cognitive Processing Therapy for Rural Combat Veterans with PTSD | $280,976 | Project to evaluate the clinical effectiveness of a telemental health modality (video-teleconferencing) for providing an evidence-based group intervention to rural OEF/OIF Reservists, National Guardsmen, and Veterans with PTSD. The long-term objective of this project is to develop an empirically sound telemental health protocol that will facilitate the extension of a manual-guided evidence-based PTSD treatment intervention to remote VA and DoD sites through video-teleconferencing. |
| Impact of a Plain Language Prostate Cancer Decision Aid on Decision Making | $894,356 | Tests the impact of a decision aid (designed to have a low reading level) on prostate cancer patients' decision-making experience and in their interactions with their physician and VA's health system. This pilot study will inform a larger, already approved study, "Impact of a plain language prostate cancer decision aid on decision making." |
| Proactive Tobacco Treatment for Diverse Veteran Smokers | $903,681 | The primary objectives of this study are to: 1) assess the effect of a proactive care intervention (PRO) on population-level smoking abstinence rates and on utilization of tobacco treatment compared to reactive/usual care (UC) among a diverse population of Veteran smokers (greater than 40 percent ethnic minority);2) compare the effect of PRO on population-level smoking abstinence rates and utilization of tobacco treatments between African American and White smokers; and 3) determine the cost-effectiveness of the proactive care intervention. |
| Video to Encourage Active Patient Participation | $100,000 | Proposed evaluation of the acceptability and feasibility of using video to encourage patients to use active participatory communication behaviors in medical interactions and to conduct a pilot test of the video among patients with poorly controlled type-2 diabetes. |
| Pilot Study of Reintegration and Service Needs for Women Veteran Mothers | $69,100 | Pilot study to deepen understanding of the concerns and stressors that accompany reintegration into civilian life for OEF/OIF Reserve and Guard woman Veterans who are or are not mothers of dependent children. To also understand the potential barriers to utilizing available support services for these same women and determine what services would provide a better fit for their needs. |

| Title | Amount | Synopsis |
|---|---|---|
| Further Development and Validation of the DRRI | $139,500 | Study to examine the relevance of content domains within existing Deployment Risk and Resilience Inventory (DRRI) scales and generate information that can be used to refine DRRI scales, as needed. The long-term goal of this project is to provide a suite of scales that will be optimally useful to researchers and clinicians. |
| Gender and Medical Needs of OIF/OEF Veterans with PTSD | $28,700 | In response to recent attention to the high rates of PTSD in returning OEF/OIF Veterans, there have been considerable efforts to characterize their mental health services needs. However, the general medical care needs of OEF/OIF Veterans with PTSD have not been characterized. The objectives of this project are to identify medical conditions associated with PTSD in women (and men) OEF/OIF returnees, stratified by age, and, among those with PTSD, identify medical conditions associated with war-zone exposure and military sexual trauma. |
| Gender and Medical Needs of OEF/OIF Veterans with PTSDII | $41,400 | In response to recent attention to the high rates of PTSD in OEF/OIF Veterans, there have been considerable efforts to characterize their mental health services needs. Core analyses have been completed documenting higher rates of a range of medical conditions in women and men Veterans with PTSD. Supplemental funds have enabled additional examination of whether this effect is even more pronounced for those with a dual diagnosis of PTSD plus a substance use disorder. |
| Examining the Diagnostic and Clinical Utility of the PTSD Checklist (PCL) | $35,500 | Project to examine the impact of these variables on the diagnostic and clinical utility of the PCL. Funding for this project will expedite the completion of our analyses and our subsequent reports. The findings will help VHA clinicians and researchers in their interpretation of PCL scores and subsequent clinical care decisions. |

| Title | Amount | Synopsis |
|---|---|---|
| Telemental Health and Cognitive Processing Therapy for Rural Combat Veterans with PTSD | $280,976 | Evaluation of the clinical effectiveness of a telemental health modality (video-teleconferencing) for providing an evidence-based group intervention to rural OEF/OIF Reservists, National Guardsmen, and Veterans with PTSD. The long-term objective of this project is to develop an empirically sound telemental health protocol that will facilitate the extension of a manual-guided evidence-based PTSD treatment intervention to remote VA and DoD sites through video-teleconferencing. |
| Impact of a Plain Language Prostate Cancer Decision Aid on Decision Making | $894,356 | Tests the impact of a decision aid (designed to have a low reading level) on prostate cancer patients' decision-making experience and in their interactions with their physician and VA's health system. This pilot study will inform a larger, already approved study, "Impact of a plain language prostate cancer decision aid on decision making." |
| Proactive Tobacco Treatment for Diverse Veteran Smokers | $903,681 | Study to: 1) assess the effect of a proactive care intervention (PRO) on population-level smoking abstinence rates and on utilization of tobacco treatment compared to reactive/usual care (UC) among a diverse population of Veteran smokers (greater than 40 percent ethnic minority); 2) compare the effect of PRO on population-level smoking abstinence rates and utilization of tobacco treatments between African American and White smokers; and 3) determine the cost-effectiveness of the proactive care intervention. |
| Video to Encourage Active Patient Participation | $100,000 | Evaluation of the acceptability and feasibility of using video to encourage patients to use active participatory communication behaviors in medical interactions and to conduct a pilot test of the video among patients with poorly controlled type-2 diabetes. |
| Pilot Study of Reintegration and Service Needs for Women Veteran Mothers | $69,100 | Pilot study deepen understanding of the concerns and stressors that accompany reintegration into civilian life for OEF/OIF Reserve and Guard woman Veterans who are or are not mothers of dependent children. To also understand the potential barriers to utilizing available support services for these same women and determine what services would provide a better fit for their needs. |

*Appendix H (IOM Recommendations 6, 7, and 8): Related VA Studies CONTINUED*

| Title | Amount | Synopsis |
|---|---|---|
| Barriers and Facilitators to PTSD Treatment Seeking | $362,117 | Study to: 1) identify barriers to and facilitators of treatment-seeking for PTSD and determine whether there are variations by gender and period of service; 2) describe Veterans' beliefs about PTSD treatment; 3) identify targets for interventions to promote appropriate treatment-seeking for PTSD; and 4) confirm and expand upon a conceptual model of PTSD treatment-seeking. |
| A Pilot of PTSD-Focused Cognitive Behavior Therapy (PFCBT) for Partner Violence | $92,673 | Proposed study to: 1) develop and standardize a group intervention for intimate partner violence (IPV) perpetration for recently separated male combat Veterans with PTSD; 2) test the efficacy of PFCBT for partner violent Veterans by conducting a small-scale randomized trial comparing 24 sessions of PFCBT with 24 sessions of supportive therapy; and 3) explore differences in participant treatment compliance and process factors across conditions. |
| Sexual Violence and Women Veterans' Gynecologic Health | $786,901 | Study to: 1) determine if the odds of current gynecologic disorders are significantly greater for sexually assaulted Veterans in comparison to non-assaulted peers; 2) identify if the presence and frequency of cofactors known to be associated with cervical cytologic abnormalities is greater in sexually assaulted Veterans when compared to non-assaulted peers; 3) determine the frequency and types of gynecologic services used by sexually assaulted women Veterans in comparison to that of non-assaulted peers; and 4) identify and compare type and frequency of gynecologic health risk behaviors in sexually assaulted Veterans with that of their non-assaulted peers. |
| Evaluation of Military Sexual Trauma Screening and Treatment | $385,700 | Project to determine: 1) patient-level and facility-level factors associated with variation in rates of MST screening, detection, and treatment; 2) modifiable practices associated with MST screening and detection; and 3) modifiable practices, patient factors and facility factors associated with utilization of MST-related treatment. |

| Title | Amount | Synopsis |
|---|---|---|
| PTSD, Anger, Cognition, and Partner Violence Among Combat Veterans | $435,740 | Proposed study to investigate: 1) the relationship between PTSD symptom severity and the components and manifestations of anger among combat Veterans; 2) the association between PTSD symptom severity and a number of cognitive deficits and biases; 3) How PTSD, anger dysregulation, and cognitive factors are associated with more partner violence perpetration among combat Veterans; and 4) the hypothesis that acute exposure to trauma-related cues will potentiate associations between PTSD symptom severity and various aspects of the anger response. |
| The Impact of Health Literacy on Racial Differences in Cancer Stage at Presentation | $965,736 | Study to determine if racial differences in the rate of advanced stage presentation for prostate, colorectal, and lung cancer can be explained by differences in health literacy, use of screening tests, or both. |
| Assessing and Addressing Patient Colorectal Cancer (CRC) Screening Barriers | $816,578 | Study to: 1) estimate the relative effect of patient cognitive, environmental, and background factors on CRC screening behavior; 2) identify factors that contribute to any disparities in CRC screening behavior by race/ethnicity or other patient characteristics; and 3) identify from these analyses priority population subgroups to target in future interventions. |
| Dissemination Evaluation of Educational Materials for Puerto Rican OIF/OEF Veterans and Families | $50,000 | Project to adapt existing education materials to help Puerto Rican (PR) OEF/OIF Veterans and their families readjust to life after returning home. This project is the critical, first step in accomplishing our long-range goal to improve the quality of life of PR OEF/OIF Veterans/families through education interventions. |
| Printed and Web-Based OEF/OIF Culturally-Relevant Family Education | $100,000 | Our long-term goal is to improve community reintegration of OEF/OIF Veterans throughout VA by creating and disseminating culturally relevant and low-literate, printed and web-based family education materials. To accomplish this long-term goal, we plan to extend our previous work in which we developed family health information for Puerto Ricans in VA's Caribbean Healthcare System. |

*Appendix H (IOM Recommendations 6, 7, and 8): Related VA Studies CONTINUED*

| Title | Amount | Synopsis |
|---|---|---|
| Translation and Cultural Adaptation of a PTSD Therapy for Hispanics | $120,300 | Project to translate therapist and client manuals of an established theoretically-based exposure therapy for PTSD and to evaluate the cultural compatibility of the translated manualized intervention and culturally adapt the theoretically-based, exposure therapy intervention manuals. |
| Telemedicine and Anger Management Groups for PTSD Veterans in the Hawaiian Island | $840,751 | Proposed study to expand upon previous pilot findings by evaluating the clinical effectiveness of providing mental health services via VTC modality as compared to the traditional in-person modality for Veterans with PTSD who reside in remote locations. |
| Impact of a Plain Language Prostate Cancer Decision Aid on Decision Making | $894,356 | Study testing the impact of a plain language decision aid (i.e., a low reading level) on prostate cancer patient's decision making experience as well as in their interactions with their physician and VA's health system. This study will also test if there are differences in receipt of active treatment between men with low vs. high literacy skills and between African American and White men. We will also test whether the decision aid is effective both for low and high literacy patients and for African American and White men. |
| A Culturally Sensitive Values-Guided Aid for End of Life Decision-Making | $861,762 | Given that the medical-technical orientation of care at the end-of-life has been severely criticized and is considered as 'poor' quality of care by some, these observed disparities may reflect yet another example of 'worse' care for minorities. Alternatively, it could represent true cultural, ethnic, or racial differences in decision-making for end-of-life care. Our study will identify these values and gain further insight into the decision-making process at the end-of-life. |
| Improving Self-Management through Facilitated Patient-Physician Communication | $51,675 | Study to: 1) test the feasibility of assessing and enrolling Veterans with poor health literacy and multiple co-morbid conditions, and physicians with poor communication skills to participate in the study; 2) test the feasibility of a one-on-one consultation between Veterans with low health literacy and a health educator focusing on communicating about self-management.; 3) simultaneously test the feasibility of a physician-based communication enhancement intervention., and 4) use the pilot data to develop an investigator-initiated research (IIR) that will test the effectiveness of the interventions in a randomized clinical trial. |

## *Appendix I. OEF/OIF-Specific Data*[8]

**TBI and Related Blast Injuries**

- Estimates of the percentage of OEF/OIF Service members returning with TBI range from 10 percent to 33 percent.
- Some long-term outcomes are apparent at or soon after the time of injury but TBIs that have no physical signs may cause serious long-term effects that can go undetected until the Service member returns home and cannot function as before

**Polytrauma**

- Frequent co-occurring problems with TBI include
  - Amputation
  - Chronic pain
  - Mental health disorders (e.g., PTSD, Depression)
  - Polytrauma (i.e., multiple injuries, head injury or cognitive disability, and lower-limb injuries)

**Mental Health Disorders**

- Major depression
  - Estimates of self-reported major depression in OEF/OIF active-duty service members range from 5 percent to 37 percent
- Post traumatic stress disorder
  - OEF/OIF Service members who experience combat exposure and those who are wounded are at higher risk than others
  - One 2006 government study estimated 17 percent of soldiers and 14 percent of Marines met PTSD screening criteria while deployed (other estimates vary)
  - Service members not identified during deployment may be identified 3-4 months (or many years) after their return Afghanistan and Iraq
  - MHS has spent more than $63.8 million in care and $13.1 million in prescription drugs for those with PTSD
  - Self-report screening, different outcome measurement, and the use of convenience samples in the extant post-deployment studies may underestimate the prevalence of PTSD and depression
  - Among 199 OEF/OIF Veterans referred to military behavioral health clinicians, those with PTSD or depression were five times as likely to report

---

888 8 Complete citations or attributions are included in the IOM chapter on Preliminary Findings.

problems with family readjustment as those who did not and almost one third of the Veterans reported that their partners were afraid of them.
    - There is a shortage of mental health professionals
    - Services available to OEF/OIF service members and veterans are poorly distributed.
- Substance abuse disorder
    - A recent study of three Army and one Marine Corps units reported that OEF/OIF deployment was associated with higher prevalence of alcohol misuse compared to pre-deployment prevalence.
    - A study of reserve and National Guard reported that personnel deployed to OEF/OIF were at increased risk for new-onset heavy weekly drinking, binge drinking, and other alcohol-related outcomes.
    - Military deployment was associated with smoking initiation and more strongly with smoking recidivism
    - No data were available on drug abuse among OEF/OIF Service members

**Deployment**

- In a survey of OEF/OIF Army spouses conducted in 2004,
    - 78 percent reported loneliness
    - Over 51 percent reported anxiety
    - Over 48 percent cited a problem with the military because of the lack of accurate information around the timing of the deployment
    - Over 42 percent reported depression
    - 41 percent reported difficult in communication with the deployed member
    - 29 percent reported difficulties in household maintenance
    - Over 23 percent reported fears about personal safety
    - 21 percent reported problems with overall health
    - 18 percent reported effects on jobs
    - 16 percent reported problems with child care
    - 12 percent reported financial problems
    - Almost 10 percent reported problems with their marriages
- Few studies focus on the normative course of reintegration
- One longitudinal study of reintegration during OIF reported that couples in a sample of reservists were preoccupied with relational communication and expectation, especially regarding independence, roles, and responsibilities.
- Since 2003, family separation has consistently been among the top concerns of Service members stationed in Iraq and Afghanistan and is more strongly related than any other concern to mental health problems
- Length of deployment appears to be positively correlated and pay grade appears to be negatively correlated with a plan for divorce on return (so far, there is little evidence that these plans are realized)

- Two small studies of OEF/OIF families suggest that symptoms of combat-related trauma are related to marital distress for both partners
- No data were found on the effects of deployments on unmarried partners or the parents and other family members of Service members
- The effects of OEF/OIF deployments on children who have parents deployed are consistent with those of earlier research, with studies on the current conflict reporting
  - Depression
  - Anxiety
  - More reactions to stress and resource losses
  - Academic difficulties
  - An increase in the use of mental health-care services
- Effects on child maltreatment and intimate-partner violence are not yet known
- Studies suggests that the unemployment rate of OEF/OIF Veterans may be higher than that of other Veterans
- DoD's unemployment compensation costs increased 75 percent from 2002 to 2004, suggesting that OEF/OIF Veterans are having difficulty transitioning to the civilian labor market. 58 percent of the increase from 2002 to 2004 is attributed to the Army reserve components
- OEF/OIF deployment reduced spousal labor-force participation almost 3 percent overall, with higher rates negatively correlated with the ages of the children.
- The relationship between deployment and earnings among reservists is not clear.

**Women and Minorities**

- Although 11 percent of all personnel deployed to Iraq and Afghanistan are women, there is little research specific to that population. Among military women in general:
  - Over 72 percent of women in one study reported having experienced sexual harassment during their military service
  - 63 percent reported experiences of physical and sexual harassment during military service
  - 43 percent reported rape or attempted rape during military service
  - Rates of pre-military trauma are higher in women than in men; one study reported 58 percent in women versus 35 percent in men
  - Among civilians, women have higher rates of depression and anxiety disorders than men. Studies of military populations posted at permanent bases have yielded similar findings.
- The distribution of U.S. casualties in Iraq for the first 12 months of conflict show racial equity for minorities
- In the military population overall, findings of differences in service delivery or outcomes associated with race or ethnicity are inconclusive.

○

**Projecting the Lifelong Burden of War**

- Historically, the number of Veterans receiving disability and pension benefits peak several decades after the war.
- As of 2008, 230,000 OEF/OIF Veterans had filed disability claims.
- The majority of claims have not yet been submitted. One study suggests that 791,000 OEF/OIF Veterans will eventually seek disability benefits.
- Unique aspects of OEF/OIF may result in significant deviations from historical trends (e.g., survivors of very severe injuries need more intensive care then the most severely wounded from prior wars).

| *Appendix J: Acronyms* | |
|---|---|
| AF | Air Force |
| AFRTS | Armed Forces Radio and Television Service |
| AL | Assisted Living |
| ALS | Amyotrophic Lateral Sclerosis |
| BAA | Broad Agency Announcements |
| BATE | Behavioral Activation and Therapeutic Exposure |
| BCT | Brigade Combat Teams |
| CBO | Congressional Budget Office |
| CBOC | Community Based Outpatient Clinic |
| CCTA | Collaborative Clinical Trial Award |
| CDC | Centers for Disease Control and Prevention |
| CDE | Common data element |
| CDMRP | Congressionally Directed Medical Research Programs |
| CHPS | Civilian Health Professions Scholarship program |
| CNS | Clinical nurse specialist |
| COLA | Cost of Living Adjustments |
| CRC | Colorectal cancer |
| CSP | VA Cooperative Studies Program |
| CSTS | Center for the Study of Traumatic Stress |
| CTF | Clinical Tracking Form |
| DCoE | Defense Centers of Excellence for Psychological Health and Traumatic Brain Injury |
| DES | Disability Evaluation System |
| HHS | Department of Health and Human Services |
| DLS | Deployment Life Study |
| DMDC | Defense Manpower Data Center |
| DoD | Department of Defense |
| DoDI | Department of Defense Instruction |
| DRRI | Deployment Risk and Resilience Inventory |
| DTI | Diffusion tensor imaging |
| DTM | Directive-Type Memorandum |
| DVBIC | Defense Veterans Brain Injury Center |
| ECCC | Early Combined Collaborative Care |
| ESP | Evidence-Based Synthesis Project |
| FOCUS-CI | Families Over Coming Under Stress-Combat Injury |
| FTEE | Full-time equivalent employee |
| FY | Fiscal year |

## *Appendix J: Acronyms (CONTINUED)*

| | |
|---|---|
| GMT | Goal management training |
| GWVI | Gulf War Veterans with illnesses |
| GWAS | Genome-wide Association Study |
| HPO | Health professions officers |
| HSR&D | Health Services Research and Development Service (VA) |
| IAMPS | International Applied Military Psychology Seminar |
| IIR | Investigator-Initiated Research |
| IB-EW | Internet based-expressive writing |
| IOM | Institute of Medicine of the National Academy of Sciences |
| IPS | Individual placement and support |
| IPV | Intimate partner violence |
| IRB | Institutional Review Board |
| IVR | Interactive voice response |
| MA | Mortuary affairs |
| MCS | Millennium Cohort Study |
| MDR | Military Health System Data Repository |
| MHEI | Mental Health Expansion Initiative |
| MHICM-RANGE | Mental Health Intensive Case Management – Rural Access Network for Growth Enhancement |
| MHS | Military Health System |
| MOMRP | Military Operational Medicine Research Program |
| MRI | Magnetic residence imagining |
| MST | Military sexual trauma |
| mTBI | Mild traumatic brain injury |
| MTF | Medical treatment facility |
| MVC | Mobile Vet Center |
| NCI | National Cancer Institute |
| NDAA | National Defense Authorization Act |
| NDI | National Death Index |
| NHRC | Navy Health Research Center |
| NIAAA | National Institute of Alcohol Abuse and Alcoholism |
| NIDA | National Institute on Drug Abuse |
| NIDRR | National Institute on Disability and Rehabilitation Research |
| NIH | National Institutes of Health |
| NIMH | National Institute of Mental Health |
| NINDS | National Institute of Neurological Disorders and Stroke |
| NP | Nurse practitioner |

## *Appendix J: Acronyms (CONTINUED)*

| | |
|---|---|
| OACT | Office of the Actuary |
| OEF | Operation Enduring Freedom |
| OHI | Office of Health Administration |
| OI&T | Office of Information and Technology |
| OIF | Operation Iraqi Freedom |
| OMHS | Office of Mental Health Services |
| OPES | Office of Productivity, Efficiency, and Staffing |
| OQP | Office of Quality and Performance (VA) |
| ORD | Office of Research and Development (VA) |
| OSD | Office of the Secretary of Defense |
| OTS | Office of Telehealth Services |
| PA | Physician assistant |
| PACT | Prazosin and Combat Trauma |
| PBRN | practice-based research network |
| PCL | PTSD Checklist |
| PCS (1) | Physical Component Summary |
| PCS (2) | Post-concussion Syndrome |
| PFCBT | PTSD-Focused Cognitive Behavior Therapy |
| PH | Psychological health |
| PHS | Public Health Service |
| PHRAMS | Psychological Health Risk-Adjusted Model for Staffing |
| PRC | Polytrauma Rehabilitation Centers |
| PRO | Proactive care intervention |
| PSA | Public service announcements |
| PT/BRI QUERI | Polytrauma and Blast-Related Injury Quality Enhancement Research Initiative |
| PFCBT | PTSD-focused cognitive behavior therapy |
| PTSD | Post traumatic stress disorder |
| QUERI | Quality Enhancement Research Initiative |
| RC01 | Research Committee 01 of the International Sociological Association |
| RCS | Office of Readjustment Counseling |
| RCT | Randomized controlled trial |
| RFA | Request for Applications |
| R/NG | Reserve and National Guard |
| rTMS | Repetitive transcranial magnetic stimulation |
| RM | Regular military |
| SAMHSA | Substance Abuse and Mental Health Services Administration |
| SBIRT | Screening, Brief Intervention, Referral and Treatment |

## *Appendix J: Acronyms (CONTINUED)*

| | |
|---|---|
| SCI | Spinal Cord Injury |
| SF-36V | The Veterans Short Form 36 Questionnaire |
| SME | Subject matter expert |
| SMI | Serious mental illness |
| SOC | Senior Oversight Committee |
| SSA | Social Security Administration |
| STARRS | Study to Assess Risk and Resilience in Service Members |
| SDQ | Strengths and Difficulties Questionnaire |
| SUD | Substance use disorder |
| T2 | DCoE's National Center for Telehealth and Technology |
| TATRC | Telemedicine and Advanced Technology Research Center |
| TBI | Traumatic brain injury |
| TEAM | Troop education for army morale |
| TRICARE | *not an acronym* (the military medical health system) |
| TBIMS | TBI Model Systems |
| TLD | Third-location decompression |
| TOP | Telemedicine Outreach for Post Traumatic Stress |
| TRMD | Treatment-resistant major depression |
| UC | Usual care |
| UK | United Kingdom |
| USAMRMC | US Army Medical Research and Materiel Command |
| USDA | US Department of Agriculture |
| USUHS | Uniformed Services University of the Health Sciences |
| VA | Department of Veterans Affairs |
| VA RR&D | VA Rehabilitation Research and Development Service |
| VAMC | VA Medical Center |
| VBA | Veterans Benefits Administration |
| VetPop | The Veteran Population |
| VHA | Veterans Health Administration |
| VISN | Veterans Integrated Service Network |
| VRP | Vocational rehabilitation program |
| VSA | Veterans Service Area |
| WVHSHG | Women Veterans Health Strategic Health Care Group |

# D

# SUMMARY OF FEDERALLY FUNDED RESEARCH RELATED TO OEF AND OIF POPULATIONS

Table D.1 lists federally funded research related to Operation Enduring Freedom (OEF) and Operation Iraqi Freedom (OIF) populations, including completed studies, ongoing studies, and studies that had missing or incomplete information such that the committee was unable to determine their status. The table is incomplete due to the difficulty in finding some of the information; however, it provides the reader with an idea of the breadth of the numerous studies that are being conducted and/or funded by the U.S. government.

**TABLE D.1** Summary of Federally Funded Research Related to OEF and OIF Populations

| End Date | Title | Study Population and Methods | Principal Investigator/Sponsor |
|---|---|---|---|
| Completed Studies | | | |
| 2008-04 | Evaluation of Two Telehealth Interventions Targeting Post-Trauma Stress in Combat Veterans: Comparing Mindfulness and Psychoeducation | The study targeted newly returned veterans from the Iraq and Afghanistan conflicts. Specifically, researchers compared the relative efficacy of an alternative therapeutic approach, a mindfulness-based treatment, with a psychoeducation treatment in reducing symptoms of posttraumatic stress disorder (PTSD) and more generalized psychiatric symptoms, while increasing quality of life. Of note, both treatment conditions consisted of two in-person sessions and six brief, weekly telephone calls. Participants were 58 veterans (29 per condition) recruited from the Department of Veterans Affairs (VA) Boston Healthcare System. Assessment occurred before and after the delivery of the intervention. It was hypothesized that while both treatments will result in improved outcomes the mindfulness intervention will promote more healing than the psychoeducation intervention (Final N = 33). | Barbara L. Niles (principal investigator)/VA |
| 2008-09 | Tracking OEF/OIF Transition from DOD to VA | The primary objectives of the study were to establish the feasibility of Department of Defense (DOD)-to-VA protected health information transfer on a local level, and to assess the rate of transition to VA from Brooke Army Medical Center (BAMC) for the cohort of BAMC patients seen during fiscal year (FY) 2002–FY2007. Cohort included 994 OEF/OIF seriously wounded warriors cared for at and discharged from BAMC during FY2002–FY2006. | Laurel Anne Copeland, VA South Texas Health Care System/VA |
| 2009-03 | Evaluation of Polytrauma Brain Injury Rehabilitation Transitional Program | Objectives of this 6-month evaluation using multimethods were to (1) identify learning needs (skills, knowledge, attitudes) of providers in the transitional program at one VA Medical Center (VAMC) as perceived by staff as well as patients and family members; (2) determine the content and processes of an educational program to meet the needs of providers; and (3) determine feasibility, test burden, and content validity of a battery of outcome measures for patients and families. | Steven G. Scott, James A. Haley Veterans Hospital/VA |
| 2009-04 | Treatment of Insomnia in Military Veterans: Phase 1 | A 4-week behavioral treatment that targets chronic insomnia (lasting >1 month) was tested in 12 service members returning from OEF/OIF. | Anne Germain, University of Pittsburgh |
| 2009-05 | Rural/Urban Differences in Service Utilization Among OIF/OEF Veterans | Data from the OEF/OIF registry and the Veterans Integrated Service Network (VISN) 16 data warehouse were used to identify OEF/OIF veterans (n = 32,164) who were enrolled in VISN 16 since September 11, 2001. Demographic, service use, alcohol use disorders, depression and PTSD screening, and pharmacy records were extracted for the 6 months following the index dates for VA first encounter. | Teresa J. Hudson, PharmD Central Arkansas VHS, Eugene J. Towbin Healthcare Center/VA |

| End Date | Title | Study Population and Methods | Principal Investigator/Sponsor |
|---|---|---|---|
| 2009-05 | Assessment of the Health Care Needs and Barriers to VA Use Experienced by Women | The National Survey of Women's Veterans (NSWV) is a nationwide telephone survey of women veterans, including both VA users and VA nonusers, with oversampling of OIF/OEF veterans. Survey items included measures of demographic and military service characteristics, health status, VA- and non-VA ambulatory care use, and determinants of and barriers to VA health care use (N = ?). | Donna L. Washington, VA Greater Los Angeles Healthcare System/VA |
| 2009-06 | Team Based Initiative Support (pilot study) | This study investigated family needs of six rural families caring for a veteran with traumatic brain injury (TBI) 1 to 5 years post-injury. Unmet needs were indentified, training about TBI and a resource book with information on TBI diagnosis, prognosis, and symptoms provided to families. | Linda Olivia Nichols, Memphis, TN/VA |
| 2009-07 | Forgiveness-Based Writing to Prevent PTSD in OEF/OIF Veterans | A forgiveness-based writing intervention was evaluated in 20 OEF/OIF veterans who recently experienced combat-related trauma. | Catherine R. Barber/South Central VA |
| 2009-08 | Visual Dysfunction in MTBI: A Comparison Group Study | In this study, 75 patients diagnosed with PTSD but with no history of mild traumatic brain injury (mTBI) completed a visual screen (assessments of visual acuity, visual field, self-reported visual function, and measures of accommodative function, vergence, pursuit, and saccades). The results were compared to data from the ongoing study of visual dysfunction in patients diagnosed with mTBI. | Gregory Goodrich, VA Palo Alto Health Care System/VA |
| 2009-08 | The Use of Anti-Oxidants to Reduce Sequela of Mild TBI (mTBI) After Blast Exposure | This study compared the effectiveness of the observation and administration of N-acetyl-cysteine (7 days) to placebo in 150 individuals with mTBI on hearing and balance function. | Michael E. Hoffer/Brooke Army Medical Center |
| 2009-09 | Motivational Interviewing to Engage OEF/OIF Veterans in Mental Health Treatment | In this study, a randomized controlled trial of 1,000 OEF/OIF veterans was used to evaluate the efficacy of telephone-administered motivational interviewing compared to informational support sessions. | Karen H. Seal/San Francisco VA |
| 2009-09 | Telephone Based Care for OIF/OEF Veterans With PTSD | In this study, 20 patients with a clinical diagnosis of PTSD were followed by a case manager for up to 6 months to evaluate the feasibility of augmenting standard PTSD treatment with Translating Initiatives for Depression into Effective Solutions (TIDES)-based telephone-based nurse-care management. | Bradford L. Felker, Puget Sound VA Health Care System/VA |
| 2009-09 | Impact of Practice Structure on Quality of Care for Women Veterans (Phase 2) | This study examined changes in how VA women's health care was organized over time, conducting analyses of VA women's health organizational surveys administered in 2001 and 2006–2007 to the census of VAMCs and large community-based outpatient clinics (CBOCs) that served 300 or more women veterans, based on prior year. | Elizabeth M. Yano, VA Greater Los Angeles Health Care System/VA |

| End Date | Title | Study Population and Methods | Principal Investigator/Sponsor |
|---|---|---|---|
| 2009-10 | The Efficacy of Virtual Reality (VR) as an Adjunct Therapy for Acute Combat-Related Post-Traumatic Stress Disorder (PTSD) in Non-Combatants | In this study, 136 service members with PTSD related to service in Iraq or Afghanistan were randomly assigned to receive either the virtual reality treatment or usual treatment. | Brenda Wiederhold/Office of Naval Research, Virtual Reality Medical Center |
| 2009-10 | Dissemination Evaluation of Educational Materials for Puerto Rican OIF/OEF Veterans and Families | A postdeployment education materials booklet was disseminated to 3,400 veterans and family members at the "Welcome Home" event in San Juan, Puerto Rico. Partners, champions, and other providers disseminated 10,326 additional booklets to Puerto Rican veterans and family members. The webpage on the VA Caribbean Health Care was accessed 263 times. | Constance R. Uphold, North Florida/South Georgia Veterans Health System/VA |
| 2009-10 | Implementation and Sustainability of VA Women's Mental Health Clinics | Researchers designed and conducted semistructured telephone interviews of a national sample of clinic directors of special women veterans' mental health programs (n = 35 VA mental health clinicians and administrators); interviewed a small pilot sample (n = 9) of women veterans based at the VA Greater Los Angeles Healthcare System to explore their needs, preferences, utilization, and experiences in seeking and obtaining VA mental health care services; conducted two focus groups of OEF/OIF women veterans (VA users and nonusers). | Elizabeth M. Yano, VA Greater Los Angeles HCS/VA |
| 2009-11 | Testing the Use of Interoceptive Exposure to Reduce Barriers to Psychotherapy | In this study, 40 male OEF/OIF veterans with combat-related PTSD randomized to either receive 4 weeks of supportive counseling or interoceptive exposure to test anxiety sensitivity and avoidance. Assessments were conducted prior to and 5 to 6 weeks after therapy. | Kevin S. Del Ben/G.V. (Sonny) Montgomery VA Medical Center |
| 2009-12 | Prazosin vs Paroxetine in Combat Stress Symptoms in OIF/OEF Returnees | This study involved a placebo-controlled 12-week clinical trial of prazosin versus paroxetine in 210 OEF/OIF veterans to evaluate efficacy and tolerability of prazosin. The study assessed trauma-related nightmares, sleep disturbance, and change in global clinical status at baseline, 6, and 12 weeks. | Elaine Peskind, VA Puget Sound Health Care System, Seattle/VA |
| 2009-12 | Implementing Integrated Care for Veterans with Serious Mental Illness | The objective of this study was to assess the organization and degree of integrated care for substance use and general medical services in Veterans Health Administration (VHA) mental health programs and to evaluate the association between underlying organizational characteristics (e.g., staffing, information technology, performance incentives), degree of clinical integration (e.g., coordination, comprehensiveness, and continuity of care), and patient-level outcomes (e.g., quality of care). | Amy M. Kilbourne, VA Ann Arbor Healthcare System/VA |

| End Date | Title | Study Population and Methods | Principal Investigator/Sponsor |
|---|---|---|---|
| 2009-12 | Effects of Performance Measurement on Healthcare Systems | The aim of this study was to develop an in-depth understanding of positive and negative unintended effects of primary care clinical performance measurement on care delivery processes, on health care providers, and on patients. Researchers conducted semistructured in-person individual interviews of staff members at four VA facilities between February and July 2009. A total of 60 interviews were conducted, including 44 with primary care staff and 16 interviews with facility administrators. | Adam A. Powell, VA Medical Center, Minneapolis/VA |
| 2010-04 | Process Quality Measures of Addiction Care: Validation and Refinement | The objectives of this study were to determine the degree of association between meeting the process of care criteria at the patient level with outcome quality measures; determine the degree of association between facility-level rates of meeting the process of care measures with outcome quality measures (e.g., average patient outcomes), structural quality measures (e.g., number of substance use disorders (SUD) beds, patient-to-staff ratios), and other process measures (e.g., adherence to clinical practice guidelines). Researchers examined three preexisting samples of VA SUD patients (n = 5,723; 3,450; and 340,000, respectively) and evaluated the degree of association between the three process-of-care quality measures and outcome quality measures (e.g., SUD symptom and psychosocial improvement) and structural quality measures. | Alex H.S. Harris, VA Palo Alto Health Care System/VA |
| 2010-04 | VA's Quality Transformation: Lessons for Evidence-Based Management | The purpose of the study was to integrate and analyze a series of highly unique data sources that span VA's reorganization launched in 1996 with Kizer's Vision and Journey for Change policy documents, starting from a pre-directive year (1993), through early (1996) and later reorganization (1999–2000). The objective was, therefore, to evaluate organizational and contextual determinants that contributed to VA's quality transformation. | Elizabeth M. Yano, VA Greater Los Angeles HCS/VA |
| 2010-05 | Benzodiazepine Receptor in PTSD | This project examined binding of the benzodiazepine receptor in Iraq combat veterans with and without PTSD and to see if it can predict which returning veterans will develop chronic PTSD. | James Douglas, Emory University Bremner/National Institute of Mental Health (NIMH) |
| 2010-05 | The Effect of EFT (Emotional Freedom Techniques) on Psychological States in a Veterans Population: A Randomized Controlled Trial | In this study, those with a PTSD-positive assessment on the PTSD Checklist-Military (PCL-M) were randomized into two groups. Control group continued to receive standard of care (SOC) from providers. Experimental group received SOC plus emotional freedom techniques coaching. Assessments were made after 6 completed sessions and after 3 and 6 months (N = ?). | Dawson Church/Soul Medicine Institute |

| End Date | Title | Study Population and Methods | Principal Investigator/Sponsor |
|---|---|---|---|
| 2010-06 | Improving Quality-of-Life and Depressive Symptoms for OEF/OIF Combat Veterans: Assessing the Benefits of Interactive, Internet-based Psychotherapy and Peer-to-Peer Support | This pilot study of potential benefit, feasibility, and safety of the Vets Prevail Program Intervention consisted of a single group (pre-/post-comparison) of 50 recent OEF/OIF veterans in the frame work of a phase 1 clinical trial (phase 1). Feasibility (adherence and satisfaction), evidence of clinical benefit, would be evaluated through changes in the following clinical self-report measures: (1) symptoms of depressed mood (Center for Epidemiologic Studies Depression Scale), (2) PTSD (PCL-M), and (3) functional status (Short Form 12), as well as changes in key attitudes toward mental health care seeking (intent to seek treatment, mental health self-efficacy, and stigma). | Benjamin VanVoorhees, Rise Consulting, LLC/Prevail Health Solutions, LLC |
| 2010-06 | Participation in PTSD: Who Starts, Who Stays and Who Drops Out | This pilot study sampled over a 1-year period veterans with no non–substance abuse mental health–related visits in the prior year who received a PTSD diagnosis (n = 20,284). Objectives were to (1) fill the gap in the PTSD treatment evidence base by ascertaining rates and extent of treatment participation among veterans for whom PTSD was recently identified as a problem; (2) identify patient, treatment, and contextual factors associated with treatment dropout or lack of followup in the 6 months following receipt of a PTSD diagnosis; and (3) identify specific targets in the PTSD treatment pathway amenable to intervention. | Michele R. Spoont, PhD, Minneapolis VA Health Care System, Minneapolis, MN/VA |
| 2010-07 | Exposure Therapy for Chronic PTSD: Efficacy and Mechanisms | In this study, 36 OEF/OIF veterans with chronic PTSD of at least 3 months duration were randomly assigned to 15 sessions of either prolonged exposure (PE) therapy or present-centered therapy. | Sheila Rauch, Ann Arbor Healthcare System/VA |
| 2010-07 | Randomized Trial of a Self-Management Early Intervention for Combat-Related PTSD | This study was a randomized trial Internet-based intervention aimed at reducing PTSD symptomatology and associated functional impairment among combat-exposed soldiers. The intervention was designed to be both efficacious in reducing PTSD symptomatology and attractive to soldiers returning from combat who are experiencing PTSD symptoms but fear seeking formal mental health treatment because of the stigma and the perceived negative career impact (N = ?). | Juesta M. Caddell, RTI/NIMH |
| 2010-08 | Development of a Family-Based, Post-Deployment Intervention | This pilot study assessed the feasibility and acceptability of the Family Intervention Telephone Tracking-Deployment Readjustment intervention in returning military personnel and their partners (N = ?). | Ivan W. Miller, Butler Hospital/NIMH |

| End Date | Title | Study Population and Methods | Principal Investigator/Sponsor |
|---|---|---|---|
| 2010-08 | MST Effects on PTSD and Health Behavior: A Longitudinal Study of Marines | In this study, relationships between military sexual trauma (MST) and respondents' functioning approximately 11 years after joining the Marines were evaluated utilizing a sample of 1,847 Marine recruits as part of a prospective longitudinal study. The objectives were to (1) identify premilitary risk factors for MST; (2) evaluate MST impact on mental health, health risk behaviors, and functional health outcomes; (3) examine PTSD severity as a mediator of MST and health risk behaviors, and between MST and functional health outcomes; (4) identify risk and resilience factors that moderate the impact of MST on health outcomes; and (5) identify risk factors for suicide. This study is the fifth wave of data collection (T5) in a longitudinal investigation of 1,847 Marines. T5 occurred approximately 10 years after recruit training. | Jillian C. Shipherd, VA Boston Healthcare System/VA |
| 2010-08 (ter-minated) | Imagery Rescripting for Posttraumatic Nightmares in Rural Operation Enduring Freedom (OEF)/Operation Iraqi Freedom (OIF) Veterans With Posttraumatic Stress Disorder (PTSD) | In this study, 7 veterans with combat nightmares and PTSD tested a technique that teaches specific skills to help improve their sleep habits and decrease the frequency and severity of their nightmares, decrease symptoms of depression and PTSD, and improve sleep quality and quantity. | Mary E. Long, DeBakey VAMC/VA |
| 2010-09 | Efficacy of Mantram Repetition on PTSD Symptoms in Veterans | This study was a randomized, controlled clinical trial to compare a mantram group intervention (6 weeks, 90 minutes per week in small groups) to a delayed treatment control group on outcomes of self-reported PTSD symptoms, psychological distress, and quality of life (N = 146). | Jill E. Bormann, VA San Diego Health Care System/VA |
| 2010-09 | Evaluation of Family Outreach Mental Health Programs for OEF/OIF Veterans | No additional information found. | Heather Reisinger, Iowa City VAMC/VA |
| 2010-09 | Pilot Test of Preference-Based Insomnia Treatment for OEF/OIF Veterans | The specific aims of the pilot test were to evaluate the feasibility of implementing preference-based insomnia treatment and examine its preliminary effectiveness in improving self-reported insomnia and daytime functioning. Twenty-six veterans participated in a one-group prepost design pilot intervention study. | Dana R. Epstein, Phoenix VA Health Care System/VA |
| 2010-09 | Placebo-Controlled Study of Mirtazapine for PTSD in OIF/OEF Veterans | In this study, 100 OEF/OIF veterans with PTSD were randomized to either mirtazapine or placebo to study efficacy and tolerance to the drug. | Lori Lynne Davis, Tuscaloosa VAMC/VA |
| 2010-09 | Supported Education for OI/EF Veterans with Disabilities | A Participatory Action Research approach was utilized via assembling a development team. The development team was tasked with conducting a needs assessment and an implementation assessment for supported education. Data was collected through focus groups with OIF/OEF veterans with self-reported symptoms of PTSD. Researchers prepared a supported education practice curriculum and implementation guidelines based on data collected (N = ?). | Marsha Langer Ellison, Edith Nourse Rogers Memorial Veterans Hospital/VA |

| End Date | Title | Study Population and Methods | Principal Investigator/Sponsor |
|---|---|---|---|
| 2010-09 | Physical and Sexual Assault in Deployed Women: Risks, Outcomes and Services | Phase 1 of this study used focus groups to refine the study interview, pilot the interview protocol, and ascertain its psychometric properties. Phase 2 involved the identification and successful interviewing of 500 women, using random sampling with stratification. The telephone interview was used to assess sociodemographic variables, trauma exposures, health history, current health status, military environmental factors (organizational and situational factors), military and VA health care and barriers to this care, and self-reported service use. | Anne G. Sadler, VA Medical Center, Iowa City/VA |
| 2010-09 | Outpatient Waiting Times, Outcomes, and Cost for VA Patients with Diabetes | This project explained the variation within the VA in how long veterans wait for outpatient care with supply and demand characteristics and examined the potential effects of waiting for outpatient care on health outcomes and health care cost. This research used VA administrative data and other publicly available Medicare and Medicaid data from the Centers for Medicare and Medicaid Services. | Steven Daniel Pizer, VA Medical Center, Jamaica Plain Campus/VA |
| 2010-09 | Predicting Post-Deployment Mental Health Substance Abuse and Services Needs | The goal of this study was to understand risk and resilience factors that predict development of a psychiatric or substance-abuse disorder and associated mental health and/or substance-abuse service use. A national, stratified random sample of 1,300 veterans enrolled for VA care served as the study sample. | Susan V. Eisen, Edith Nourse Rogers Memorial Veterans Hospital/VA |
| 2010-09 | Treatment of OEF/OIF Veteran Neuropsychiatric Outcomes Following TBI | Website intervention was developed for OEF/OIF veterans and their families to treat veteran and family stresses from neuropsychiatric/behavioral consequences of complicated mild TBI (cm-TBI). The feasibility and acceptability of the websites was tested via a random controlled trial, which enrolls 25 cm-TBI veterans assigned in a 2 (treatment as usual [TAU], n = 10):3 (intervention, n = 15) ratio. | Armando J. Rotondi, VA Pittsburgh Health Care System/VA |
| 2010-09 | Measuring and Improving Sustainability in Mental Health System Redesign | This research project was designed to examine the issue of sustainability as it relates to the VA Mental Health Systems Redesign (MHSR) initiative. The project had three specific objectives: (1) Describe the array of systems redesign projects and their outcome measures that had been started in the first phase of the MHSR project. (2) Use the 10-item British National Health Service Sustainability Index to (a) describe the variability in sustainability factors across VISNs and facilities; (b) describe the predictors of sustainability index scores for the various projects; and (c) predict outcome measures and their sustainability for individual projects. The model posits that sustained change is related to ten metrics that can be group as process, organization, and staff factors, which are included in the sustainability index. (3) Interview a random sample of systems redesign team members, including VISN 2 and 12 leadership, facility-level leadership, and clinical and administrative staff, to better understand the factors that facilitate and impede change and sustainability. | Dean D. Krahn, MD, William S. Middleton Memorial Veterans Hospital, Madison/VA |

| End Date | Title | Study Population and Methods | Principal Investigator/Sponsor |
|---|---|---|---|
| 2010-09 | CSP 575—PTSD Genomewide Association Study of OEF/OIF Deployed Military Personnel: Phase I (Feasibility Study) | The PATRIOT research project was designed to identify possible genetic variations that may influence risk for combat stress reactions. The study was completed in two stages: (1) feasibility study to test out the study process and (2) use the results from the feasibility study as a guide for the structure of the second study. The second part of the study will aim to identify genes that may contribute or protect against PTSD (N = 20,000). | Murray B. Stein and Joel Gelernter/VA |
| 2010-10 | Advanced MRI in Blast-Related TBI | The purpose of this study was to examine the usefulness of magnetic resonance imaging (MRI) scans in predicting memory loss, attention deficit, depression, or PTSD in 100 active-duty military personnel serving in Iraq or Afghanistan with TBI and other injury control 6 to 12 months postinjury. | David L. Brody/Washington University School of Medicine |
| 2010-10 | Online Interventions for Female OEF/OIF Reserve/National Guard War Vets | Phase 1 of this study identified a random sample of 137 OEF/OIF Reserve/National Guard (R/NG) service women from a five-state Midwest area who returned from deployment in Iraq or Afghanistan in the prior 12 months. Phase 2 involved 37 follow-up telephone interviews with a trained coordinator who also provided information about VHA resources and facilitated access to care as indicated. The long-term goal was to improve R/NG servicewomen's knowledge about their own postdeployment adjustment and improve their willingness to access VA mental health care. | Anne G. Sadler, VA Medical Center, Iowa City/VA |
| 2010-10 | Innovative Practices for Psychological Health and TBI | This study identified and evaluated the effectiveness of DOD-sponsored programs designed to support psychological health and TBI among service personnel and their families. | Robin Weinick, RAND Corporation/DOD |
| 2010-12 | Treatment of Moderate to Mild Cognitive Dysfunction Caused by Traumatic Brain Injury (TBI) With Hyperbaric Oxygen Therapy (HBOT) | In this study, 50 OIF/OEF individuals with chronic mild to moderate TBI were assigned to an intervention (100% oxygen at 2.4 ATA in three 30-minute periods separated by 10 minutes of breathing air at 2.4 ATA; ATA = atmosphere absolute) or sham arm. Assessments (computer based cognitive tests) conducted pre-exposure, after 15 HBOT, and 6 weeks post-HBOT. | Robert S. Michaelson/San Antonio Military Medical Center |
| 2010-12 | Combined Exposure Therapy and D-Cycloserine vs Placebo for Posttraumatic Stress Disorder | In this study, 40 participants with 9/11-related or Iraq War–related PTSD were assigned to one of two programs—both included Virtual Reality Exposure Therapy and standard cognitive-behavioral therapy techniques. One group received cycloserine (seromycin), and one group received a placebo. | JoAnn Difede/Weill Medical College of Cornell University |
| 2010-12 (terminated) | PTSD Symptom Reduction by Propranolol Given After Memory Activation | In this study, 76 OEF/OIF veterans meeting *Diagnostic and Statistical Manual of Mental Disorders*, 4th Edition (DSM-IV) criteria for chronic PTSD were randomly assigned to the propranolol or placebo drug condition. Six memory reactivation sessions were immediately followed by administration of propranolol or placebo. Assessments were conducted immediately after and 6 months after the treatment sessions. | Scott P. Orr, VA Medical Center, Manchester/VA |

| End Date | Title | Study Population and Methods | Principal Investigator/Sponsor |
|---|---|---|---|
| 2010-12 | Blast-Related Health Problem Identification and Polytrauma Taxonomy | This 2-year population-based study characterized the OEF/OIF experiences with polytrauma and blast-related injuries (PT/BRI) among the 10,000 current members of the Florida National Guard. The purpose of project was to be able to modify the natural history of these blast-related injuries, minimizing the adverse sequelae and maximizing recovery. | Steven G. Scott, James A. Haley Veterans Hospital/VA |
| 2010-12 | Identifying Potential Demand for VA Rehabilitation Services for OEF/OIF Veterans | The objective of this research was to improve access to rehabilitation services for OEF/OIF veterans with spinal cord injury (SCI), TBI, and amputations. Researchers identified those geographic areas and their injured OEF/OIF veteran cohorts that have the greatest potential demand for VHA rehabilitation services. Researchers used Geographic Information System tools previously applied to both the VHA TBI population and, more recently, to the FY2003 and FY2004 OEF/OIF traumatically injured veterans who used VHA services. | W. Bruce Vogel, North Florida/South Georgia Veterans Health System/VA |
| 2011-00 | A Needs Assessment of Returning Veterans and their Families in NY State | The objective of this project is to assess the physical health, mental health, and social service needs of veterans and their family members residing in New York State. | Terry Schell, RAND Corporation |
| 2011-01 | Risperidone Treatment for Military Service Related Chronic Post-Traumatic Stress Disorder | In this study, 400 veterans with the diagnosis of military-related PTSD were enrolled at 20 VAMC hospitals over a 2-year period. Patients were randomized in a double-blind manner to risperidone or placebo. Comparison between groups were made at 6 months. | John H. Krystal, VA Connecticut Health Care System/VA |
| 2011-01 | Effects of Escitalopram on Autonomic Reactivity in Post Traumatic Stress Disorder Among Veterans of Operation Enduring Freedom and Iraqi Freedom (OEF/OIF) | In this study, researchers studied if taking escitalopram normalized heart rate variability and decreased (or no effect implying a lack of serious cardiac side effects), including QT variability in veterans with PTSD. Primary outcome measures were to (1) investigate the effects of escitalopram on cardiac vagal function as measured by R-R interval variability, especially in the high-frequency (0.15–0.5 Hz) band in OEF/OIF veterans with PTSD [time frame: 12 weeks; designated as safety issue: Yes]; and (2) investigate the effects of escitalopram on an absolute or relative decrease in cardiac sympathetic function and serious cardiac side effects as measured by QT interval variability in OEF/OIF veterans with PTSD (N = 30). | Sriram Ramaswamy, VA Nebraska Western Iowa Health Care System/VA |
| 2011-02 | Applying Rapid Assessment Process to Health Outreach to OIF/OEF Veterans | In this study, participants were recruited from key stakeholder groups within the 22nd VISN geographic area: (1) OEF/OIF veterans; (2) OEF/OIF veteran's social contacts important to their health care seeking; and (3) outreach, policy, and administrative personnel from the VA. Semistructured interviews were performed with outreach staff, policy and administrative personnel, and veteran's social contacts. OEF/OIF veterans were to participate in focus groups and complete a short survey (N = ?). | Patrick E. Link, VA Greater Los Angeles Healthcare System/VA |

| End Date | Title | Study Population and Methods | Principal Investigator/Sponsor |
|---|---|---|---|
| 2011-03 (with-drawn) | Early Intervention for PTSD in Iraqi Veterans | In this study, 160 OIF veterans who returned from Iraq in the past 6 months and who meet criteria for early PTSD were randomized to receive either paroxetine or placebo. PTSD symptoms, brain markers, neuropsychological testing of memory, and cortisol response to an Iraq-related traumatic script before and after the intervention were assessed. | Doug Bremner, Atlanta VA Medical and Rehab Center, Decatur/VA |
| 2011-03 | Evaluation of TBI Screening Processes and Healthcare Utilization | The aims of this study were to examine factors associated with receipt of the TBI clinical reminder (CR) and the association between the results of the TBI CR, veteran characteristics, and subsequent VA health care utilization and costs. | Bridget Smith, Edward Hines, Jr. VA Hospital/VA |
| 2011-03 | Identifying Patterns of BMI Change in OEF/OIF Veterans | The objective of this pilot proposal was to identify patterns of body mass index (BMI) change in veterans returning from Afghanistan (OEF) and from Iraq (OIF). Researchers created and analyzed a longitudinal database using VA electronic record data (N = 16,656). | Patricia Hirt Rosenberger, VA Connecticut Healthcare System West Haven Campus/VA |
| 2011-03 | Mission Reconnect: Promoting Resilience and Re-Integration of Post-Deployment Vet | In this study, 40 veterans and their chosen partners participated in focus groups and workshops and to test prototype materials with the overall goal of producing a multimedia educational intervention that will support OEF/OIF veterans and their partners with instruction in cognitive and behavioral processes at home. | William B. Collinge, Collinge and Associates/NIMH |
| 2011-03 | Perspectives on Enhancing Family Involvement in Treatment for PTSD | This study involved approximately 160 participants (80 veterans and 80 family members). Researchers used qualitative methods to identify the needs and preferences of OIF/OEF veterans and family members and assessed the implications of study findings for program design. Researchers conducted individual and group interviews in Little Rock and Oklahoma City with 40 male veterans. Researchers conducted separate individual and group interviews in Little Rock and Oklahoma City with 40 female veterans and with 80 family members of participating veterans in those cities. Interviews addressed perceived needs, desires for family involvement in treatment, types of services that are attractive/unattractive, elements of alternative approaches to meeting needs that are attractive/unattractive, as well as logistic considerations (e.g., timing and frequency of meetings, mode of meeting, child care). Researchers used the techniques of constant comparison and content analysis to analyze interview data (N = 160). | Ellen P. Fischer, Central Arkansas VHS Eugene J. Towbin Healthcare Center/VA |
| 2011-03 | Psychophysiological Reactivity to Identify and Treat Veterans at Risk for PTSD | No additional information found. | VA |
| 2011-03 | Treatment of Comorbid Insomnia in Military Veterans | In this study, 40 OEF/OIF returnees were randomized to either the brief behavioral treatment of insomnia intervention or to information control condition. Sleep measures, as well as measures of PTSD, anxiety, depression, and perceived physical health, were measured. | Anne Germain, University of Pittsburgh/NIMH |

| End Date | Title | Study Population and Methods | Principal Investigator/Sponsor |
|---|---|---|---|
| 2011-03 | Using Stimulator to Enhance Cognitive Recovery after Brain Injury | The goal of this study was to determine whether participants with a history of mTBI and/or PTSD and self-reported driving difficulties perform more poorly than healthy controls on an assessment of driving abilities and to examine the association between cognitive and behavioral symptoms with driving abilities (N = ?). | Melissa Amick/VA |
| 2011-03 | Understanding and Meeting the Needs of Informal Caregivers to Improve Outcomes for Traumatic Brain Injury Patients with Polytrauma | This was a mixed-method, cross-sectional, observational study. Next of kin for veterans discharged from four VA Polytrauma Rehabilitation Centers were mailed a questionnaire that included demographic information; objective burden; instrumental, social, cognitive resources, and resiliency factors available; caregiver; caregiver and family outcomes; and patient health and functioning outcomes. | Joan M. Griffin, VAMC Minneapolis/VA |
| 2011-03 | Health Care Use and Costs of Veterans with Neurotrauma | The primary objective of this study was to examine VA, Medicare, and Medicaid utilization and costs for veterans with neurotrauma. The study was retrospective, and included available VA, Medicare, and Medicaid demographic, utilization and cost data starting in calendar year 1999 (includes OEF/OIF) (N = ?). | Bridget M. Smith, Edward Hines, Jr. VA Hospital/VA |
| 2011-03 | Promoting Implementation of My Health*e*Vet Among Veterans with SCI/D | The goal of this study was to understand the issues associated with implementing a campaign to promote use of the My Health*e*Vet (MHV) system among veterans with spinal cord injury or disorder (SCI/D) and their VA SCI/D health care providers and to assess the effectiveness of two different promotional campaign strategies. Data sources and analysis activities included semi structured interviews and questionnaires administered to veterans with SCI/D and VA SCI/D health care providers at both centers and the use of Computerized Patient Record System (CPRS) data to examine changes in in-person authentication rates before and after the promotional campaigns (N = ?). | Timothy Patrick Hogan, Edward Hines, Jr. VA Hospital/VA |
| 2011-03 | Adapting Coordination of Care Measures to Assess Polytrauma Care | In Phase 1 of the study, researchers modified an existing structural integration measure for use in the Polytrauma Network Site (PNS) clinic context, which was reviewed by a PNS clinic director to ensure adequacy. The refined measure was then administered to the other 21 PNS clinic directors. Information obtained from Phase 1 informed the Phase 2 coordination measures. These instruments were administered to two focus groups comprised of PNS clinic core providers and staff to which the PNS clinics make referrals. Staff provided feedback on how to improve the surveys. Based on these results, in Phase 3 researchers created a Web-based coordination survey and administered it to providers at 10 randomly selected PNSs. The psychometric properties of the coordination scales were then assessed. | Terri Krangel Pogoda, VA Medical Center, Jamaica Plain Campus/VA |

| End Date | Title | Study Population and Methods | Principal Investigator/Sponsor |
|---|---|---|---|
| 2011-03 | Survey of the Organizational Structure of the Physical Therapy Service in VHA | The specific aims of this pilot project, achieved through a collaborative effort between VA clinicians, service administrators, and researchers, were to (1) develop a survey instrument that is useful for administrative and research purposes and designed to identify administrative and operational characteristics hypothesized to influence quality and outcomes of care for patients treated by physical therapists, (2) gather pilot data from a subsample of service managers, and (3) revise and finalize the survey instrument. | Patricia L. Sinnott, VA Palo Alto Health Care System/VA |
| 2011-04 (with-drawn, did not obtain IRB approval) | A Pilot Study Using Gradual Virtual Reality Exposure Therapy and D-Cycloserine (DCS) for Treatment of Combat-Related Psychological Trauma in Burn Service Members | Feasibility of using gradual virtual reality exposure therapy and DCS in the management of PTSD symptoms in four burned OIF/OEF service members was examined. | Kathryn M. Gaylord/U.S. Army Institute of Surgical Research |
| 2011-04 | A Psychophysiologic Study of Weakening Traumatic Combat Memories with Post-Reactivation Propranolol | In this study, 66 OEF/OIF veterans with combat-related PTSD were randomly assigned to one of two groups: postreactivation propranolol or nonreactivation propranolol. Subjects in the nonreactivation propranolol group received propranolol in the absence of traumatic memory reactivation. Subjects randomized to the postreactivation propranolol group received matching placebo capsules. | Roger K. Pitman/ Massachusetts General Hospital, VA |
| 2011-04 | Printed and Web-Based OEF/OIF Culturally-Relevant Family Education | The goal of the study was to develop a model for developing and disseminating Spanish- and English-language OEF/OIF family health information throughout VISN8. The study was to (1) conduct an implementation project in the U.S. Virgin Islands to refine and adapt the study's methods by creating printed and Web-based health information that are written in the English language at a low literacy level and tailored for a unique cultural group and (2) use the lessons learned in Puerto Rico and the U.S. Virgin Islands to plan and develop a service-directed project to address the diverse informational needs of predominant cultural subgroups in VISN8. | Constance R. Uphold, North Florida/South Georgia Veterans Health System/VA |
| 2011-05 | Internet Self-Help Program for Major Depressive Disorder in Spouses of Combatants | This was a pilot study of spouses of veterans with major depressive disorder who will provide feedback on an existing cognitive-behavioral Internet program shown to be efficacious in treating depression. The modified program was tested against the existing program in a randomized trial (N = ?). | Bentson H. Mcfarland, Oregon Health and Science University/NIMH |
| 2011-05 | PTSD Symptoms and Alcohol Problems: Vulnerability and Resilience Factors | This study explored the relationships among traumatic symptoms, vulnerability (impulsivity) and resilience factors (emotional intelligence), and alcohol use and problems among recent returning OEF/OIF veterans (N = ?). | Raluca M. Gaher, University of South Dakota/NIAAA |

| End Date | Title | Study Population and Methods | Principal Investigator/Sponsor |
|---|---|---|---|
| 2011-05 | A Computer Adaptive Test to Measure Community Reintegration | This was a field study of 400 veterans, including (1) 100 veterans under the age of 60 who were observed to have good community reintegration, i.e., those with housing stability and steady employment, (2) 100 veterans under the age of 60 who are homeless and/or chronically unemployed, and (3) 200 OIF/OEF veterans. | Linda J. Resnik, PhD, MS, VA Medical Center, Providence/VA |
| 2011-05 | Gender Differences in Mental Health Treatment Needs and Service Use | Researchers conducted telephone interviews and medical records reviews on 100 VA New Jersey patients (50 men and 50 women) randomly selected from a Decision Support System (DSS) list of patients who screened positive for PTSD in the last 3 years. The questionnaire consisted of mixed and open-ended response items exploring mental and physical health and VA treatment experiences. | Anna Kline, VA New Jersey Health Care System/VA |
| 2011-05 | Implementing Alcohol Counseling with Clinical Reminders: Barriers and Facilitators | The purpose of this study was to identify facilitators and barriers to effective use of alcohol-related clinical reminders (CRs). A secondary purpose was to refine methods in preparation for a national evaluation. This study was an observational, qualitative study of the way clinicians interact with CRs at nine outpatient clinics within VA Puget Sound. VA clinicians were recruited and verbally consented. Four researchers took notes as they observed clinicians interacting with CRs. Notes were transcribed and analyzed qualitatively using template analysis based on an a priori coding template that was derived from Greenhalgh's implementation model. Overall, 58 clinical staff (25 registered nurses, 26 licensed practical nurses, 7 health technicians), and 21 providers (16 medical doctors, 5 nurse practitioners) caring for 166 patients were observed. | Emily C. Williams, VA Puget Sound Health Care System/VA |
| 2011-05 | Service Utilization and Barriers to Care for Veterans in Rural and Urban Settings | This was a planned pilot population-based mail survey study to compare random samples of 100 rural vs 100 urban veterans in the state of Hawaii known to have barriers to care in rural regions. Aims of the study were to determine if veterans in rural communities perceive more community stigma than those located in urban areas and determine the relationship between individual, institutional, and community stigma-related factors in predicting health care utilization among rural and urban veterans. | Julia Whealin, VA Pacific Islands Health Care System, Honolulu/VA |
| 2011-06 | The Effectiveness of FMPO in Improving the Quality of Care for Persons with Severe Mental Illness | The study tested the effectiveness of Family Member Provider Outreach (FMPO)—an innovative, structured, brief and manualized family engagement intervention for veterans with severe mental illness (SMI). In this randomized controlled trial of 240 VA outpatients with SMI, patients were randomized to receive the FMPO intervention or usual services. Baseline and 6-month assessments were completed with all participants. | Lisa B. Dixon, Baltimore VAMC VA Maryland Health Care System/VA |
| 2011-06 | Characterization and Care Coordination of Polytrauma Patients | The purpose of this retrospective chart review study was to describe the short-term durability of functional outcomes for veterans with TBI. A secondary objective was to identify factors that may limit functional independence and are associated with poor outcomes (N = ?). | David Cifu, Boston DVBIC/VA |

| End Date | Title | Study Population and Methods | Principal Investigator/Sponsor |
|---|---|---|---|
| 2011-06 | Manualized Treatment for Veterans with Military Sexual Trauma | The purpose of this study is to evaluate the effectiveness of cognitive processing therapy (CPT) versus present-centered therapy (PCT) in treating current post-traumatic stress symptoms associated with sexual assault that occurred while veterans were serving in the military (N = 170). The study objectives will be met by three levels of hypotheses. Hypotheses focus on the primary outcome (PTSD symptoms), confirmatory outcomes (depression symptoms, quality of life), and exploratory outcomes (cost and utilization). Based on the results of the study, researchers intend to produce an educational CD-ROM, which will include a training manual to educate practitioners on the use of the more effective treatment with veterans. | Alina Suris, PhD, VA North Texas Health Care System, Dallas |
| 2011-06 | Preventive Web-Based Intervention for Spouses of Traumatized Military Personnel | Spouses of veterans with PTSD provided feedback on interactive Web-based technologies that provide education about PTSD and coping strategies (N = ?). | Bentson H. McFarland, OR Health and Science University/NIMH |
| 2011-06 | Relationships and PTSD Study: Detection of Intimate Partner Violence | To examine intimate partner violence (IPV) documentation practices, Phase 1 of this study reviewed every note in the medical record over 5 years for a random sample of 507 veterans enrolled into PTSD treatment. Researchers determined whether an IPV perpetration assessment was documented and, if so, when, which clinic, what provider discipline, and how IPV was detected. Study Phase 2 used a nonexperimental design with 460 veteran/partner dyads recruited from a stratified random sample. Subjects completed paper and pencil instruments and participated in structured interviews. Researchers sought to determine if IPV can be reliably discriminated based on PTSD severity, relationship mutuality, early IPV exposure, and/or substance abuse (discriminant analysis). To determine if these indicators are associated with providers' detection of IPV, logistic regression was to be used (N = 441 couples). | April A. Gerlock, VA Puget Sound Health Care System/VA |
| 2011-06 | Combat, Sexual Assault, and Post-Traumatic Stress in OIF/OEF Military Women | This study had a cross-sectional design with two sequential phases. Phase 1 included focus groups to refine the current study interview specific to regular military populations. Phase 2 involved the identification and successful interviewing of 669 regular military service women who completed a telephone interview that assessed sociodemographic variables, trauma exposures, health history, current health status, military environmental factors (organizational and situational factors), military and VA health care and barriers to this care, and self-reported service use. | Anne G. Sadler, VA Medical Center, Iowa City/VA |

| End Date | Title | Study Population and Methods | Principal Investigator/Sponsor |
|---|---|---|---|
| 2011-06 | Behavioral Couples Therapy Implementation in SUD Specialty Care | In this study, program directors and VISN SUD representatives were be contacted for each of the 21 SUD outpatient programs implementing Behavioral Couples Therapy (BCT), as reported on the FY2008 Drug and Alcohol Program Survey (DAPS; n = 19) or identified by the treatment developer (n = 2). Five sites that have successfully implemented BCT and five sites that have been relatively unsuccessful ("high" versus "low" adopters) were be the focus of this evaluation. Three key informants from each of the 10 sites were interviewed. The interview and survey data were complemented with preexisting data from the DAPS and the National Patient Care Database. | Elizabeth V. Gifford, VA Palo Alto Health Care System/VA |
| 2011-06 | Treatment Preferences and Barriers in OIF Soldiers with mild TBI and/or PTSD | The primary objective of the study was to examine the receipt of best practices and to identify barriers to PTSD treatment among veterans with a history of mTBI. Specifically, the primary aims were to (1) describe the rehabilitation and mental health treatment history, with a focus on receipt of best practices, among OIF deployed veterans with a history of mTBI and/or PTSD and (2) better understand PTSD treatment seeking among veterans with and without a history of mTBI. | Shannon M. Kehle, PhD, VA Medical Center, Minneapolis/VA |
| 2011-07 | Randomized Trial of an Online Early Intervention for Combat PTSD in Primary Care | A randomized, controlled trial of 160 service members with PTSD compared an Internet-based, nurse-assisted, cognitive behavioral self-management program to usual care alone with follow-up at 6 and 12 weeks. | Charles Engel/NIMH |
| 2011-07 | Barriers to Mental Health Care Among OIF/OEF Veterans | Objectives of this study were to (1) compare and contrast psychologically symptomatic veterans who do utilize mental health services with symptomatic veterans who do not utilize mental health services and evaluate the link between subjective barriers to mental health care and actual utilization of behavioral health services in veterans returning from Iraq and Afghanistan and (2) analyze the relationship between beliefs about mental health (subjective barriers to care, psychotherapy, medication, and attributions) and mental health care utilization. Researchers recruited veterans from the Primary Care Clinic or the Mental Hygiene Clinic (N = ?). | Ilan Harpaz-Rotem, VA Connecticut Healthcare System West Haven Campus/VA |
| 2011-07 | Assessing Implementation of Post-Deployment Integrated Care: Pilot Project | This 15-month pilot project studied clinic planning, implementation, and organizational arrangements for six clinics established within VA's Post-Deployment Integrated Care Initiative (PDICI). The study documented and characterized (1) the introduction of PDICI clinics into individual VA health care delivery facilities and (2) the clinics' structure and organizational arrangements. The project identified key factors leading to different implementation processes and organizational arrangements and assessed selected impacts of different implementation processes and organizational arrangements. | Tamar Wyte and Brian Mittman/QUERI RRP, VA |
| 2011-08 | A Cognitive Enhancer May Facilitate Behavioral Exposure Therapy for Veterans with PTSD | In this study, 150 OIF veterans with PTSD were randomly assigned to one of three groups: virtual reality exposure (VRE) therapy and D-cycloserine, VRE therapy and alprazolam, or VRE therapy and placebo. | Barbara O. Rothbaum, Emory University/NIMH |

| End Date | Title | Study Population and Methods | Principal Investigator/Sponsor |
|---|---|---|---|
| 2011-08 | Mobile Enabling Technology to Promote Adherence to Behavioral Therapy | The mobile application iHeal was used by 25 returning combat veterans with PTSD and/or substance abuse to determine whether the physiological changes detected are predictive of posttraumatic stress or drug cues. | Edward W. Boyer, University of Massachusetts Medical School, Worcester/NIDA |
| 2011-08 | Reintegration: The Role of Spouse Telephone BATTLEMIND Pilot Study | In this study, 60 spouses of service members participated in 12-hour-long structured telephone support groups focusing on education, coping skills, and support targeting readjustment postdeployment. | Linda O. Nichols, Memphis VAMC/VA |
| 2011-08 | Theory-Driven Mixed-Methods Evaluation of PTSD Treatment Implementation in VA | Quantitative and qualitative assessments of more than 250 mental health providers in residential PTSD treatment settings (n = 40). The overarching goal was to characterize and assess the implementation process of the two evidenced-based psychotherapies for PTSD, PE, and CPT. The proposed study was conducted in partnership with the Northeast Program Evaluation Program, which monitors all VA mental health programming nationwide, and the National Center for PTSD, which oversees the dissemination of PE and CPT nationally among VA providers. | Joan Cook, Yale University/NIH (OD) |
| 2011-08 | Web-Based Behavioral Intervention For Returning Veterans with Risky Alcohol Use | In this study, 200 returning veterans were randomly assigned to either an initial intervention group or a delayed intervention group to evaluate the efficacy of the Web-based intervention to reduce alcohol use, alcohol problems, and PTSD symptoms. | Terence M. Keane, Boston University Medical Campus/NIH (OD) |
| 2011-08 | Stigma, Gender, and Other Barriers to VHA Use for OEF/OIF Veterans | The primary objective of this project was to examine the contribution of individual, institutional, and most importantly, stigma-related barriers, to VA health care. A secondary objective was to document unique barriers to VA care for women and men. Phase I involved focus groups with OEF/OIF veterans, six focus groups (48 participants). For Phase II, mail surveys incorporating barrier measures and addressing health care use were administered to a nationally representative sample of OEF/OIF veterans (N = 1,000). | Dawne S. Vogt, VA Medical Center, Jamaica Plain Campus/VA |
| 2011-09 | Pain, Psychiatric Disorders, and Disability Among Veterans With and Without Polytrauma | In this study, data on pain and emotional problem prevalence, associated impairments, and barriers to care and community reintegration was assessed in 600 OEF/OIF service members with and without polytrauma. | Michael E. Clark, James A. Haley Veterans Hospital/VA |
| 2011-09 | Accessible Website Design for Cognitive Impairment | The overall goal of this project was to use a group of persons with cognitive impairments to explore website interface design effectiveness, and develop a set of empirically based interface design guidelines to create accessible websites for a population of persons with cognitive impairments. Specifically, the project focused on persons with schizophrenia/schizoaffective disorder (N = ?). | Armando Rotondi, University of Pittsburgh/VA |
| 2011-09 | Cerebrospinal Fluid Neuropeptide Y in PTSD | No additional information found. | VA |

| End Date | Title | Study Population and Methods | Principal Investigator/Sponsor |
| --- | --- | --- | --- |
| 2011-09 | Treating Insomnia and Nightmares After Trauma: Impact on Symptoms and Quality of Life | In this study, 80 participants with PTSD who meet diagnostic criteria for both insomnia and recurring nightmares were randomly assigned to one of two treatment groups to examine whether the addition of sleep treatment decreases PTSD symptoms and improves overall clinical outcomes. | Sean P.A. Drummond, University of California, San Diego/NIH, NINR |
| 2011-09 | Outcomes and Correlates of Suicidal Ideation in OEF/OIF Veterans | This multisite, mixed-methods study was conducted at three VA facilities (Portland, Houston, and Indianapolis) and involved the collection of quantitative data from local facility databases and collection of qualitative information from interviews of 45 veterans screened for suicidal ideation. | Steven K. Dobscha, VA Medical Center, Portland/VA |
| 2011-09 | Prescription Drug Abuse and Addiction Among Active Duty Service Members | This study intended to identify patterns of prescription misuse to characterize its potential impact on military readiness and to make recommendations regarding the needed programs to prevent and treat misuse. Data were from electronic health records and from drug testing. | Diana D. Jeffrey, Center for Healthcare Management Studies/funder unknown |
| 2011-11 | VA Facility Determinants of Racial-Ethnic Variations in Quality of Care | In this study, global, summary, and individual quality indicators and measures were used to identify high disparity sites and their modifiable characteristics associated with disparities. Objective were to identify modifiable VA facility-level characteristics associated with quality of care for specific racial-ethnic minority groups, and to do so within the context in which VA facilities deliver care. | Donna L. Washington, VA Greater Los Angeles Healthcare System/VA |
| 2011-11 | Neurobiological Correlates of PTSD During REM Sleep | The overarching aim of this Exploratory/Developmental Research Grant Award (R21) was to explore the neurobiological correlates of PTSD during rapid-eye-movement sleep by using state-of-the-science positron emission tomography sleep imaging. This observational study allowed researchers to gain insight into the differences in sleep and waking brain mechanisms between veterans with PTSD and those without PTSD (N = 24). | (No PI information)/ University of Pittsburgh |
| 2011-12 | National Guard Outreach and Linkage to Treatment | In this study, investigators conducted semistructured interviews with 25,000 soldiers, buddies, and National Guard leadership to develop and pilot test survey items relevant to implementation; develop and pretest survey items relevant to soldier symptomatic and functional status; conduct a small feasibility study to determine response rates and veteran willingness to allow access to linkable Post-Deployment Health Assessment/Post-Deployment Health Reassessment data and health services data; and construct a merged, de-identified longitudinal dataset comprised of postdeployment health assessment and reassessment data, MHS/TRICARE, and VA services data from National Guard soldiers in Michigan and comparison states of Indiana and Ohio. | Marcia T. Valenstein, Ann Arbor VA HCS/VA |

| End Date | Title | Study Population and Methods | Principal Investigator/Sponsor |
|---|---|---|---|
| 2011-12 | Evaluation of VA's TBI Clinical Reminder and Secondary Level Evaluation | The purpose this study was to determine the clinical validity and reliability of the VA's TBI Clinical Reminder and the Comprehensive TBI Evaluation used to screen for mTBI. Examining the reliability of the two screens determined whether they are dependable. Verifying the clinical validity was important because valid screening and evaluation of mTBI leads to accurate diagnosis and timely treatment. Accurate screening also improves clinical efficiency and ensures that resources are provided to those who need them most. The project findings are expected to advance the science of screening and diagnosis of a mTBI event (N = 456). | Judi L. Babcock-Parziale/VA |
| 2011-12 | Sleep Disturbance in OEF/OIF Veterans with PTSD: A CVD Risk Factor | No additional information found. | VA |
| 2011-12 | The Effect of Acupuncture on PTSD-Related Insomnia | This clinical, single-site, randomized, controlled trial consisted of OIF/OEF veterans with PTSD-related insomnia assigned to group auricular acupuncture, sham control, or true control. The sample size was 20 per group. | Michelle Kennedy Prisco, VA Medical Center, DC/VA |
| 2011-12 | Pilot of Acupuncture to Improve Quality of Life in Veterans with TBI and PTSD | The objective for this pilot project was to determine the efficacy of adjunctive acupuncture for improving quality of life and function and alleviating comorbidities associated with TBI and PTSD in service members injured in the current wars. OIF/OEF veterans who screen positive for TBI or PTSD and were treated with a 12-week standard individualized acupuncture method compared to veterans randomly assigned to standard care alone. Outcomes were measured by the veteran's SF-36 at 6-, 12-, and 24-week follow-ups (N = 50). | Thomas W. Findley, East Orange Campus of the VA New Jersey Health Care System/VA |
| 2011-12 | Central Auditory Processing Disorders Associated with Blast Exposure | The incidence of central auditory dysfunction in war fighters exposed to high-explosive blasts while serving in combat have not been clearly determined. The objectives of this study were to determine whether central auditory processing (CAP) disorders are associated with exposure to high-explosive blasts. This study also examined the incidence, magnitude, and timing of spontaneous recovery of CAP function from blast exposure. The information provided by this study will help guide clinicians in both the military and VA health care systems regarding the likelihood of central auditory processing disorders in soldiers returning from deployment and suggest some clinical rehabilitative strategies for the treatment of these patients with CAP deficits. Subjects took part in a battery of audiological tests meant to evaluate the function and status of the auditory system. These tests are similar to those carried out routinely in audiology clinics and included behavioral tests of pure tone hearing, speech perception, and central auditory function and electrophysiological testing of the middle ear and of the central auditory system (N = 200). | Marjorie R. Leek, VA Medical Center, Portland/VA |

| End Date | Title | Study Population and Methods | Principal Investigator/Sponsor |
|---|---|---|---|
| 2012-03 | Evaluating a Peer Visitor Program for OIF/OEF Veterans with Polytrauma | The goal of this study was to train OIF/OIF veterans with multiple injuries to be peer visitors, i.e., volunteers who visit more recent OIF/OEF veterans and provide support. Researchers evaluated the effectiveness of the training and evaluated any benefits that volunteer peer visitors and the recipients of peer visitors might experience as a result of participating in peer visitation (N = 50). | Rhonda M. Williams, VA Puget Sound Health Care System/VA |
| 2012-03 | Assessing and Reducing Post-Deployment Violence Risk | In this study, 1,000 OEF/OIF veterans were surveyed at baseline and at 1 year about violent behaviors; 300 veterans and a member of their family were to be interviewed at baseline and at 1 year about violence, substance use, family adjustment, PTSD, and employment status. | Eric B. Elbogen, University of North Carolina Chapel Hill/NIMH |
| 2012-03 (ter-minated) | Neural Correlates of Early Intervention for PTSD | In this study, 160 service members returning from Iraq with early PTSD were randomized to receive paroxetine or placebo for 3 months with repeat imaging and assessments. After this, they were treated with open-label paroxetine for 3 months followed by repeat imaging and assessments. 80 healthy service members who did not deploy to OIF and 80 health service members who deployed will serve as controls. | James D. Bremner, Emory University/Atlanta Research and Education Foundation |
| 2012-03 | Brain Markers of Treatment Response in PTSD | In the context of an open-label 12-week clinical trial of paroxetine, this study performed pre- and posttreatment functional MRI (fMRI) of amygdala reactivity, ventral medial prefrontal cortex (vmPFC) response, and amygdala-vmPFC interactions ("connectivity") during processing of threat/fearful face stimuli and reappraisal-based regulation of negative affect in 80 veterans returning from OEF/OIF, all of whom had been exposed to moderate-severe combat trauma, including 40 with PTSD and 40 without PTSD. | K. Luan Phan, University of Michigan/VA |
| 2012-03 | Preventing PTSD Related Functional Impairment in Veterans | No additional information found. | VA |
| 2012-03 | The Effects of Explosive Blast as Compared to Post-Traumatic Stress Disorder on Brain Function and Structure | This study examined the neural consequences of blast exposure by comparing the functional and structural brain characteristics of 180 OIF National Guard soldiers who returned from deployment who have blast injury, blast injury and PTSD, PTSD, and no blast injury or PTSD (45 demographically similar subjects in each group). | Scott R. Sponheim/Minnesota Veterans Research Institute |

| End Date | Title | Study Population and Methods | Principal Investigator/Sponsor |
|---|---|---|---|
| 2012-03 | Imaging and Cognitive Correlates of Blast TBI in OIF/OEF Combat Veterans | The primary objective of this study was to characterize white matter integrity using diffusion tensor imaging (DTI), as well has functional activity using fluoro-2-deoxy-d-glucose (FDG) positron emission tomography (PET) and continuous fMRI in combat veterans exposed to blast wave. The secondary objective was to examine the relationship between white matter integrity and functional imaging findings to neuropsychological function and to activities of daily living (functional assessment and quality of living questionnaires). In the study, 48 OEF and OIF combat veterans who have sustained mTBI following blast injury were matched with a group of 48 OIF/OEF veteran controls (by age, education, and sex). | Effie M. Mitsis, James J. Peters VAMC/VA |
| 2012-03 | An Exploratory Survey of My Health*e*Vet Authenticated Users and Usage | This study followed 250 newly authenticated veterans for 6 months. Baseline data included health literacy, demographics, patient activation measure, Internet access, internet use, e-Health literacy, report of the authentication process and source of information about MHV. The 6-month follow-up included MHV self-report usage, MHV experience, and MHV Login data. | Susan S. Woods, VA Medical Center, Portland/VA |
| 2012-03 | Imaging-Genetics of PTSD in OEF/OIF Veterans | This study leveraged the substantial investment of the Mid-Atlantic Mental Illness Education and Clinical Center to acquire a large database of OEF/OIF veterans to investigate the influence of genes on the development of PTSD using neuroimaging phenotypes. Broadly, the three specific aims of the study integrated advanced methods in brain imaging and human genotyping to identify new genes associated with PTSD and understand the role these genes play in brain function. The first aim was to perform fMRI studies on OEF/OIF veterans with PTSD (n = 80) and trauma exposed controls (n = 80) in a working memory task and emotion-processing task to identify brain regions of differential activation. The second aim was to assay a targeted list of five candidate genes based on biological plausibility in working memory and emotion processing. The third aim was to analyze the genotype information from Aim 2 and brain activation information from Aim 1 to study the interaction of genotype, brain activation, and PTSD severity in dorsal frontoparietal regions and ventral frontolimbic regions. In this manner an imaging-genetics approach is expected to help identify genes associated with PTSD. | Rajendra A. Morey, Durham VAMC/VA |
| 2012-04 | Rehabilitation Strategies to Reduce Violence and Anger in TBI and PTSD | No additional information found. | J.C. Beckham, MIRECC Assistant Director, Genetics Research |
| 2012-04 | Treatment of Insomnia in Military Veterans: Phase 2 | This study examined sleep and daytime symptoms of psychiatric distress in 40 participants randomized to the Brief Behavioral Treatment of Insomnia for Military Veterans group (face-to-face visits on weeks 1 and 3 and telephone appointments on weeks 2 and 4) or the control group (received two brochures on insomnia). Follow-up assessment was conducted 6 months posttreatment in responders. | Anne Germain/University of Pittsburgh |

| End Date | Title | Study Population and Methods | Principal Investigator/Sponsor |
|---|---|---|---|
| 2012-04 | Extinction of Fear Memories with Glucocorticoids in Veterans with PTSD | There were two aims of this study. Aim 1 was to examine the effects of glucocorticoid administration following traumatic memory reactivation on psychiatric symptoms in veterans with combat-related PTSD. Aim 2 was to examine the effects of glucocorticoid administration following traumatic memory reactivation on physiological responses to veterans' personal combat memories (N = ?). | Alina Suris, VA North Texas Health Care System/VA |
| 2012-04 | Reengineering Systems for the Primary Care Treatment of PTSD | The immediate objectives of this study were to implement collaborative care in five VA primary care clinics to facilitate the management of PTSD and evaluate the effects on patient outcomes, provider knowledge and behavior, and costs. Across five VA sites, 195 patients with PTSD who are not receiving mental health care were randomized to receive 3CM or usual care. They were assessed prior to treatment and 3 and 6 months following treatment initiation. | Paula P. Schnurr, VA Medical and Regional Office Center, White River Junction, VT/VA |
| 2012-04 | Cognitive Assessment of Veterans After Traumatic Brain Injury | In this 4-year prospective cohort study, researchers looked at TBI profiles for clinically meaningful patterns of deficits related to injury status, which were then used as predictors of community participation and quality of life with hierarchical set regression analyses. 500 OIF/OEF veterans were recruited VISN-wide from the OIF/OEF registry, allowing for 40% attrition at each step. | Kerry T. Donnelly, VA Western New York Healthcare System at Buffalo/VA |
| 2012-04 | Access to Treatment and Outcomes for Veterans with Substance Use Disorders | This study was a retrospective observational cohort study of patient-level administrative data extracted from VA, Medicare, and Medicaid records over the period from January 1, 2001, to December 31, 2005. These data were augmented by program-level survey data from the VA Drug Abuse Program Survey and the National Survey of Substance Abuse Treatment Services. Objectives were to describe patterns and trends in fiscal, supply, wait time, and utilization variables; estimate the relationship between fiscal variables, the supply of treatment, and utilization of VA treatment; estimate the relationship between access to local treatment and health outcomes for veterans with substance use disorder diagnoses. | Steven Daniel Pizer, VA Medical Center, Jamaica Plain Campus/VA |
| 2012-06 | Validation of Brief Objective Neurobehavioral Detectors of Mild TBI | In this study, 100 OEF/OIF veterans (70 with mTBI and 30 without) were administered the Brief Objective Neurobehavioral Detectors test to determine its validity. | Julie C. Chapman, DC VAMC/VA |
| 2012-06 | Outreach Intervention for OIF Veterans to Promote Use of Mental Health Services | The goal of this study was to determine which beliefs predict behavior health treatment initiation among returning veterans with combat-related behavioral health disorders. Questionnaires and telephone interviews were used to assess which veterans initiated treatment (N = ?). | Tracy A. Stecker, Dartmouth College/NIMH |
| 2012-06 | Family-Enhanced Cognitive Behavioral Therapy for Comorbid PTSD and Alcohol Abuse | In this study, 15 veterans with family member/significant other involvement were randomized to compare a cognitive-behavioral skill-based intervention for comorbid alcohol use disorder (AUD) and PTSD to an individual coping skills treatment for AUD. | Meghan E. McDevitt-Murphy, University of Memphis/NIAAA |

| End Date | Title | Study Population and Methods | Principal Investigator/Sponsor |
|---|---|---|---|
| 2012-06 | Increasing PTSD Treatment Engagement Among Returning OEF/OIF Veterans | The effectiveness of a brief, individualized cognitive-behavioral intervention to promote entry into PTSD treatments was tested in 250 veterans who screened positive for PTSD postdeployment. | Tracy A. Stecker, Dartmouth College/NIMH |
| 2012-06 | Longitudinal Study of PTSD, TBI, and Functional Impairment Among OEF/OIF Veterans | This study analyzed and disseminated results from existing longitudinal data from more than 1,000 individuals previously deployed to the OEF/OIF conflicts. The baseline sample was recruited using geographically targeted, random-digit dialing and captures a wide range of individual characteristics, including all branches of service. The baseline sample included more than 300 respondents who had probable PTSD or major depression and more than 400 who experienced a probable TBI during deployment. Follow-up interviews were completed in October 2009 on these participants, approximately 18 months after baseline data collection. The project would provide funds to enable additional research using this longitudinal data. Specifically, the project addressed three broad aims: (1) document the magnitude of the mental health problems facing individuals previously deployed for OEF/OIF, (2) investigate the relationship between PTSD and postconcussive symptoms, and (3) identify the factors that inhibit service utilization for individuals with mental health problems. | Terry Schell, RAND Corporation/NIMH |
| 2012-06 | Biomarkers for Marine PTSD Risk and Resilience | The objective of this study was to identify gene-based biomarkers of PTSD in an effort to better understand the biological factors related to the risk of developing PTSD and the resilience as represented by resistance to development of PTSD. The study had two specific aims as follows. Specific Aim 1: Identify gene-expression-based biomarker profiles of PTSD risk and resilience in peripheral blood mononuclear cells. Specific Aim 2: Identify changes in gene-expression-based biomarker profiles of risk and resilience in peripheral blood mononuclear cells. | Ming T. Tsuang, University of California, San Diego/NIMH |
| 2012-06 | Accelerated Resolution Therapy (ART) for Psychological Trauma | The purpose of this study was to (1) evaluate how effective Accelerated Resolution Therapy (ART) is in treating symptoms of psychological trauma among non-active-duty veterans who served in OIF or OEF in Iraq and in Afghanistan or other combat conflicts and (2) learn if there is improvement in symptoms of psychological trauma (such as bad memories, anxiety, depression, and guilt) after receiving ART (N = 80). | Kevin Kip, University of South Florida/VA |
| 2012-07 | A Placebo-Controlled Trial of D-Cycloserine and Exposure Therapy for Combat-PTSD | The primary aim of this project was to examine whether administration of D-cycloserine (DCS), a partial N-methyl-D-aspartate (NMDA) receptor agonist that has been shown to facilitate fear extinction, enhances the therapeutic benefit of exposure-based cognitive-behavioral therapy (CBT) in OEF/OIF veterans with PTSD. 68 OEF/OIF veterans with PTSD were randomly assigned to CBT plus DCS or CBT plus placebo. Assessment interviews were conducted by independent evaluators and self-report occurred at pretreatment, posttreatment, and at the 3- and 6-month follow-ups. | Brett T. Litz, VA Boston Health Care System/VA |

| End Date | Title | Study Population and Methods | Principal Investigator/Sponsor |
|---|---|---|---|
| 2012-08 | Aripiprazole Augmentation of Antidepressants in PTSD | Evaluate the therapeutic potential of aripiprazole augmentation to a stable antidepressant regimen for reducing PTSD symptoms, cognitive symptoms, psychotic symptoms, and depressive symptoms in veterans (n = 48) with PTSD. [NOTE: Information provided to committee does not mention if specific to OEF/OIF.] | Christine E. Marx/Durham VA Medical Center |
| 2012-08 | Supporting Education Goals of OIF/OEF Veterans with PTSD: Pilot Process and Outcome | In this study, 40 OEF/OIF veterans with PTSD were randomly assigned to either a group that received weekly supported education intervention or a group that received services as usual plus an hour of attentive intervention not focused on education. | Marsha Langer Ellison, Edith Nourse Rogers Memorial Veterans Hospital, Bedford/VA |
| 2012-08 | PROJECT VALOR: Development of a PTSD Population Registry for Veterans | A longitudinal registry of 1,600 male and female service members was created to study the natural history of PTSD. The cohort included combat-exposed men and women with PTSD deployed to OEF/OIF, combat veterans without PTSD, and veterans who were not deployed to OEF/OIF. Data were collected from administrative databases and electronic medical records and a self-administered questionnaire and semistructured diagnostic telephone interview. The study was designed to evaluate clinical course of PTSD, psychosocial correlates, and health outcomes. | Terence M. Keane/Boston VA Research Institute |
| 2012-08 | Personalized Drinking Feedback Interventions for OEF/OIF Veterans | Primary purpose of this study was to test the effectiveness of a computer-delivered Personalized Drinking Feedback (PDF)-only intervention at preventing hazardous alcohol-use and alcohol-related problems among OEF/OIF veterans. A secondary aim was to examine potential mediators and moderators of intervention effectiveness. Subjects were randomized to either a PDF-only or educational information condition and completed measures of alcohol use, alcohol-related problems, and other alcohol-related variables at baseline, 1-month, and 6-month follow-up. Analyses of follow-up between-group differences while controlling for baseline values were used to determine the efficacy of the PDF-only intervention. | Matthew P. Martens/University of Missouri–Columbia, NIAAA |

| End Date | Title | Study Population and Methods | Principal Investigator/Sponsor |
|---|---|---|---|
| 2012-08 | Alcohol Use and Associated Problems Among Veterans and Student Service Members | This study examined the prevalence and correlates of military veterans'/student service members' alcohol use and abuse following (re)entry into college. It specifically explored whether student veterans' alcohol-related cognitions and patterns of use differ from those of their nonmilitary peers, as well as whether they also experienced a greater proportion of negative outcomes (mental health, social, and academic) as a result of their alcohol use. The sample included 354 students (195 veterans/student service members; 68 Reserve Officers' Training Corps students; 91 civilian students). Data collection involved Internet-based surveys addressing alcohol-related expectancies, beliefs, consumption patterns, as well as mental health (e.g., including depression, psychological distress, PTSD) and academic (grade point average, major, academic self-efficacy, locus of control) related correlates. Individual (e.g., combat exposure), interpersonal (e.g., social support), and institutional (e.g., campus alcohol culture) predictors of alcohol use were also to be explored. | Shawn David Whiteman, Purdue University/sponsor unknown |
| 2012-09 | Evaluation of Stepped Care for Chronic Pain in Iraqi/Afghanistan Veterans | The purpose of this study was to determine if a stepped-care intervention makes pain symptoms better and reduces activity limitations because of pain. Researchers compared the stepped-case intervention to usual care in 300 OEF/OIF veterans with chronic and disabling musculoskeletal pain to evaluate the impact of the intervention on pain-related disability, work function, psychological distress, and other outcomes. | Matthew J. Bair, Richard Rodebush VAMC/VA |
| 2012-09 | Adjunctive Biofeedback Intervention for OIF/OEF PTSD | In this study, 30 OIF/OEF veterans receiving care for PTSD at CBOCs were randomized to a 24-week course of StressEraser or usual care. Follow-up clinical assessments were conducted at 12 and 24 weeks. | Timothy Kimbrell, Central AR VHS/VA |
| 2012-09 | PTSD Couples Therapy | The goal of this study was to test the efficacy of a novel couple-based PTSD treatment, called Structured Approach Therapy (SAT), by randomly assigning 130 OEF/OIF veterans and their spouses to either a 12-session SAT program or to a 12-session PTSD Family Education comparison condition. The efficacy of the two treatment conditions were ascertained by obtaining measures of PTSD severity, marital functioning, and community functioning prior to treatment, immediately after treatment, and 3 months after the last treatment session. | Frederick Sautter, Southeast Veterans Healthcare System, New Orleans/VA |
| 2012-09 | Regional Anesthesia Military Battlefield Pain Outcomes Study | This was an observational study of 500 OEF/OIF soldiers with 1+ mangled or amputated limbs who were aggressively treated with regional anesthesia for pain control vs receiving standard treatment for pain control. Prospective data collection, evaluation 2 years after start of rehabilitation, and medical record information was collected retrospectively. | Rollin McCulloch Gallagher, Pain Management Service/VA |
| 2012-09 | Development of a Quality of Life Tool for Deployment Related TBI | Qualitative data obtained from focus groups of veterans and VA providers (n = 600) was used to develop a psychometrically sound tool to measure health-related quality of life applicable to wounded warriors with deployment-related TBI. | Shirley Groer, James A. Haley VA Hospital/VA |

| End Date | Title | Study Population and Methods | Principal Investigator/Sponsor |
|---|---|---|---|
| 2012-09 | Telemental Health and Cognitive Processing Therapy for Rural Combat Veterans with PTSD | In this study, 126 combat reservists, National Guard members, or veterans with PTSD were randomized to receive Cognitive Processing Group Therapy via videoteleconference (experimental) vs in person (control). Assessments were conducted at baseline, midtreatment, immediately, and 3 months and 6 months posttreatment. | Leslie A. Morland, PSYD VA Pacific Islands Health Care System/VA |
| 2012-09 | Couples Treatment of PTSD in OEF/OIF Veterans | In this study, 130 OEF/OIF veterans and their spouses were randomly assigned to either a 12-session structured approach therapy program or to a 12-session PTSD family education program. Efficacy of the two treatments was assessed. | Frederick Sautter, SE Veterans Healthcare System, New Orleans/VA |
| 2012-09 | Daily Fluctuations of PTSD Symptoms and Alcohol Use Among OEF/OIF Veterans | In this study, 168 OEF/OIF veterans with combat-related PTSD who endorse risky drinking behavior received cell phones connected to an Interactive Voice Response system that provided daily prompts to report on PTSD and alcohol use for 28 days. | Paige Ouimette, Syracuse VAMC/VA |
| 2012-09 | Executive Functioning in OEF/OIF Veterans with Traumatic Brain Injury | A comprehensive battery of tests and diffusion tensor brain imaging was conducted in OEF/OIF veterans with mTBI to document impairments in cognitive skills (N = ?). | J.V. Baldo, VA Northern California Health Care System/VA |
| 2012-09 | PTSD-Focused Relationship Enhancement Therapy for Returning Veterans and Their Partners | In this study, 440 couples were randomly assigned to receive either PTSD-Focused Relationship Enhancement Therapy or Support Therapy to prevent the perpetration of intimate partner aggression. | Casey T. Taft, National Center for PTSD, Boston VAMC/CDC |
| 2012-09 | Randomized, Placebo-Controlled Trial of the Dopamine-B-Hydroxylase (DBH) Inhibitor, Nepicastat, for the Treatment of PTSD in OIF/OEF Veterans | In this study, approximately 120 outpatient OIF/CEF veterans with PTSD were randomized to either nepicastat or placebo in a 6-week randomized clinical trial. | Carlos Berry/Tuscaloosa Research and Education Advancement Corporation, VA |
| 2012-09 | The Neuropsychology of Blast-Induced Traumatic Brain Injury | No additional information found. | VA |
| 2012-09 | Long-Term Outcomes in Burned OEF/OIF Veterans (LOBO) | This study used data from U.S. Army Institute of Surgical Research (USAISR)/BAMC databases and patient surveys to compare the rate of functional recovery for three cohorts (survivors of combat burn, combat non-burn trauma, and civilian burns) discharged from the USAISR Burn Center or the BAMC Trauma Center (N = ?). | Valerie Ann Lawrence, VA South Texas Health Care System/VA |
| 2012-09 | Marine Resiliency Study | The objective of this program was to complete a series of three prospective, longitudinal, interrelated projects that seek to better understand risk and resilience in a cohort of ~2,500 Marines bound for Iraq or Afghanistan. | Dewleen Baker, VA San Diego Healthcare System/VA |

| End Date | Title | Study Population and Methods | Principal Investigator/Sponsor |
| --- | --- | --- | --- |
| 2012-09 | Mindfulness and Self-Compassion Meditation for Combat Posttraumatic Stress Disorder: Randomized Controlled Trial and Mechanistic Study | This study compared a 16-week psychotherapy group for PTSD involving mindfulness and self-compassion meditation with a more standard form of group psychotherapy known as present-centered group therapy. Both therapies were conducted at the VA Ann Arbor PTSD clinic by VA psychotherapists. (The study was also approved by the Institutional Review Board of the VA Ann Arbor.) Combat veterans were randomly assigned to either the meditation or the standard group psychotherapy. All patients will also receive fMRI brain scans before and after the therapy, as well as assessment interviews before, at 8 weeks, and immediately posttherapy, and at 3-month and 6-month follow-ups. Saliva cortisol and measures of attention were also obtained at each assessment (N = 80). | Israel Liberzon, University of Michigan/VA |
| 2012-09 | A Brief Educational Intervention to Improve TBI Screening Outcomes | This research study was designed to learn about veterans' understanding of mild TBI and the VA TBI screening process. All OEF/OIF veterans who came to one of the study-related clinics for TBI screening were invited to participate. An educational handout on TBI was given to half of the participants along with their TBI screening. The other half of the participants had the usual TBI screening without the educational handout. Veterans enrolled in the study were asked to answer a 5–10-minute research questionnaire (N = 1,500). | Jessica L. Hamblen, White River Junction VAMC/VA |
| 2012-09 | Evaluating the VA's Assessment of Military Sexual Trauma in Veterans | A qualitative in-person interview study was completed by recruitment of a random sample of 90 men and women stratified across four sites: Iowa City VA Health Care System, VA Pittsburgh Health Care System, Miami VA Medical Center, and Philadelphia VA Medical Center. Initial recruitment steps occurred by sending mailed letters of invitation to a random sampling of potential participants stratified by whether they answered MST screening questions in the clinical setting affirmatively or not. Those who expressed interest in the study by calling study personnel were administered the Sexual Experiences Questionnaire (SEQ), a comprehensive sexual harassment/assault measure used by the DOD with tens of thousands of active-duty service members. SEQ responses were used to characterize and direct recruitment of potential participants into true MST positive, false MST negative, and true MST negative subgroups. In-person interviews and analyses of resultant qualitative data will explore the different subgroups' understandings of the screening questions as well as of federal definitions of sexual harassment/assault. | Anne G. Sadler, Iowa City VAMC/VA |

| End Date | Title | Study Population and Methods | Principal Investigator/Sponsor |
|---|---|---|---|
| 2012-09 | Photovoice as an Educational Intervention to Improve Care of OEF/OIF Veterans | The primary aim of the project was to establish feasibility of Photovoice with OEF/OIF veterans. The secondary aims of the study were to explore preliminary effectiveness of Photovoice as an educational intervention to (1) increase health communication self-efficacy and decrease social anxiety for veteran participants and (2) positively impact attitudes and knowledge of VA leadership, providers, and staff as relates to the experiences and needs of OEF/OIF veterans. Findings from the pilot study will inform the design of a multisite study of Photovoice as an educational intervention for veterans and VA providers/staff, including identification of appropriate outcome variables and data collection tools. The broad, long-term objective of the work is to improve the quality and equity of care for OEF/OIF veterans. | Jennifer Gala True, Philadelphia VAMC/VA |
| 2012-09 | Identifying Opportunities for Targeted Interventions via My Health*e*Vet | Objectives of this study were to (1) create an eHealth QUERI database linking clinical data (e.g., ICD-9-CM codes) and key patient-level demographics for all veterans who obtained care in VA in FY2010 to current, with data on MHV registration and In-Person Authentication, use of MHV for prescription refills, and use of MHV for secure messaging; (2) characterize use of MHV across disease categories and patient demographics. Researchers will focus on the most prevalent or high priority diagnoses and conditions among veterans. Researchers propose to specifically target conditions of interest to the nine disease-specific QUERI centers; and (3) use facility-level data to create graphic displays of variations in authentication and use, in general and by condition, that can be used by MHV coordinators and Patient Aligned Care Teams when planning marketing of MHV and by QUERIs in determining ways to employ MHV in implementation of interventions. | Cynthia Ann Brandt, VA Connecticut Healthcare System West Haven Campus/VA |
| 2012-09 | Strength at Home Couples Program | The purpose of the project was to develop and test a couples-based relationship enhancement group intervention for married or partnered OEF/OIF/Operation New Dawn (OND) veterans to prevent the perpetration of intimate partner aggression (IPA) among participants. Specific aims of this project were to (1) develop and standardize Strength at Home Couples Group for male combat veterans, including the development of a clinician-friendly intervention manual detailing Strength at Home Couples Group, along with intervention adherence measures and therapist training and certification procedures; (2) test the efficacy of Strength at Home Couples Group for OEF/OIF/OND veterans by conducting a multiple-site randomized trial comparing 10 sessions of Strength at Home Couples Group to 10 sessions of a supportive group therapy condition; and (3) explore differences in compliance and process factors across conditions (N = 440). | Casey T. Taft, National Center for PTSD, VA Boston Healthcare, and Tracie Shea, Providence VAMC/VA |

| End Date | Title | Study Population and Methods | Principal Investigator/Sponsor |
|---|---|---|---|
| 2012-09 | Modifiable Risk and Protective Factors for Suicidal Behaviors in the U.S. Army | Four institutions collaboratively conducted an epidemiologic study of mental health, psychologic resilience, suicide risk, suicide-related behaviors, and suicide deaths in the U.S. Army. The case-control study examined OEF/OIF veterans who made nonfatal attempts, relatives of soldiers who committed suicide, and carefully matched controls. Blood or saliva samples would also be collected. The aim is to find risk and protective factors. It is the largest study on mental health and suicide (50 million). | Robert J. Ursano/NIMH |
| 2012-09 | Validation of Modified DRRI Scales in a National Sample of OEF/OIF Veterans | The primary objective of this project is to conduct a systematic empirical investigation of modified Deployment Risk and Resilience Inventory (DRRI) scales in a sample of OEF/OIF veterans. In Wave I, the original DRRI items and any items that have been modified or added will be administered to a nationally representative sample of 600 OEF/OIF veterans. In Wave II, finalized DRRI scales and health measures will be administered to a second sample of 400 OEF/OIF veterans. | Dawne S. Vogt, VA Boston Healthcare System Jamaica Plain Campus, Jamaica Plain, MA/VA |
| 2012-10 | A Head-to-Head Comparison of Virtual Reality Treatment for Post Traumatic Stress Disorder | This randomized, head-to-head study compared 40 PTSD patients treated with Virtual Reality Exposure Therapy to 40 PTSD patients treated with Augmented Exposure Therapy (control). | Robert N. McLay/U.S. Naval Medical Center, San Diego |
| 2012-10 | Women Veterans Cohort Study | Researchers collected data on OEF/OIF women (n = 163,812) veterans who had enrolled in VHA and who had at least one visit within 1 year of last deployment and matched them to male controls in an Health Services Research and Development Service (HSR&D) cohort and followed them longitudinally in order to determine the effect of sex on health services utilization and costs and health outcomes. The study replicated and built on methods used for the nationally recognized Veterans Aging Cohort Study. | Cynthia Ann Brandt, VA Connecticut Health Care System/VA |
| 2012-10 | Simulation Based Planning Model for Mental Health Care Services | Researchers developed a simulation-based planning model incorporating patient flow and provider and staff workflow between and within mental health clinics at a large VAMC. The objective was to provide a capacity planning and resource allocation tool to improve quality measures related to resource utilization and timely access to mental health services. | Bradley N. Doebbeling, Richard Roudebush VAMC/VA |
| 2012-10 | An Evaluation of the Blue Button Feature of My Health*e*Vet: Veteran and Provider Use and Satisfaction | The main objective of this study was to determine the factors that contribute to the adoption and meaningful use of the Blue Button feature in users of My Health*e*Vet (N = ?). | Carolyn L. Turvey, Iowa City VAMC/VA |

| End Date | Title | Study Population and Methods | Principal Investigator/Sponsor |
|---|---|---|---|
| 2012-10 | Providing Mental Health Services to Operation Iraqi Freedom (OIF)/Operation Enduring Freedom (OEF) Veterans: Provider Perspectives | The purpose of this study was to gather information from VISN 19 Denver VA mental health professionals regarding their perspectives of necessary resources to provide best-practice mental health service to OIF/OEF veterans. Specifically, this study aimed to describe provider perspectives regarding the following: (1) clinical needs of OIF/OEF veterans; (2) collaboration and referral processes; (3) barriers to providing optimal treatment to this cohort; (4) provider needs and resources that may improve service delivery to this cohort; (5) provider perspectives regarding psychiatric outcomes in this cohort; and (6) professional satisfaction. Semi-structured interview regarding provider experiences of providing mental health treatment to OIF/OEF veterans. The interview took approximately 1 hour to complete and was conducted one time with each participant (N = 30). | Gina M. Signoracci, VA Eastern Colorado Health Care System/VA |
| 2012-11 | Adjunctive Pregnenolone in Veterans with Mild TBI | In this study, cognitive, PTSD, and depressive symptoms were evaluated in 40 OEF/OIF veterans with mTBI randomized to receive pregnenolone or placebo for 10 weeks. | Christine E. Marx, Durham VA/Durham VA Medical Center |
| 2012-11 | Supporting Military Caregivers: Phase 1 | No additional information found. | Rajeev Ramchand and Terri Tanielian, RAND Corporation/ Elizabeth Dole Foundation |
| 2012-12 | Cognitive Behavioral Treatment of Posttraumatic Stress Disorder Enhanced by Virtual Reality for Individuals with PTSD and Substance Abuse | In this study, 11 individuals with comorbid PTSD and substance abuse resulting from the attacks of September 11, 2001, or from military service in Iraq were treated with cognitive behavioral therapy enhanced with the use of a virtual environment. | JoAnn Difede/Weill Medical College of Cornell |
| 2012-12 | Strength, Pain, and Function in OIF/OEF Amputees: A Nurse-Managed Program | In this study, 60 OEF/OIF amputees were randomly assigned to either the nurse-managed neuromuscular electrical stimulation rehabilitation program or to the Walter Reed Army Medical Center amputee protocol to assess gait, quality of life, functional performance, and residual and phantom limb pain. | Laura A. Talbot, Sara Breckenridge-Sproat, and Michael Rosenthal/UNC-Charlotte, Walter Reed National Military Medical Center and Naval Medical Center, San Diego |
| 2012-12 | TBI Screening Instruments and Processes for Clinical Follow-Up | In this study, the TBI Clinical Reminder Screen was evaluated for reliability and validity in 210 OEF/OIF veterans. | Rodney D. Vanderploeg/VA |

| End Date | Title | Study Population and Methods | Principal Investigator/Sponsor |
|---|---|---|---|
| 2012-12 | A Comparison of CPT vs PCT for Veterans | In this study, 10 male OEF/OIF veterans with combat-related PTSD were randomized to cognitive processing therapy or present-centered therapy. The veteran were assessed at pre-, post-, 3-month, and 1-year follow-ups. | Kathleen Chard, Cincinnati VA MC/VA |
| 2012-12 | Bright Light: An Adjunct Treatment for Combat PTSD | In this study, 70 OIF/OEF veterans with PTSD were randomly assigned to one of two 4-week treatments (45 min/day): (1) bright light exposure or (2) a negative ion generator. Clinical assessments, as well as self-reported measures of PTSD, anxiety, depression, and sleep, were assessed. | Shawn D. Youngstedt, WJB Dorn Veterans Hospital/VA, University of South Carolina |
| 2012-12 | Evaluation of Approaches to Auditory Rehabilitation for Mild TBI | In this study, effectiveness of FM use and/or auditory training for OEF/OIF veterans with mTBI was examined in a randomized clinical trial of 132 veterans. | Gabrielle Saunders, Portland VAMC/VA |
| 2012-12 | Breaking the Cycle IV: Military PTSD (MPTSD) Treatment Study | The study compared the efficacy of Trauma Affect Regulation: Guide for Education and Therapy (TARGET) vs the best validated psychotherapy for adults with PTSD, PE. Male military personnel and veterans suffering with PTSD and problems with anger after returning from military service in Afghanistan (OEF) and/or Iraq (OIF) were participants. The goal was to determine if a present-centered psychotherapy that teaches skills for emotion regulation and does not require retelling of traumatic memories is as efficacious as the trauma memory-focused PE psychotherapy (N = 80). | Julian Ford/ University of Connecticut Health Center |
| 2012-12 | Examining the Implementation of Evidence-Based Psychotherapy for Veterans with PTSD | The specific objectives of the study were to<br>1. Determine the current use of PE and Cognitive Processing Therapy (CPT) for the treatment of PTSD within the PTSD Clinical Teams (PCTs) in VISN 1.<br>2. Examine how contextual factors contributed to implementation of PE and CPT in VISN 1.<br>a. Explore VISN 1 PCT providers' view of the evidence supporting the use of PE and CPT (research, clinical experience, patient experience, and local data).<br>b. Explore VISN 1 PCT providers' view of their context (culture, leadership, and evaluation).<br>c. Explore VISN 1 PCT providers' view of the facilitation activities of PE and CPT (purpose, role, and skills/attributes).<br>d. Determine what factors (if any) are unique to the implementation of evidence-based psychotherapies. Attempt to map any newly identified factors onto the existing implementation frameworks and develop measures to account for these characteristics. | Bradley V. Watts, White River Junction VAMC and Regional Office/VA |

| End Date | Title | Study Population and Methods | Principal Investigator/Sponsor |
|---|---|---|---|
| 2012-12 | A Comparison of CPT vs PCT for Veterans | In this study, all-male OEF/OIF veterans were screened for their appropriateness for the study by phone screen and then by an assessment technician. The participants were assessed at pre-, post-, 3-month, and 1-year follow-up. The assessment technicians were blind to the participant's condition. CPT is a 12-week long individual psychotherapy treatment shown to be effective at reducing PTSD and related symptoms for survivors of various types of traumas, including combat. PCT is a supportive counseling treatment that has been utilized as an alternative to waitlist control in VA cooperative studies of PTSD (N = 47). | Kathleen Chard, Cincinnati VAMC/VA |
| 2012-12 | Amino Acid Supplementation in Recovery From Traumatic Brain Injury | In this study, investigators have shown that even 1 year after injury, plasma valine, an essential amino acid (EAA), was markedly reduced in patients with TBI compared to healthy controls. The investigators speculated that low plasma valine concentration contributes to chronic fatigue after TBI, since valine and tryptophan compete for the same transporter into the brain, and a low plasma valine concentration will allow more tryptophan to be transported. As a consequence, increased brain tryptophan will increase serotonin production, which may significantly contribute to the development of fatigue. Thus, the investigators tested if restoring valine concentration in persons with TBI may reduce fatigue perception and improve physical and neuropsychological function. Further, the investigators have previously shown that EAA intake has an anabolic effect in healthy young and elderly individuals. However, no data are currently available in persons recovering from TBI. Thus, the investigators also tested if EAA and/or valine can improve muscle mass in patients with TBI (N = 45). | Elisabet Borsheim/ University of Texas, Galveston |
| 2012-12 | Mental Health Seeking and Help-Seeking of Returning Veterans in Rural Community Colleges | Using a sample from eight public community colleges in Arkansas (N = 1,000, including 500 veterans), researchers fielded a Web-based survey to collect and analyze data to address the following specific aims: (1) estimate the prevalence of depression, PTSD, TBI, substance misuse, and suicidal ideation among the student veteran population and compare it to the broader student population of community colleges; (2) estimate the prevalence of help seeking among the student veteran population and compare it to the broader student population of community colleges; and (3) identify the most salient barriers to help seeking among student veterans. The long term goal of the researchers' agenda is to develop a screening and linkage intervention for OEF/OIF veterans attending these underserved community colleges. | Justin B. Hunt, University of Arkansas Medical School/NIMH |

| End Date | Title | Study Population and Methods | Principal Investigator/Sponsor |
|---|---|---|---|
| 2012-12 | Identifying the Needs of OEF/OIF Veterans and Their Families: TBI and Co-Occurring Behavioral Health Issues | The focus of this project was on qualitative data collection to facilitate product development, including assessment and treatment guidelines to improve non-VA community mental health care for OEF/OIF veterans with TBI and co-occurring behavioral health issues within the state of Colorado. In addition to the development of assessment and treatment guidelines, other products developed through this study included a training and accompanying toolkit, which may be used for annual educational training of mental health providers (N = 90). | Lisa Brenner, VA Eastern Colorado Health Care System/ VA |
| Complete | Review of Literature and Best Practices for Promoting Resilience | No additional information found. | Lisa Meredith, RAND Corporation/ DOD |
| Complete | Evaluation of VHA Mental Health Services | No additional information found. | Katherine Watkins, RAND Corporation/ VA |
| Complete | Examining the Well-Being of Children of Deployed Military Personnel | No additional information found. | Anita Chandra, RAND Corporation/ National Military Family Association |
| Complete (awaiting DOD approval as of 09/2012) | Needs of Servicemembers and Their Families for Information on Traumatic Brain Injury (TBI) | No additional information found. | Andrew Parker, Lisa Meredith, RAND Corporation/DOD |
| 2013-03 | Improving Quality of Care Through Improved Audit and Feedback | This research compares how leaders of high-, low-, and moderately performing VA Medical Centers use clinical performance data from VA's External Peer Review Program as a feedback tool to maintain and improve quality of care. Qualitative, grounded theory analysis of up to 60 interviews with primary care, facility, and VISN leadership of high-, moderate-, and low-performing facilities (http://www.ncbi.nlm.nih.gov/pubmed/22607640). | Sylvia J. Hysong, Michael E. DeBakey VAMC |
| Ongoing Studies | | | |
| 2013-01 | Telemedicine Outreach for Post Traumatic Stress in CBOCs | The objective of this proposed effectiveness study is to evaluate a telemedicine intervention to improve PTSD outcomes in CBOCs without onsite psychiatrists. Approximately 400 veterans will be recruited from nine CBOCs in VISN 16 and 22. Veterans screening positive for PTSD and those already in active treatment will be recruited. | John C. Fortney, Central Arkansas VHS Eugene J. Towbin Healthcare Center, Little Rock/ VA |

| End Date | Title | Study Population and Methods | Principal Investigator/Sponsor |
|---|---|---|---|
| 2013-02 | The Efficacy of Stellate Ganglion Block as PTSD Therapy: A Pilot Study | This pilot clinical trial is studying the efficacy of a stellate ganglion nerve block in veterans to reduce the symptoms of PTSD in relatively long-standing (Vietnam era) or relatively recently induced PTSD (from deployment in Afghanistan or Iraq as part of OEF, OIF, and OND (N = 12). | Michael T. Alkire, Long Beach VA Healthcare system/Southern California Institute for Research and Education |
| 2013-02 | Implementation of Diabetes Performance Measures: Focus on Unintended Consequences | Using a random sample drawn from 25 VAMCs, investigators will conduct telephone interviews from the VA Pittsburgh Healthcare System using both closed- and open-ended questions with 750 African American, Hispanic, and white veterans as well as a small sample of other minority veterans (Asian, Pacific Islander/Native Hawaiian, or American Indian/Native Alaskan). This mixed-methods design allows for the examination of the direct, mediated, and/or moderated associations of race/ethnicity on satisfaction outcomes. The open-ended questions will provide data for a formal qualitative analysis of both reasons for satisfaction and dissatisfaction with VA health care and ways to improve VA care that are culturally sensitive. Finally, random effects modeling of coded qualitative data will be used to formally estimate and test racial/ethnic differences. Because the random effects modeling uses open-ended, qualitative data this statistical analysis allows this study to go beyond reliance on preestablished satisfaction items and instead capture very specific reasons for satisfaction and dissatisfaction with VA health care as described by the veterans themselves. | Laura J. Damschroder, VA Ann Arbor Healthcare System/VA |
| 2013-03 | Mental Health and Service Utilization Among Reserve and National Guard Forces | The study will document psychopathology, health risk behavior, and mental health service utilization among National Guard and to identify personal factors (e.g., sociodemographic factors, social supports), reserve and National Guard involvement (e.g., length of time in service, unit cohesion, extent of training, rank, separation from family/loved ones), and life circumstances (e.g., integration of regular work circumstances) that are associated with both stage-sequential psychological morbidity and trajectories of psychological morbidity over time among reserve and National Guards when accounting for combat exposures (e.g., international deployment, active-duty combat) and other traumatic event experiences (N = ?). | Sandro Galea, Columbia University Health Sciences/NIMH |
| 2013-03 | Telemedicine Outreach for Post Traumatic Stress in CBOCs | The objective of this effectiveness study was to evaluate a telemedicine intervention to improve PTSD outcomes in CBOCs without onsite psychiatrists. Approximately 400 veterans were recruited from nine CBOCs in VISN 16 and 22. Veterans screening positive for PTSD and those already in active treatment were recruited. | John C. Fortney, Central Arkansas VHS Eugene J. Towbin Healthcare Center/VA |

| End Date | Title | Study Population and Methods | Principal Investigator/Sponsor |
|---|---|---|---|
| 2013-03 | Access to Care for Veterans with Chronic Lower Limb Wounds | This project will identify a retrospective cohort of VISN 20 veterans with incident lower limb wounds in FY2007. It will then characterize the level of organized wound care present in each VHA VISN 20 facility at the midpoint of FY2007, April 1, 2007 and determine, for this sample their actualized access to care, the complexity and healing trajectory of their wounds, and the time to wound healing (N = ?). | Gregory J. Raugi, VA Puget Sound Health Care System/ VA |
| 2013-03 | Neural Correlates of PTSD in Veterans with Blast-Related Traumatic Brain Injury | The aim of this study is to determine neural biomarkers that can differentiate mTBI, and mTBI with PTSD. In the short run, researchers may be able to develop a more exact model for the neural effects of these disorders in the veteran population (N = ?). | Alan N. Simmons, VA San Diego Healthcare System/ VA |
| 2013-03 | Web Intervention for OEF/OIF Veterans with Mental Health Problems | The primary purpose of this study was to (1) develop an innovative, Web-based intervention for OIF/OEF veterans that addresses mental health, barriers-to-care, and treatment participation issues to facilitate healthy recovery; (2) develop video illustrations to facilitate learning of educational material; (3) develop thorough evaluation mechanisms to assess knowledge change relevant to common symptoms, healthy coping strategies, and access-to-care issues; (4) conduct a series of focus groups to guide development and refinement of intervention content; and (5) preliminarily evaluate the intervention using thematic semistructured interviews with a small sample of OIF/OEF veterans recruited via mental health specialty clinics within the Ralph H. Johnson VAMC and affiliated CBOCs. | Kenneth J. Ruggiero, Ralph H. Johnson VAMC/VA |
| 2013-03 | Examining Telehealth Applications for Evaluation of Mild TBI | The long-term goal of the study is to improve the quality of life of veterans who have mTBI and other related conditions by developing a service-directed proposal to facilitate implementation of telehealth strategies to perform comprehensive TBI evaluations (CTEs). The specific aims are to (1) characterize approaches to using telehealth to provide CTEs; (2) examine the association between patient characteristics and use of telehealth to perform the CTE and outcomes associated with telehealth; (3) convene an expert panel and develop recommendations to facilitate the implementation of telehealth strategies to provide comprehensive TBI evaluations; and (4) conduct a preliminary cost analyses of the intervention to provide the foundation for the cost analyses for future larger interventions (N = ?). | Bridget M. Smith, Edward Hines Jr. VA Hospital/VA |
| 2013-03 | Exploring Deployment Stress and Reintegration in Army National Guard Chaplains | The purpose of this 2-year pilot study is to explore the impact of deployment on the psychosocial and health characteristics and reintegration of military chaplains, specifically those of the Army National Guard. This pilot will serve as the foundation for subsequent investigations of chaplains from multiple branches of the military (N = 266). | Karen Besterman-Dahan, BS, James A. Haley Veterans Hospital/VA |

| End Date | Title | Study Population and Methods | Principal Investigator/Sponsor |
|---|---|---|---|
| 2013-03 | Veterans' Experiences Using Secure Messaging on My Health*e*Vet | The primary aim of this project is to describe veterans' experiences when using the secure messaging (SM) feature on My Health*e*Vet. Objective 1: Describe veterans' beliefs, attitudes, and perceptions toward using SM. Objective 2: Describe the user patterns and trends of Veterans when using SM. Objective 3: Identify the barriers to and facilitators for using SM. Objective 4: Identify strategies for overcoming barriers to using the SM feature on My Health*e*Vet Regarding the research design, this mixed-methods descriptive study will utilize in-person qualitative interviews, usability testing of the SM feature on MHV; SM secondary data analysis, and 3-month follow-up interviews. Purposive sampling will be used to identify a sample of 30–40 veterans who have been personally authenticated for the SM feature on MHV. Quantitative data will be summarized with descriptive statistics to describe sample characteristics. Researchers will examine frequency counts and proportions to provide a descriptive picture of the usability. Using Morae software, a usability analysis will be conducted to analyze and interpret the patterns and trends of veteran testing data. | Jolie N. Haun, James A. Haley Veterans' Hospital, Tampa, FL/VA |
| 2013-03 | PE-Web: Online Training for VA Providers in Prolonged Exposure for PTSD | The objectives of this study are to (1) develop PE-Web, a Web-based VA provider-training protocol in PE, (2) conduct a RCT to examine the utility of PE-Web as a VA provider-training resource, (3) examine fidelity to and knowledge of PE in relation to provider variables (e.g., theoretical orientation, demographics, etc.), and (4) obtain data on website usability, satisfaction levels, and Web-usage patterns (e.g., time to completion of PE-Web, viewing frequency for each video, etc.) for purposes of guiding improvements to the PE-Web protocol. Researchers will use randomized controlled trials methodology to examine the utility of PE-Web as a refresher course for VA providers who had previously attended a 4-day workshop as part of the PE dissemination initiative, a national effort funded by the Office of Mental Health Services in VHA Central Office. Researchers will recruit 100 providers from a national list of VA providers participating in initiative. After completing a baseline assessment, participants will be randomized to one of two conditions: PE-Web refresher training or no refresher. | Kenneth J. Ruggiero, Jr., Ralph H. Johnson VAMC/VA |
| 2013-04 | Working with Veterans Organizations to Encourage Use of My Health*e*Vet | Abstract is under review as of September 14, 2012. | Jeffrey C. Whittle, Clement J. Zablocki VAMC/VA |
| 2013-05 | Cognitive Rehabilitation of OIF/OEF Veterans with Cognitive Disorder | In this study, 280 OEF/OIF veterans with cognitive disorder resulting from mTBI will be randomly assigned to either the cognitive strategy training group or the usual care group to evaluate its efficacy. | Daniel M. Storzbach, (Portland VAMC)/VA |

| End Date | Title | Study Population and Methods | Principal Investigator/Sponsor |
|---|---|---|---|
| 2013-05 | Interventions Online to Facilitate Post-War Access of Reserve and National Guard Servicewomen | Abstract is under review as of September 14, 2012. | Anne G. Sadler, Iowa City VA Health Care System/ VA |
| 2013-05 | Access to Care for Veterans with Chronic Lower Limb Wounds | The goals of this study were to (1) identify and characterize an urban and a rural cohort of VISN20 veterans with at least one complex chronic lower limb wound in FY2007 and (2) determine whether rural and urban veterans with chronic lower limb wounds were equally likely to receive evidence-based good wound care, organized wound care, and coordinated wound care. Researchers also planned to compare clinical outcomes, including time to healing and amputation, across groups. A cohort of unique veterans with chronic lower limb wounds at each primary care site in VISN20 was identified. | Gregory J. Raugi, VA Puget Sound Health Care System Seattle Division/VA |
| 2013-05 | Internet-Based Smoking Cessation for OEF/OIF Veterans | The objectives of this study are to (1) evaluate the impact of an Internet-based smoking cessation intervention on rates of abstinence from cigarettes (self-reported 7-day point prevalent abstinence) at 3-month and 12-month posttreatment follow-ups; (2) evaluate the impact of an Internet-based smoking cessation intervention on reach of smoking cessation treatment; (3) evaluate the relative cost-effectiveness of the standard specialty care intervention to the Web-based intervention. Proposed is a two-group design in which 410 smokers will be randomized to receive one of the following: (1) VA Specialty Smoking Cessation Treatment control, which includes all the elements associated with enrollment in a VA specialty smoking cessation clinic including group counseling, individual telephone counseling, self-help materials, and smoking cessation aids including choice of pharmacotherapy; or (2) Internet-based counseling intervention that includes membership to a Web-based smoking cessation treatment program, QuitNet, and access to nicotine replacement. | Patrick S. Calhoun, Durham VAMC/VA |
| 2013-05 | Telerehabilitation for OIF/OEF Returnees with Combat-Related Traumatic Brain Injury | In this study, benefits and limitations of Internet-based rehabilitation (i.e., telerehabilitation) will be evaluated in 85 veterans with TBI. | Kris Siddharthan, HSR&D/RR&D Center of Excellence/VA |
| 2013-06 | PTSD Hyperarousal Symptoms Treated with Physiological Stress Management | In this study, 50 volunteers with at least moderate hyperarousal will be randomized to treatment consisting of five sessions of individual physiological relaxation training with electromyographic feedback and with capnographic feedback over a 4-week period or to a 2-month waiting period after which they also may receive this therapy. The waiting-list group and a nonanxious control group will be tested psychophysiologically twice at the same interval as the patients before and immediately after treatment. | Walton Roth, VA Palo Alto Health Care System/VA |

| End Date | Title | Study Population and Methods | Principal Investigator/Sponsor |
|---|---|---|---|
| 2013-06 | Spouse READI (Resilience Education And Deployment Information) Post Deployment Telephone Support Groups | This 12-month study is for spouses or significant others of service members who have returned from Afghanistan or Iraq. This study will determine if participating in a telephone discussion group offering education, skills building, and support will help increase postdeployment adjustment. There will be 225 spouses recruited for this study. Each telephone discussion group will meet 12 times during 6 months. The 1-hour calls will be semistructured conference calls with education, training in coping skills and cognitive restructuring, and support. | Linda O. Nichols and Jennifer L. Martindale-Adams, Memphis VAMC and University of Tennessee Health Science Center/VA |
| 2013-06 | Urogenital Symptoms, Depression and PTSD in OEF/OIF Women Veterans | Objectives of this study are to (1) define the prevalence and 1-year incidence and remission rates of urogenital symptoms, especially urge urinary incontinence and urinary frequency, in a representative population of OEF/OIF women veterans; and (2) identify the impact of depression and PTSD symptoms, a history of sexual assault, and deployment-related factors on the prevalence and 1-year incidence of urogenital symptoms, especially urge urinary incontinence and urinary frequency (N = 2,127). | Catherine S. Bradley, MD, MSCE, VA Medical Center, Iowa City |
| 2013-06 | CBT for Nightmares in OEF/OIF Veterans | In this study, 160 OIF/OEF veterans with insomnia will be randomized to one of two talk therapies with the intent to reduce posttraumatic nightmare frequency and distress. | Richard Ross, Philadelphia VAMC/VA |
| 2013-06 | Complicated Family Reintegration in OEF-OIF Veterans | The purpose of this study is to understand better how war-related psychiatric symptoms of OEF/OIF veterans may interfere with family reintegration and family functioning. This study will test whether difficulties with family reintegration account for the impact of psychiatric symptoms on overall family functioning over time. The quantitative aspect of the study will be a nontreatment two-wave (baseline and 12-month follow-up) clinical assessments of military veterans (target n = 220 with complete data) and their family members recruited within 2 years of their return from OEF/OIF deployments. | Steven L. Sayers, VA Medical Center, Philadelphia/ HSR&D |
| 2013-06 | Functional Outcomes in OEF/OIF Veterans with PTSD and Alcohol Misuse | This longitudinal study aims to better understand the functioning of returning OEF/OIF veterans over time and to identify potentially malleable resilience factors associated with higher levels of functioning. A total of 300 returning OEF/OIF veterans will be followed for a 1-year period. Veterans will complete a baseline assessment, followed by three follow-up assessments (two self-report assessments mailed at 4 and 8 months post-baseline and a 1-year in-person follow-up assessment that repeats many of the baseline clinician-administered assessments). Multiple functional outcomes will be evaluated, including occupational, family, social, and physical functioning. | Sandra Morissette, Central Texas Veterans Health Care System-Waco/ VA |
| 2013-06 | Internet-Based Smoking Cessation for OEF/OIF Veterans | In this study, 410 OEF/OIF veteran smokers will be randomized to receive either an Internet-based smoking cessation intervention and nicotine replacement therapy or referral to receive usual VA care. | Patrick Shields Calhoun, Durham VAMC/VA |

| End Date | Title | Study Population and Methods | Principal Investigator/Sponsor |
|---|---|---|---|
| 2013-06 | Characteristics and Treatment Preferences of Women Veterans with Insomnia | Abstract is under review as of September 14, 2012. | Jennifer Martin, VA Greater Los Angeles Healthcare System/VA |
| 2013-07 | Intensive Treatment of Chronic Pain and PTSD for OEF/OIF Veterans | The primary objective of this study is to evaluate the efficacy of an intensive integrated treatment for OEF/OIF veterans with comorbid chronic pain and PTSD. A secondary objective is to examine potential mechanisms of action that might account for improvements in pain or PTSD. Third, exploratory analyses will be conducted to assess the relationship between participation in treatment and cognitive functioning (N = 102). | John Otis, VA Boston Health Care System, Jamaica Plain/VA |
| 2013-07 | Evaluation of the Veterans In-home Program for Veterans with TBI and Families | The study will enroll 100 veterans with war-related TBI and a designated family member or partner. Veterans will be outpatients of the polytrauma service of the PVAMC. The VIP will be tested using a randomized two-group wait-list design in which participants are assigned to either the 3-month intervention or a usual care control condition. All are evaluated at baseline and 3 months (T2). Primary aims are to (1) establish acceptability and preliminary effectiveness for the impact of the intervention on functioning and community integration in TBI patients at 3 months and (2) evaluate VIP's acceptance by veterans using both project evaluations and focus group discussion. Secondary aims are to (1) establish VIP's acceptability and preliminary effectiveness on caregiver burden and mood and (2) assess its acceptability to family members using project evaluations and focus groups discussions. | Laraine Winter, Philadelphia Research and Education Foundation/National Institute of Child Health and Human Development |
| 2013-08 | Initial Randomized Controlled Trial of Acceptance and Commitment Therapy (ACT) for Distress and Impairment in OEF/OIF Veterans | The study is a randomized, controlled trial of Acceptance and Commitment Therapy as compared to control psychotherapy, present-centered therapy, for individuals with distress and impairment who deployed as part of OEF/OIF (N = 158). | Ariel J. Lang, PhD, University California, San Diego/Veterans Medical Research Foundation |
| 2013-08 | Military to Civilian: RCT of an Intervention to Promote Postdeployment Reintegration | In this study, 1,152 OIF/OEF veterans are randomized to one of the following three intervention groups: (1) Internet-based expressive writing, (2) Internet-based control writing, and (3) no writing/TAU. Self-report measures of psychological symptoms, psychosocial functioning, and life satisfaction at measured at baseline, 3 months, and 9 months. | Nina A. Sayer (Minneapolis VAMC)/DOD |

| End Date | Title | Study Population and Methods | Principal Investigator/Sponsor |
|---|---|---|---|
| 2013-08 | Cognitive Processing Therapy for Combat-Related PTSD | The first purpose of this study is to compare group-administered Cognitive Processing Therapy-Cognitive-only version (CPT-C), an evidence-based treatment for PTSD, to Present Centered Therapy in order to determine whether the results of CPT exceed those of receiving a therapy that focuses on current problems rather than past trauma in a group format. A second purpose is to conduct a randomized controlled trial to compare group and individual CPT-C for the treatment of PTSD in OIF/OEF military personnel (N = 400). | Patricia A. Resick, National Center for PTSD/VA Boston Healthcare System |
| 2013-08 | Examining Alcohol Use After Combat-Acquired Traumatic Brain Injury | The three research aims of this study are to (1) compare the postdeployment drinking behaviors for service members who experienced a TBI to those who did not, (2) examine the relationship between experiencing a TBI and postdeployment drinking-related negative consequences, and (3) examine the possible meditational effect of PTSD on the relationship between having experienced a TBI and the two outcome variables (drinking behaviors and negative postdeployment consequences). To analyze these research aims, this study will use the 2008 Department of Defense Survey of Health Related Behaviors among active-duty military personnel, a worldwide population-based assessment. The survey was self-administered and anonymous with a response rate of 71.6 percent. The proposed study is a quasi-experimental design. The study sample includes a cohort of service members with a recent combat deployment (past year) and at least 6 months postdeployment before completing the survey (over 4,000 respondents), allowing the study to examine postdeployment drinking behaviors and consequences. The study will use multivariate linear and logistic regressions to assess the relationship between experiencing a TBI and (1) drinking behaviors and (2) negative consequences, as well as path analysis to examine whether PTSD mediates the relationship between TBI and drinking behaviors and negative consequences. | Rachel S. Adams, Brandeis University/ National Institute on Alcohol Abuse and Alcoholism (NIAAA) |
| 2013-09 | CSP 566—Neuropsychological and Mental Health Outcomes of OIF: A Longitudinal Cohort Study | Follow up with the U.S. Army soldiers who took part in the Neurocognition Deployment Health Study (NDHS), also called "Prospective Assessment of Neurocognition in Future Gulf-deployed and Gulf-Nondeployed Military Personnel: A Pilot Study." Examine any enduring effects of war on mood and stress symptoms, thinking and reaction skills, and different aspects of day-to-day life (such as work and daily activities). Results from previous participation in the NDHS will be compared to the new information that will be obtained. A subset of 200 participants will also be invited to complete some of the thinking and reaction time tasks that were done as part of previous NDHS participation (N = 817). | West Haven VA Connecticut Healthcare System/ VA |

| End Date | Title | Study Population and Methods | Principal Investigator/Sponsor |
|---|---|---|---|
| 2013-09 | Linking National Guard Veterans with Need to Mental Health Care: The Buddy to Buddy Program | This study aims are to (1) evaluate the implementation of the B2B (buddy-to-buddy) program to inform ongoing program modifications and facilitate future dissemination efforts, (2) assess whether the B2B program increases mental health and substance use treatment initiation and treatment retention among returning National Guard soldiers, and (3) explore whether the B2B program improves mental health symptoms, deceases hazardous alcohol use, and improves soldier well-being (N = 35,000). | Marcia T. Valenstein, MD, AB, VA Ann Arbor Healthcare System/ VA |
| 2013-09 | Neural Substrates of Cognitive Control in Traumatic Brain Injury | No additional information found. | VA |
| 2013-09 | Prazosin and Combat Trauma PTSD (PACT) | This 26-week randomized double-blind placebo-controlled study is designed to demonstrate both short-term efficacy and long-term effectiveness of prazosin for PTSD (N = ~326). | Murray Raskind, Elaine Peskind, VA Puget Sound Health Care System/VA |
| 2013-09 | Developing a Computer-Adapted Test for PTSD | Objectives the study are to (1) create and test a PTSD Computer-Adapted Test (CAT) that will be useful for assessing the presence and severity of PTSD symptoms at a given point in time following traumatic exposure, and longitudinally over time to monitor course and/or outcomes of treatment; (2) develop a static, short-form PTSD assessment instrument composed of the most discriminating and informative items for use in situations where computer administration is not practical; (3) validate both the CAT and short forms using three other widely used paper-and-pencil self-report measures of PTSD severity as well as clinical diagnoses; and (4) assess sensitivity to change over time for both versions of the instrument. Researchers will administer the items to a sample of 1,000 veterans, stratified by age/cohort (Vietnam, OEF/OIF) and gender (N = ~1,100). | Susan V. Eisen, Edith Nourse Rogers Memorial Veterans Hospital, Bedford, MA/VA |
| 2013-09 | Engaging Homeless Veterans in Primary Care | In this study, investigators are conducting a multisite prospective randomized controlled trial in which 280 homeless veterans from the Providence and New Bedford areas not currently engaged in primary care will be randomized to receive either a personalized health assessment/brief intervention-based or usual care (social work/housing focused) outreach. Baseline assessments will include demographics, medical, mental health and substance use comorbidities, health seeking behavior, readiness for behavior change, and motivation for health care. Serial assessments at months 1 and 6 will assess evolving readiness and motivation as well as changes in homeless status (sheltering, employment/income, etc.). Actual utilization of services will be assessed using the CPRS electronic medical records. | Thomas P. O'Toole, Providence VAMC/ VA |

| End Date | Title | Study Population and Methods | Principal Investigator/Sponsor |
|---|---|---|---|
| 2013-09 | Psychotherapy Treatment of Deployment-Related PTSD in Primary Care Settings | The purpose of this study is to evaluate cognitive-behavioral therapy (CBT) for deployment-related PTSD that can be used by behavioral health consultants working with service members in the primary care clinic. CBT is a well-researched, very effective individual (one-to-one) treatment that is designed to help people to directly deal with traumatic events they have suffered in the past, including combat. Many service members prefer to see behavioral health providers in primary care rather than the mental health clinic. The researchers hope to learn if a brief treatment for PTSD in primary care can be just as useful as more traditional treatment given in the mental health clinic. This study will enroll approximately 45 participants overall; with approximately 30 participants at Wilford Hall Medical Center or BAMC, and 15 participants to be enrolled at the South Texas Veterans Health Care System over a period of 1 year. | Lisa Kearney, Jeffrey Cigrang, Diana Dolan, Laura Avila/University of Texas Health Science Center at San Antonio, Brooke Army Medical Center, Wilford Hall Medical Center, South Texas Veterans Health Care System |
| 2013-09 | Behavioral Activation for PTSD, Depression Treatment in OIF/OEF Veterans | In this study, OIF/OEF veterans with PTSD or PTSD and major depressive disorder will be randomized to behavioral activation and usual VA care treatment groups to determine efficacy (N = ?). | Amy W. Wagner, VA Medical Center, Portland/VA |
| 2013-10 | Vestibular Consequences of Blast-Related Mild Traumatic Brain Injury | Four subject groups of veterans complaining of dizziness/imbalance will be studied to determine the effects of mTBI and blast exposure on the central nervous system and vestibular system. | Faith Wurm Akin (James H. Quillen VAMC)/VA |
| 2013-10 | Stepped Enhancement of PTSD Services Using Primary Care (STEPS UP): A Randomized Effectiveness Trial | The overall objective of this study is to test the effectiveness of a systems-level approach to primary care recognition and management of PTSD and depression in the military health system. More specifically, the investigators will test the effectiveness of telephone care management with preference-based stepped PTSD/depression care—STEPS UP—as compared to Optimized Usual Care (N = 1,500). | Charles C. Engel, Walter Reed National Military Medical; Robert M. Bray, RTI International; Lisa Jaycox, RAND Corporation/DOD |
| 2013-11 | Information Processing Modification in the Treatment of PTSD | In this study, 96 OEF/OIF veterans with PTSD will be assigned to receive a computer-delivered attention-modification program designed to enhance attention disengagement from threatening stimuli or to a placebo condition. | Nader Amir/San Diego State University |
| 2013-11 | The Mission Connect Mild TBI Translational Research Consortium's Integrated Clinical Protocol | In this study, 200 mTBI subjects randomized to the treatment arm of the phase II drug trial of atorvastatin 7 days postinjury vs placebo. A Rivermead Post-Concussion Symptoms Questionnaire will be administered at 3 months after injury. | Claudia S. Robertson/Baylor College of Medicine |

| End Date | Title | Study Population and Methods | Principal Investigator/Sponsor |
|---|---|---|---|
| 2013-12 | Neuropsychological Screening of OEF/OIF Veterans in VA Primary Care | The goal of this study is to investigate the extent to which the VA TBI screening process may fail to detect or accurately identify the source of cognitive dysfunction and other postconcussive symptoms, limiting VA clinicians' ability to optimally communicate, triage, and provide targeted services for OEF/OIF veterans. | Karen Seal, San Francisco VAMC/VA |
| 2013-12 | Prolonged Exposure for PTSD Among OIF/OEF Personnel: Massed vs Spaced Trials | In this study, 210 OEF/OIF personnel will be randomly assigned to receive a 10-session PE therapy over 2 weeks or 10 sessions over 8 weeks. | Edna B. Foa/ University of Pennsylvania |
| 2013-12 | Telephone Cognitive Behavior Therapy for OEF Veterans with Pain | This primary aim of this study is to investigate the effectiveness of telephone Cognitive Behavior Therapy (CBT) in the management of chronic pain with OEF veterans enrolled in VA primary care clinics. The secondary aim of the study is to determine moderator and mediating factors by which telephone CBT facilitates pain management and successful adjustment of OEF/OIF veterans to chronic pain (N = 150). | Timothy Carmody, PhD, VAMC, San Francisco/VA |
| 2013-12 | The Effect of Goal Management Training with Mild TBI Veterans | This study will test the effect of Goal Management Training (10-week group therapy that teaches strategies to improve individual's ability to complete everyday tasks) on 12 OEF/OIF veterans with mTBI. Measures will be reported after each session and at 1-month follow-up. | Julia Waid-Ebbs, North Florida/South Georgia VHS/VA |
| 2014-03 | Innovative Service Delivery for Secondary Prevention of PTSD in At-Risk OIF-OEF Service Men and Women | This study has two primary objectives: (1) to develop, implement, and evaluate a treatment program (Behavioral Activation and Therapeutic Exposure, BATE) for OIF and OEF veterans with PTSD symptoms and (2) to determine whether or not this program delivered via telepsychology will be as effective as in-person treatment. Secondary objectives include determining (a) which treatment modality is more effective in terms of process variables (e.g., treatment satisfaction, session attendance), (b) which treatment modality is more cost-effective, and (c) whether treatment effects differ across race and gender. Study participants will be randomized to two treatment conditions, BATE will be delivered via telepsychology (BATE-T) and in-person (BATE-IP) (N = 200). | Ronald Acierno, Ralph H. Johnson VAMC; Thomas Uhde, Medical University of South Carolina/DOD |

| End Date | Title | Study Population and Methods | Principal Investigator/Sponsor |
|---|---|---|---|
| 2014-03 | Treatment Strategy for Alcohol Use Disorders in Veterans with TBI | The objectives of this study are to determine (1) whether the presence of prefrontal brain damage will be associated with poorer response to the Intensive Outpatient Treatment (IOP), (2) if valproate is more effective than naltrexone to treat alcohol use disorder (AUD) in this group of patients with severe psychiatric comorbidity and TBI exposure, and (3) if completion of the IOP will be associated with good psychosocial outcomes at 6 months follow-up. This is a double-blind active-controlled randomized clinical trial. Patients will be evaluated at baseline, followed weekly for 12 weeks, and evaluated at 6 months. The study's primary outcome variable will be time to relapse to heavy drinking. Secondary outcome measures will include proportion of heavy drinking days, severity of PTSD symptoms measured by the Clinician-Administered PTSD Scale, severity of depressive symptoms measured by the Hamilton Depression Rating Scale, and psychosocial outcome measured by the Community Integration Questionnaire (N = ?). | Ricardo E. Jorge, Iowa City VAMC/VA |
| 2014-03 | A Structured Communication Tool to Improve OEF/OIF Veteran Care | The specific aims for this proposed 2-year pilot are to (1) modify an existing computerized structured communication tool called DIALOG to reflect the mental health treatment needs of OEF/OIF veterans and enhance implementation procedures based on principles and strategies of cognitive-behavioral therapy; and (2) complete a randomized pilot for 32 OEF/OIF veterans and their mental providers to generate preliminary data supporting the study's hypotheses that use of the modified and enhanced DIALOG tool will (a) improve mental health treatment engagement as defined by increased likelihood of attending a subsequent mental health appointment following index use of the tool and (b) result in a decrease in veteran reported unmet needs, more positive ratings of treatment satisfaction, and improved ratings of quality of life (N = ?). | Richard W. Goldberg, Baltimore VAMC/VA |
| 2014-03 | The Influence of Posttraumatic Stress Disorder on Perceptions of Injury | The primary aim of this study is to examine whether the impact of PTSD on injury perceptions is different for those with a history of mTBI compared to those whose injuries are non-TBI-related. Using a 2x2 factorial design, the present study seeks to compare injury perceptions among four well-defined groups of veterans: (1) those with mTBI and current symptoms and co-occurring PTSD; (2) those with mTBI and current symptoms and no PTSD; (3) those with non-TBI physical injury and current symptoms and co-occurring PTSD; (4) and those with non-TBI physical injury and current symptoms and no PTSD (N = ?). | Nazanin H. Bahraini, VA Eastern Colorado Health Care System/VA |

| End Date | Title | Study Population and Methods | Principal Investigator/Sponsor |
|---|---|---|---|
| 2014-03 | Implementing Collaborative Care for Depression Plus PTSD in Primary Care | The objective of this study is to use a collaborative process to implement the Translating Initiatives for Depression into Effective Solutions (TIDES)/PTSD model in two primary care (PC) clinics and further develop methods for implementing veteran-centered care management that would facilitate spread of the VA's national tool kit for integration of mental health services into veteran-centered PC teams. An expert panel will be used to prioritize adaptations based on pilot study findings, as well as identify specific aims for tool production. Local stakeholders will participate in a tailoring process specific to each clinic. Staff at each clinic will be trained in the customized TIDES/PTSD model, and implementation support will occur in regular collaborative sessions. Evaluation questions will address feasibility of implementing the TIDES/PTSD model in PC clinics, contextual factors influencing the implementation, acceptability of this model, and the ability to integrate relevant clinical outcome tools into routine care. The influence on access and processes of care will be assessed, as well as exploring influence on clinical outcomes. Data sources will include clinical data collected in the usual process of care and qualitative interviews with stakeholders (N = ?). | Bradford L. Felker, VA Puget Sound Health Care System/VA |
| 2014-03 | Racial/Ethnic Variation in Family Functioning Post-Deployment | For this study, investigators will employ a mixed-methods design. Participants will consist of white, black, and Hispanic OEF/OIF veterans who have returned from deployment for no less than 3 months and their significant others (15 dyads per group). A clinical/demographic data form will be used to collect participants' clinical, demographic, and veterans' service history information. The Family Assessment Device will be used to collect individual family members' perceptions on seven dimensions of family functioning (N = ?). | Ivette M. Freytes, VHA/VA |
| 2014-03 | The VA Women's Overall Mental Health Assessment of Needs (WOMAN) | The goal of this project is to build on the Women's Overall Mental Health Assessment of Needs (WOMAN) study by adding an emphasis on gender-sensitive access to mental health care and explore the role of patient activation and engagement in women veterans' access to mental health care. Specifically, the objectives of this project are the following:<br>1. Assess potential gender-sensitive dimensions of access to mental health services;<br>2. Validate indicators of gender-sensitive access by examining the associations of the access dimensions to utilization and quality;<br>3. Examine the associations of patient activation with mental health care utilization, quality, and gender-sensitive access.<br>The WOMAN study is a nationwide telephone survey of approximately 4,000 women veteran VA health care users to determine the prevalence of a wide range of mental health symptoms and conditions among women in VHA and to assess mental health care needs and utilization. | Rachel Kimerling, VA Palo Alto Health Care System/VA |

| End Date | Title | Study Population and Methods | Principal Investigator/Sponsor |
|---|---|---|---|
| 2014-04 | Genomic Predictors of Combat Stress Vulnerability and Resilience | The goal of this project is to identify such factors by (1) studying a prospectively assessed, systematically phenotyped population to discover factors that predict development of PTSD and (2) indentifying gene-by-environment interactions. The San Diego Marine Resiliency Study is an ongoing, prospective study of >2,500 U.S. Marines bound for combat deployment to Iraq or Afghanistan, with the goal to identify factors that predict development of PTSD. Each Marine is evaluated predeployment on an array of psychosocial, psychophysiological, and biophysiological phenotypes and then followed by longitudinal assessments postdeployment. | Caroline M. Nievergelt, University of California, San Diego/NIMH |
| 2014-04 | Stress and PTSD Among OEF/OIF Soldiers and Their Spouses | The proposed investigation is an initial test of this possible mechanism linking PTSD, marital strain, and risk of cardiovascular disease. Specifically, it will assess the association of PTSD and cardiovascular reactivity (CVR; i.e., increases in heart rate and blood pressure) during potentially stressful marital interactions. Researchers will examine CVR in both veterans (with and without PTSD) and their spouses, as well the recovery of these cardiovascular stress responses following potentially conflictual marital interactions. These relations will be tested via several specific aims. The primary aim of the proposed investigation is to evaluate the differential physiological impact of negative marital interactions on OEF and OIF veterans, with and without PTSD, and their spouses. | Catherine M. Caska, University of Utah/NIMH |
| 2014-05 | A Brief Intervention to Reduce Suicide Risk in Military Service Members and Veterans—Study 2 (SAFEMIL) | The goal of this study is to evaluate the efficacy of the safety planning intervention on suicide ideation, suicide-related coping, and attitudes toward help seeking for hospitalized military personnel at high suicide risk. The investigators will randomize 186 patients to one of two conditions: Safety Planning for Military (SAFE-MIL) or Enhanced Usual Care (E-CARE). The SAFE-MIL condition (intervention) will consist of three targeted suicide prevention components including (a) structured risk assessment; (b) strategies to increase coping with suicidal thoughts and urges in order to reduce suicide risk; and (c) problem solving and motivational enhancement to increase acceptability of mental health treatment and maximize likelihood for postdischarge utilization of health services. The E-Care will consist of the usual care patients receive at an inpatient facility during their hospitalization in addition to assessment services provided by independent evaluators who work directly with our research team. Primary outcomes include suicide ideation, suicide-related coping, and acceptability and initiation of mental health care and substance use treatment in the 30 days after hospital discharge. Patients in both conditions will be assessed on the dependent measures at the time of hospital admission (i.e., baseline), at the time of discharge (Follow-Up Interval 1 [FU-1]), at 1 month (Follow-Up Interval 2 [FU-2]) and at 6 months (Follow-Up Interval 3 [FU-3]). | Marjan Holloway, Henry M. Jackson Foundation for the Advancement of Military Medicine |

| End Date | Title | Study Population and Methods | Principal Investigator/Sponsor |
|---|---|---|---|
| 2014-05 | Effectiveness of a Web-Enhanced Parenting Program for Military Families | The goal of this study is to advance research on family-based substance use prevention for reintegrating OEF/OIF personnel by examining whether an Oregon Parent Management Training prevention intervention, enhanced with e-technology and adapted for combat-deployed families' needs, will reduce risk behaviors associated with youth substance use by improving parenting, child, and parent adjustment. The program's feasibility and acceptability will be examined, and subsequently a randomized controlled trial of the 14-week group program and Web enhancement will be conducted with 400 families from the Minnesota Army National Guard. Families with 6–12-year-old children will be followed over 2 years to examine program effects. | Abigail Gewirtz, University of Minnesota, Twin Cities/NIH |
| 2014-05 | Prolonged Exposure (PE) for PTSD: Telemedicine vs In Person | In this study, 226 OIF/OEF veterans diagnosed with PTSD will be randomized to examine effectiveness measured in terms of symptoms, patient satisfaction, and costs (baseline, posttreatment, and 3- and 6-month follow-ups) of PE therapy delivered via telemedicine vs PE therapy delivered in person. | Ronald E. Acierno (Ralph H. Johhnson VA MC)/VA |
| 2014-06 | Effects of Mindfulness-Based Cognitive-Behavioral Conjoint Therapy (MB-CBCT) on Post-Traumatic Stress Disorder (PTSD) and Relationship Function | The purpose of this study is to develop a treatment intervention that combines mindfulness meditation with cognitive behavioral therapy for PTSD to be taught to veterans diagnosed with PTSD and their partners. This study will examine the effects of this integrated intervention on PTSD symptoms and intimate relationship functioning of OEF and OIF veterans. | Louanne Whitman Davis, Richard Roudebush VAMC, Indianapolis VA/VA |
| 2014-06 | A Placebo-Controlled Augmentation Trial of Prazosin for PTSD | In this study, 210 OIF/OEF soldiers and veterans with war zone trauma were randomized to prazosin or placebo to evaluate the efficacy and tolerability of prazosin augmentation in the treatment of PTSD trauma-related nightmares, sleep disturbance, global function/sense of well-being, and other clinical features and comorbidities of PTSD. | Murray Raskind/ Seattle Institute for Biomedical and Clinical Research |
| 2014-06 | First Longitudinal Study of Missed Treatment Opportunities Using DOD and VA Data | This study investigates the substance abuse and psychological outcomes of receiving early identification and linkage to behavioral health care in a cohort of Army members returning from OEF/OIF, merging MHS and VA data to create previously unavailable data sets. The study involves a quasi-experimental design, with longitudinal data files and statistical models of deployment-related factors and military health services on the odds of long-term poor substance abuse outcomes, poor psychological outcomes (e.g., PTSD, depression), thoughts of harmful behavior, and attrition from the Army. These analyses will provide operationally actionable data useful to quality improvement programs in the MHS and VA on urgent issues requiring clinical and policy attention. | Mary Jo Larson, Brandeis University, National Institute on Drug Abuse (NIDA)/DOD |

| End Date | Title | Study Population and Methods | Principal Investigator/Sponsor |
|---|---|---|---|
| 2014-06 | Integrated CBT for Co-Occurring PTSD and Substance Use Disorders | The purpose of this study is to assess the safety and practicality, feasibility, and efficacy of Integrated CBT (ICBT) for co-occurring PTSD and substance use disorders within the OEF/OIF/OND veterans population, as delivered by routine clinicians at the VA. The efficacy of ICBT will be tested among 64 veterans who screen positive for both disorders and are randomly assigned to either ICBT or standard treatment. | Mark McGovern, Darthmouth College; NIDA |
| 2014-06 | Psychological Stress and Risk of Cardiovascular Disease (CVD) | In this study, a database of more than 200,000 veterans returning from Iraq and Afghanistan will be used to compare CVD incident rates in those with and without PTSD. In addition, (1) a pilot prospective study will be conducted to examine established and novel CVD risk factors in a group of older veterans and civilians without known CVD and (2) an ancillary study of 820 men and women with known CVD will be conducted to determine what mechanisms link PTSD and recurrent CVD events. | Beth Cohen, University of California, San Francisco/NHLBI |
| 2014-06 | Veteran Interactions with VA Primary Care Prior to Suicide | The proposed study directly responds to the HSR&D mental health priority to improve identification and treatment of suicidality by aiming to identify what opportunities may exist in VA primary care settings to intervene with veterans at high risk for suicide. This retrospective descriptive and case-control study will link National Violent Death Reporting System Data from 10 states with VA administrative data to identify veterans who completed suicide from 2005 to 2009 who received VA primary care in the year prior to death. Researchers will review medical records, describe the primary care received by veteran suicide decedents, and identify potential gaps in identifying and addressing suicide risk. | Steven K. Dobscha, Portland VAMC/VA |

| End Date | Title | Study Population and Methods | Principal Investigator/Sponsor |
|---|---|---|---|
| 2014-07 | Use and Abuse of Prescription Opioids Among OEF/OIF Veterans | This study has two aims. Aim 1 is to use univariate statistics to characterize clinical and demographic characteristics of four groups of veterans in VA care: (1) opioid users, (2) chronic users, (3) chronic opioid users with pharmacy profiles suggestive of opioid misuse, which is termed "possible opioid misuse" here, and (4) individuals with diagnosed substance abuse/dependence. Aim 2 is to use event history analysis and multilevel models to assess geographic variation and identify patient (sociodemographic and clinical) and treatment (clinical settings) factors associated with (1) chronic use, (2) possible use, (3) discontinuation of chronic opioid use among veterans with chronic opioid use, and (4) OUD diagnosis in veterans with possible opioid misuse and in veterans with chronic opioid use. Aim 3 is to use trend analyses to investigate rates of chronic use, possible misuse, discontinuation of chronic opioid use, and diagnosed OUDs in the 3 years prior to the release of the pain directive and guidelines (FY2008–FY2010) with rates in the first full 3 years after the release of the directive and guidelines (FY2011–FY2013). Researchers will utilize secondary data analysis of 6 years of VA administrative data (FY2008–FY2013), with separate analyses for OEF/OIF veterans and all veterans. | Teresa Jo Hudson, University of Arkansas for Medical Sciences/NIDA |
| 2014-07 | Novel Treatment of Emotional Dysfunction in PTSD | The objective of this study is to determine if adding repetitive transcranial magnetic stimulation prior to Cognitive Processing Therapy significantly alters measures of arousal in individuals with combat related PTSD and improves clinical outcome. The investigators have assembled a multimodal human performance laboratory including 64-channel EEG and repetitive transcranial magnetic stimulation system. These resources combined with the neuroimaging capabilities of the Advanced Imaging Research Center at University of Texas Southwestern and skilled Cognitive Processing Therapy practitioners will be used in this study. The study involves 16 visits over the course of roughly 16 weeks with a 6-month follow-up assessment via telephone (N = 100). | John Hart, Jr., University of Texas, Dallas/DOD, University of Texas Southwestern Medical Center |
| 2014-07 | Integrated Cognitive Behavioral Therapy for Co-Occurring PTSD and Substance Use Disorders | The purpose of this study is to assess the safety and practicality, feasibility, and efficacy of ICBT for co-occurring PTSD and substance use disorders within the OEF/OIF/OND veterans population, as delivered by routine clinicians at the VA. ICBT is a non-exposure-based, manual-guided individual or group therapy. Primary Outcome Measures are decrease from baseline in clinician-administered PTSD Scale score (PTSD symptom severity) at 3 months and at 6 months (N = 80). | Mark P. McGovern, Dartmouth-Hitchcock Medical Center |

| End Date | Title | Study Population and Methods | Principal Investigator/Sponsor |
|---|---|---|---|
| 2014-07 | Enhancing Exposure Therapy for PTSD: Virtual Reality and Imaginal Exposure with a Cognitive Enhancer | The purpose of this study is to test the differences between four active treatment conditions for combat-related PTSD: virtual reality exposure therapy or prolonged imaginal exposure therapy (PE), both with D-cycloserine or placebo, as well as to examine predictors for PTSD and response to treatment in active-duty military personnel, veterans, and civilians who served in Iraq and Afghanistan (N = 300). | JoAnn Difede, Weill Medical College of Cornell University; Barbara Rothbaum, ABPP Emory University; Skip Rizzo, University of Southern California/Weill Medical College of Cornell University |
| 2014-08 | Web-Based CBT for Substance Misusing and PTSD Symptomatic OEF/OIF Veterans | This study has two aims. Aim 1 is to develop an interactive, Web-based psychosocial treatment for OEF/OIF veterans with hazardous or problematic substance use and PTSD symptoms. Aim 2 is to evaluate the efficacy of the Web-based intervention with OEF/OIF veterans with hazardous or problematic substance use and PTSD symptoms. Researchers plan to conduct a controlled trial in two primary care VA treatment centers. Participants will be randomized to two groups: (1) TAU, reflecting the model of treatment provided to most OEF/OIF veterans (n = 81) or (2) TAU plus the Web-based CBT intervention (n = 81). Primary outcomes will be (1) number of heavy drinking days and/or number of days of illicit or nonprescribed drug use in the past 30 days; (2) quality of life; and (c) PTSD symptoms. Aim 3 is to evaluate the cost and cost-effectiveness of the Web-based intervention plus TAU relative to TAU alone. | Andrew Bruce Rosenblum, National Development and Research Institutes/NIAAA |
| 2014-08 | Phase IV Study of Cognitive Rehabilitation Effectiveness for Mild Traumatic Brain Injury | This is a prospective, randomized, control treatment trial of cognitive rehabilitation for OEF/OIF service members with a history of mTBI and persistent (3–24 months post-injury) cognitive complaints. Subjects will be recruited from consecutive patient referrals to the TBI Service at SAMMC-North. Patients who meet eligibility criteria and consent to participate in the treatment trial will be randomly assigned to one of four 6-week treatment arms of the study. Subjects will be evaluated prior to the start of treatment and at 3, 6, 12, and 18 weeks following the initiation of the study. The total number of patients to be studied is 160 (maximum), which is approximately 20 patients per month (N = 160). | Douglas B. Cooper/Brooke Army Medical Center |
| 2014-09 | Genetic and Environmental Risk/Resilience Factors for PTSD in OEF/OIF Veterans | The purpose of this study is to examine the genetic and environmental determinants of risk and resilience to PTSD in OEF/OIF combat veterans. This is an evaluation only study and participation will last 1 to 2 days (N = ~800). | Bekh Bradley, Emory University/NIMH |

| End Date | Title | Study Population and Methods | Principal Investigator/Sponsor |
|---|---|---|---|
| 2014-09 | Neuropsychological and Mental Outcomes of OIF: A Longitudinal Cohort Study | In this study, 817 OEF/OIF veterans will be surveyed by mail/Internet/phone about mood, stress symptoms, etc. Approximately 200 will randomly selected from the larger group to take part in an in-person assessment which involved taking a small subset of neuropsychological tasks. | Jennifer J. Vasterling, VAMC, Jamaica Plains/VA |
| 2014-09 | Identifying and Validating Complex Comorbidity Clusters in OEF-OIF Veterans | This project establishes a line of inquiry examining patterns and trajectories of comorbidity, risk factors, and patient outcomes in OEF/OIF VA patients using a team comprised of VA, Army, Air Force, and Navy investigators. Identification of comorbidity clusters and their trajectories will provide insight for clinicians and policy makers to project future population characteristics and resource needs and determine how VA health care resources should be organized and delivered for this cohort of veterans. Examination of the relationship between coping patterns, social support, and comorbidity trajectories may provide the opportunity to develop interventions aimed at improving coping, social integration, and support. In both cases, such interventions offer the promise of utilizing health promotion to augment clinical care in line with VA goals for patient-centered care. | Mary Jo Pugh, South Texas Health Care System, San Antonio, TX/VA |
| 2014-09 | Neuropsychological Screening of OEF/OIF Veterans in VA Primary Care | The long-term goal of this study is to promote early accurate detection and appropriate triage for postconcussive symptoms in OEF/OIF veterans to prevent long-term disability. The short-term goal of this proposal is to investigate the extent to which the VA TBI screening process may fail to detect or accurately identify the source of cognitive dysfunction and other postconcussive symptoms, limiting VA clinicians' ability to optimally communicate, triage, and provide targeted services for OEF/OIF veterans. Researchers will assess the feasibility of conducting integrated primary care–based screening for a history of mTBI, postconcussive symptoms using the Neurobehavioral Symptom Inventory and objective cognitive dysfunction using the brief, computer-administered Automated Neurocognitive Assessment MetricsTM in conjunction with postdeployment mental health screening (N = ?). | Karen H. Seal, Veterans Affairs Medical Center San Francisco/VA |

| End Date | Title | Study Population and Methods | Principal Investigator/Sponsor |
|---|---|---|---|
| 2014-09 | RE-INSPIRE: Rich-Context Evaluation of INSPIRE | RE-INSPIRE is a prospective, longitudinal, and mixed-methods study of context embedded within an existing randomized-controlled trial. The Consolidated Framework for Implementation Research serves as the study's conceptual framework. This study will collect context-related data through annual site visits at all 12 VA facilities, semistructured phone interviews, and ongoing document/artifact capture. In addition, seven standardized measures will be administered to assess contextual factors at the level of individual, team, clinical microsystem, and facility: the Team Development Measure, the Competing Values Framework Measure, the Utrecht-9 Work Engagement Survey, the Baldridge Series Measures on Organizational Commitment to Quality Improvement, the Local Management Support Survey, the Clinical Microsystem Assessment Tool, and the Change Orientation Measure. | Edward J. Miech, Richard L. Roudebush VAMC/VA |
| 2014-10 | Psychophysiology of Prolonged Exposure for PTSD With/Without Yohimbine | In this study, 60 OEF/OIEF veterans with PTSD were randomized to receive yohimbine 1 hour before first imaginal exposure in PE therapy vs placebo. Physiological responses and self report of PTSD-symptom improvement will be measured at 0 weeks, 15 weeks, and 27 weeks. | Peter W. Tuerk (Ralph H. Johhnson VAMC)/VA |
| 2014-10 | Racial and Ethnic Disparities in Satisfaction with VA Care | Using a random sample drawn from 25 VAMCs, researchers will conduct telephone interviews from the VA Pittsburgh Healthcare System using both closed- and open-ended questions with 750 African American, Hispanic, and white veterans as well as a small sample of other minority veterans (Asian, Pacific Islander/Native Hawaiian, or American Indian/Native Alaskan). This mixed-methods design allows for the examination of the direct, mediated, and/or moderated associations of race/ethnicity on satisfaction outcomes. | Susan L. Zickmund, VA Pittsburgh Healthcare System/VA |
| 2014-11 | Mindful Yoga Therapy as an Adjunctive Treatment for PTSD Among OEF/OIF Veterans: A Pilot Study | The primary objective of this study was to establish the safety and acceptability of Mindful Yoga Therapy as an adjunctive treatment for PTSD among OEF/OIF/OND veterans. The study also sought to establish preliminary efficacy of Mindful Yoga Therapy for reduction of symptoms of PTSD and explore heart rate variability as a mechanism of therapeutic action (N = 30). | Rani Desai, Connecticut Healthcare System/VA |
| 2014-11 | Comparing Virtual Reality Exposure Therapy to Prolonged Exposure in the Treatment of Soldiers with Post Traumatic Stress Disorder (PTSD) | This study is evaluating the efficacy of virtual reality exposure therapy (VRET) by comparing it to PE therapy and a waitlist group for the treatment of PTSD in active-duty soldiers with combat-related trauma. The investigators will test the general hypothesis that 10 sessions of VRET or PE will successfully treat PTSD, therapeutically affect levels of physiological arousal, and significantly reduce perceptions of stigma toward seeking behavioral health services (N = 538). | Gregory A. Gahm, Defense Centers of Excellence; Greg Reger, Defense Centers of Excellence/National Center for Telehealth and Technology, The Geneva Foundation |

| End Date | Title | Study Population and Methods | Principal Investigator/Sponsor |
|---|---|---|---|
| 2014-12 | PTSD, TBI, and Neuropsychological Factors in Partner Violence Among Veterans | The primary objective of this study is to test the hypotheses that (1) TBI and executive functioning deficits will be positively and uniquely associated with higher physical and psychological intimate partner violence (IPV) severity and (2) TBI and executive functioning deficits will moderate the impacts of PTSD symptoms and cognitive deficits/biases on the IPV outcomes. Participants will be 150 male OEF/OIF veterans over the age of 18 who have been married or cohabitating with a partner for at least 1 year. | Casey T. Taft, VA Boston Health Care System/VA |
| 2015-01 (sus-pended) | Adjunctive Pregnenolone in PTSD and Depression in OEF/OIF Veterans | This study is an 8-week randomized, placebo-controlled clinical trial of pregnenolone administered adjunctively to TAU in 80 OIF/OEF veterans with PTSD and depression. | Victoria M. Payne/ VA |
| 2015-01 | Eye-Movement Recordings in the Diagnosis of Traumatic Brain Injury | This study examines the use of eye movement recordings to provide a reliable diagnostic of previously undiagnosed mTBI in OIF/OEF veterans (N = ~50). | Jonathan Jacobs, Cleveland VAMC/VA |
| 2015-01 | TBI and PTSD Comorbidity in OIF/OEF Veterans: Prevalence and Predictors | No additional information found. | Kathleen Carlson, Oregon Clinical and Translational Research Institute/VA |
| 2015-04 | Integrated Treatment of Operation Enduring Freedom/Operation Iraqi Freedom Veterans with Post-Traumatic Stress Disorder and Substance Use Disorders | The intervention, called "Concurrent Treatment with Prolonged Exposure" (COPE), represents a novel treatment that integrates cognitive-behavioral therapy for SUDs with prolonged exposure therapy for PTSD. In earlier studies with civilians, COPE has demonstrated efficacy in reducing alcohol and drug use severity, PTSD symptoms, and associated mental health problems (e.g., depression, anxiety). In this hybrid Stage Ib/Stage II study, researchers will (1) use a manualized, well-tolerated behavioral treatment for SUDs and PTSD (COPE); (2) employ a two-arm randomized between-groups experimental design (COPE versus a modified TAU; and (3) examine standardized, repeated dependent measures of clinical outcomes and process variables at five time points (pre-, mid-, and posttreatment and 3- and 6-month follow-up) (N = 90). | Sudie E. Back, Medical University of South Carolina/Medical University of South Carolina |

| End Date | Title | Study Population and Methods | Principal Investigator/Sponsor |
|---|---|---|---|
| 2015-04 | Neural Correlates of Cognitive Rehabilitation in Posttraumatic Stress Disorder | The longitudinal research design for this project will be a three factor mixed factorial design with between subject factors of PTSD (+PTSD × –PTSD) and cognitive remediation (learning-based cognitive training [LBCT] × nonlearning training [NLT]) and the within subject variable of time tested (pretraining, posttraining, 3-month follow-up). In this study, 40 participants will be enrolled in four groups of 10 each: (1) +PTSD/LBCT, (2) +PTSD/NLT, (3) –PTSD/LBCT, and (4) –PTSD/NLT. All groups will receive 40 hours of computerized training. Outcomes will be measured at baseline (i.e., pretreatment), after an average of 8 weeks of treatment and at 6 months posttreatment. The active treatment is the Posit Science visual cognitive remediation paradigm (i.e., InSight), while the control treatment will utilize games face valid for cognitive training. This study will examine the effects of a standardized cognitive rehabilitation program on neurocognitive functioning and brain functional activation in OEF/OIF veterans with PTSD (N = 40). | Brian Schweinsburg, VA Connecticut Healthcare System, Yale University/VA |
| 2015-05 | Integrated Treatment of OEF/OIF Veterans with PTSD and Substance Use Disorders | The proposed study will test the feasibility and preliminary efficacy of an integrative behavioral intervention for the treatment of co-occurring SUDs and PTSD modified for use among U.S. military personnel (including National Guard and reservists) who have served in OEF/OIF. The intervention, called "Concurrent Treatment with Prolonged Exposure" (COPE), represents a novel treatment that integrates cognitive-behavioral therapy for SUDs with prolonged exposure therapy for PTSD. In this hybrid Stage Ib/Stage II study, researchers will (1) use a manualized, well-tolerated behavioral treatment for SUDs and PTSD (COPE); (2) employ a two-arm randomized between-groups experimental design (COPE versus a modified TAU; and (3) examine standardized, repeated dependent measures of clinical outcomes and process variables at five time points (pre-, mid-, and post-treatment and 3- and 6-month follow-up). | Sudie E. Back, Medical University of South Carolina/ NIDA |

| End Date | Title | Study Population and Methods | Principal Investigator/Sponsor |
|---|---|---|---|
| 2015-05 | Predicting Treatment Response Using Psychophysiologic Reactivity Measures | The specific aims of the study are to (1) evaluate the clinical utility of psychophysiologic reactivity measures to predict overall PTSD symptom response among OEF/OIF/OND veterans receiving treatment for PTSD and (2) evaluate the clinical utility of psychophysiologic reactivity measures to predict psychosocial functioning and health-related quality of life response among OEF/OIF/OND veterans in treatment for PTSD. Develop psychophysiologic, neuropsychological, and/or self-report models to predict PTSD symptom response to pharmacotherapy, psychotherapy, and combined pharmacotherapy/psychotherapy. Investigators will divide psychophysiologic reactivity predictors into two groups: heart rate variability and attentional bias (eye gaze tracking and modified Stroop). Investigators will collect observational and longitudinal data from a treatment-seeking sample of 50 OEF/OIF/OND veterans with PTSD recruited from the Central Arkansas Veterans Healthcare System Mental Health Clinics (N = 50). | John Spollen, MD, Central Arkansas Veterans Healthcare System/VA |
| 2015-06 | Stress-Induced Drinking in OEF/OIF Veterans: The Role of Combat History and PTSD | The proposed clinical laboratory project will use a three-group design. The target OIF/OEF population will have no trauma exposure (control group), combat trauma exposure without PTSD, and combat trauma exposure with PTSD. This project will use a well-established clinical laboratory paradigm of stress induction employed by the group, the Trier Social Stress Test (TSST), to investigate the role of a history of exposure to combat trauma on reactivity to the TSST and on stress-induced voluntary drinking. First specific aim examines the effect of combat trauma history on stress reactivity, using subjective, neuroendocrine, and physiological measures of stress. The second specific aim will examine the effect of combat trauma history on subsequent drinking behavior and subjective response to alcohol using established procedures in a clinical laboratory paradigm (N = ?). | Ananda B. Amstadter, Medical University of South Carolina/NIAAA |
| 2015-07 | Exposure Therapy for Veterans with PTSD and Panic Attacks | This study is the first systematic investigation of a time-limited, multicomponent cognitive-behavioral treatment for veterans with specific comorbid anxiety problems. The purpose of the first phase of the study is to evaluate the feasibility and acceptability of the multicomponent cognitive-behavioral treatment in an open trial. The purpose of the second phase of the study is to evaluate the effectiveness of the multicomponent cognitive-behavioral treatment in comparison to standard PTSD treatment in military personnel returning from active duty (N = ?). | Ellen Teng, Michael E. DeBakey VAMC/VA |

| End Date | Title | Study Population and Methods | Principal Investigator/Sponsor |
|---|---|---|---|
| 2015-08 | Veteran Reintegration, Mental Health and Substance Use in the Inner-City | The specific aims of the project are as follows:<br>• Aim A—Substance use. To understand changes over time in substance use (including illegal drugs, psychotherapeutic drugs without a prescription, alcohol, and tobacco), problem use, treatment experiences, and barriers to treatment among veterans returning from Afghanistan OEF/OIF to the inner city.<br>• Aim B—Mental health disorders. To document the path to mental health problems (especially PTSD, consequences of TBI and depression) among OEF/OIF veterans returning to the inner city, as well as factors that promote or impede resilience and effective use of treatment.<br>• Aim C—Civilian reintegration. To identify successful coping strategies that promote healthy, productive reintegration to civilian life in the inner city, as well as personal problems, unproductive behaviors, and social forces that challenge veterans with regard to family, HIV infection/risk, work, and community life. | Andrew L. Golub, National Development and Research Institutes/NIAAA |
| 2015-08 | Central Auditory Processing Deficits Associated with Blast Exposure | This research team has established that recently blast-exposed soldiers show differences from controls on tests of central auditory function. This project will (1) develop a more accurate estimate of the prevalence of central auditory dysfunction among veterans exposed to blasts over the past 10 years, (2) identify the functional outcomes associated with abnormal performance on tests of central processing, and (3) improve understanding of the ways in which blast-exposure resembles and differs from both the normal aging process and non-blast-related TBI in terms of performance on tests of central auditory processing (N = 200). | Frederick Gallun, Portland VAMC, Portland, OR/VA |
| 2015-08 | Homeless Solutions in a VA Environment (H-SOLVE) | The objectives of this study are to (1) identify organizational facilitators and barriers to implementation of Housing First in a VA context through qualitative data collection among four VA facilities that are currently adopting this approach, in contrast to four VA facilities that are not adopting Housing First; (2) provide a manual identifying manipulable service elements for VA facilities seeking to implement Housing First programs with the use of presently available housing vouchers; (3) compare homeless vulnerability indicators (homeless chronicity, homelessness immediately preceding referral, health diagnoses, utilization history) among veterans served through more traditional homeless veteran programs at four VA sites, in contrast to veterans served at four VA sites that have implemented a Housing First approach; and (4) assess whether VA-based Housing First programs achieve results that are superior to conventional programs in regard to housing. | Stefan G. Kertesz, VAMC, Birmingham, AL/ VA |

| End Date | Title | Study Population and Methods | Principal Investigator/Sponsor |
|---|---|---|---|
| 2015-09 | Integrated vs Sequential Treatment for PTSD and Addiction Among OEF/OIF Veterans | The investigators hypothesize that veterans in the integrated conditions will show greater reductions in substance abuse and PTSD symptom severity at the end of treatment and at 6- and 9-month follow-ups. The investigators further hypothesize that offering veterans PE therapy at the onset of treatment in the integrated condition will leader to greater retention and satisfaction than in the sequential treatment design (N = 200). | David W. Oslin, University of Pennsylvania/VA |
| 2015-09 | Improving PTSD Outcomes in OIF/OEF Returnees: A Randomized Clinical Trial of Hydrocortisone Augmentation of Prolonged Exposure Therapy | This study seeks to examine the efficacy of hydrocortisone administration in the augmentation of the therapeutic effects of PE therapy, an empirically tested treatment shown to be effective in the treatment of PTSD. The augmentation builds on both the translation of neuroscience findings demonstrating the effects of glucocorticoids on learning and on empirical clinical findings from other investigators demonstrating beneficial effects of glucocorticoids in reducing traumatic memories in trauma-exposed persons (N = 60). | Rachel Yehuda, James J. Peters VAMC/Mount Sinai School of Medicine |
| 2015-09 | Diagnosing mild TBI in VA and Active Duty Military Patients Using MEG and DTI | There are three specific aims in the proposed study. The first aim will investigate the diagnostic value of the integrated magnetoencephalography (MEG)-diffusion tensor imaging (DTI) approach in VA and active duty patients with mTBI by detecting neuronal injuries (locus of the injury as well as affected neuronal networks) not visible with conventional neuroimaging methods (e.g., computed tomography [CT] and MRI). Preliminary data show that pathological MEG slow-waves, reduced MEG functional connectivity, and reduced DTI anisotropy are characteristics of axonal injury due to tissue shearing and stretching in mTBI, with markedly better sensitivity than CT/MRI in diagnosing individual mild TBI patients. The second aim is to study the neurophysiological basis of the cognitive impairments using N-back working memory MEG task in active-duty and VA patients with mTBI. The third aim will study the relationship between post-concussive symptoms, cognitive deficits as measured by neuropsychological exams, and the neuroimaging measurements with MEG and DTI in VA and active-duty patients with mTBI. To achieve these aims, the study proposes to develop new imaging analysis tools: frequency-domain VESTAL for accurately localizing pathological MEG slow-waves; Dual-core Beamformer for reliably obtaining the neuronal networks with reduced functional connectivity using MEG under the condition of poor signal to noise ratio; and a platform for integrating the functional MEG findings in the gray matter with structural DTI findings in the white-matter fiber tracts (N = ?). | Mingxiong Huang, VA San Diego Healthcare System/VA |
| 2015-09 | Measuring Quality of Life in Veterans with Deployment-Related PTSD | Abstract is under review as of September 14, 2012. | Stephen Lee Luther, James A. Haley Veterans' Hospital, Tampa, FL/VA |

| End Date | Title | Study Population and Methods | Principal Investigator/Sponsor |
|---|---|---|---|
| 2015-10 | Neural Markers and Rehabilitation of Executive Functioning in Veterans with TBI and PTSD | Although the relationship between combined TBI/PTSD diagnoses and postdeployment adjustment problems has been demonstrated, there has been little research into clinical interventions designed to reduce the severity of cognitive and affective symptoms in veterans with both TBI and PTSD. Therefore, the investigators propose a randomized clinical trial involving a cognitive rehabilitation intervention that targets improved executive functioning, with the participation of n = 100 veterans diagnosed with both TBI and PTSD (n = 50 in experimental group and n = 50 comparison). | Eric B. Elbogen/ University of North Carolina, Chapel Hill |
| 2015-10 | Brain Training to Enhance Frontal Lobe Reasoning in Soldiers and Civilian Adults with TBI | This study is being done to improve the ability to diagnose and to achieve higher levels of functional recovery in soldiers and civilians who have suffered either mTBIs or moderate-to-severe TBIs at chronic stages of brain recovery (greater than 12 months). This study will examine short-term effects of treatment on cognition and real-life outcomes in soldiers and civilians with TBI. Participants will undergo neuropsychological testing posttraining (10 weeks) as well as 3 months posttraining (N = 100). | Daniel Krawczyk/ The University of Texas, Dallas, University of Texas Southwestern Medical Center |
| 2015-10 | Brain Training to Enhance Frontal Lobe Reasoning in Soldiers with TBI | This study is being done to improve the ability to diagnose and to achieve higher levels of functional recovery in soldiers and civilians who have suffered either mTBIs or moderate-to-severe TBIs at chronic stages of brain recovery (greater than 12 months) (N = ~100). | Daniel Krawczyk/ University of Texas, Dallas |
| 2015-12 | Randomized Trial of Sertraline, Prolonged Exposure, and their Combination for Post-Traumatic Stress Disorder (PTSD) in Operation Enduring Freedom/Operation Iraqi Freedom (OEF/OIF) | This study aims to compare the effectiveness of two proven treatments for PTSD: PE, sertraline, and their combination. In addition, the investigators are examining predictors of response to these two treatments and how PTSD symptoms, thoughts, and biological factors may be changed by such treatments. In addition, the investigators will examine acceptability of each treatment and reasons for ending treatment. PTSD symptoms as measured by the Clinician Administered Posttraumatic Stress Disorder Scale (N = 441). | Sheila Rauch, VA Ann Arbor Healthcare System/ VA |

| End Date | Title | Study Population and Methods | Principal Investigator/Sponsor |
|---|---|---|---|
| 2016-01 | Accuracy and Validity of ICD9 Codes for PTSD in Veterans | The purpose of this study was to examine the validity of three algorithms tested against medical chart evidence for two different types of basic research questions (1) which definitions best predict for a diagnosis of PTSD and (2) which definitions best predict for the receipt of medication treatment for PTSD. Investigators will use electronically stored medical record data to examine 600 veterans, 300 with PTSD and 300 without any administrative data evidence for PTSD. Charts will be reviewed specifically to determine whether the treating providers' presented evidence of either the identification of PTSD or treatment for PTSD. Data will be extracted using a structured chart abstraction form and will be done by trained research assistants with formal psychological training. Medical record evidence of the identification of PTSD and/or treatment of PTSD will be gathered and then scored based on a 5-point Likert scale indicating the degree of certainty that PTSD was being actively monitored and/or treated. | Thad Abrams, MD, Iowa City VAMC/ VA |
| 2016-03 | Improving PTSD Service Delivery for Veterans with Severe Mental Illness | The aim of this study is to compare the efficacy of PE for PTSD plus TAU (PE+TAU) relative to TAU alone using a randomized, between groups, repeated measures design. In this study 156 ethnically/racially diverse male and female veterans with PTSD and SMI will be recruited from the Charleston VA and affiliated CBOCs during the study time frame. Veterans will be randomized 1:1 to one of two conditions: PE+TAU or TAU. The active intervention phase is 12 weeks. Veterans randomized to TAU will receive support services through the VA, potentially inclusive of case management, psychotropic medication management, and/or supportive counseling, and veterans randomized to PE plus TAU will receive 12 weekly sessions of PE in addition to TAU. All participants will be assessed at baseline, 6 weeks, posttreatment, and at 3 and 6 months. | Anouk L. Grubaugh, Ralph H. Johnson VAMC/VA |
| 2017-04 | Neuroimaging and Cognitive Correlates of Repetitive Blast-Related mTBI | This study will address some of these gaps in the literature by evaluating the neural underpinnings of persisting cognitive difficulties in veterans with a history of repeated blast-related mTBI. Specifically, preliminary research involving OEF/OIF veterans with a history of blast-related mTBI has found evidence of both reduced working memory on neuropsychological measures and cerebellar abnormalities that are visible on neuroimaging. A large-scale brain system that includes both cortical and cerebellar components is involved in verbal working memory, and this Career Development Award will enable the investigation of the functional and structural integrity of that system. Two complementary neuroimaging methodologies (resting state functional connectivity fMRI and diffusion tensor imaging) will be used to investigate the functional connectivity of the cerebral components of this network with the cerebellar components and the integrity of the white matter tracts that physically mediate this connectivity. | Kathleen Pagulayan, VA Puget Sound Healthcare System |

| End Date | Title | Study Population and Methods | Principal Investigator/Sponsor |
|---|---|---|---|
| 2020-01 (estimate) | Millennium Cohort Study | This study will evaluate the long-term health effects of military service, including deployments. About 150,000 current participants are expected, with low response rates. | Nancy F. Crum-Cianflone, Naval Health Research Center, San Diego, CA/DOD |
| Awaiting ARI approval and Army data for sampling (as of 09/2012) | The Soldier's Life Study (Expansion to Deployment Life Study) | No additional information found. | Terry L. Schell, RAND Corporation/ U.S. Army |
| Data collection and analysis under way (as of 09/2012) | Welcome Back Veterans Performance Monitoring Center | No additional information found. | Terri Tanielian and Laurie Martin, RAND Corporation/ McCormick Foundation |
| Data collection and analysis under way (as of 09/2012) | Informing the Department of Defense Strategy on Prevention of Suicide by Members of the Armed Forces | No additional information found. | Rajeev Ramchand, RAND Corporation/ DOD |
| Awaiting IRB approval (as of 09/2012) | Preventing and Managing Prescription Drug Misuse Among Military Personnel | No additional information found. | Rosalie Pacula, RAND Corporation/ DOD |
| Preparing IRB application (as of 09/2012) | Family Resilience in the Military | No additional information found. | Sarah Meadows, RAND Corporation/ DOD |

| End Date | Title | Study Population and Methods | Principal Investigator/Sponsor |
|---|---|---|---|
| Preparing IRB application (as of 09/2012) | Framework for Quality Assessments of Department of Defense Traumatic Brain Injury and Psychological Health Systems of Care | No additional information found. | Carrie Farmer, RAND Corporation/ DOD |
| Preparing IRB application (as of 09/2012) | Stigma Reduction Efforts in the Department of Defense | No additional information found. | Joie Acosta, RAND Corporation/DOD |
| Preparing IRB application (as of 09/2012) | Availability and Efficacy of Military-Culture Appropriate Psychological Health Treatment for Geographically Distant Service Members and Their Families | No additional information found. | Ryan Brown and Grant Marshall, RAND Corporation/ DOD |
| Preparing IRB application (as of 09/2012) | Sleep in the Military: An Evaluation of Military Programs and Policies | No additional information found. | Regina Shih and Wendy Troxel, RAND Corporation/ DOD |
| Phase I Complete; Phases II and III expected early 2013 | Review of DOD Suicide Prevention Programs | No additional information found. | Rajeev Ramchand, RAND Corporation/ DOD |
| Recruit-ment under way (as of 09/2012) | Systematic Treatment Engagement for Posttraumatic Stress Disorder Using Primary Care (STEP-UP) | No additional information found. | Lisa Jaycox, RAND Corporation (in partnership with RTI International, Uniformed Services University, and the Deployment Health Clinical Center/ Congressionally Directed Medical Research Program |

| End Date | Title | Study Population and Methods | Principal Investigator/Sponsor |
|---|---|---|---|
| Baseline recruitment completed among three services, follow-up waves ongoing (as of 09/2012) | The Deployment Life Study | This study is examining how deployment affects the health and well-being of military families over the course of 3 years. The success of military operations depends not only on the preparation of service members, but also on the preparation of their families—a concept known as family readiness. This study, which is being conducted by the RAND Corporation, will help researchers learn more about the skills and tools that military families need in order to handle the stresses associated with deployments. | Benjamin Karney and Terri Tanielian, RAND Corporation/ DOD |
| Several reports available on RAND website, several others forth-coming | Innovative Practices to Support Psychological Health and Well-Being | No additional information found. | Carrie Farmer, RAND Corporation/ DOD |
| Studies with Missing or Incomplete Information* | | | |
| NA (Award Amount: $1,134,157) | Identification of Abuse and Health Consequences for Military and Civilian Women | In this study, a random sample of 2,000 military women screened for intimate partner abuse; 200 cases and 200 controls selected for in-depth interviews and medical record reviews. The civilian comparison sample of 2,000 women enrolled in Kaiser Permanente HMO. Interview data will include a lifetime history of abuse and opinions about domestic violence screening and reporting. | Jacquelyn C. Campbell (Johns Hopkins University)/DOD (CDMRP) |
| NA (Award Amount: $1,874,879) | Health Status of Military Women in the Total Force | A survey will be mailed to active-duty Army, Air Force, and Guard/reserve personnel in all military branches. Data will be combined with comparable data from a survey of active-duty Navy and Marine Corps personnel under way by the Naval Health Research Center. | Robert M. Bray (Research Triangle Institute)/DOD (CDMRP) |

| End Date | Title | Study Population and Methods | Principal Investigator/Sponsor |
|---|---|---|---|
| Unknown | The Wellbeing of Army Personnel in Dual-Military Marriages | The central hypothesis of the proposed research is that individuals in dual-military marriages are exposed to unique stressors and benefits in the work and family domain and that those in dual-military marriages who receive little or no support from either domain will experience both negative health and lower subjective feelings of well-being. The proposed research will utilize interviews and surveys. Since there is little empirical research examining dual-military marriages, a qualitative research design (interviews) (Phase I) will be used to examine potential relationships between variables. Phase II of the study will consist of survey administrations. Questionnaires will be administered to individuals who are currently in dual-military marriages and those who have previously been in a dual-military marriage. | Ann Huffman, Northern Arizona University |
| Unknown | Identifying Military and Combat-Specific Risk Factors for Child Adjustment: Comparing High and Low Risk Military Families and Civilian Families | This proposal seeks to extend the current investigation of identifying risk and resilience factors in children ages 3–7 of military families with a combat-deployed parent by (1) surveying civilian families so as to identify those risk and resilience factors specific to a military family and (2) surveying military families with a parent deployed in a support/noncombat role so as to identify those risk and resilience factors specific to high-risk deployments. Researchers predict that military families with a high-combat exposure deployed parent will show unique parent and child risk factors in comparison to military families with a low-combat exposure deployed parent and civilian families. Using a similar survey as with this ongoing work with military families, researchers will assess 200 civilian families with children ages 3–7 from the greater Watertown, New York, area. The study will also survey 200 military families from deployed support brigades of Fort Drum, New York. | Julie Wargo-Atkins, University of Connecticut, Storrs |
| Unknown | Post-Traumatic Stress Disorder In-Home Therapy Clinical Trial Award | This study will evaluate the feasibility and efficacy of a treatment delivery method that could help overcome these barriers to care and make effective PTSD treatment more accessible to underserved military personnel and veterans. It will evaluate one of the leading treatments for PTSD, a form of counseling known as Cognitive Processing Therapy, when delivered in service members' and veterans' homes, either through in-person therapist visits or via the technology of telebehavioral health, as compared to standard, face-to-face treatment in a therapist's office. | Alan Peterson, University of Texas, Health Science Center at San Antonio |
| Unknown | Using Complementary and Alternative Medicine (CAM) to Promote Stress Resilience in those with Co-Occurring Mild TBI and PTSD | The project utilizes a placebo-controlled, randomized, single-blind design to determine acupressure's efficacy at improving mental health and stress reactivity in veterans with co-occurring mTBI and PTSD. Veterans returning from deployment in Iraq or Afghanistan will be recruited and after informed consults is obtained, each will be screened for study eligibility, including the presence of mTBI and comorbid PTSD (N = ?). | Theresa Hernandez, University of Colorado Boulder/ unknown funding source |

| End Date | Title | Study Population and Methods | Principal Investigator/Sponsor |
|---|---|---|---|
| Unknown | Structural and Functional Neuroimaging Studies of Combat Veterans | Objectives of this study are to evaluate changes in brain function in recent combat veterans that may be related to PTSD or postconcussive syndrome (N = 260). | Eric M. Wassermann, National Institute of Neurological Disorders and Stroke (NINDS)/ NINDS |
| Unknown | A Clinic-Based Intervention to Promote Veteran Enrollment in My Health*e*Vet | Abstract is under review as of April 20, 2012. Additional information not found. | Steven R. Simon, BS, MD, VA Boston Healthcare System Jamaica Plain Campus, Jamaica Plain, MA |
| Unknown | Testing and Evaluation of a Predeployment Stress Inoculation Training Program (PreSTINT) | This study proposes to test and evaluate a group-based, combat-relevant, predeployment stress inoculation training (PreSTINT) program designed to help deploying personnel better cope with combat-related stressors and reduce the negative behavioral effects of trauma exposure. The PreSTINT program includes an educational component in which two arousal reduction techniques are presented. During a virtual reality simulated mission, soldiers are trained to control excessive arousal levels while focusing on the mission at hand. Their speed and accuracy in responding to threats as well as their ability to focus and maintain attention are assessed. Two phases of study will test and evaluate the effectiveness of the PreSTINT training program. The effectiveness of the PreSTINT program for arousal and attentional control will undergo testing in year 1, and its ability to reduce postdeployment distress will be examined in years 2 and 3. | Laurel Hourani, RTI/funder unknown |
| FY 2011 Award Amount: $260,100 | Using Complementary and Alternative Medicine (CAM) to Promote Stress Resilience in those with Co-Occurring Mild TBI and PTSD | The proposed project will utilize a placebo-controlled, randomized, single-blind design to determine acupressure's efficacy at improving mental health and stress reactivity in veterans with co-occurring mTBI and PTSD. Veterans returning from deployment in Iraq or Afghanistan will be recruited and after informed consults is obtained, each will be screened for study eligibility, including the presence of mTBI and comorbid PTSD. | Theresa Hernandez, Institution Receiving Award: University of Colorado, Boulder Program: DMRDP |

*The committee was not able to accurately group these studies into the other two categories.

# APPENDIX E

# INDIVIDUAL ETHNOGRAPHIC ASSESSMENTS OF SIX COMMUNITIES

Westat conducted a series of ethnographic assessments for the Committee. The communities visited include: Jacksonville, North Carolina; El Paso, Texas; Watertown, New York; Lakewood and Lacey, Washington; Georgetown, South Carolina; and Little Falls, Minnesota. This appendix contains each of those individual assessments and Chapter 7 provides a summary and conclusion regarding the impact of military deployments on communities.

# Understanding the Community Effects of Multiple Military Deployments

## Case Study Reports

# Jacksonville, North Carolina

Case Study Report

# Impacts of Multiple Deployments: Jacksonville, North Carolina

## OVERVIEW

This report presents the study team's findings from a weeklong site visit (April 18–25) to Jacksonville, North Carolina, a midsized city on the coast that is adjacent to Marine Corps base Camp Lejeune. A key finding from this location was that multiple deployments appear to have had little effect on the overall local economy. Many interviewees attributed this to Project CARE, a Chamber of Commerce–initiated effort to mitigate negative community effects from deployments by providing support to service members' families, communicating with businesses, and promoting a positive community spirit toward the military. Community members spoke of their concerns that additional mental health care services are needed both on base and in the community, where some service members prefer to seek help. They also spoke of the need for more federal resources to address infrastructure problems in the community related to the growing military population.

**Data Sources**

- Chamber of Commerce
- Churches
- City Government
- Fire and Police Chiefs
- Health Department
- Jacksonville Jamboree
- Kindergarten Readiness Program
- Onslow County Partnership for Children
- Recreation and Parks Department
- School Board and Transition Counselors
- Social Services Department
- United Way

## GEOGRAPHIC ORIENTATION

### Community: Jacksonville, North Carolina

Jacksonville, North Carolina, lies on the eastern shore of the state in Onslow County and adjacent to the southern Outer Banks and is contiguous with both Marine Corps Base Camp Lejeune and Marine Corps Air Station New River. According to the 2010 Census, Jacksonville's population of 70,1451 represents an increase of about 5% over the 2000 population. Demographically, 9.7% of the population of the city is age 5 or younger, compared with 6.6% for North Carolina and 6.5% for the United States. Only 5.4% of Jacksonville residents are age 65 years or older, compared with 12.9% for North Carolina and 13.0% for the United States. Jacksonville also has a proportionately larger male population than the rest of the state or country, at 58.8% of the population. The young age distribution and high proportion of males are likely due to the presence of the Marine Corps in the community.[1]

Race and ethnicity trends in Jacksonville are similar to those in the state of North Carolina, with 67.7% reporting their race as white, 20% reporting their race as black, and 13% reporting Hispanic or Latino origin. Home ownership rates in Jacksonville are disproportionately

[1]All population statistics are from the 2010 Census and the American Community Survey (http://quickfacts.census.gov/qfd/states/37/3734200.html). As will be noted throughout this report, Jacksonville officials and other community members do not believe these figures accurately represent the local population.

low (38.8%) when compared with the rates for North Carolina (68.1%) and the United States (66.6%). The median household income in Jacksonville during the years 2006–2010 was $42,469, compared with $45,570 for North Carolina and $51,914 for the United States.

### Military Installation: Camp Lejeune

Camp Lejeune is home to the largest concentration of Marines and U.S. Navy personnel in the world and currently encompasses 156,000 acres. The base was established in 1941 to meet the need for an East Coast amphibious training facility and has grown over the years to train men and women to fight wars in the Pacific Islands, Korea, Vietnam, Kuwait, Afghanistan, and Iraq. Several satellite facilities offer infantry training and serve as the home of the amphibious assault Marines and vehicles, the Marine Corps Engineer School, and the Coast Guard's Port Security Training Detachment. The Marine Corps Air Station New River, a helicopter base, is also located in Jacksonville.

According to its website, Camp Lejeune is the "Home of Expeditionary Forces in Readiness," and troops from the base have played a crucial role in both Operation Iraqi Freedom (OIF) and Operation Enduring Freedom (OEF). The author of an August 2010 article from the *Jacksonville Daily News* explains how "the contribution of the corps—with a heavy emphasis on the efforts of Camp Lejeune-based troops—played a vital role in rounding a corner in the war and securing a victory pennant."[2] As one city official recounted:

> I have a vivid memory . . . after everything took place and 9/11 became apparent, there were some announcements made as to how we were going to be impacted . . . we were going to be the first ones in.

Since 2003 when the first U.S. troops entered Iraq, Jacksonville has been faced with a steady stream of deployments. Members of the Social Services Department explained how the deployment patterns have changed over time:

> [Deployments are] more frequent than they used to be. . . . [They] used to be a little longer, would go a year or 18 months, but then they'd be back for at least a year or 2 years . . . now they are gone anywhere between 6 and 9 months, they are here a couple of months, and then they are gone again for the same amount of time. [Social services representative]

Many of the troops deployed to Iraq and Afghanistan from Camp Lejeune are infantrymen, and the base has suffered a high proportion of troop deaths compared with other military installations.

### Relationship Between Community and Military Installation

The relationship between the base and the community is best described as *dichotomous.* Although there are extremely close ties between the base and both the city and the county, in other regards the military and civilian worlds are separate. The close ties are noticeable

[2] See http://www.jdnews.com/articles/success-82029-iraq-vital.html.

everywhere: Military families may live on base but shop, work, and send their children to school in the county school system; military members may live on base or in civilian housing and purchase goods and services in the city or county; civilian contractors and other business people provide goods and services to the base; and civilian staff work on the base. Military and civilian personnel, such as police officers and firefighters, respond to emergencies together and occasionally train together on or off the base. Military personnel may serve as volunteer coaches for school or community sports teams.

The areas of separation, though not as immediately apparent, are equally widespread. Military or military-affiliated status confers a set of rights and privileges that is not shared by those without military status. A social service professional pointed out, for example, that women who are in relationships with service members but are not legally married cannot seek services on base. Conversely, a military member who obtains a restraining order against an abusive spouse through military channels will find that the restraining order cannot be enforced off base because it is not recognized in a civilian jurisdiction.

The base is the main economic driver in the area, with effects felt both in the city and throughout Onslow County. One Jacksonville Chamber of Commerce member said that the "entire market is the base." According to the *Camp Lejeune 2012 Base Guide,* the base and surrounding community are home to an active duty, dependent, retiree, and civilian employee population of more than 180,000 people and the base contributes more than $3 billion each year to the local economy in payroll, contracts, construction, and other services. The economic and social effects are mixed:

Positive effects of the military presence include

- Source of income and employment (e.g., as the leading employer in Onslow County, the Marine Corps Community Services employs more than 2,200 civilians at Camp Lejeune),
- Strong consumer base, and
- Source of civic pride and cultural continuity.

Negative effects of the military presence include

- Traffic congestion and strains on infrastructure,
- Overreliance on one source of income, which decreases the level of available employment opportunities,
- Prevalence of high-risk behaviors associated with hosting a large population of young men and women (e.g., drinking and driving), and
- Need to provide social services beyond those available on base to those who do not have access.

Historically, Jacksonville saw a substantial drop in its population during the first Gulf War as dependents left to return to their families for support during deployments.

> In the first Gulf War . . . a lot of people broke their leases because they thought that war was going to be an incredibly long period of time . . . they picked up and went back home to be with their loved ones. [City official]

> In that time period, Jacksonville pretty much emptied out. Not only did the service members leave, but a lot of their dependents left as well. [Community college representative]

In an effort to prevent this flight from reoccurring, the Onslow County Chamber of Commerce put an innovative program called Project CARE in place. This effort, which was activated several times starting in 2003, combines the efforts of various local government, military, Chamber of Commerce, and community organizations to provide support to families of deployed services members, assist businesses in dealing with the deployments, and increase community spirit toward the military. Project CARE was cited by many interviewees as a successful strategy to mitigate the potential negative effects of multiple deployments:

> I think the community as a whole . . . made it important to let the dependents know during the second Gulf War that they could stay here, that people in the community cared about them and were going to take care of them. It made a very big difference. Jacksonville certainly didn't clear out. [City official]

This intervention has helped to create social and economic stability in Jacksonville throughout the OIF/OEF engagements.

## EFFECTS OF DEPLOYMENT ON THE COMMUNITY

### Economic Impacts

Multiple deployments appear to have had no discernible effects on the broad, community-level economy. Interviewees regularly described the local economy as robust and benefiting from the nearby presence of Camp Lejeune. There were suggestions that deployments may cause microlevel economic shifts (e.g., increased storage unit rentals before deployments, increased large-item purchases by young soldiers upon return from deployment), but interviewees did not indicate multiple deployments to be behind these small-scale rhythms.

#### Overall Commerce

As suggested above, the overall economy in the area has seen continued growth, strong military incomes, a good business climate, and relatively low unemployment rates. As of March 2012, unemployment rates were lower in Jacksonville and Onslow County (8.7% and 8.4%, respectively) than in North Carolina (9.7%) and the United States as a whole (9.1%) (http://data.bls.gov). Pay and housing allowances to military families have spurred a construction boom in homes, apartments, retail stores (including major consumer goods such as furniture and cars), restaurants, hotels, child care facilities, and ancillary services such as barbershops and storage facilities. Jacksonville officials noted that there is a large amount of construction work being done on base, and the restaurants in town are always full.

> Every restaurant in town has a long line . . . hotels are packed . . . over the past several years there has been a lot of construction and work on base, and that has put a lot of construction workers . . . into our community. . . . [Emergency services representative]

Some of these businesses experience cyclical ups and downs related to deployments. For example, barbershops see less business during deployments, but storage facilities flourish. In addition, the Basic Allowance for Housing (BAH), hazard pay, and savings while overseas tend to make the military-affiliated population stronger consumers than civilians are. Spikes in spending for consumer goods can probably be linked to deployment cycles, with young single service members reportedly making large purchases (e.g., cars, motorcycles) upon return from the combat theater. Importantly, the change in deployment cycles (shorter duration, but more frequent) was perceived by some respondents to have helped reduce the impact on the local economy:

> They're only gone for 6 to 9 months now; it doesn't hit the economy within the county as hard as it used to when they deployed for a year at a time. . . . [Social services representative]

For the most part, the data suggest that the community has been insulated from the national economic recession. Some interviewees did note one probable effect of the recession, namely, that many family members of deployed Marines have moved to Jacksonville to help the nondeployed spouse because they themselves are unemployed and thus able to relocate.

> We've been seeing a lot of family members relocate here . . . to help them take care of the kids . . . and once they've been here for 3 or 4 months, they start getting into the job market . . . it's not a short-term thing, it's a long-term thing. [Chamber of Commerce member]

Although the supports are undoubtedly welcomed by the nondeployed spouse, unemployed relatives can put an extra strain on family finances. And if these family members do find work, they often end up being underemployed, as discussed below.

The community also has been spared an economic blow in that the Department of Defense has not chosen to pursue any large-scale Base Closure and Realignment (BRAC) actions at the base. The only BRAC action taken at the base to date is the closing of the brig in an effort to consolidate correctional facilities in the mid-Atlantic Region.[3] Although several respondents mentioned that the Marine Corps plans a gradual drawdown of service members, to date this has not significantly affected the area and business leaders say it will likely take place over the nextseveral years.

Although the economy of the area remains fairly robust, economic conditions for individuals can vary:

[3] See http://www.jdnews.com/news/brac-14971-lejeune-gombar.html.

**Single Marines** receive hazard pay, housing allowances, and other benefits; are typically economically stable; and can afford to make major purchases such as cars and furniture upon their return from deployments.

**Civilians** may experience more dire economic situations, social services may be stretched because of the alleged Census undercount that affects federal funding for local programs (see below), high-paying jobs are scarce, housing is expensive, and consumer goods like cars may be high-priced because local businesses set their prices relative to the military salaries:

> When I purchased my car, I went to Wilmington because I can't buy in Jacksonville . . . the prices in Jacksonville are significantly higher . . . they know they are going to get those young military guys who have all this pocket change. [Community member]

**Military families'** economic situations may depend on their number of dependents, employability of the "at-home" spouse, and their skills in managing money.

**Unofficial military dependents** (e.g., girlfriends and children) can experience more economic stresses depending on available jobs and how much the military member is willing and/or able to support them.

Family spending cycles may be related to deployments. For example, the number of pregnancies increases dramatically when Marines return from overseas, potentially resulting in increased spending for health care and, ultimately, food, clothing, and other items needed for the new family member.

**Labor Supply and Employment**

Military activities have had a significant effect on high turnover of the labor supply in Jacksonville and Onslow County, but this must be seen as a result not necessarily of deployments, but of regularly scheduled Permanent Change of Station (PCS) rotations. One member of the Chamber of Commerce representing a large national retailer told us that each year about 4% to 5% of his staff members ask for "hardship transfers" to other national locations because of a family member's PCS transfer. Representatives of child care facilities, the hospitality industry, automotive sales, and city government all reported that military-affiliated employees have a lot of turnover and it is difficult to replace good staff members who leave:

> You get some really good ones, and you know they are going to leave one day and you just hate it . . . our office manager . . . we are just dreading the day when she leaves and how we are going to replace her. [Chamber of Commerce member]

> There's about 700 volunteers for fire and rescue in the county. I'd say about 85 to 100 of those are direct military connected, and that is a constant revolving door in that area. They'll be here for a while and then they'll leave for deployments. [County EMS representative]

> It has been a struggle these last couple of years trying to keep staff, and we've tried to be as consistent as possible because with the kids dealing with transition at home, we want them to at least be able to come to the Rec site and see familiar faces. [Recreation and Parks Department representative]

> It's almost like if I could ask two nonlegal interview questions, it would be are you pregnant, or are you a spouse of an active duty military, because I know what is going to happen. [Health Department representative]

The Onslow Police and Fire Departments are particularly prone to seeing turnover because many of their staff members are affiliated with the military. Among paid staff, they said, Police Department members are about 50% retired military; paid Fire Department staff members are about 20% retired military. They see turnover of about 15% per year. A representative of the County Health Department said turnover is a major problem in the Health Department as well, where many positions require specialized, long-term training and have licensure and certification requirements. For example, a nurse specializing in treating sexually transmitted diseases may require up to 2 years of training in order to function independently in the position; if staff members are prone to leave every 3 years, it is difficult for the county to justify the cost of such trainings.

Deployments also directly affect the labor supply. During the Health Department and Police/Fire Department interviews, interviewees mentioned that local employers must be flexible in terms of spouses' issues during deployment, such as finding child care and spending time with active duty spouses before and after deployments. One interveiwee told us that following one return from deployment, 19 of 20 waitresses at one restaurant became pregnant. For employers, it is illegal to ask a potential employee if they are married to a Marine or if they are pregnant, so businesses are forced to be flexible to accommodate military families to meet their staffing needs:

> A girl that works for us, her husband was just injured, that's a major thing. For childcare, they are the only one at home [and we] just have to work with them on their schedules. [Chamber of Commerce member]

> [As an employer, we're sensitive . . . you've got a mom who is weeping, or it was just really hard to come in the day after she put her husband on the bus. . . . [Mental health representative]

In addition, and as suggested previously, deployments and PCS transfers together contribute to a scenario where underemployment is common. Unlike communities with universities or large-company headquarters that draw long-term residents who are highly educated, Jacksonville is focused on providing goods and services to the highly transient base population and to civilians in and around the city. Many local residents are underemployed in low-pay, semiskilled retail or service jobs. Underemployment disproportionately affects military dependents and individuals moving to Jacksonville to support their families; these people are more likely to have higher skills than the local job market can accommodate:

> A lot of them are coming from larger cities where there's a lot of hi-tech or tech or manufacturing firms. So when they get here, we don't have the same firms and we definitely don't have the same pay scales that they have. [Chamber of Commerce representative]

> I think the issue for us is underemployment. . . . We are so heavily reliant upon retail sales. . . . We have seen a decline in the ability to be self-sufficient in that even though you may be . . . employed, you still require economic assistance to maintain family stability. [Social services representative]

Thus, even though the overall unemployment situation in Jacksonville and Onslow County looks good, findings from the site visit suggest that multiple deployments have potentially exacerbated an already dynamic labor market by contributing to high staff turnover rates, increasing the need for employers to make periodic accommodations for military spouses, and leading to a high underemployment rate among extended members of military families.

**Housing Market**

Continued overbuilding of the housing stock was a topic of concern to almost everyone interviewed. As one city official explained, the "housing market is soft because it's been overbuilt." The BAH is high enough for many Marines to purchase homes or rent recently constructed apartments. This has created a strong housing market that has had several effects.

- Growth in areas outside the city has put severe pressure on infrastructure and EMS services:

  > The city taxpayers bear the burden . . . [we] need resources for infrastructure and road improvements . . . funding for that would be really helpful. [EMS representative]

  > . . . infrastructure . . . we are way behind the 8-ball on that. . . . [Chamber of Commerce representative]

- Home and apartment prices are driven by the BAH, putting adequate housing well out of reach for many nonmilitary individuals and families:

  > The housing that is being built is really being built to those housing allowances. [Chamber of Commerce member]

  > I can't afford to live in Onslow County, I'd love to. I work here . . . but I can't [afford it]. . . . [Community member]

  As a result, individuals and families that do not receive the BAH may spend a high proportion of their income on housing, leaving them in danger of having insufficient funds for food, gasoline, medical care, and other necessities. This situation leads to higher demand for social services.

- Because large builders can price new homes competitively with older homes, military personnel preparing for a PCS may not be able to sell their homes, especially if the home is not brand new:

  > [There have] . . . been a lot of people who are affected by the lower property values and a significant number of new built houses. People, if given the choice, want to buy new instead of buying old. [City official]

  A Marine told us he is preparing for a 2-year assignment in another region of the United States. Because he and his family own an older home, they have been unable to rent or sell it. His wife and young son will stay in Jacksonville while he moves to another state, creating a State-side situation that is, in his words, "essentially a 2-year deployment."

Many respondents expressed concern about the future of the real estate market in the area, especially in light of a housing construction plan that is, in the words of Colonel Lecce, the base commanding officer, "the largest in this base's history," as stated in a 2011 letter to Military.com (http://www.military.com/opinion/0,15202,231435,00.html). This new base construction plan will result in nearly 700 new homes, for a total of more than 5,000 homes *on base* by 2013. In response to the increased availability of on-base homes,

> [The Marines] are making [service members] move back on base because their occupancy rate is so low . . . and they are building with taxpayer dollars and [those houses] cannot sit empty. [Chamber of Commerce representative]

This may result in a severe drop in housing prices off base and cause a negative ripple effect in the local economy.

**Changes in Population Size**

Census data indicate that the population of Jacksonville has increased by 5.1% between 2000 and 2010. City officials and Police and Fire Department representatives, however, discussed their belief that the Census numbers are inaccurate because they do not count deployed military members as part of the local community. More specifically, the Census enumerates overseas soldiers as "deployed," not in the locations where they were last stationed[4]:

> The rules for Census counting impacted on us, because of the deployments . . . financially and otherwise . . . it is because of a rule established from the fallout from Vietnam and doesn't account for the current way that we deploy our forces. . . . [City official]

[4] For more information, see: www.census.gov/hhes/veterans/about/faq.html#Q9 and http://www.mcclatchydc.com/2011/02/07/108265/census-undercount-of-overseas.html#storylink=cpy.

> From a resource standpoint, that has probably hurt us more than anything in the past 4 or 5 years. [EMS representative]

Several respondents told us they believe that, despite the official Census count, the community has shown substantial growth in recent years. A Health Department official provided data showing a 30% increase in the military population from 2000 to 2012. A child care provider reported that at least half the population is affiliated with the military and that even with a downsizing of the military, the city will still have a larger population than before the Gulf War. This is partly due to the trend for extended family members to relocate to Jacksonville. A school board member told us that last year, 18,000 local Marines were deployed. The County Health Department told us that the population of Onslow County is approximately 170,000 and of these, 27% are active duty and 18% are retirees. Counting family members/dependents, close to 70% to 80% of the population is affiliated with the military.

## Information and Communication

### Open Discussion of Deployment-Related Issues

The military is very much on everyone's mind in Jacksonville, according to all interviewees, and that level of understanding is what makes Jacksonville feel like home for so many military families:

> You don't want to hang the yellow ribbon on the trees in your front yard if you are the only one in the neighborhood whose husband is deployed . . . but they couldn't tell because everyone had yellow ribbons. [City official]

City government officials pointed out the symbolism of Jacksonville's Beirut and Vietnam War memorials. Local media sources, such as the *Jacksonville Daily News* (JDN), continually report on items of interest to military-affiliated individuals and families. The JDN website includes a "Lejeune Deployed" blog that publishes news and photos from deployed units and links to specific unit webpages; they also have a reporter assigned to cover the military. A targeted online newspaper, *The Globe,* is published by a private company but dedicated to the military reader. Other local and countywide news sources, such as television news programs, provide Marine-related news. Also, *Lejeune Underground* and *Lejeune Yard Sales* are two local online bulletin boards where individuals can exchange news and seek help and advice from peers.

Community events also serve as a venue for passing along information about the military. For example, the first annual Jacksonville Jamboree, a community fair widely publicized throughout Onslow County, hosted booths for organizations specifically dedicated to military-related issues as well as booths for the general community. Booths included

> **P.S. Charities**, which was raising money to build an accessible home for a veteran with triple amputations and severe burns sustained from an IED blast in Afghanistan;

**Paws for Veterans**, which was promoting their efforts to provide therapy dogs for veterans with PTSD, TBI, or mobility issues; and

**A chiropractic practice** where military members could discuss their medical and chiropractic needs with the clinic's staff.

These issues are being seen as both challenges for all those involved and opportunities for the area to retain its population and provide the services residents need.

**Sources of Information for Military Families**

Military members and their families may find out about resources in a number of ways. The base offers predeployment and postdeployment briefings to service members and their families; targeted briefings such as the Kindergarten Readiness program, which focuses on ways families can prepare for sending their children to school; and information on supportive resources. Representatives of programs such as the FOCUS project (Families OverComing Under Stress™), Relocation Assistance Program, and Exceptional Family Member Program will sometimes attend these targeted briefings and set up tables with program materials and staff members to answer questions. For example, the FOCUS project provides resiliency training to military families and children and teaches practical skills to meet the challenges of deployments and reintegration. Family members can also contact the base Family Readiness Program to discuss specific needs.

Outside the base, military members and families obtain information about community resources through a variety of sources. For example, and as noted previously, Project CARE has been activated at times of high deployments to make a communitywide push to inform military families of the resources available to them.

> The city helped to organize an effort called the Caring Communities Committee that was to try to help provide some services to persons of deployed families. With the Chamber, we institutionalized that into the Community Action Readiness Effort, which memorialized that caring communities program. . . . [City official]

During more "normal" times, two Marines told us, wives of Marines like to use online social networking to find answers to their needs. This statement was reinforced by a mental health care provider who told us that "brochures don't work for 18- to 20-year-olds; we have stopped printing them, it's a waste;" and "on paper, young women are connected to services, but don't have real connections." The mental health care provider believes this is a generational phenomenon linked to the popularity of cell phones and Facebook. This may also be tied to what one Marine wife told us, that she believes it is difficult for Marine wives to talk to each other about their problems when their spouses differ in rank.

Shared-interest organizations, such as churches, also appear to play a key role in supporting military family members. Church members, for example, often are aware of the challenges being experienced by military families within their congregations, and they can offer resources from within the church membership.

## Information Sources for Civilians

The Jacksonville Chamber of Commerce and city officials are very committed to supporting information flow between the base and the community, especially to business members. The city receives biweekly reports from the base on the number of Marines to be deployed and who will return from deployments, and it disseminates this information to aid local businesses in planning. According to one Chamber of Commerce member, these updates "are well received and help our businesses not be taken by surprise by a large influx of people." She was not aware of any other such services in Jacksonville to provide updates on projected deployments and returns. Civilians receive general information on resources through the local media; at community fairs such as the Jamboree; and through friendships at work, church, and recreational groups.

# Community Health

As discussed in more detail below, existing physical and behavioral health challenges have intensified since the OIF/OEF deployments began, and some new problems have emerged. Demand for mental health services has increased, according to Chamber of Commerce members, and city officials noted that they are seeing more homeless veterans. The demographics of homeless veterans reportedly are also changing:

> A significant number of those veterans were single, and a surprising number of them were female and . . . had family members with them. [City official]

A United Way representative told us that the population of homeless veterans has increased 70% in the past few years. According to one mental health provider, the deployments "created a lot of stressed young women glued to CNN." Overall, the need for more mental health services was emphasized, especially as the community braces for the return of troops with severe physical and behavioral health issues that they will experience for the rest of their lives.

## Mental and Behavioral Health

Almost all interviewees concur in noting a growing demand for mental health services in the community.

> Mental health . . . [is] one of the biggest areas and issues wholeheartedly for the families. . . . [Chamber of Commerce member]

> There is a lot of need for counseling and they're not gonna go on base. I don't care how many times you tell them it's not going to affect their career, there is a pervasive urban legend [that seeking mental health services will affect one's career]. [Mental health provider]

Individuals are experiencing symptoms whether or not they have received a mental health diagnosis. A Health Department representative described a situation where the county had moved away from providing direct services and now provides only referrals. As a result, the Onslow Memorial Hospital emergency room became overwhelmed with mental health cases, which strained resources:

> The emergency room was just inundated with mental health type patients . . . you're bogging down an emergency system . . . with mental health patients that are very time-consuming, that prevent you from handling that heart attack . . . but that person needs their needs met and you are not able to meet them in a 15-minute, in-and-out emergency room visit. [Health Department representative]

Mental health difficulties express themselves in a variety of ways. These include

> **Prescription drug use and abuse:** A mental health care provider told us that prescription drug use is huge and people use these drugs "like candy" and they have "huge amounts of medications in cabinets." In response, she has seen a rise in people seeking alternative therapies in order to reduce their reliance on pharmacologic agents:
>
>> I've known people who just pay out of pocket and go on their own [to a chiropractor or for acupuncture] because they are tired of taking the pills, can't function on the pills, don't want to be addicted to the pills. . . .
>
> This provider indicated a need for educational services to help people overcome their addictions to prescription drugs.
>
> A social services representative added that military spouses are also showing high levels of addiction to prescription drugs:
>
>> One of the biggest things we've seen, especially with military spouses, is prescription drug use. . . . A lot of them have their own prescriptions, are misusing those prescriptions, are shopping with different doctors, different pharmacies to get those prescriptions.
>
> **Illegal substance use:** The Chamber of Commerce and County EMS representative noted an increase in the use of SPICE (synthetic marijuana) and bath salts (synthetic methamphetamine). They worked with the base to get statistics on this and went to the state legislature to outlaw these substances. According to representatives of the School Board, this problem is not isolated to adults; many children in Jacksonville are dealing with substance use issues as well.
>
> **Automobile accidents:** Accidents originating from reckless driving, driving under the influence, and substance use have increased, according to County EMS, Jacksonville Police, and the Health Department. The county EMS representative noted that Marines come back from deployments with an "adrenalin addiction, addicted to driving fast." He noted that the area has the highest rate in the state of accidents based on substance use, and the second-highest crash rate in the state.

> In 2002 we went from 10 or 11 DUIs to . . . 484 last year . . . that was one thing we did see, prior to a deployment, people would get intoxicated. A lot of times we would take 'em straight to the base. [EMS representative]

> When they're deployed that adrenalin is constantly there for them, and they come back, and they need it, it's like an addiction. [Chamber of Commerce member]

**PTSD:** A social services representative noted that "countless families have been dissolved because of untreated PTSD." Individuals self-medicate for PTSD with pharmaceuticals or alcohol and do not want to disclose their problem. A Health Department representative told us PTSD has never been seen at such high rates, and we are seeing how it affects employability and risk-taking behavior:

> With the rapid succession, there has been no time to debrief, or to reintegrate with your family . . . or seeking services . . . it continues to be a double-edged sword for that service member, fearful that their career will inadvertently be harmed. [Social Services representative]

**Suicide attempts:** County EMS and police representatives both discussed the rise in suicide attempts, and a Health Department representative described an increase in gun accidents:

> We had two officer-assisted suicides where the people charged the officer with guns, and we've seen some other suicides. . . . [EMS representative]

> We've had a lot of fatalities from gun accidents . . . you've got military guys . . . and it's really hard to always know what exactly is going on in those situations . . . he was cleaning his gun, but was he? [Health Department representative]

**Traumatic brain injuries** and the concomitant **cognitive difficulties:** These conditions are affecting young veterans' abilities to plan for their futures:

> You've got a lot of 22, 23, 24-year-olds getting out of the military that joined right out of high school . . . gonna get out with the GI bill and go to college. . . . Well, depending on their cognitive abilities when they get out, they can't. [Mental health provider]

Despite this array of reported problems, it is important to note that interviewees did not necessarily link these issues to *multiple* deployments. Three deployments to an installation "behind the lines" may have no effect on a service member, whereas a single deployment to a "hot" combat zone may have a profound impact on a Marine. Some of the behavioral changes noted by interviewees may simply be the result of an American military at war.

**Family Challenges**

Interpersonal difficulties and violence also arise from untreated mental health issues. According to data from the Police Department, there was a 15% increase in calls for emergency services between 2008 and 2011. These interpersonal issues include

**Child abuse:** A police official, the County EMS representative, and a mental health provider all told us they see child abuse reports originating in parental anxiety, depression, and anger issues:

> Some of the most significant maltreatment issues and abuse are military affiliated. [Mental health provider]

The call volume on these kinds of cases increases each year. According to the Police and Fire Departments, there has been a 73% increase in child abuse and neglect in the last 2 years. Prescription drug abuse by nondeployed spouses undoubtedly has added to these numbers.

**Spousal abuse:** Domestic violence reports and police calls have greatly increased. A social services respondent said that it is possible to tell when deployments end and when Marines are back because their caseloads increase:

> There are tremendous reintegration problems that are causing havoc for families. . . oftentimes the report may be domestic violence, but once you dig a little deeper you can see how gravely the children are impacted. [Social services representative]

**Separation and divorce:** A mental health provider told us she is now getting calls from more senior members of the military and officers: "They're tired and never thought they'd need counseling, but now their families are falling apart."

**Violent acts:** The police representative told us of recent acts of violence conducted by Marines, including a man stabbing dogs in his house.

> We've seen some other things that are quite disturbing. . . . We had another Marine who was intoxicated, sitting on top of his roof with an M4, pointing it at people. . . . Those kinds of things we have seen on an occasional basis. [EMS representative]

**Physical Health Issues**

Physical problems are also on the rise. One respondent mentioned that many Marines are coming back from overseas with significant hearing loss, or orthopedic injury and pain that will disqualify them from obvious postmilitary career choices.

> They are probably not going to be a firefighter or police officer . . . depending on their joint injuries . . . and back injuries. . . .

A staff member at the chiropractic practice booth at the Jacksonville Jamboree confirmed this, saying that older military members are almost completely disabled at 38 or 40 years old and are living in constant pain. Following deployments, the Health Department representative also sees many cases of sexually transmitted diseases among Marines at the county STD clinic, as well as cases of travel-related illnesses such as malaria and tuberculosis at their communicable disease clinic.

**Children's Issues**

Children of both military and civilian families are affected by the mental and physical health difficulties experienced by military families. Representatives of the Recreation and Parks Department told us that the friends of military children are always moving away and it is hard on them. Their fathers are home for only short periods of time between deployments and cannot get too reattached when they are home. Returning Marines may not be able to reintegrate into the family easily; they are "trained to wake at a pin-drop and come back to 2-year-olds jumping on [the] bed in the middle of the night." Or, for example, they are trained to yell at fellow Marines to get the job done and keep them safe, and use the same approach to talk to their kids and their teachers;

> or you get a dad who's freshly back from Afghanistan . . . [and] the past year [he] has been yelling at a Marine because he is going to die if he doesn't pay attention to the IED. [Now his] child is failing math and [he] comes across the table [at the teacher] . . . it's just difficult for the faculty. [School system representative]

Often, even when military members are not deployed, they are still away from home on trainings as much as if they were deployed; this creates added stress for the spouse.

Physical health issues also arise among military families. For example, one provider reported seeing cases of mumps among children from the base because their parents do not have them vaccinated as a result of either frequent relocation or differing vaccine schedules by state. Overall, there is a young parent population in Jacksonville. According to one mental health provider, the average age of mothers delivering their first child at Onslow Memorial Hospital is 23, and at the Naval Hospital it is 20. One school representative estimated that 75% of military children in the area are in fifth grade or below. Other child-related issues include the fact that no systems are in place to prevent both parents from being deployed at once if they are both active duty. In these circumstances, unique custody arrangements need to be put in place. For example, a representative from a local child care facility reported that one of the teachers and her husband took in and helped raise two of her students whose parents had been deployed. "We are the only family that the parents have," she said.

The school representatives to whom we spoke told us that, on base schools, they see mental health issues with younger populations, such as a second-grader with suicidal thoughts, and middle school substance use. In one school, 40 of 400 middle school students were investigated for substance use. Substance use, depression, anxiety, and anger issues are heightened not just for the children, but for their parents as well:

> We've seen a lot of attendance issues with that, at least aboard the base schools . . . mom is depressed and doesn't get out of bed, so she doesn't get the kids ready for school… [School system representative]

Representatives of the Recreation and Parks Department told us that "younger kids deal by outbursts, teens are more inward until they are set off, ADHD is on the rise, and kids lash out physically." The city police representative told us he sees a correlation between deployments and juvenile crime. We also met a church-going parent whose 8-year-old son was recently diagnosed with PTSD.

The Onslow Partnership for Children is one organization focused on improving children's lives. The partnership is home to a Child Advocacy Center, parent education classes, and a multitude of services to support the area's children. In addition, the school system employs military transition counselors and school liaisons to help children with military-related stresses. The PEERS program is also available to military families and offers free drop-in child care, parenting classes, and an adolescent parenting program.

## Community Competence

Throughout Jacksonville and Onslow County and on base, there is a wealth of resources available to help military and civilian families and individuals cope with the stresses of deployments. On the macro level, agencies communicate regularly: "We don't duplicate efforts," said one city official. "We work hand in hand with MCCS." For example, the city has regular meetings of service agencies to help streamline efforts for veterans, and the Local Inter-Agency Children's Council meets monthly to coordinate efforts.

On the interpersonal level, individuals and families are quite connected as well. Word-of-mouth networks through churches, online forums, and other groups help to connect people with informal services (e.g., child care assistance, financial, or around-the-house support).

> As soon as anything happens, people just show up . . . word of mouth, Facebook . . . everyone is comfortable doing that with one another. [School system representative]

> I think it's more word of mouth now. I think there still is that group of people who are saying, "Oh, contact them, they helped me through this" and I hear a lot through my church. [Social services representative]

### Eligibility Requirements

Services on base are available to service members and their dependents. According to the *2012 Camp Lejeune Base Guide,* these services include, but are not limited to, car service, banks, child care, restaurants, shopping, schools, libraries, employment assistance for families, new parent support programs, marriage preparation workshops, religious education, substance abuse prevention and counseling, and hospital, dental, and health clinics. Base services are not available to civilians, and we heard that military members and their dependents sometimes choose to seek services off base, especially for mental health issues. Certain city and county programs have income eligibility requirements that place these services out of reach for military families whose wages are too high to qualify. In addition, partners who are not legally married cannot access base services and must rely on the county; this is a far-reaching issue according to many service providers.

> We have a lot of pregnant girls. . . . I know they are military connected in some way . . . they don't tell us that, but then if you get into asking about the absent parent a lot of times they tell us it's a Marine and they don't know who it is. . . . Most of our pregnancies, if they are single, are Marine related in one way or another. [Social services representative]

> Most people are not getting married until later in life, so we've got a young active duty lance corporal who is here, and his girlfriend follows him here, and she receives no benefits, she's not able to go on base. . . . [Health Department representative]

One social service provider estimated that one third of pregnant women they see are connected to the military in some way. Without established paternity, however, neither the mom nor the child is eligible for base services.

**Barriers to the Provision of Services**

Although there is a wide array of services available to Jacksonville residents, it is still possible for individuals to fall through the cracks. According to a mental health provider, there was a recent death of an infant in Jacksonville. The mother was an active duty spouse whose husband was deployed. She ran out of formula and started feeding water to her baby, who then developed nutrition-related health issues and subsequently died. This mental health provider explained how it is difficult to figure out how to reach a mom like this who had so many services available to her.

> That was a young mom who was eligible for a variety of services . . . how do you reach that new mom who is so overwhelmed . . . or didn't know how to connect with someone who could help her. . . . [Mental health provider]

Additional barriers to service provision include

- Fear of damage to career,
- Lack of awareness of services,
- Pride/take care of own problems,
- Too much "drama" on base, and
- Confidentiality concerns.

In addition, many services designed to help military families and individuals during deployments are tied to grants that may end as the drawdown in troops begins. For example, the military transition counselors in the school system are funded through a Department of Defense

Education Activity (DoDEA) grant that started in 2009. These positions were initially funded to help students deal with deployments, but they now help with reintegration and assist children in working through confusing issues to them, such as one that a school official described: "Daddy yells at me a lot and I don't know why." These staff positions have filled a major gap in services, and the school system is working to ensure that funding for these positions continues.

### Social Capital

Many interviewees explained that compassion fatigue has not been a large problem for the community. "It's been a constant level of support," said one city official. Reportedly, support for the troops has become "a way of life" ever since the 1983 Beirut bombing; the Beirut memorial is the largest military memorial constructed with private funds and was viewed as a testament to the community's commitment to the troops. Although Jacksonville as a community is still very committed, some interviewees felt that many residents are not as emotionally engaged as they might have been earlier in the war efforts:

> Sometimes I think there is a tendency, especially in a large military town where it's the norm, . . . sometimes people are . . . kind of calloused to that . . . there is a lot of support, but sometimes people get calloused and desensitized to it because everybody is going through it. . . . [Health department representative]

Overall, however, there was a sense that individual families are "very networked" and there is a strong commitment in the community to fundraising to help each other with projects and hardships, as described by these school system representatives:

> We had a parent who had a back injury, and her husband was deployed, and she had three kids and couldn't pick her kids up from school . . . and the principal and the faculty got together and paid for child care to get kids to stay until a neighbor could pick them up. [School system representative]

Our findings suggest that the largest source of informal support was the faith-based community. According to one pastor, "It is amazing what church can do for those families." He described the challenges faced by one active duty spouse with five children whose husband is on his seventh deployment. When this woman sought services on base, she was told by one program that the situation with her family was "too severe" and they would have to go to the command; she did not want the family's issues to bring her husband home and jeopardize his career. The pastor said that the church "bent over backwards" to help this woman and her family get the supports they needed. Another church member believed that it was nice to have the church to go to, they are mostly military and "understand, but without the drama." One pastor said the church can offer confidentiality and immediate supports "without the red tape." Churches in Jacksonville offer the following services:

- Military luncheons,
- Men's PTSD support group,
- Deployed member support group,
- Care packages, and
- Financial, respite, and household support.

One pastor explained how one of his parishioners sought PTSD support from a facility in another state and said he never would have had the courage to go if he had not started attending the PTSD support meetings the church offered. This pastor explained his belief that "certain things, only God can do," and his aim was "for these men to be restored to wholeness," because "they shouldn't be doomed to nightmares and being forever shattered." This same pastor explained how one church member decided to stay in Jacksonville during her husband's deployment solely because of the deployed member support group. Her family "thought she was crazy" and did not understand why she chose to stay during the deployment.

The strength the church gives to service members and their families both at home and when deployed is evidenced in a letter sent to and shared by a pastor we met with. In a letter to the pastor from the battlefield, written on a piece of cloth, this service member said, "Thank you for all that you have done for me and my wife [redacted] and all that you continue to do for our community . . . my extended thanks to the support group for the care package that I just received, the timing was perfect . . . it is difficult to be positive 100% of the time but I find a well of strength when I look to God."

## SUMMARY OF STRENGTHS AND CHALLENGES

### Model Programs and Services

- **Project CARE** successfully maintained and strengthened the city of Jacksonville's population, even during deployments.
- The city's agencies and services are well networked and communicate regularly.
- The **Chamber of Commerce** regularly alerts businesses of upcoming deployments and returns.

### Needs and Challenges

- **Mental health services** were touted by many interviewees as the largest current and anticipated need for the community. Individuals' concerns about the perceived adverse effect of help-seeking on the service member's career was cited as a significant barrier to service.
- **Infrastructure** improvements are needed to keep up with the growing population. Because of how the Census Bureau counts service members (they are counted as part of the U.S. overseas population and not Jacksonville's), interviewees said the region is not receiving adequate federal resources to support the expanding population.

### Suggestions from the Community

- Increase the focus on mental health and service availability.*
- Continue to build partnerships among the  city, county, and base.
- Create transition programs for returning troops.

- Address child custody issues during deployments.*
- Increase access to prescription drug use education.
- Continue funding wartime programs (e.g., transition counselors at schools).
- Increase funding for Family Readiness Groups.
- Address Census issues to support emergency services and infrastructure development.*
- Improve employment and assimilation opportunities for spouses seeking work.

*Suggestions noted with an asterisk were cited by multiple respondents.

# El Paso, Texas

## Case Study Report

## Impacts of Multiple Deployments: El Paso, Texas

### OVERVIEW

Fort Bliss, a massive Army training installation for armored units and infantry, is located in the northeastern part of El Paso, Texas, and, along with the adjacent White Sands Missile Range, stretches north into New Mexico. During a study team site visit (May 8–13, 2012), representatives from El Paso provided their perspectives on the impacts of multiple deployments from Fort Bliss on their community. Site visit findings indicate that as a result of Base Realignment and Closure (BRAC) decisions, Fort Bliss growth has had a huge, positive impact on El Paso's local economy. Potential impacts from multiple deployments were not readily discernible by interviewees. The greatest concern expressed by community members was the need for more mental health services for service members and their families. Although the area is rich in informal services and supports, the capacity of the formal service delivery system was described as "strained" even for civilians, let alone military-affiliated individuals. Children's services were called out as an area of increasing need.

### GEOGRAPHIC ORIENTATION

#### Community: El Paso, Texas

El Paso is situated in the westernmost corner of Texas, bounded on the north by New Mexico and on its south, just across the Rio Grande, by the Mexican city of Juarez (Figure 1). The city is bisected from south to north by the Franklin Mountains, whose dry, rugged peaks stretch northward some 15 miles and rise in places to an altitude of more than 7,000 feet.[1] El Paso's landscape is also visibly marked by its location in the Chihuahuan Desert: Light brown sandy soil hosts few plants, and tumbleweeds are common. City residents' "lawns" are similarly arid, with some sporting a thin layer of small, dark brown rocks to create a more consistent appearance.

**Data Sources**

- City government
- Chamber of Commerce
- El Paso Independent School District (EPISD) Administration and Faculty
- County Domestic Relations Office
- Churches
- Rotary Club
- Social Service organizations
- United Way
- Fort Bliss Garrison Command
- Fort Bliss MWR
- Military families
- El Paso Police Department
- Ethnographic observation

El Paso and Juarez combined include more than 2 million people. Together they represent a single metropolitan area, which is clearly evident at night when city lights south of El Paso stretch as far as the eye can see. In numerous respects, the border at the Rio Grande is simply another local geologic feature and not a political

[1] See http://www.geo.utep.edu/pub/lemone/1301/franklin_mts.html.

boundary: 80% of El Paso's 650,000 residents, for example, self-identify as Hispanic.[2] Traditional Mexican food can be found throughout the city, Spanish is so commonly spoken among El Paso residents that city council meetings have a Spanish interpreter in addition to an American Sign Language (ASL) interpreter, and thousands of residents from Juarez make daily commutes across the river. In other respects, however, the border clearly demarcates two dramatically different lifestyles. For several years in a row, El Paso has been one of the safest U.S. cities with a population over 500,000, a designation the study team heard about during almost every interview. In 2010, for example, there were only five homicides in the city. In contrast, Juarez has received notoriety as one of the most dangerous cities in the world outside of a declared war zone because of a flare-up of drug cartel–related violence.[3] In Juarez in 2010, 3,075 residents were murdered, a number that sits in stark contrast to its sister city across the river. As a result of a murder rate of more than eight persons per day, there has been an exodus from Juarez. Since the drug wars began in 2008, an estimated 250,000 people—possibly twice that number—have emigrated from Juarez.[4] From El Paso's perspective, the border has become a one-way valve: People are still coming into El Paso from Mexico,[5] but the State Department has warned Americans against crossing into Juarez.

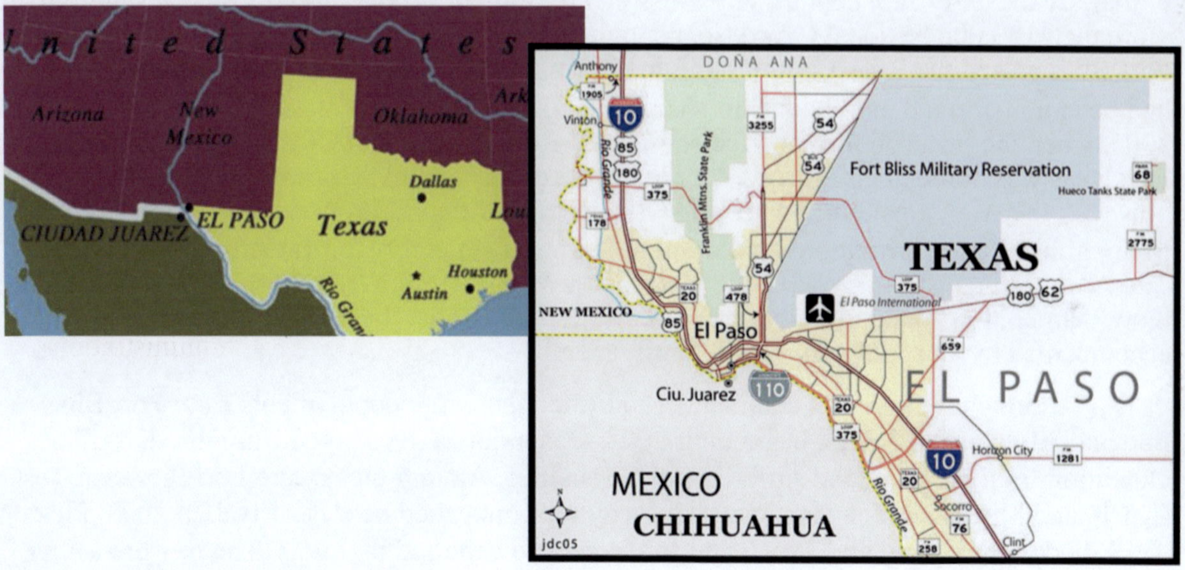


**FIGURE 1** El Paso geographic orientation.

What is happening in Juarez is germane to this report, for there is recognition throughout El Paso that posttraumatic stress disorder (PTSD) is not unique to the soldiers who are returning from their fourth or fifth deployment to Iraq or Afghanistan. Some counselors who work with soldiers with PTSD indicated they needed no additional training because they are already serving traumatized families from Juarez; at least one school faculty member directly compared the experiences of children in military families with those of some of the children fleeing Mexico, noting that the latter have often witnessed the death of a parent. Also, as discussed later in this

---

[2] See http://quickfacts.census.gov/qfd/states/48/48141.html.

[3] See http://www.chron.com/news/nation-world/article/Ciudad-Juarez-passes-2-000-homicides-in-09-1593554.php.

[4] See http://borderzine.com/2010/08/exodus-from-ciudad-juarez-impacts-el-paso-economy.

[5] See "Bridging a Gap Between Fear and Peace," *New York Times,* Feb. 15, 2011: A8 of the New York Edition (also available at: http://www.nytimes.com/2011/02/15/world/americas/15juarez.html).

report, the El Paso Police Department received training from Fort Bliss personnel on crisis situations and PTSD, but department leaders also told us that their concerns about their officers encountering community members with PTSD extended to the Spanish-speaking immigrants. In short, the city is working to address the harmful effects of PTSD, but is doing so because it is host to two large and potentially traumatized populations.

### Military Installation: Fort Bliss

With 3.2 million acres, the Fort Bliss installation is larger than the state of Rhode Island; it is home to the country's largest unrestricted airspace and is the second largest restricted airspace (Washington, DC, is the largest). Because of its position on the border with Mexico, El Paso has long held strategic significance for the United States. After the end of the Mexican-American War (1848), which solidified U.S. annexation of Texas from Mexico, a military garrison was established in the greater El Paso area. Although the post's exact location shifted several times in its first 50 years, the foundation of what is today Fort Bliss was settled by 1893.

Although the installation was initially developed to maintain security along the southern border, by the early 20th century Fort Bliss had developed a more global focus. The area hosted more than 100,000 National Guard troops in the middle of the First World War, and by WWII Fort Bliss hosted the largest cavalry unit in the United States. By the end of that war, Fort Bliss had been transformed into the nation's largest facility for anti-aircraft training.[6] Indeed, up until 2005, when the installation was affected by Base Realignment and Closure (BRAC) decisions, Fort Bliss was home to the Army's Air Defense Artillery (ADA). As a result of BRAC, however, the ADA was sent to Fort Sill, Oklahoma, and Fort Bliss was converted into a massive training installation for armored units and infantry, most notably the 1st Armored Division.[7] The Army estimates that by 2013 the installation will have gone from hosting 13,000 soldiers to more than 33,000 young infantrymen. It is also estimated that these soldiers will be accompanied by an additional 30,000 family members.

Although the garrison commander indicated that large deployments from Fort Bliss to Iraq and Afghanistan did not begin until 2008, area units were engaged from the start of Operation Iraqi Freedom and suffered early casualties. Among them were Lori Piestewa, Jessica Lynch, and Shoshanna Johnson, whose convoy was ambushed near Nasiriyah in 2003. Piestewa was killed in the attack, and Lynch and Johnson were captured by Iraqis. The *El Paso Times* estimated that more than 25,000 soldiers have been deployed from the installation over the course of the last 9 years of war, accounting for nearly 240,000 total deployments. As one service provider told us: "You don't know anybody who's only been deployed once. It's multiple, multiple deployments."

#### Effects of BRAC

The BRAC-related changes, as described above, have had a marked impact on El Paso. Interviewees repeatedly commented on the rapid population growth, which has necessitated the

[6] See https://www.bliss.army.mil/Secure/Military/MaDBDE/SECURE/DoD,%20DA,%20AD%20Mil/Welcome%20Packet/Fort%20Bliss%20History.pdf.

[7] For more on the BRAC decisions about Fort Bliss, see http://www.globalsecurity.org/military/facility/fort-bliss.htm.

development of an infrastructure capable of supporting such a large influx of residents. The Chamber of Commerce estimated that the BRAC changes brought more than $5 billion into the local economy, an addition that several said effectively allowed the city to weather the recession. As part of this investment, El Paso and Fort Bliss collaborated to build the world's largest inland desalinization plant, which is located on Fort Bliss property. The desalination plant afforded the post access to a brackish groundwater bolson that would have otherwise been unusable. Consequently, the post does not draw on the desert city's water supply.

More important than their focus on the construction, however, was civilian interviewees' assessment of the changing characteristics of on-post personnel. Numerous interviewees described the installation as now having a "different type of soldier" as a result of BRAC:

> When I was growing up, especially air defense artillery kids, for the most part we were pretty well-behaved kids . . . back when I was growing up it was an honor and a privilege to serve in the Army and there were very high standards. You couldn't have certain tattoos showing in areas, your hair had to be a certain way, and, I mean, that's just how it was. People kind of respected that code. . . . After 9/11, especially when we started to really deploy, it just seemed like, I don't think we had enough in the military and it just seemed like they were really pulling in anybody who wanted to join. Unfortunately, some of those people do not have the cleanest backgrounds, and I think that kind of came out a little. The kids have changed, they're a little bit rowdier and parents have changed, they're a little bit more crass and they're impatient and it's "I'm military, my husband/wife is serving, I deserve X, Y, Z." I feel like it wasn't as prestigious as it used to be. [Social services provider]

> I've seen the transition from only having sergeant major academy children there to a different type of soldier. . . . So we have grown and there is a difference in the structure, in the dynamics. [What's the difference?] . . . The family structure with the sergeant major family is a little bit more disciplined, more structured. As a family unit, there's a little bit more organization. With the younger soldier, I'm not seeing the educational background, there's not as much discipline or structure in the family. I don't know if it's because the soldier is out more, deployed more, I'm not sure. But the family dynamic is not as stable as when we had only the sergeant major children. I saw something very different. [School faculty member]

> Our prior military community . . . was air defense artillery. That's a completely different set of educational skills, a higher level of education, a different—may I say, social class of soldier. . . . It's very cerebral . . . even the lowest level soldier was trained to fight through video technology. . . . We now have shipped off air defense artillery and brought in armored divisions. . . . And armored division soldiers and infantry soldiers are trained to pull triggers. There's a lower level of education . . . and remember when people are chosen, when they're given their jobs in the military, they're chosen based on their background and their skills. . . . So we have a lot of kids who've been shipped into El Paso who maybe are not as educationally advanced and have not had some of the same economic benefits as soldiers that we previously had. It's a different social class of

soldier. And I hate to say it, but it's a reality. The numbers, the impact on the community is significant. . . . [Attorney]

Importantly, roughly 70% of the soldiers stationed at Fort Bliss live off post. Military families live throughout El Paso, but the largest concentration of military residences is directly west of the post, in the neighborhood called "the Northeast," and south of the post. Many veterans also live in the northeastern area of the city. Partly as a result of the BRAC-related enhancement of the transportation infrastructure, some military families have chosen recently to locate throughout the city and even in somewhat-distant locations, such as Socorro and Horizon City. At the suggestion of Mayor John Cook, however, the study team focused on City Council Districts 2 and 4, the areas immediately adjacent to the post that would most likely be affected by multiple deployments.

### Relationship Between Community and Base

In certain respects, El Paso is the ideal location for young troops preparing for the wars in Iraq and Afghanistan. Several community members pointed out, for example, the similarities between the local terrain and what the soldiers face when they deploy to one of these two combat theaters. The photographs in Figure 2 illustrate the similarities.

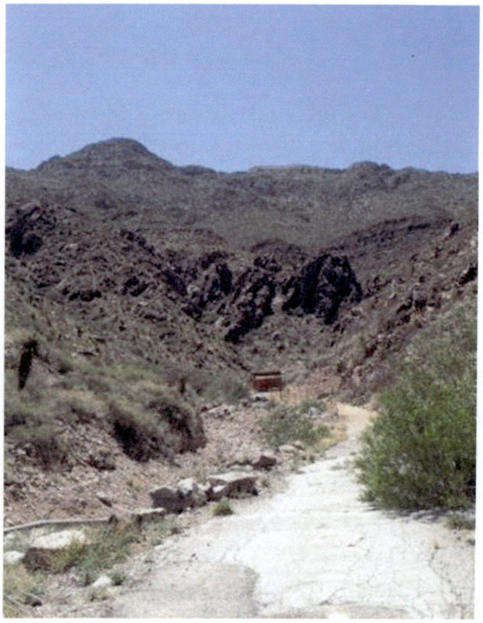

McKelligon Canyon, El Paso

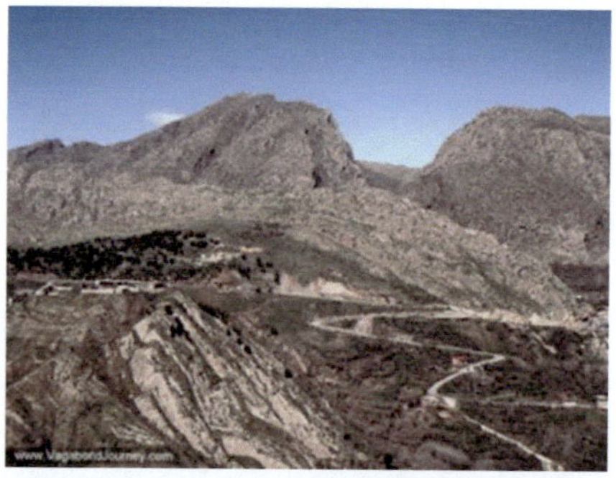

Iraq

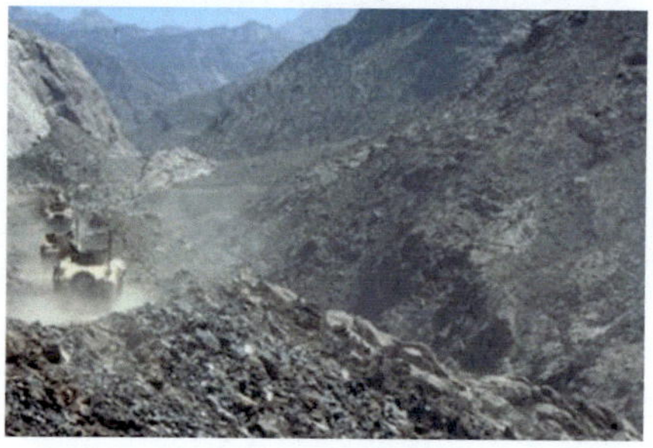

Afghanistan

**FIGURE 2** Similar landscapes.

What makes the area ideal, however, also creates its own set of problems. Reminders of the desert landscape are seen from the post and in the front yards of nearly every home. The rocky Franklin Mountains are within plain view of the post. At least three interviewees pointed out that the landscape is so similar to what soldiers face overseas that just getting up in the morning and looking out the window can trigger an individual's PTSD. One interviewee remarked that his stepson, who has been deployed three times, often struggles with driving in the area because of its unfortunate similarity to what he faced in theater.

The landscape also led to a small dustup between City Council District 2 Representative Susie Byrd and the Fort Bliss Garrison Command. District 2, located directly west and south of Fort Bliss, is home to McKelligon Canyon, a popular recreational area where the photograph in Figure 2 was taken. Representative Byrd reported receiving complaints from constituents that the Army was not using the canyon only for training, but at one point had closed the area to the public in order to carry out an exercise. Numerous discussions reportedly ensued before the command was willing to acknowledge that the military had overstepped its bounds. Our understanding is that the area continues to be used for Army training, but that improved communications have prevented any additional problems from arising between soldiers and city residents.

One of the few general complaints we heard from civilians, which came from a couple of interviewees, was that military families sometimes convey a sense of entitlement simply because of their army affiliation. Examples all involved situations where a military-affiliated individual—often the wife—requested that standing rules be broken because of their relationship with the Army. Overall, though, residents interviewed by the study team perceived their community to be quite welcoming to the military and appreciative of the sacrifices made by service members and their families. Not only did stores throughout the city post signs advertising discounts for military members, but numerous businesses displayed photographs of, or mementoes from, service members out of respect for the men and women who had passed through their community on the way to war. Anecdotally, the study team heard about individuals in restaurants picking up the tabs for service members. Parents in the Socorro School District were delighted when the District had "Purple T-shirt Day," during which students and staff all wore purple T- shirts to show solidarity with the military.

Several military-affiliated individuals the study team talked to offered a counter perspective, perceiving the community appreciation as superficial, at best. One observer said:

> Politically, it's very well received. I think that you'll find areas and pockets where . . . what I've witnessed far too often is, it's politically correct to say, "Welcome and we're glad you're here." But I think in their heart a lot of people are kind of holding their nose [*sic*] at the same time. It's not as genuine as I'd like it to be.

As an example, a military spouse described how a friend's husband shattered both ankles in an IED blast and the couple was trying to get a wheelchair ramp built to their apartment. Our interviewee said that if the ramp does not work out, the couple will have to relocate, but the complex manager is refusing to let them break the lease without paying a "couple hundred dollars" penalty. She reported that the Family Readiness Group (FRG) had come through with the money for the penalty, but she was dismayed by the manager's attitude:

> I'm thinking, to me, her husband was fighting for you . . . and you can't even forgive that couple hundred dollars? That's another example of unsincere [*sic*] gratitude.

When individuals associated with the Fort Bliss Garrison Command were presented with the above apartment manager example, the command pointed out that there is a strategy in place not only to help young families in such situations (the FRG), but also to ensure that the business owner does not have to suffer financial consequences because of what's happening to soldiers and their families. They also reiterated the post's extensive collaborative efforts with the city that are intended to mitigate any potential negative effects of the post on the community at large, including the physical disabilities that might result from combat. Incidents such as the one with the apartment are clearly frustrating to the Army families; nevertheless, it is perhaps just these kinds of situations that might lead civilian community members to perceive a sense of entitlement among their military neighbors.

## EFFECTS OF MULTIPLE DEPLOYMENTS ON THE COMMUNITY

### Economic Impact

Interviewees described numerous, large-scale changes to the El Paso economy in recent years, including infrastructure growth (e.g., highway construction), increased commerce, and residential expansion into outlying areas east of the city. Because of the large infusion of capital into the region resulting from BRAC decisions, however, interviewees were unable to tie any of these changes to multiple deployments.

#### Commerce

Overall, and as suggested above, we were unable to link impacts on the El Paso general economy to multiple deployments. One business leader suggested that this was by design:

> From the business sector [perspective], [the multiple deployments are] relatively benign. [If] there are some negative impacts, I haven't had anybody articulate that to me. I haven't seen it personally. But I think the reason is because as there's a deployment occurring there's also a circular motion occurring where troops are coming back. . . . It used to be where we would see a deployment then we would feel the impact because the families would go home and so all of a sudden the grocery stores weren't as busy, clothing stores, the shopping centers . . . we don't see that so much anymore because a lot of families stay here. . . . Part of the reason for that is the community is extremely welcoming. Soldiers with families who actively engage in the community, they see a genuine, a sincere approach toward "You're part of our community and you're welcome here and we want to support you."

The BRAC-prompted growth at Fort Bliss reportedly buffered El Paso from the recession, but accommodating the growth required substantive changes in El Paso's infrastructure, particularly in housing and transportation. Though bounded by New Mexico to the north and Juarez to the southwest, expansion went outward. Along with new housing were shopping developments, located primarily on the west side of El Paso and on the southeast along I-10, stretching into adjacent towns such as Horizon City and Socorro. In contrast, the team observed aging, often neglected, structures from the 1960s or earlier in established neighborhoods in downtown El Paso and the Northeast, adjacent to Fort Bliss. These areas seem to have changed very little as a result of BRAC-related growth.

**Housing**

When BRAC was first announced, Fort Bliss projected an average stay in El Paso of 7 years for a service member. Although there was a housing shortage on post,[8] El Paso, with nearly 5,000 houses standing empty in 2005, had the capacity to readily absorb the newcomers and their families. Soldiers coming to the installation, however, have been a younger and more mobile cohort than expected, and were reported to have neither the resources nor the stability to purchase single-family homes. The result, according to city leaders, is that El Paso's housing market has required an increase in rental housing, a type of housing the team was told had never really existed in the city. To encourage building this new type of housing, the Chamber of Commerce brought together the post, the city government, and developers. The city also instituted incentives that allowed developers to secure loans more easily. So great is the need for rental housing that even though developers continue to work hard to meet the demand, as one city leader put it, "We can't build them [the units] fast enough."

**Transportation**

Since 2003, El Paso has invested $1.5 billion in several major transportation projects. Notable additions include the 601 spur that connects Highway 375 and Highway 54 and has six off-ramp exits onto Fort Bliss. The Highway 375 "loop" has been expanded, and two major freeway interchanges (or "spaghetti bowls") have been built. These transportation improvements have allowed military families to live farther away from post and still have manageable commutes to the post. Growth has increased, particularly in the west side of El Paso and in Horizon City and Socorro, which are suburban towns southeast of El Paso. Long-time residents complain about the increased traffic.

**Job Opportunities**

Despite the BRAC-related growth, El Paso's poverty rate remains well above the national average. In 2010, 24% of El Pasoans lived in poverty, compared with 15% nationwide.[9] El Paso struggles to find good-paying jobs for its permanent residents. In March 2012, El Paso's unemployment rate was 9.5%,[10] above the national rate of 8.2%.[11] Moreover, El Paso's business community is structured on low-wage labor; many of the region's largest private employers are minimum-wage call centers. Many military spouses we spoke with said they could not find good-paying jobs, and instead choose to volunteer, especially if they have children at home. Business leadership envisions opportunities that leverage technological advancements driven by Fort Bliss, such as energy improvements and metal bending that can absorb the expected influx of retiring soldiers into El Paso. Fort Bliss aims to be a net-zero installation in energy, waste, and water by 2018.[1]

---

[8] The study team was told that the wait time to get into housing on post is at least 2 years.
[9] American Community Survey, U.S. Bureau of the Census, 2010.
[10] See http://www.elpasotimes.com/news/ci_20442789/el-paso-unemployment-rate-unchanged-march?source=rss.
[11] See http://www.bls.gov/news.release/pdf/empsit.pdf.

## Information and Communication

Civic and military leaders described several formal communication channels that have been established to ensure the timely and accurate flow of information about deployments to the civilian community. Civilian recipients included the business community, educators, and law enforcement. Information about the availability of particular services and supports in the community was said to occur through informal channels (e.g., word of mouth) rather than through more formal communication mechanisms.

El Paso leaders repeatedly pointed out the importance of good communication between the community and the post. Fort Bliss has been part of the El Paso community for more than a century, and the city values the contributions of the military to the city. At the same time, community leaders recognize challenges associated with military culture. These leaders have made concerted efforts to build bridges with Fort Bliss, and Fort Bliss, in turn, has responded. Below are just two comments we heard regarding communication as the key to mitigating any potential negative effects of the post and of multiple deployments:

> We integrate directly into Fort Bliss. We have breakfast every month with the commanding general. He tells us what he needs and we tell him what we think—it's communication. You have to integrate into the post. You can't let the walls and the gates keep you outside. And it has to be a two-way street. The military has a mindset as to how they will be received by the community, and they get here and they aren't the first to reach out to us. We reach out to them, every time we get a new garrison commander . . . we overtly reach out to say, "We want you to know we're here for you, let's get together." They brief at our monthly Board meeting—we have a segment of the meeting dedicated to Fort Bliss briefing our board. [Chamber of Commerce member]
>
> Communication is critical, whether it be what's happening at the school, construction on the post, new families coming in, dates when they anticipate growth to happen, deployments, reintegrations, all those things . . . and we'll continue to accommodate them . . . we feel like it's part of our community and so we'll continue to work with them. [School administrator]

The Greater El Paso Chamber of Commerce plays an important role in brokering conversations between the city government and the post. In addition to having the garrison commander present an update about the post at the Chamber's monthly meetings, the Chamber has an Armed Services Division that serves as the liaison between Fort Bliss and the business and regional communities and advocates for Fort Bliss initiatives at all levels of government. It is through these mechanisms that the city becomes aware of upcoming issues related to deployments that will affect the city and, in conversation with the post, can identify strategies to address them.

Also, the El Paso mainstream media prominently features stories of public interest about Fort Bliss. Several major media outlets—including the *El Paso Times,* the local ABC news affiliate, and the local Fox news affiliate—have sections on their website dedicated to military news. As an example of the media attention El Paso pays to the stories involving the military, the study team's site visit generated front-page coverage from these news outlets,[12] and during the course of the team's stay in El Paso, several community members with whom the team had unscheduled interviews said they recalled hearing about the study on the local news. In addition, Fort Bliss publishes the *Fort Bliss Monitor,* a free weekly newspaper that is readily available to civilians and service members throughout El Paso.

Representatives from the El Paso Independent School District (EPISD), which runs all of the schools located on Fort Bliss, described early challenges they faced related to deployments. The school districts depend on reliable, accurate communication from the base about deployments and their anticipated impact on schools. Shortly after BRAC, for example, conversations with Fort Bliss led the EPISD to prepare for a large influx of soldiers and family members, including school-age children. The soldiers, however, deployed shortly after arriving and did not bring their families. The families arrived later. This situation presented forecasting challenges and underscored the need for ongoing communication with Fort Bliss about deployments and their anticipated impact on public schools.

All nine El Paso school districts participate in the Fort Bliss Process Action Team with military leadership and military parents. This coalition serves as a conduit of information between the community and the post, addresses questions related to command turnover, and gives incoming command information about the school districts and their activities. This coalition has improved communication flows between the post and the school districts and eased the transition between commands on post. Through this improved communication, the post has also alerted the districts to Department of Defense (DOD) grant opportunities for additional programs at schools that benefit all children.

In the schools, teachers require day-to-day information about military activities, such as deployments that will affect students in their classrooms. To address this need, EPISD instituted a Military Family Liaison Program in its schools with large populations of students from military families. Military liaisons are entry-level positions, often held by military spouses or veterans. The liaisons interface with the post, military families, and the teachers and counselors. They help school staff understand military culture, notify them about upcoming deployments or returns, and help defuse challenges that arise, such as students' transitioning to a new school or giving extrasupport to students whose parents are deployed.[13] This highly regarded program has been adopted by DOD schools in Germany as a best practice.

One of the biggest challenges in El Paso is not the availability of community services, but the ability to connect people in need with the appropriate services (see the Community Competence section). Interviewees said that "word of mouth" is one of the primary means of communication, but that it is not the most effective approach. The team learned of at least two efforts to address this challenge. The Northeast coalition is an organization of approximately 200 schools, elected officials, agencies, community organizations, and the post to link services and identify ways to identify existing capacities. In the field of public education, the Fort Bliss

[12] Selected local news coverage of our visit: http://www.elpasotimes.com/news/ci_20570359/ep-joins-study-effects-deployment; http://www.kvia.com/video/31030911/index.html; http://www.kfoxtv.com/news/news/new-study-shows-how-afghan-war-impacted-soldiers/nNzBY.

[13] More information about the EPISD Military Family Liaison Program is available at http://www.episd.org/_schools/mil.php?KeepThis=true&TB_iframe=true&height=290&width=350.

Process Action Team is a coalition of Fort Bliss military leadership, military parents, and school administrators from nine local school districts that informs members of current activities and plans for upcoming education needs.

## Community Health

### Service Member Behaviors

Community members described numerous behaviors by service members that were the cause of significant concern. First and foremost, they said, were issues related to the operation of motor vehicles, including an increased number of arrests for driving while intoxicated (DWI). Respondents debated whether the DWIs were simply the result of an influx of young soldiers ("That's what young men do") or because soldiers were self-medicating with alcohol to quell the symptoms of deployment-induced PTSD. Regardless, the garrison command was alerted to the problem, and the *Fort Bliss Monitor*, the local military newspaper, displayed on page 2 the number of DWI arrests the previous week by unit, as well as the total number of arrests for each unit for the year as a whole.

Numerous interviewees spoke about reckless driving and the number of deadly high-speed crashes by service members, particularly on motorcycles. Interviewees did *not* say that these crashes were the result of multiple deployments per se, but suggested that service members returning from deployment may simply be looking for an adrenaline rush. Nevertheless, the behaviors were a cause for community concern.

There were also quiet discussions about an increased number of suicides by returning service members. The study team did not receive hard numbers from anyone, and the police did not perceive an increase in relation to multiple deployments. Nevertheless, it was a concern expressed by community members to the team.

Finally, there was a perception that soldier-on-soldier community violence had increased. A few weeks prior to the site visit there had been a shooting in a bar frequented by military personnel on Dyer Street (adjacent to the post) that resulted in the death of a service member and injury to two others.[14] Interviewees also reported that a couple of the bars frequented by service members had been closed recently because of violent incidents. Interestingly, when interviewees were recounting the perceived increase in community violence, they tended to refer to thesesame, few incidents. The relatively low crime rate and the fact that these events were tied to "the different type of soldier" suggest that these events do not happen regularly, but rather that a rare negative incident may take on heightened relevance in the public imagination.

### Health of Military Families

Although the above behaviors by service members were hard for interviewees to link to multiple deployments, they were profoundly concerned about the toll these deployments are exacting on young families. Two features of the deployments in particular were cited as problematic: the many times these service members are being asked to deploy and the lack of

[14] See http://www.kvia.com/news/30224247/detail.html.

sufficient reintegration time for families before the service member is deployed again. Numerous interviewees described the challenging family dynamics created by the rapid and multiple deployment cycles. One spouse, who was working in a counseling setting and whose husband had deployed numerous times, offered the following description:

> It just shifts the whole dynamics of the home, because here you are as a spouse, you have control of your kids and the household and the yard and the bills and everything, and here comes the soldier who's supposed to be the king of the castle and you're wanting to give it back to him, but you're not. How much do you keep? How much are you wanting to give back knowing that he's going to be gone in a few months again. And then your kids are like, "Well, ok, who do I ask now? Who's boss now? Now that dad's home do I ask Dad, do I ask you? What?"

A counselor at another facility, whose son and his wife were both in the Army, made a similar statement, noting in particular the effects on the children:

> It's very hard, and when there are multiple deployments—you get, how long before he knew he was leaving? There's not even time for the soldier to recoup, much less the family, and when the kids know this they don't even have the opportunity to think "Let's get comfortable" because they're on their guard—"I want to be prepared, I don't want to get hurt again."

Despite the shortening of the deployments (from well over a year down to 9 months or fewer), the continued need for combat troops in Afghanistan has led to more rapid rotations. One young spouse described the transition period between her husband's seventh and upcoming eighth deployment:

> [My husband] just returned in December from a deployment and they're deploying again in June. So for us, we lacked reintegration time. My husband returned on November 27th and found out December 22nd that he was leaving again. So although we've had time in between there, they've attended training, things like that, been in the field, and while he has been home for 5 months, that reintegration time was taken away from us. So for us, we honestly didn't tell the kids for a couple months because we wanted them to experience that reintegration time and to have that weight lifted off their shoulders.

Interviewees expressed significant concern about how the children of military families are faring. The family upheaval associated with the repeated deployment of one parent was problematic, but several individuals noted additional challenges faced by children from single-parent households as well as households in which both parents were service members:

> With dual or single-soldier families, you have kids that don't even have their own room—they go live with a relative or a friend . . . teenagers have to go live with a friend. Could you imagine living with a teenager you don't know? I mean, I didn't even like living with my own kids when they were teenagers! I can't imagine bringing someone else in who's going through the stress of having a deployed parent and you're trying to be

> a surrogate. There's a lot of, "I don't even get my own room because both my parents are deployed right now and I'm living at grandma's." [Counselor]

> The room situation is interesting because when we were both deployed my daughter ended up staying with a family member and didn't have her own room, and that above everything else [upset] her. She went from being an only child to one of five and not having a place of her own. And what I noticed, too . . . there was more resentment towards me as a mother than there was towards her dad as a father. It was almost expected that the father would do that type of thing, but as a mother, I abandoned her. [Parent]

Some interviewees viewed the youth as "resilient," noting that their tendency to handle these changes with aplomb and even provide assistance to other children struggling with similar situations. Others, however, were not so convinced:

> I had one soldier explain to me, "Is it [being] resilient or detachment? Detachment is a way to cope, but that's kind of scary. And I wonder 5 years down the line, 10 years, what are we going to see?"

Others suggested that the resilience might be superficial at best. One counselor said, "Sometimes the hostility overshadows everything for me on a day-to-day basis with these kids."

Just as important is the distress these deployments are causing for the spouse who is left behind to take care of the household. One interviewee, herself a military spouse, offered the following description of the problem:

> We're sort of missing a piece of our population to some degree in that the spouses have this emotional burden that is this bubble that is beyond comprehension right now. . . . And that's a whole other piece that I don't know if you guys have looked at that all yet . . . the extent to which a huge piece of the population that— it's sort of this "stuck" situation that we as the spouse are in because we have to always tell our soldier, "Don't worry, we got it, Honey, you go. We got it." And no matter what's happening we're not allowed to talk about that because he has to be safe downrange. And to our kids—"Don't worry, we got it! We got you, we got me, we got Dad, we got it all!" And it's affecting our spousal population to a huge, huge degree. And although the resources are out to get the counseling and things like that, right now we're so busy being stellar . . . that we're not going after it. We're not seeking the support that *we* need right now because we don't have time to seek that. We're too busy being stable . . . we're too busy with our feet on the ground that we don't have the chance to crumble.

In sum, the El Paso community appears to be seeing an occasional "burst" of adverse effects from multiple deployments in the form of DWIs, bar violence, and so forth. But the bigger challenges are in the homes, where each family is struggling to cope with a set of issues that not only change with each deployment, but compound over time. And because 70% of these families are living in the greater El Paso area, and those whose children are attending public schools attend El Paso–run schools, these issues ultimately will find their way into the broader community.

## Community Competence

Between the offerings on post and in El Paso, there are many services available to service members and their families. School administrators have a long relationship with the post and, as deployments increased, instituted new strategies to anticipate upcoming needs at the system and school levels. However, many other El Paso community services remain underused. As one military spouse put it, "There are so many options, it's difficult to choose." Despite this wealth of services, El Paso residents noted a lack of sufficient behavioral health facilities on post and in the community. Each of these service areas is discussed below.

### Education Supports

Educators described numerous efforts to ensure that military-affiliated students who attend public schools receive the services and supports they need to cope with multiple deployments. One of the most important efforts, they believed, was the use of military "liaisons" in the public schools, that is, military-affiliated individuals (usually spouses of service members) who can help translate military culture and its stressors to school faculty. These individuals also function as an in-school source of support for youth who need to discuss their problems with an adult.

Training efforts are also being undertaken to increase teacher and counselor awareness of deployment-related issues with students in their schools. In partnership with Fort Bliss, EPISD counselors are invited to "soldier for a day" trainings where they learn "military speak" and find out about behavioral issues to expect in children of service members experiencing multiple deployments. Also, Fort Bliss is working with the University of Texas at El Paso to develop a curriculum to train teachers about working with students from military families so that teachers will be prepared to understand the ways in which deployments—indeed, multiple deployments—may adversely affect military students.

### Behavioral and Mental Health Services

Interviewees described mental health services as the greatest need in the community. Long wait times exist for services on post, and interviewees voiced concern about the lack of available mental health facilities in the community, especially with the projected increase in need with the drawdown of troops. Within military health care, military leaders noted that military support systems for active duty service members and veterans had waiting lists. Psychiatric careis a particular area of need in El Paso. In Texas, psychologists cannot prescribe medications; therefore, people in need of additional mental health care must obtain referrals for psychiatrists. Waiting times to get an appointment to see a psychiatrist can be several months.

To help reduce the wait times, between 2007 and 2010 the San Antonio Federation partnered with The Dallas Foundation and the Permian Basin Area Foundation to establish the Texas Resources for Iraq-Afghanistan Deployment (TRIAD) Fund. The goal of the grants was to support Texas-based military families affected by deployment to Iraq or Afghanistan. More than $11.9 million in grants was made to Texas community organizations, including 14 in El Paso. Grantees included mental health providers, food banks, and children's services. These grants have been important in building behavioral health capacity and expanding community resources for military families.

Other programs are still in early development, but indicate El Paso's efforts to expand mental health capacity. In addition to a 24-hour suicide prevention hotline, Emergence Health Network offers peer support groups to service members and their families. The program draws funds from a Texas-based program, and facilitators receive 40 hours of training prior to leading the groups. Fort Bliss Morale, Welfare and Recreation (MWR) Program supports Emergence Health Network, and it in turn sponsors events on post to promote its services.

Interviewees noted that there have been efforts to expand behavioral health capacity on Fort Bliss itself to meet the needs of service members who have been deployed multiple times. Although well intended, they said, the effort has had some unanticipated negative effects. One is that service members reportedly have been required to leave their community providers and receive behavioral health services on post. Community counselors worried that individuals who truly need assistance may be reluctant to follow through with military-provided care out of fear that it may have a negative effect on their military careers. Many service members and their families seek counseling off post, they said, explicitly to avoid this problem.

The second effect of the capacity building on post has been to reduce capacity in the community provider agencies. More specifically, several interviewees said that the military can pay mental health providers much higher salaries than can community-based agencies; this has resulted in a "brain drain" in the community as counselors leave their agency positions to take a job at Fort Bliss. These vacant positions also were hard to fill because of this same salary differential.

**Law Enforcement**

There was general community concern about the behaviors of service members returning from deployment, including reckless driving, driving while intoxicated, bar fights, and other public disturbances. Concerns were also expressed about more serious negative behaviors, including suicides, hostage situations, domestic violence, and situations requiring the use of crisis management teams. Although these more serious negative behaviors rarely occur, the team heard that when they do occur they get "sensationalized" in the press. Nevertheless, Fort Bliss and El Paso law enforcement have collaborated to increase awareness of possible issues in the community that are triggered by PTSD. The following programs are examples of the types of collaborative efforts we heard about during our visit:

**Veterans Court.** Veterans Court is a specialty court akin to a drug or mental health court.[15] Under the program, combat veterans or active-duty service members who find themselves in the civilian criminal justice system receive assistance from mental health counselors, court administrators, and veterans' advocates. Participants must have a

[15] See http://www.texaspolicy.com/pdf/2009-11-PB22-VeteransCourts-ml.pdf.

service-related disability such as PTSD, traumatic brain injury (TBI), or severe depression. El Paso County has had a Veterans Court since September 2010, but in February 2012, the program was expanded to two subprograms for felony and misdemeanor cases.[16]

**PTSD Training.** Fort Bliss worked with the El Paso Police Department to train police officers to recognize situations that might have a mental health component and to try to stabilize the situation long enough for the department's crisis management team to arrive on the scene. Situations envisioned by the police ranged from a traffic citation that might rapidly escalate to a crisis situation, such as a service member taking someone hostage or threatening to commit suicide. It is important to note, however, that the department's awareness that officers might be encountering mental health issues in the community stemmed not solely from the soldiers stationed at Fort Bliss, but also from citizens fleeing the drug violence in Juarez.

**Domestic Relations/Legal Issues**

The study team heard from numerous interviewees that multiple deployments are having a significant negative impact on the family structure. In part, they observed a tendency for young people who have known each other for a relatively short time to enter into marriage just prior to deployment. A local attorney offered the following observations:

> We've been hearing about people getting married without knowing the other person. [One soldier on leave for 2 weeks in the United States] met a girl in a bar, fell in love . . . they were married, he went back to Afghanistan, they had a baby . . . and now they're getting divorced. And this is PTSD issues, shrapnel from IEDs, he's been blown up three times in IED incidents, he's had horrible [experiences, such as] stuffing intestines back into the guy that was driving . . . he was [this soldier's] best friend throughout basic camp, throughout their first deployment. And so he comes home . . . he drinks all the time. She doesn't know him; his personality is such that he just blows up. And it scares the snot out of her. Well, of course, she doesn't know him!

The weak foundation of this and similar relationships, she believed, was unable to withstand the strains of one or both partners deploying multiple times. She also gave us a list of the following observations of how multiple deployments are affecting military families that she sees:

1. Increased marriages between service members; increased marriages between service members and nonservice members with weak relational foundations;
2. Approximately 40% increase in parent-child [court] orders between service members, and between service members and local residents, after deployment;
3. Increase in the number of parent-child orders entered in local courts with one or both parents leaving the jurisdiction (impact on child) with little or no understanding of the

[16] See http://www.elpasotimes.com/news/ci_19958322.

result of such a move on the child-support case;

4. Increase in the number of administrative writs of withholding issued to DFAS [Defense Finance and Accounting Services]; service member separated from active duty-Reserve status and delinquent child support case; and
5. Increase in the number of long-distance child-support orders with one or both parents (and children) leaving the El Paso jurisdiction.

In short, it is easy for young people to enter into marriage, interviewees said, but much harder for them to get out of one, particularly when children are involved. Issues of child custody, visitation, and payment of child support are additionally challenging across state lines. Challenges related to divorce and child custody could also be exacerbated when service members seek assistance from Judge Advocate General (JAG) attorneys who are not necessarily familiar with Texas family law, as well as by service members' attempts to avoid paying lawyers' fees by using LegalZoom to get the paperwork to file for divorce. We heard of at least two interventions in El Paso that are designed to mitigate these challenges:

- The HEROES Program (Help Establishing Responsive Orders and Ensuring Support for children in military families), which is run through the Texas Office of the Attorney General, helps service members with child custody disputes across state lines.[17] It is supported in part by the Department for Health and Human Services Administration for Children and Families. The program has been operating since 2008.

- The El Paso County Domestic Relations Office worked with the Fort Bliss JAG office to train JAG lawyers on Texas child custody law and pro se divorce. They also worked with the Fort Bliss Morale Welfare and Readiness office on seminars about military and the law.

## Social Capital

Community members described an array of informal supports and services for service members and their families. Sources of such supports ranged from the faith community, mutual interest groups, and the community at large.

### Faith Community

One source of support is the faith community. On a church-by-church basis, the community is providing whatever services they can. We interviewed the leadership of one church, for example, that had adopted a unit as part of a larger community effort—the AUSA/Bradley Strong Foundation (described below). This congregation and its leadership were moved to take action specifically because of the repeated deployments of soldiers from the post:

> We consciously three and a half years ago, as a staff, saw the deployments and what they were doing to the families. So, on a staff planning meeting for the next year we said, "We're going to do everything we can to reach out to our military community and meet them where their need is." [Church leader]

[17] See http://www.acf.hhs.gov/programs/cse/pubs/2011/csr/csr1112.pdf.

This church has an extensive counseling ministry that reportedly is overwhelmed by service members coming back from combat with a whole array of challenges. Some of the issues require individual counseling, such as service members who are addicted to alcohol, drugs, or pornography. And yet many of the marriages also need support. One of the church counselors we interviewed indicated he was currently working with a young couple that had been married only a few months. The now-husband had been deployed once before they got married, but he would soon be heading out for his second deployment. "They've had no chance to establish a life as husband and wife," the counselor said, and he expressed concern about the ability of that relationship to endure over the long term.

Given the practical time limitations of the site visit, the team did not hold a group discussion at another church in the area. We did attend services at two different churches in the Northeast area, however, and observed very little in the way of military connections (one church had a photograph of apparently the only service member in the congregation who was currently deployed). We also spoke with another church that was working with military families struggling with the effects of multiple deployments, but doing so on a case-by-case basis. As this pastor explained, "We try to treat them normal, not segregated in any way, so they have the opportunity to be part of the community . . . and get out of the military culture on base." That being said, we cannot say that there are no other churches within the area that are providing significant supports to members of their congregation who are being affected by multiple deployments. Indeed, given the large number of houses of worship in the El Paso community, there undoubtedly are other congregations that offer relevant services and counseling to these families.

**AUSA/Bradley Strong Foundation**

The community is also supporting service members and their families through the AUSA/Bradley Strong Foundation. The Foundation, which has the backing of the Chamber of Commerce, describes itself as a "bridge" between El Paso and the installation. The website[18] offers a message of hospitality for the military that is similar to what we heard from numerous civilian interviewees:

> The City of El Paso has a great love for Soldiers and respects their commitment to serve our great nation. We view their assignment to Fort Bliss as an opportunity for the community to welcome them into our home, "*Mi casa es su casa.*" The Bradley Chapter is one of the primary organizations in El Paso that helps the local community understand the culture of the Army. We help El Paso citizens and businesses understand the joys and challenges of service in the greatest Army in the world. For Soldiers and their family members coming to El Paso for the first time, the Chapter attempts to provide them with a taste of the rich 400-year history of El Paso and its culture.

Through this program, sponsors—including churches, defense contractors, and ice cream companies—are linked with a unit at Fort Bliss ostensibly to provide a link between the unit and the community while the unit is stationed in El Paso as well as deployed overseas. The sponsor also connects with the FRG affiliated with the particular unit and provides support for the family members while the unit is deployed. Although the program may be helping to better integrate the

[18] See http://www.ausabradleychapter.com/info.php?pnum=3.

soldiers and their families into the community, activities are up to the individual sponsor. And sponsors may not necessarily be offering supports specifically related to the effects of multiple deployments. For example, none of the spouses with whom we spoke made any mention of their unit sponsor when recounting where they can go to find services or supports to deal with the stresses accumulating after four, five, or six deployments.

**Mutual Support Networks**

The study team did see some evidence of various informal mutual support networks throughout the community. For example, while dining out one afternoon, the team was seated next to two tables of motorcycle riders, all of whom sported a back-of-the-jacket patch that read: "Combat Veterans Association." Most of these diners were young men, all of whom had "Iraq" or "Afghanistan" combat patches on the front of their outer wear. Further research indicated that the Combat Veteran Motorcycle Association (CVMA) is a nationwide group of riders who advocate peer-to-peer supports. Chapter 23-2, which is based in El Paso, is one of seven Texas-based chapters of CVMA.[19]

Peer support is also available through other venues. As mentioned earlier, Emergence Health Network, one of the few behavioral health providers in the city, is establishing peer-to-peer support groups for active duty service members and for female service members specifically. Not only are the support groups held off post, but they are not affiliated in any way with either Fort Bliss or the Department of Veterans Affairs (VA); consequently, we were told, active duty service members can feel more secure that their participation will not get to their commanders. Emergence is also developing spouse support groups that are structured to avoid some of the common issues we heard described about the Family Readiness Groups (FRGs). For example, several interviewees described the "drama" associated with spouse groups on post in terms similar to the quote below:

> The FRG is helpful to many and for many it's their worst nightmare. A lot of it is the ranking—"What rank is your husband? My husband has more rank than yours so you don't have the say." That sort of stuff.

In the current spouse groups at Emergence, there reportedly is no disclosure of rank in a concerted effort to avoid the discord that would result.

Hearts Apart, a program run through the Fort Bliss Army Community Service, also offers support to families with a deployed soldier. They run a support group and organize activities several times a month for families of service members stationed at Fort Bliss. At Thanksgiving, for example, they organized a group meal at Cattleman's Steakhouse, a popular restaurant on the outskirts of the city. Although run by the installation, Hearts Apart received a TRIAD grant that allowed them to expand services to more than 300 families.

The city is also host to many of the more familiar veterans associations, such as the Veterans of Foreign Wars (VFW) and the American Legion. Prior to the site visit, a Vietnam veteran told the study team during a telephone interview that the younger service members do

---

[19] See http://combatvet.org.

not engage with these organizations because, he believed, "they feel they can take care of whatever issues emerge on their own." An evening visit to a VFW post in the Northeast, however, revealed a mix of young service members and older veterans. The degree to which veterans of the Iraq and Afghanistan wars feel comfortable seeking support from organizations like the VFW remains to be explored. Similarly, the degree to which Vietnam-era veterans are comfortable supporting these young soldiers remains unclear. The study team spoke with one Vietnam veteran who characterized his cohort's ambivalence as follows:

> I came back from both tours in uniform and the second time I caught a lot of crap getting off the plane and was spit on. And I wanted to talk my devils away, I wanted to talk about it, I wanted to explain to somebody what I was feeling. Nobody wanted to hear what I had to say! I took everything I felt . . . and put it in a box, wrapped it in chains, and buried it in my mind. Today people say, you know, "Oh, thanks for your service. Let me buy your meal. We appreciate what you're doing."' So what you've got are essentially two groups—you've got the disgruntles, "They never did it for me, so I ain't gonna do it, screw them guys!" Or, like me, "Thank god the attitude is changing! And it didn't happen for me, but I'm glad it's happening to somebody else and let me help it happen."

**Online Supports**

In addition, and perhaps consistent with the young age of this group of service members and their families, numerous interviewees reported seeking support through Internet-based channels. Each of the FRGs, for example, has its own Facebook page, and spouses can contact each other through that venue outside of the regular meeting times. The then-garrison commander, Colonel Joseph Simonelli, also started a Facebook page ("Colonel Joe Wants to Know") that was serving as an information and support forum for military-affiliated individuals.[20] Colonel Simonelli stated that the El Paso media as well as service providers in the city regularly log in to the site to keep abreast of any issues that may be arising. He said that when the page was first started, individuals would post about a problem they were having and he would tackle the issue immediately. Now "it's taken on a life of its own," as the posters are taking it upon themselves to help out their fellow soldiers and families and frequently offer recommendations based on their own experiences. Of note, though, is that most of the posts were about day-to-day challenges at Fort Bliss, not about how to deal with the effects of multiple deployments. This broader focus is not surprising, given that this is a public forum.

Facebook was not the only avenue for online communication. We also heard from a young woman who said she regularly goes to her church website to post requests for prayers for her husband, who is currently deployed to Afghanistan. The church's minister, who was participating in the same discussion, indicated that although the discussion group we held was the first time he had met this woman in person, he does see her prayer requests and every week the group says a special prayer for her spouse. Although these and numerous other virtual connections may be unsatisfying to an older cohort, the young soldiers currently stationed at Fort Bliss are intricately familiar with online social networking and may be finding numerous sources of support there to cope with the stresses caused by multiple deployments.

[20] On May 24, 2012, Garrison Commander Brant Dayley established a new Facebook page *Tell It To Col D*, that continues the model established by his predecessor: https://www.facebook.com/TellittoColD.

### Retired Veterans as Support

Finally, and as noted elsewhere in this report, El Paso is home to a large population of retired veterans who have been through combat and fully appreciate the sacrifices made by these soldiers and their families. The study team had numerous opportunities to engage these individuals informally (e.g., brief discussions after the District 4 weekly community breakfast and the Northeast Rotary Club), and all expressed their concern about the toll these rapid deployment cycles had taken on service members and their families. As one retired service member said, "We never had to go through anything like what they're going through." Some of the Army spouses may have questioned whether the community was "genuine" in its support of their partners' service, but the study team was left with the impression that, at least among retired veterans (if not the broader community), there is tremendous empathy for what these service members and their families are being asked to endure.

## SUMMARY

In many ways, El Paso and Fort Bliss are working well together under difficult circumstances. Though they do not always see eye-to-eye, they share a mutual respect, and both post and community are making concerted efforts to work with each other.

### What's Working

The El Paso community is welcoming to military families and makes earnest attempts to show appreciation for their service. Symbols of the town's appreciation of the military are all around—on Franklin Mountains, on Wal-Mart storefronts, and at the local liquor store. Businesses of all types make efforts to offer discounts to military families.

The relationship between post and city is reinforced by established communication mechanisms. Fort Bliss interacts with the city and Chamber of Commerce, the school districts, and community leadership. Through coalitions and regular meetings, there are ongoing opportunities for city stakeholders to learn about deployments, changes on post, or other factors that may affect the community. These coalitions also offer an opportunity for conflict resolution, when needed.

For service members and their families, several programs in El Paso were mentioned as making a positive impact and defusing some of the challenges introduced by deployments.

- **The AUSA/Bradley Strong Foundation** sponsorship of units connects individual service members to local community organizations and is a tangible way for local organizations to connect with the units on post and show appreciation for their service.
- **TRIAD grants** increased the service capacity of community organizations. In 2010, when Fort Bliss knew their services would be under strain, the post referred service members to these grantees.
- **The HEROES program**, managed by the Texas Office of the Attorney General, helps service members navigate the complex legal terrain of child custody disputes across state lines.

- **Hearts Apart,** run by the Fort Bliss Army Community Service, builds friendships and eases the stress and demands on the family during times of separation.
- With a cohort of families accustomed to seeking out solutions online, **"Colonel Joe Wants to Know,"** started by the former garrison commander and now transformed by the new garrison commander as **"Tell It to Col. D,"** is an example of effective digital community building using Facebook. This online page, run by the garrison commander's office, is a bulletin board for community events, answers routine day-to-day questions posted by military families, and also connects families in need with appropriate services. It effectively makes the garrison commander accessible to those on and off post.
- Although faced with the significant challenges of a large transitory population, limited tax base, and overcrowding, the EPISD has instituted strategies such as the **Military Family Liaison Program** and **counselor training** that bridge the gaps between community and post. These trainings raise awareness with teachers and counselors of the challenges faced by military families and offer best practices in how to help families deal with these stressors. The liaisons help the teachers and counselors address day-to-day military-related challenges that may adversely affect a child's behavior in the classroom.

**Needs and Challenges**

Leaders perceived an urgent need to increase **behavioral health capacity.** Community leaders and El Pasoans working in the health sector identified civilian mental health services, especially psychiatric care, as a broader area of need in El Paso. As indicated in the "Community Orientation" section of this report, families fleeing the violence in Juarez are also coming into the city with trauma from what they have witnessed across the broader. And with the upcoming drawdown in troops, leaders observed there would be an increase in need for mental health services that would exceed the capacity of current systems.

Many service members reportedly are also **reluctant to seek care.** Conditions such as PTSD or depression may be hard for the individual to recognize, and help-seeking behavior may run counter to messages of resilience and toughness coming from command. Although military policy states that accessing mental health care services cannot be considered when making promotions, we heard that there is still concern about the potential fallout from seeking mental health services. Many soldiers fear that the chain of command will learn that they sought psychological care and that such knowledge would place their military career or retirement at risk. Military spouses are also reluctant to seek care or divulge too much information because they do not want to damage their spouses' careers. Mental health providers and church leadership spoke of the need to provide a "safe space" for service members. Staff at one mental health organization, well aware of these concerns, said the counselors who work with soldiers stagger the appointments to ensure that service members do not encounter each other in the parking lot.

Interviewees also said the **families at home are subjected to considerable stress** during the deployment process. During predeployment they prepare for the time away, and that preparation often includes protracted trainings that require the service members to be away from home. During deployment, spouses are in essence single parents, managing family responsibilities, home, and work on their own. When their service member spouses return, they must work with them to renegotiate household division of labor and act as a support as the service member attempts to readjust to a noncombat setting. The rapid pace of redeployment, they said, ultimately disrupts all attempts the family is making to settle into the "old normal" life, and for some, the "new normal" is simply untenable.

Community members identified **underserved constituencies** of military families for whom additional supports may be needed. Fathers whose wives deploy contend with the challenges associated with being single fathers, but may also have additional social challenges because they are performing nontraditional family roles. These men may be less likely to reach out to established military support mechanisms such as FRG activities, which are mostly attended by women. Conversely, women who have been deployed may encounter gender-associated challenges in theater (e.g., sexual assault) and they may not receive the support they need from the current military support systems. Moreover, as they reintegrate, military mothers may face different challenges in reestablishing bonds with children and their routines at home. Finally, we heard from several interviewees about the strains placed on children in single-parent households or in households where both parents are deployed at the same time.

**Suggestions from the Community**

The community offered suggestions for possible improvements or next steps that may help address the needs associated with multiple deployments. For many community members, recommendations emerged from their assessment that the multiple deployment strategy is problematic for families and children. **They desired wider recognition from the public and from the Army that the multiple deployments were having adverse effects on many families and children.**

Concerns were voiced about anger and hostility issues in children, and attachment disorders for children whose parents deploy while they are still babies. Those we interviewed relied on anecdote and personal observation for these negative impacts. To build an evidence base of the long-term effects, the community suggested a **longitudinal study of the behavioral health of children** with parents who experienced multiple deployments.

Finally, the community underscored the importance of **maintaining good communications** between city and the post as the command leadership changes. During our visit, Fort Bliss was preparing for a change in garrison command. City leaders wondered how receptive the incoming garrison commander would be to working with them, and what efforts they would have to undertake to maintain the relationships they had previously established with the leadership on post.

# Watertown, New York

## Case Study Report

# Impacts of Multiple Deployments: Watertown, New York

## OVERVIEW

This report summarizes findings from Westat's ethnographic site visit (May 12–18, 2012) to Watertown, New York. The study goal was to assess impacts on the Watertown community from multiple deployments to Operation Iraqi Freedom (OIF) and Operation Enduring Freedom (OEF) from neighboring Fort Drum, a large Army installation. Interviews with Watertown government, business, and community leaders and other community representatives include the following highlights. Fort Drum has experienced both large growth and many deployments in recent years, and it was difficult for interviewees to identify community effects stemming solely from deployments. Positive effects from the military presence have included economic stimulus for the area and a large supply of health care providers available to all residents. Interviewees said, though, that multiple deployments have contributed to a tight housing market, a shortage of mental health care services (especially for children), and new demands on school staff. Residents would like more information about posttraumatic stress disorder (PTSD) to recognize symptoms and provide appropriate responses. An integrated military/civilian community promotes strong resident support for deployed service members and their families.

**Data Sources**

- Community members
- Chamber of Commerce
- Churches
- City government employees
- Emergency service providers (i.e., fire, police, emergency medical personnel)
- Community college
- Regional partnership organizations
- Social service organizations
- Behavioral health organizations
- Hospitals
- Local businesses
- Media and the arts
- Observation
- Secondary sources (e.g., news articles, Internet videos, survey results provided by respondents)

## GEOGRAPHIC ORIENTATION

### Community: Watertown, New York

Watertown is a small city in rural upstate New York located approximately 70 miles north of Syracuse and 30 miles from the Canadian border. It is the seat of Jefferson County, which has a population of 116,229, including 27,023 Watertown residents and 12,955 Fort Drum residents. The tri-county area of Jefferson, St. Lawrence, and Lewis Counties covers 5,223 square miles, with a population of 241,128.[1]

The terms Greater Watertown and "North Country" (and less frequently, "Drum Country") were used by interviewees and secondary sources[2] to define the community (Figure 1).

[1] See http://quickfacts.census.gov.

[2] E.g., see http://www.drumcountry.com/index.cfm.

This report focuses on the city of Watertown, where most of our interviewees are employed, and the surrounding villages and towns of Jefferson County, where many of them live.

Historically, Watertown has been relatively homogeneous with regard to race and ethnicity; the city and county are predominantly white. A few interviewees mentioned that military families have had a diversifying effect. We were informed that poverty is an issue in the community and confirmed that the median household income is lower in Watertown than in the state of New York and the United States.

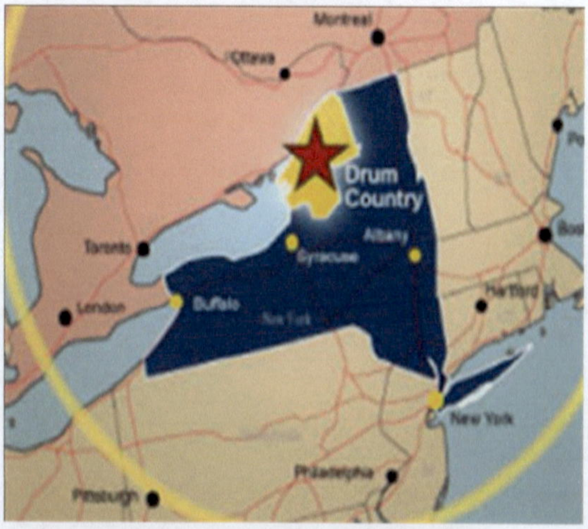

**FIGURE 1** Community orientation.

The community has experienced extensive growth and development in recent years as a result of the approximate doubling of the active duty personnel assigned to Fort Drum in 2004–2005. The community has formed two homegrown nonprofit organizations to identify and address military-civilian challenges: the Fort Drum Regional Liaison Organization (FDRLO), which grew out of a committee formed in the1980s, addresses community planning generally and any specific issues as they arise; and the Fort Drum Regional Health Planning Organization (FDRHPO), which focuses on meeting physical and behavioral health needs. The boards of both organizations represent the local civilian and military communities.

Although our visit occurred during a temperate spring week, most persons the team interviewed mentioned long winters and lake effect snowfall averaging more than 112 inches per year as characteristic of the region. Multiple interviewees also described how the region's harsh climate can create adjustment, transportation, and home maintenance challenges for newcomers, especially military families from warmer climates. Several of them described how the community helps those struggling to adjust to regional and other challenges, pointing out how its culture is reflective of "small town attitudes" and a willingness to help anyone in need.

## Military Installation: Fort Drum

Fort Drum is home to the 10th Mountain Division (Light Infantry) and other units (Figure 2). It was primarily a training camp until 1984–1985, when it was designated as home to the reactivated 10th Mountain Division. The 10th Mountain Division was described by several interviewees as "the most deployed force" in the country. Two respondents separately commented, "they are either gone or training to go." The post is responsible for the mobilization and training of almost 80,000 troops annually, including Reserve and National Guard members. The post covers 107,265 acres. The division includes four brigades, including aviation, a sustainment brigade, and associated companies including engineering, ordinance, and public affairs. The installation also supports Air Force units, Army and Navy Reserve, and some cross-branch training.

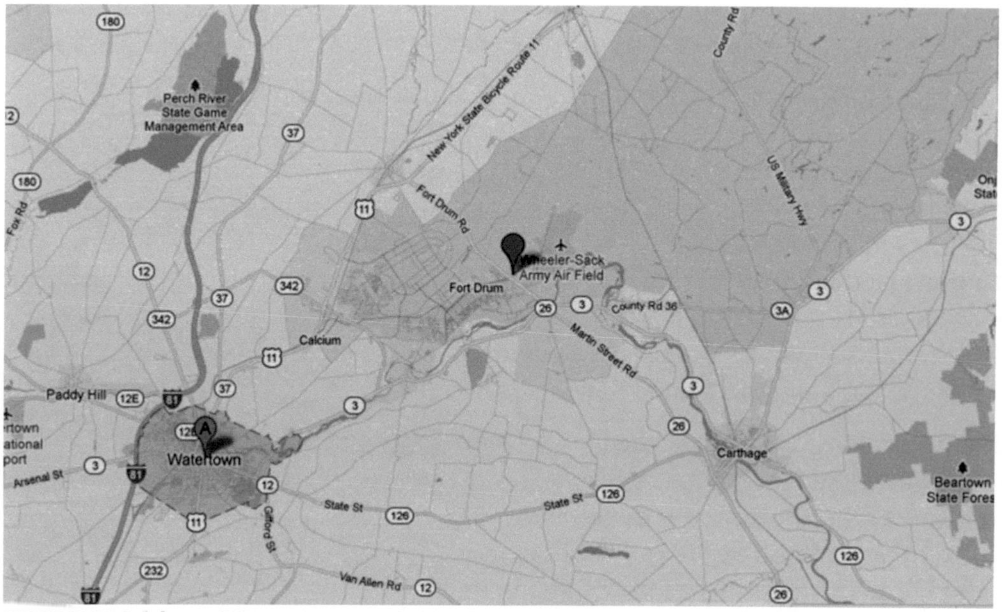


**FIGURE 2** Map of Watertown and Fort Drum. (Source: Google Maps.)

According to our interviewees and publicly available information, the role of the 10th Mountain Division in OEF/OIF theaters has been continuous but variable since October 2001. Early on in OEF/OIF, soldiers were deployed by brigade for tours longer than 1 year, but now smaller units (e.g., battalion or company) are deployed for shorter times. Deployments have included cavalry, light infantry, field artillery, signal and intelligence, and combat aviation.[3] A 2007 article in the *Army Times* describes how 10th Mountain Division's 2nd Brigade out of Fort Drum

> has served the most time on the battlefield since 2001 . . . . The brigade is in its 14th month of an extended 15-month tour—"the most-deployed brigade in the U.S. Army," he noted. On its return home, which should be completed over the next several weeks, it will have served 40 months overseas since December 2001.[4]

### Relationship between Community and Post

An overwhelming majority of interviewees described the social and economic relationship between Watertown's civilian community and the military as positive, supportive, and symbiotic. It was reported to have been strained in the 1980s and early 1990s by perceptions among long-time residents that soldiers were receiving unfair economic advantages. A civilian and long-time resident of the area explained:

> A lot of the local people—and I say a lot because I witnessed it—were very negative about the military coming, primarily for what it would do to their small town. . . . Now it's much better. But . . . a lot of military were mistreated because people were resentful if

[3] See http://www.drum.army.mil/2ndBCT/Pages/History_lv2.aspx.
[4] See http://www.armytimes.com/news/2007/10/ap_mountaindivision_home_071005.

> they [military] received percentage-off discounts for anything from buying cars, to dinner out, to hotels. [Social services provider #1, spouse of a veteran]

A variety of interviewees reported that the relationship is now quite good, both professionally and personally, across multiple aspects of community life. The intentional integration of Fort Drum personnel and their families with the civilian community for housing, schooling, and medical and social services was cited by several community members as the underlying reason for this exceptionally close civilian/military partnership. Respondents also described an affective bond between the two communities:

> I just think that the rest of the country just doesn't get it . . . that, "We're at war?" . . . I just don't think they get it. And we get it. . . . We get it when Mary's husband is getting deployed and I know she's going to be scared every day. . . . I just think the whole community feels these things. How can we not? This is our community—our friends, our neighbors . . . we are so closely integrated that there is . . . no one here who is not working with a military spouse. . . . Every time you see a casualty, you think, you know that is somebody's somebody. . . . But, it's kind of a strange thing because I also think it makes us a united community. [Regional partnership organization representative, civilian]

## EFFECTS OF DEPLOYMENT ON THE COMMUNITY

It was not always possible for interviewees to tease out the effects of multiple OEF/OIF deployments from increases in population because of the significant growth of Fort Drum over the past several years. Overall, the most visible positive effects of a large military presence in the Watertown and Jefferson County community are support for the economy and the increased availability of general and specialist medical care for entire community, which we heard about from a variety of interviewees. Nearly every interviewee also connected the continued mutual support among soldiers, military families, veterans, and the civilian community to multiple deployments.

Numerous interviewees said the greatest negative effects of multiple deployments include a shortage of behavioral health care services (particularly for children), added demands and stressors on school staff, and a small number of apparently isolated, high-profile violent crimes speculated (but not confirmed) to be related to soldiers' deployment experiences.

### Economic Impact

Multiple persons with whom the team spoke suggested that any potential economic impact on the community from multiple OEF/OIF deployments may have been buffered or masked by the simultaneous growth of the post and surrounding community. Many of them also stated they could not differentiate between the impact of multiple deployments and major growth, which began in 2004–2005, as well as external factors nationwide (i.e., the recession).

**Commerce**

Although there have been fluctuations in the types of businesses serving the community over time, with more chain restaurants and retailers near the Interstate Highway and fewer family-owned businesses in town, interviewees were not able to tie this specifically to multiple deployments. Several interviewees did identify small boosts in select businesses shortly after large numbers of soldiers returned to Watertown after deployment. Deployment cycles reportedly had more of an economic impact in the early years of OEF/OIF, with deployments lasting up to 18 months and larger numbers of soldiers deploying at the same time. In recent years, however, with smaller numbers of troops deploying at the same time, economic impacts are less noticeable. Changes consistently reported with demobilization include increased hotel and restaurant business, demand for home rental and purchase, and increased purchases of big-ticket items among returning soldiers, particularly those soldiers who are young and single. At the same time, several interviewees reported younger soldiers often lose large down payments on major purchases when they are unable to make monthly payments. This affects their credit ratings and may adversely affect their careers.

**Housing**

Most interviewees found it difficult to differentiate the housing impact of the growth of Fort Drum since 2004–2005 from that of multiple deployments. However, a few remarked that the ongoing shortage of available housing units is felt most sharply with large demobilizations, forcing people into hotels that are often booked to maximum capacity. Several interviewees told us that some military families relocating to the area are willing to rent or buy whatever is available. One respondent described how this urgent process can lead to disappointment:

> And you'd get people who buy houses sight unseen. . . . Some of them were over in Iraq and Afghanistan still, but they were coming back to this area . . . they'd buy the house. And pictures of the inside that they saw over the Internet or from the realtor's site looked great, but when you actually look at the house in the neighborhood, it didn't warrant the price that they're paying. [Local government employee and spouse of retired military member]

We were also told that when service members deploy and their property is left vacant, they often neglect to arrange for maintenance during their absence (e.g., turning off their water during the winter months) or fail to pay mortgages and/or property taxes. This reportedly puts a strain on local government offices as they attempt to locate service members or their families to help resolve these issues.

**Public Services**

Interviewees reported that the demand for public services also changes with the deployment cycles. This includes requests for marriage licenses and ceremonies, real estate transactions, property tax collections, water/sewer usage, trash services, and roadway usage. Several interviewees mentioned increases in sales tax revenue resulting from these boom times, commensurate with decreases during larger deployments. Multiple interviewees also reported problems with increased traffic volume after large numbers of troops demobilize, particularly along the new commercial corridor near the Interstate Highway.

**Jobs**

There was no clear consensus at the macro level regarding employment and labor challenges connected to multiple deployments. Several community members indicated that soldiers bring skilled, hard-working spouses and sometimes young adult children who enrich the local labor pool. Veterans and retired military, including those who had been deployed in OEF/OIF, were also reported by several respondents to provide specialized and reliable labor that may not otherwise be available in the community. One resident described how deployment cycles and employment patterns coincide:

> When we need more workers, [it's] because folks are home and everybody's going out to eat and everybody's buying. It's also the time when the spouses are here and they're all living here and they need more jobs. . . . I can tell you—local businesses love it when they're all home. [Regional partnership organization representative, civilian]

## Information and Communication

Interviewees said that military issues, including deployment-related topics such as welcome- home ceremonies, are frequently discussed in the Watertown community. More detailed information, however, such as how to access particular services or how to identify PTSD symptoms, was reported to be much more challenging to find.

**Public Discussion of Deployment-Related Issues**

Local news media, including the *Watertown Daily Times* and *Watertown News 7* television, routinely cover deployment-related topics, such as welcome home celebrations and efforts to support soldiers and their families. Conversely, there is little evidence of town hall meetings or other events specifically intended to discuss potential deployment-related issues in the community or how to respond to them. Interviewees offered mixed perspectives on the need for additional communication. One of them told us, "I don't have any specific contacts with the military . . . at Drum. And like I said, the only way I know that there's people deployed or people coming home is by watching the news. So we don't get any special bulletin." [Emergency services provider]. In contrast, another interviewee reported regular communication between him and his military counterpart:

> As far as Fort Drum, my interactions with them is sometimes several times a week. . . . We communicate via phone and email on a regular basis—3 to 4 times a week, and more if necessary. He does alert me to times that they are expecting deployed troops home. We have discussed posttraumatic stress syndrome at length. [Emergency services provider, civilian]

Many family challenges related to deployment have been vetted through the docudrama *In My Shoes,* performed several times in Watertown area schools, on Fort Drum, and on a nearby college campus. This play was written in the words of and performed by military teenagers and includes their views on the effects of their parents' deployments. The play was mentioned by several interviewees as an important opportunity to increase awareness and understanding within the community, and to collectively address a broad set of issues affecting military families and civilians in the community. For example, in these lines from *In My Shoes,* one teen describes how she feels about lost time resulting from multiple deployments:

> I used to be like, the biggest daddy's girl in the world, like, I would prefer being with my dad. But now, I really prefer being with my mom. Maybe it's because he's missed, uh, 4 years of my life, but he's back from deployment now. . . . He's never gonna get that back, and, it's just, it's hard. [Garrett, from *In My Shoes*]
>
> And a civilian teen, who participated in the production of the play, shared her feelings in a CNN interview about how her involvement has changed her views:
>
> I've been here my whole life. I've known nothing but being a civilian in a military world. . . . It was weird to see it from their angle for once. I thought everyone had a mom and dad always there.[5]

Information about the play has been published by local and national media sources and is currently in production for broadcast on local television.

**Information Sources for Military Families**

The post has extensive information about services available to military members and their families, including a downloadable welcome package. Family Readiness Groups (FRGs) are available to all military members and their families, and can be an important source of information and support. Many interviewees also identified schools as a valuable resource, particularly through efforts such as the Military and Family Life Consultants (MFLCs) program (described in the Community Competence section). In addition, there are informal networks within the community that reach out to military families, or are available to those that seek them out. However, some of the most important resources, such as behavioral and mental health information related to deployment, were not always readily available in locations most frequented by those in need or by their families. For example, one interviewee described a search for information about deployment-related behavioral health:

> I am shocked by how little information is out on post about PTSD. . . . I was already seeing things that worried me before the guys came back from deployment, so I actively went around looking for information that I could bring to the FRG Leaders. . . . The first place that I went to was the local chapel because typically . . . people will go to their chaplain for help because it feels like it's not part of the chain of command. It's a safe place. The chaplains really didn't know anything about PTSD and they didn't have any resources and they were shocked that I was asking. . . . The second place I went to was the clinic. . . . There was nothing to be found there about PTSD. The only information I could find about PTSD was in the behavioral health center . . . they had a lot of

[5] America's anomaly: The place where war is a constant, http://www.cnn.com/2011/10/07/us/afghanistan-fort-drum/index.html.

> information. But how many people go there? [Social services provider and spouse of active duty military member]

### Information Sources for Civilians

The challenges related to multiple deployments and sacrifices made by military members and their families were mentioned very generally in a variety of community contexts, including the Armed Forces Day luncheon sponsored by the Greater Watertown-North Country Chamber of Commerce, the FDRHPO Annual Meeting, and during the course of several interviews. A few persons mentioned reading about potential issues related to multiple deployments in the newspaper or research literature. A few interviewees in law enforcement, health care, social services, and the faith community also mentioned regular information exchange with the post. In addition, several interviewees who provide key services reported receiving training in identifying and responding to the hidden wounds of war. One of them said:

> We routinely have meetings between state police, the sheriffs, and myself and military police. When there is a soldier they're worried about, they share that with us. . . . We had a Ph.D. from the Fort Drum Behavioral Science come and talk to a group of 40 people in law enforcement and medical staff about posttraumatic stress . . . to help us basically understand it and to try to defuse it. [Emergency services provider, civilian]

In general, community members do not seem to be talking formally about issues of greatest concern regarding OEF/OIF deployment. However, community members articulated common impressions regarding potential challenges associated with multiple deployments—specifically, behavioral and mental health issues and criminal activity—some of which they explicitly said they heard on the news. They described the perceived impacts on their community as more dramatic than experts in the community reported them to be. Several interviewees mentioned that community members could benefit from being trained more broadly in addressing potential problems associated with multiple deployments. In addition, many of them emphasized that information on deployment-related issues (e.g., PTSD) should be more proactively disseminated.

## Community Health

### Physical Health Issues

Physical health care for soldiers, their families, and the general community was not described as being challenged by multiple deployments. Instead, through the efforts of medical practices throughout the Army and civilian communities, as well as the influence of a local health planning organization, the quality of general and specialty care throughout the region was reported to be exceptional, particularly for a rural area.

### Behavioral and Mental Health

Behavioral health issues, such as depression, anxiety, substance abuse, PTSD, and suicide were identified by multiple respondents as one of the most serious negative effects of multiple deployments. Many described how multiple deployments put an overwhelming strain on military personnel, their families, and behavioral health services in the community. One mental health provider noted how "greater demand for services has increased stress levels" among service provider staff:

> The average service member has experienced four deployments and some as many as eight. . . . The stress on both the service member and families . . . [has] led to numerous behavioral health issues, which has increased the demand on our services. [Medical/behavioral services]

One social service provider described how a behavioral health issue stemming from combat can shock family members and friends, particularly when the signs are delayed, which can also present a treatment challenge:

> It's sad, because I think multiple deployments gives more opportunity for more and more issues with the people who are in combat. . . . [Talking about the spouse of a friend of his] One of [the husband's] deployments involved some very graphic, horrendous human suffering. And some of the things that he had to do really affected him. . . . It didn't manifest until . . . he'd been home for his 9 months' stint . . . because it was like a year out, then 9 months home, a year out, then 9 months home. He went back. . . . And they ended up sending him back. He . . . [had] terrible, terrible issues, to the point where he was cutting himself and doing all kinds of crazy things. [Social services provider, spouse of veteran]

Another military spouse told us that when Army spouses try to talk to a physician about their struggles related to a spouse's deployment, they are offered medication as a "quick fix" and an opportunity is lost:

> The other thing I don't like and I saw it happened time and time again when I went in to doctor on post. . . . They would always ask, "How are you feeling?" I was always very frank. "Some days I'm feeling great, and some days, oh, I've been crying." You know, you just go through those stages. And the first thing I was always offered were antidepressants. . . . And I would say, "No, I don't want antidepressants. I'm just sad at the moment. I'll get through it." But I was shocked to find out how many women take them up on antidepressants. . . . I had a fascinating conversation in the car one day. There were seven us in a car going down to a women's conference. . . . Come to find out, that six of the seven of us were on antidepressants. And these were young women. These were 20-year-olds. And I get it—they are tired of feeling unhappy and this kind of shuts off their emotions, but they're given nothing [else] . . . no counseling. And so they get used to feeling no emotions. [Social services provider and spouse of active duty soldier]

**Suicide**

Although there is evidence that suicide is a deployment-related issue at Fort Drum, it has not overtly affected the civilian community. According to the Watertown TV news station, "Fort Drum saw its highest level of active-duty suicides in almost a decade . . . seven Fort Drum soldiers took their own lives in 2011 . . . that makes 31 suicides among Fort Drum soldiers since 2003."[6] Suicide of soldiers was mentioned by several community members as a particular issue of concern associated with multiple deployments. One army spouse described the post's effort to reduce the incidence of suicide and suicide attempts:

> They know what their purpose is overseas. . . . And when they come home . . . they're lost. . . . There's a lot of suicide. They've only been back since November. And a lot of suicide watches with our guys. And they're not allowed to go anywhere for 2 weeks after being home . . . they are deliberately kept local so that an eye can be kept on them to make sure they're getting their feet under them before they're allowed to go out of the area. [Social services provider, spouse of active duty service member]

Although suicide is a concern for the community of Watertown, it seems that most, if not all, military-related suicides are confined to the post. We found no evidence of deployment-related suicides in Watertown. As one emergency service provider told us, "I have read in the paper that military suicides are up. I don't know of any in the city of Watertown . . . in the last 6 years." [Emergency service provider]

**Family Issues**

Several interviewees confirmed marital problems were a negative consequence of multiple deployment cycles, but also noted that family challenges are confounded by those faced by military families in general, including frequent moves and long periods of separation. Some interviewees suggested that the duration of deployment in combination with the level of associated risk is a better indicator of the extent to which deployments affect service members and their families and in what ways. One military spouse explained how the most recent deployment was very different than previous ones:

> Previous to this particular deployment, I didn't notice it [signs of PTSD] because of the jobs that he had previous to this one. His first tour out . . . was a civil affairs thing, and they were . . . not really in the line of fire. . . . His second tour . . . he never fired his weapon one time. . . . This [third] time . . . was scary. His job was to take a bullet before the colonel did. . . . So this time, I've really noticed quite a bit. Noises get him. We were just in Washington, D.C. . . . and we got out of the car and he's doing one of these things—looking [and] scanning constantly . . . he's tense and I could feel it in his body and I could see it in his arms and I said, "Sweetheart, calm down. It's ok. Nobody is trying to kill us." . . . He had to sit down on a bench. He's like, "I can't do this . . . I don't know what's wrong. I don't know if it's the smells. I don't if it's the number of people. I don't know if it's all the faces. I don't know, but I can't do this." And he was unglued for the rest of the day. . . . My kids had never seen this. My 15-year-old was just like, "Dad, what's wrong?" My 11-year-old was just beside himself. He was like, "Daddy, did we do something wrong? You didn't want to go to the zoo with us?" [He responded] "No buddy. I wanted to. I just couldn't do it." That was really hard because that's never happened before. That was really difficult. [Medical/behavioral services provider and spouse of active duty service member]

[6] See http://www.wwnytv.com/news/local/Fort-Drum-Sees-Highest-Level-Of-Active-Duty-Suicides-137775573.html.

**Children's Issues**

An overwhelming majority of interviewees expressed concern about the impact of multiple deployments on military children. One respondent summarized her feelings about the impact on the Watertown community:

> I think multiple deployments have put an ungodly amount of stress on our military . . . it has been really, really hard in these past 2 years, because you see families breaking apart. You see the cost to our children. . . . And there's no mental health that is directed towards our children. There's none. I mean, they have MFLCs, and I'm telling you, the MFLCs are [the] best things since sliced bread. . . . Most public schools have MFLCs in the schools. Private schools do not. . . . There's nobody for those kids to talk to. They are under an extraordinary amount of pressure. They see things, you know, that kids shouldn't see. [Social services provider, spouse of active duty member]

Another respondent echoed this sentiment, but acknowledged some improvements in deployment cycles during OEF/OIF that may reduce some of the stress experienced by military children:

> I think multiple deployments are hard. I think since they went down from 18-month deployments, it's better. The 18 months was just . . . too much [Respondent got a little teary eyed at this point]. So it's better that they went down from that. I think if they went back to 9 months, it would be way better. I think that it's hard on the families. It's hard on children. [Regional partnership organization representative, civilian]

Importantly, several interviewees pointed out civilian children are also affected by multiple deployments, in particular those attending schools with high percentages of enrolled military dependent children with parents deploying to OEF/OIF theaters. These civilian children often share in grief experienced by their friends, as explained by one civilian resident:

> When a 9-year-old has a best friend, and their dad gets deployed and they're sad, their friend is sad with them. Personally, I don't think that's a bad thing. You know, I think that learning different cultures and different ways of life is a good thing for kids and is a good thing for families. I think when we have causalities is when it's a . . . hard thing. . . . Obviously, Fort Drum is heavily deployed and we have casualties regularly. [Regional partnership organization representative, civilian]

Teenagers in the community, those from both military and civilian families, have knowledge of the OEF/OIF combat theater in general and are sometimes aware of incidents before they make the news. Civilian adolescents serve a supportive function to their friends who are anxious about the safety of a deployed parent and the frustrations associated with repeated absences for deployment. Several interviewees told us that military families are more likely to stay in Watertown during deployment or after the conclusion of military service if their children are in high school or college, in part because of the bonds the teens have formed with civilian peers. Respondents also mentioned that the community's children, both military and civilian, are both more empathetic and also more resilient because of their exposure to the challenges of repeated deployments. Still, we were told by a few interviewees that many teens know more about fatalities than they can effectively handle without adult assistance or a constructive outlet. The docudrama *In My Shoes* was reported by several interviewees to serve as a very important opportunity for teens in the community, both from military and civilian families, to express themselves. One interviewee emphasized that importance:

> *In My Shoes* has . . . [given] a voice to kids. . . . They need more [opportunities] . . . where these kids have a voice about what their experiences are on a regular basis. [Social services provider and spouse of former activated and deployed military Reserve member].

The impact of multiple deployments on civilian teens in the Watertown community was highlighted in a CNN piece that featured the play:

> Amy Lapp, 17, dressed in an Army uniform for her role in *In My Shoes.* Her best friend, Aurora Adams, was one of the military kids who talked about her father, Mark Adams, a chief warrant officer who has deployed several times. Amy saw her friend agonize when a chopper went down in Afghanistan. There was every chance that it might have been her father. "I cry with her," Amy says. "I let her talk and vent as much as possible. I think: 'What if that were my father?'"[7]

Interviewees explained that school faculty and staff, particularly in primary schools, face the added stressors of working with an ever-changing list of students, some of whom leave mid-year when one or both parents deploy, while others appear from another military post before or after a parent's deployment. On return from deployment, parents were reported by school personnel to be "too quick to anger" over little issues like scheduling changes, which in turn affects the children.

**Law Enforcement and Domestic Relations**

Several community members suggested a possible relationship between increases in crime and multiple deployments, but others were unable to make that connection. For example, one leader in the business community stated:

> I'm not sure if it's directly related to the military . . . [Is the] crime rate . . . a little bit higher? People you know basically say yes. . . . There's significant change in the crime rate and of those individuals they may be military family or military dependent. . . . When they're back from deployment . . . we did see more military families needing services . . . some mental health services, intervention when there was physical, emotional abuse within the family. Things like that. [Business leader and former social service provider, civilian]

Implying that crime levels were not associated with multiple deployments, one veteran who is employed at Fort Drum suggested that a particular community leader "would give the line that

---

[7] America's anomaly: The place where war is a constant, http://www.cnn.com/2011/10/07/us/afghanistan-fort-drum/index.html.

crime goes down during a deployment and goes up after one comes home." Despite perceptions among some community members regarding increases in crime and deployment cycles, representatives of emergency services and social service agencies felt uncomfortable drawing conclusions about any relationships between multiple deployments and increases in crime or domestic violence. One of them indicated that Watertown had around 1,800 domestic incidents in the past year, but pointed out that "a little over 10% would somehow be related to the military and that is not abnormal." [Emergency services provider, civilian]

Another community member seemed to understand the stress of deployments on military families, but could not link this to patterns of domestic violence:

> Sometimes, when the troops return, we might see a little spike in domestic violence incidents. But on the whole, it stays level. [Social services provider, civilian]

Law enforcement representatives reported that from 2009 to date, there were five high-profile violent crimes in Watertown and three others in surrounding communities that involved military or their family members. These include a young veteran convicted of killing an adoptive infant, a female soldier who stabbed another in a bar fight, and two armed robberies by a wounded soldier seeking pain killers. We were told these incidents were possibly deployment related, but law enforcement was not aware of any connection between these cases and the deployment histories of those involved.

## Community Competence

Between offerings on post and in the surrounding community, there are many services available to address the challenges presented by multiple deployments. Medical providers and schools have long-standing relationships with the post that have allowed them to institute new strategies as needs arise. Although there are many comprehensive and targeted services available, including some that are free of charge, there are still gaps. Moreover, several interviewees pointed out that these resources are helpful only if people are aware of them and ask for them. In addition, interviewees from the business and health care sectors expressed concern that younger, single soldiers who are not involved in the civilian community may be particularly at risk after deployments.

The needs of the military associated with the multiple deployments, combined with military reliance on civilian medical care and regional collaboration, have prompted a variety of improvements in general and an increase in the specialized medical care available to service members (pre- and postdeployment), military families, and civilians. Recognized interdependence in medical care, education, and economic well-being appears to have enhanced community resilience associated with multiple deployments. The study team was assured in multiple interviews and informal conversations with health care providers that many challenges associated with multiple deployments have been met through the collaborative efforts of military and civilian providers in the region. Two major challenges in this community are an insufficient number of behavioral health care providers, particularly for children, a need that is clearly tied to multiple deployments, and the 70-mile distance for treatment through the Department of Veterans Affairs (VA), for which the connection to multiple deployments is less clear.

## Education

Because there are no schools on Fort Drum, schools in the community have borne a large responsibility for monitoring all children for ill effects of deployment and counseling them about loss and grief. Indian River Central School District has absorbed the largest number of military families: Overall, approximately 66% of the students are children from military families; at two individual elementary schools, they make up more than 80% of the student population.

Several interviewees described how area schools provide support for military and civilian children affected by multiple deployments. Counselors, teachers, and administrators with military/family experience and special school-hosted programs are also available. It appears that schools have become a very important support system to military children, as noted by one school administrator:

> When a soldier dies in combat, [the] FRG gives us information before the official notification. We know quickly. It's outstanding. We coordinate quickly to help the family. . . . A counselor goes into the classroom when the child is pulled from class. That counselor talks to the class. . . . Another counselor, sometimes with a parent, talks to the child. The child goes back to class. . . . The child is out 1 or 2 days for the funeral and . . . back in the classroom with their peers. It's where they want to be. [Educator]

Among the programs implemented in schools to help those affected by multiple deployments, the most frequently mentioned was the Military Family Life Consultants (MFLCs) program. MFLCs have been trained to confidentially address family issues related to multiple deployments and are available to provide information, support, and guidance to all students, parents, teachers, and school staff, regardless of military affiliation.[8] Despite these and other efforts implemented in schools to help children affected by multiple deployments, several interviewees emphasized that more is needed, both in schools and throughout the community. For example, although most large public schools in the area have MFLC programs, we were told that parochial schools and smaller school districts either have few or no MFLCs available to address deployment-related issues.

Jefferson Community College (JCC) was said to provide important services to the community. For example, one college representative explained that the college is working to train more health care professionals, both to meet local service needs and to provide career opportunities for military and civilian residents. At least two interviewees specifically boasted that JCC has increased the size of its registered nurse program and currently offers a nationally ranked program with a 98% first-time board passing rate. JCC reportedly provides courses at Fort Drum, counselors who are knowledgeable about military benefits, a military lounge on campus in Watertown, an inexpensive child care facility, and flexibility in completing courses that are interrupted by deployment or associated stressors.

---

[8] See http://www.ircsd.org/students.cfm?subpage=27341.

## Physical Health Services

Fort Drum and the Watertown area provide a multitude of medical health services to active duty service members, veterans, family members, and community members affected by multiple deployments. Medical services on the post include primary care, a small obstetrician/gynecological clinic, some behavioral health care services, an urgent care clinic, and a specialized recovery unit for wounded soldiers. Within the Jefferson County community, respondents reported that military and civilians have access to primary care, a growing array of specialty care, urgent care, and emergency medical services. The two major hospitals are located in Watertown and Carthage.

Several interviewees described the quality of medical care available in the region as exemplary, and many attributed this high quality to the partnership established between the civilian and military medical communities through the FDRHPO. Because Fort Drum has no hospital on post, service members and their families receive the majority of their health care from civilian doctors. Interviewees emphasized that the military has tried very hard to work with the community to ensure minimal disruption and enhanced medical services for military and civilians alike by infusing money into the civilian hospitals. Consequently, they expressed the view that both military and civilian patients receive top-notch advanced care that is rare, if not nonexistent, in most rural areas.

We also were told that medical practitioners are among the most informed members of the community about what to expect regarding soldiers' needs before and after deployments. Interviewees, including a former manager of a medical specialty practice, told us that they offer more "ASAP" appointments and extended hours immediately before deployments to accommodate the military population. In addition, others are on alert regarding what to expect and when. One person explained how medical organizations prepare for returning deployments:

> [Military and civilian medical personnel meet regularly] . . . so that they can talk about what's happening. What are the challenges? What are the expectations? Who came home from where? And when are we expecting the 90-day [post-deployment] glow to wear off? And what is our plan? And how are we going to work on these things? What kind of training do we need to get done out there? [Regional partnership organization representative, civilian]

## Behavioral and Mental Health Services

One of the greatest negative effects of multiple deployments in the community that was articulated was an increased need for behavioral health care, particularly for children. Only one location in the area, Watertown's Samaritan Medical Center, has an inpatient behavioral health care unit. Many interviewees emphasized this as an issue, and one mentioned waiting lists as long as 6 months for military families and other civilian members of the community. All behavioral health care for military families at Fort Drum is provided in the civilian community.

One person expressed concerns about the lack of community preparedness for dealing with mental health issues that may result from multiple deployments:

> They bring the military guys right from Iraq, drop them off, and go. Do they know anything about our community? Some of them are just coming here for the first time. We are seeing a big [in]flux of PTSD, the calls for family disturbances that we have never seen before. . . . I don't think we are as prepared for the mental part of it as much as we should be. . . . There are a lot of mental issues that none of us really know how to deal with in the community. [Local government employee and spouse of retired military member]

Others expressed more optimism in this area:

> On a positive note, one thing that I have learned through contacts at Fort Drum is that when units come back from deployment, everybody does go through a prescreening for mental-health-type issues . . . they take a pretty active approach to it. Do they get to everybody? And is everybody coming back that's having problems honest with the interviewers? I don't know the answer to that, but I would guess maybe not. But I also know that Samaritan Medical Center . . . [is] there for people that need assistance. . . . Can more be done? I'm sure you can always do more. . . . But I think when things get presented to them, they try to address it. [Emergency services provider, civilian]

Some interviewees reported that there is still some stigma associated with seeking mental health services. One of them was adamant that even a spouse seeking behavioral health services could adversely affect the military member's career:

> If your husband's looking to get promoted, and you as the wife goes and gets help with some mental health issues—for your husband that could affect his promotion. They'd like to say it doesn't, but it does. [Social services provider and spouse of a veteran]

Other interviewees, however, suggest the situation has improved in recent years. One person explained how her husband set an example for his unit:

> My husband is a rock. . . . Nothing shakes him. . . . He, himself, out of his own accord, made an appointment to go to behavioral health. . . . And he's done it for himself . . . and the other reason he did it was to show his soldiers that there was no shame in doing so. If he did it, then they can do it. So his boys have all . . . made the appointments. . . . It is diminishing greatly—the stigma of it. [Medical services provider and spouse of active duty soldier]

**Social Services**

A wide variety of social services are available to military personnel and their families both on the post and in the greater Watertown community. The Jefferson County Department of Social Services (Jefferson County DSS) offers the following services to Jefferson County residents who meet eligibility criteria: volunteer income tax preparation; temporary financial assistance for shelter, fuel and basic needs; medical assistance through participating providers; food stamps; child support enforcement services; custodial care for adults; adult services, including in-home services and transportation; and family and child services to "enhance the preservation of family life."[9] It also compiles a newsletter describing available services and events that is available on the county website.

Specialized social services are also available from private agencies, including the following:

- The Jefferson County Victim's Assistance Center has a 24-hour telephone hotline that can connect victims of sexual assault or domestic violence to emergency shelter services and provide emotional support, information, and referrals. The agency offers individual and group counseling and support groups and a child advocacy center that provides services to child victims and nonoffending family members. The agency also provides community outreach and preventative training and has two advocates at Fort Drum to build rapport and increase accessibility.
- Transitional Living Services of Northern New York (TLS) is a private not-for-profit agency that provides residences, supported housing, and homeless and case management for the mentally ill population. Its 24-hour emergency crisis hotline is available to all community members, including military, and callers can remain anonymous.
- Disabled Persons Action Organization (DPAO) provides developmentally disabled children and adults in Jefferson County and Lewis County with a variety of services geared toward helping families cope with the stress of caring for their disabled loved ones. Its Snoezelen room for sensory stimulation was identified by an interviewee as a unique resource for service members with PTSD.

The limitations of local recordkeeping systems to track data on military affiliation and deployment status may hide issues related to multiple deployments in the community. Several interviewees in key positions indicated that it was difficult to assess whether or not problems could be connected to deployments, simply because many providers do not routinely identify and monitor military or deployment status. One first responder explained:

> Unfortunately, we don't have a mechanism to track whether someone is in the military, related to a military person, or here on behalf of Fort Drum. There [is] just no way for us to track that. But there are times that we are aware of that. . . . I have one, two, three, four, five cases that I would share with you as being [military related]. Two involved deaths, two were shootings, and three others were shooting-assault type situations. And it worries me because guns are involved. [Emergency services provider, civilian]

In sum, there are multiple points at which people can be connected to formal services, and those who provide social services are familiar with a variety of what's available and can provide contact information. In addition, many individual members of this small community were reported to be informed and eager to help those in need find appropriate services. Most agree that there is room for improvement in services that may be required as a result of multiple deployments, but we heard about and witnessed individuals and organizations serving as leaders in addressing key deployment-related needs in one or more sectors of the community.

---

[9] See http://www.co.jefferson.ny.us/index.aspx?page=115.

## Social Capital

Outside of services provided directly by the military, there is a range of efforts to support deployment-related issues. Three organizations are mentioned on the army.mil community covenant page for Fort Drum, namely, the Association of the U.S. Army (AUSA), the Adopt a 10th Mountain Platoon Program, and FDRLO. These organizations, which are linked to the Army but not funded by it, were also commonly mentioned by interviewees as informal supports to which community members can turn to minimize or address issues related to multiple OEF/OIF deployments.

Membership in AUSA, a private nonprofit organization, is available to all individuals, as well as to companies that wish to show support for Army communities. AUSA supports several programs that were specifically mentioned by interviewees. These include Adopt a 10th Mountain Platoon, which, like similar programs around the country, gets local organizations to send care packages to deployed soldiers. Interviewees said what makes this program unique is that every unit deployed from Fort Drum has had a sponsor, and it is not uncommon for organizations to hold events with soldiers before or after a deployment.

Many interviewees also cited Operation Yellow Ribbon, a partnership between Fort Drum leaders and North Country communities, as an important informal support. The organization encourages the display of yellow ribbons and the 10th Mountain Division insignia throughout the civilian community to recognize soldiers' service and, as appropriate, to signify retail discounts. During our visit, we observed yellow ribbons displayed on many businesses, faith and service organizations, and government office buildings.

Also present is an involved faith community, which was described as interconnected and a significant source of deployment-related support. Several interviewees mentioned that a meeting held in November 2010 between civilian clergy and military chaplains was a key to addressing issues around multiple deployments for military and their families, as well as the community as a whole.[10]

Online social networks were also seen as an important set of informal supports for connecting people about important issues. One Army spouse said that she set up a private group on the Facebook website to connect soldiers under her husband's command and, at home, the units' spouses and adolescent children. She described it as a way to get pictures of important community events, such as school graduations, to soldiers in the field so that they could remain connected. Other persons mentioned online bulletin boards (such as craigslist.org "rants and raves") as sounding boards used by a handful of individuals—military, veteran, and civilian—to vent and communicate about a range of community issues.

Several interviewees suggested that it would be an improvement to provide something constructive in the community for young soldiers—the 18- to 20-year-olds—to do off duty, perhaps including athletics or another activity that allows them to connect to one another and/or to civilians. Two interviews also highlighted the need to provide additional support to those soldiers coming back from deployment "to no one, while everyone else hugs their wives and

[10] See http://www.watertowndailytimes.com/article/20101118/NEWS03/311189981/-1/NEWS.

kisses their kids," or worse, to a process server handing them divorce papers. One community member expressed an understanding of the struggle faced by single soldiers returning to Fort Drum after deployment:

> If you're a younger person in the military . . . the single soldiers . . . [there's] such a stigma . . . with mental health . . . there needs to be something more there for soldiers to . . . invest in. So that when they're back here or back from deployment, there's a purpose. . . . Lord only knows what they see. . . . So to be able to come back and be a part of something . . . if you don't have your family here. [Business leader and former social service provider, civilian]

## SUMMARY

Watertown, the surrounding area of Jefferson County, and Fort Drum are working effectively, although not seamlessly, to support a blended community in the wake of significant growth of the post since 2004–2005. Civilian and military leaders have made joint progress in addressing challenges in the community associated with multiple deployments. Meeting the unmet needs and supporting community strength will require continued collaboration and creative problem solving.

### What's Working

For the most part, the Watertown area is very supportive of Fort Drum soldiers and their families. In the face of challenges associated with post expansion and related community growth, the civilian and military communities in Watertown and surrounding Jefferson County appear to have cultivated a mutually respectful and beneficial partnership. Symbols of the community's appreciation for Fort Drum soldiers and their families is evident; yellow ribbons and the 10th Mountain Division insignia appeared on road side signs, on banners on buildings, and on flyers in store front windows.

- The **city's agencies and services are well networked** and communicate regularly among one another. Several key agencies communicate regularly with and receive training from experts associated with Fort Drum, notably regarding policing, EMS, schooling, housing, and counseling in the faith community.
- **Adopt a 10th Mountain Platoon** has ensured that every company is connected to a sponsor to receive letters and care packages when deployed, as well as optional social networking and support before and after deployment.
- The **Fort Drum Regional Health Planning Organization** connects civilian and military medical providers and records, as well as providing military families with information about local health care options.
- The locally written and performed play ***In My Shoes*** offers adolescents from both military and civilian families the opportunity to express and discuss their feelings about multiple deployments and initiate a series of community conversations about their experiences and needs.

## Needs

- **Mental health services,** particularly for children, were identified by many interviewees as the largest current and anticipated need for the community, in part because of national shortages.
- The **long duration of deployments and short time back home** to relax and reconnect between missions pose stressors on soldiers and families that affect social networks and community resilience over time.
- Efforts to **identify soldiers** who may return from deployment without family or other social supports present were requested. Programs may be needed to connect or reconnect these individuals to community resources.
- More **proactive information** throughout the community about what families and civilians might expect from returning soldiers over time (e.g., PTSD) and how best to address their needs is needed. In addition, community agencies might provide more data about trends to inform and dispel any incorrect perceptions about, for example, crime among returning soldiers.
- **Continued communication and planning** is imperative to ensure that collaborative efforts supporting positive civilian-military connections persist.

## Suggestions from the Community

- Integrate medical records and benefits systems between DOD and VA.*
- Proactively provide more/visible information about potential mental health needs associated with deployments to help reduce the stigma in the community and help the community respond effectively to posttraumatic stress issues.*
- Provide young soldiers with mandatory counseling on better use of their money.*
- Make seed money available for creative collaborative solutions to the challenges that face military communities.*
- Provide constructive activities in the community for 18- to 20-year-old soldiers to do off duty, perhaps including athletics or a business that allows them a space to connect to one another and/or to civilians in the community.*
- Rotate MFLCs in schools less often; they need time to build rapport.
- Involve soldiers and their spouses more deeply as leaders in education systems to help bridge the gap between the challenges faced by the military and civilian communities and identify potential solutions.
- Support artistic outlets, particularly those that provide constructive outlets for children, and foster communication between the military and civilian communities.*

*Suggestions noted with asterisks were cited by multiple interviewees.

# Lakewood and Lacey, Washington

Case Study Report

# Impacts of Multiple Deployments: Lakewood and Lacey, Washington

## OVERVIEW

Joint Base Lewis-McChord (JBLM), home to about 45,000 active duty service members, is located about an hour south of Seattle, Washington. During a week-long site visit (May 16–22, 2012) to two nearby cities—Lakewood and Lacey—representatives from both communities provided their perspectives on the diverse effects of multiple deployments on their cities.

As in other sites, interviewees were not able to determine if recent changes in the local economy (primarily large-scale growth) were related to multiple deployments or Base Realignment and Closure (BRAC) decisions. A joint planning partnership between JBLM and Lakewood has been established to manage this growth over time. Community members and mental health providers alike did report a recent increase in posttraumatic stress disorder (PTSD) symptoms among returning service members, as well as other behavioral health issues that have potential long-term effects for the communities. Many believed these issues to be a result of the multiple deployments of service members to Iraq and Afghanistan. School representatives also reported behavioral problems among younger children from military families, as well as some negative experiences with stressed military parents. In response, school district leaders are working closely with the command to implement school-based programs to support military families and students. A major identified need is for more behavioral health services for military families, both on base and in the community.

**Data Sources**

**Lakewood, Washington**

- City Government (City Manager and Asst. City Manager)
- Department of Economic Development
- South Sound Military and Communities Partnership
- Department of Human Services
- School District Superintendents
- Mental Health Providers
- Public Health Administrator
- Faith-Based Housing & Social Services Provider
- Boys and Girls Club
- YMCA
- Police Department
- Lakewood City Council Member
- Realtor Group
- Hospital Administrator
- Kiwanis Club
- Armed Forces Day Events at JBLM
- Ethnographic Observation

**Lacey, Washington**

- City Government (Mayor and City Manager)
- Department of Recreation and Parks
- Police Department
- School District Administrator
- Lacey Spring Fair
- Ethnographic Observation

## GEOGRAPHIC ORIENTATION

### Community: Lakewood, Washington

Lakewood is located in Pierce County, about an hour south of Seattle. Originally settled in 1849 by the U.S. Army, the city evolved during the 20th century into an urban region outside of Tacoma and was incorporated as a city in 1996. Lakewood borders the northern edge of JBLM, which includes the National Guard's Washington State headquarters at Camp Murray (Figure 1). The layout of the city is an urban/suburban model with pockets of rural areas, some of which surround a lake community that was established as a resort area in the early part of the 20th century. The city is a popular area for sportsmen and tourists. Census data for 2010 indicate that Lakewood has a population of about 60,000 residents, most of whom are English speaking and under the age of 55.[1] Approximately 44% of Lakewood households are married couples living together, and about 30% have children under the age of 18. Lakewood officials said that about 10% of Lakewood residents are active duty military living off base.[2]

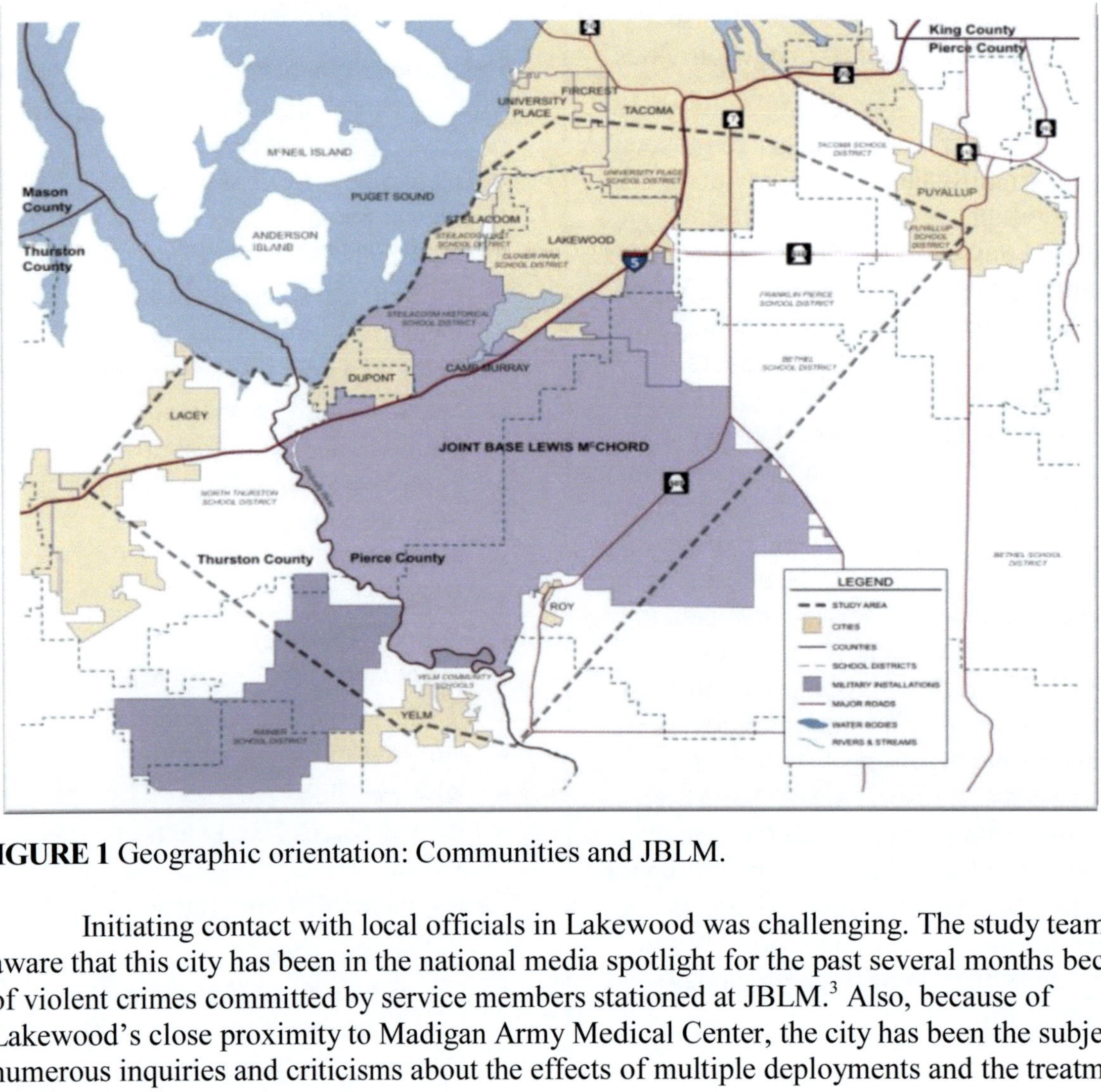


**FIGURE 1** Geographic orientation: Communities and JBLM.

Initiating contact with local officials in Lakewood was challenging. The study team was aware that this city has been in the national media spotlight for the past several months because of violent crimes committed by service members stationed at JBLM.[3] Also, because of Lakewood's close proximity to Madigan Army Medical Center, the city has been the subject of numerous inquiries and criticisms about the effects of multiple deployments and the treatment of

[1] See also http://www.cityoflakewood.us/community/about-lakewood.

[2] This was validated by a regional population distribution chart the team received during its interview with the Lacey City Manager.

[3] Examples of media coverage include the following: "Home Base of Accused Soldier Has Faced Scrutiny," New York Times, March 13, 2012. (http://www.nytimes.com/2012/03/14/us/more-scrutiny-of-lewis-mcc); "Branding a Soldier with 'Personality Disorder,'" New York Times, February 24, 2012 (http://www.nytimes.com/2012/02/25/us/a-military-diagnosis-perso), "Madigan Team Reversed 40 Percent of PTSD Diagnoses," *News Tribune*, March 21, 2012 (http://www.thenewstribune.com/2012/03/21/v-printerfriendly/2076608).

service members who have been diagnosed with PTSD. After the study team did make contact with local officials, team members learned that city officials have been fielding calls from the media on a daily basis, leading them to become wary of granting interviews and reluctant to discuss issues related to JBLM. When one nongovernment interviewee was told how difficult it had been to make contact with the city, she laughed and knowingly said, "Yep, circling the wagons." Study findings suggest that Lakewood is a community that is proud and supportive of service members and their families, all of whom are woven seamlessly into the larger fabric of the city. Limiting outsiders' access to the city is simply one more way in which Lakewood supports its military residents.

**Community:**
**Lacey**

Lacey, Washington, is located in northern Thurston County, about a 10-minute drive west of JBLM on Interstate 5 (I-5). Although Lakewood originated as an offshoot of Tacoma, Lacey was established as a suburb of Olympia, the state capital. According to 2010 Census data, most Lacey residents are white, English-speaking, and under the age of 45. A little more than 50% of city households in 2010 were married couples living together, and nearly 35% of those households had children under the age of 18. Lacey does not physically border JBLM; however, data received from the Lacey City Manager's Office indicated that 16% of the city's approximately 42,000 residents are active duty personnel. Lacey has a regional reputation for being family-friendly and is known to attract service members and their families.

Lacey, in the words of one local official, is "*South of the River*" and physically separated from Lakewood and most of JBLM by a bridge. Making contacts with officials in Lacey proved to be a relatively simple task and officials were willing to speak with the study team about the impacts of the deployments on this city, which has not received the media attention experienced by Lakewood. City officials noted that although a high number of military families live in Lacey, it has not been stigmatized around the issue of PTSD the way Lakewood has been:

> Many of the families as well as the single service men have said that people "North of the River" do not welcome them into their community. They said that's not true of Lacey. People that move here, who come into Lacey say, "This community is different than any other we've lived in. People like us here, they're not antimilitary, there's no perceived bias that we have PTSD or that we're bad people. People accept us, they welcome us . . . our neighbors are friendly." [City official]

**Military Installation: Joint Base Lewis-McChord**
**(JBLM)**

JBLM is the largest military installation in the western United States, covering more than 415,000 acres. It was formally established as a joint base on October 1, 2010, through the merging of Fort Lewis (Army) and McChord Air Base (Air Force) under BRAC decisions.[4] An Army-led joint base garrison provides all installation functions to the Army, Air Force, Navy,

[4] See http://www.lewis-mcchord.army.mil.

and Marine Corps Services that operate on base. In addition to the estimated 45,000 active duty personnel assigned to JBLM, there are about 7,500 civilians and Department of Defense employees and another 5,000 contractors who work on base.

In 2011, the South Sound Military and Communities Partnership (SSMCP)[5] conducted a "Community Needs Survey of Joint Base Lewis-McChord Personnel and Families" in collaboration with JBLM Garrison Command.[6] The purpose of the study was to provide the SSMCP, JBLM, and local communities with a demographic profile of JBLM personnel and military families living in the area and to identify needs for services and supports. These needs would be targeted for improvement to keep up with the expected growth at the installation in the coming years. Among the approximately 3,250 survey respondents, 66% were active duty service members or their spouses. The 2011 survey included questions relevant to this ethnographic study of the region:

- 40% of service members had been stationed at JBLM for a year or less. Only 35% of service members had been assigned to JBLM (on the current tour) for 3 years or longer. Length of stationing at JBLM tended to be longer for Air Force service members (4+ years) than for Army service members (3 or fewer years).
- 77% of active duty respondents had been deployed at least once since September 2001, and one-third of them had been deployed three or more times. The number of deployments tended to be slightly higher for service members in the Air Force (3+ deployments) than for Army soldiers.
- Nearly 40% of service members stationed at JBLM said they had been deployed within the past 2 years.

Most interviewees seemed aware that multiple deployments are the norm for service members, with several government and community leaders saying they had heard of individuals receiving orders to go on their fourth, fifth, and sometimes sixth deployments. Local leaders also suggested that the time between deployments seems to be getting shorter, especially for those in Special Forces (e.g., sniper squadrons). A social service provider offered the following observation:

> I think when a civilian sees a 20–40 something soldier in uniform or finds out that they are a veteran, it is just assumed by the civilian that the veteran has been deployed multiple times. I think most people find it rare to meet a soldier who has not deployed in
> support of conflicts over the past decade and the younger the solider or veteran appears to be, the more deployments are assumed.

Several interviewees also discussed the return of about 10,000 service members from two Stryker brigades during the summer of 2010 and how the influx of a large number of people in such a short time affected the region. Figure 2 depicts a bar graph extracted from the 2010 JBLM Growth Coordination Plan that shows the patterns of deployments and returns for Army

[5] The SSMCP is described in more detail later in the report.

[6] See http://jblm-growth.com/sites/default/files/JBLM%20Survey%20Report%20Final.pdf

service members stationed at JBLM between 2004 and 2010.[7] During 2009 and 2010 in particular, the region clearly experienced several fluctuations in its population as a result of large-scale deployments to the wars in the Middle East.

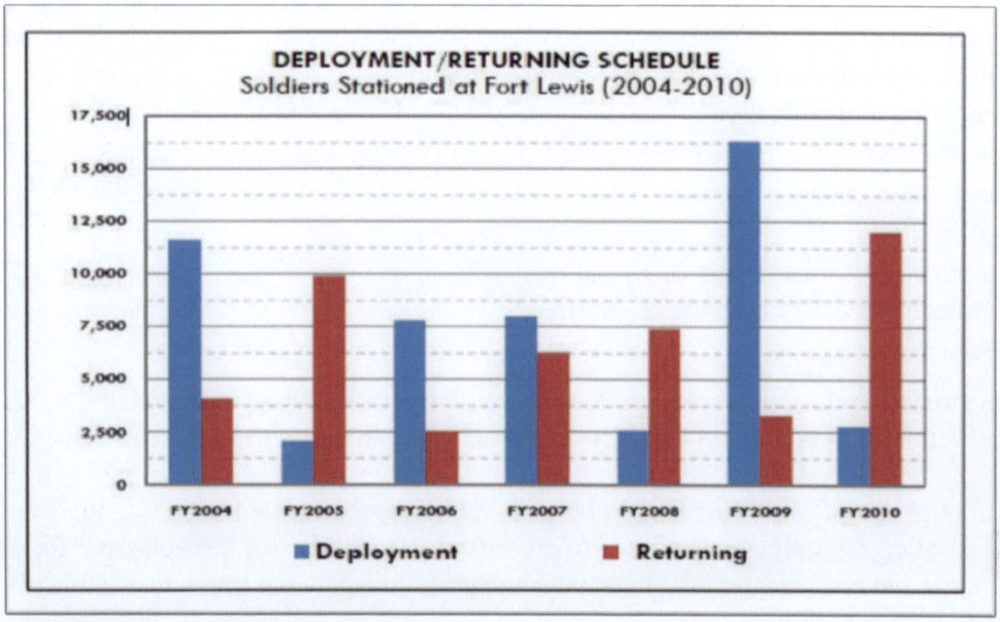


**FIGURE 2** Deployment/returning schedule JBLM 2004–2010.

**Relationship Between Communities and Base**

Interviews and observations suggest that service members and their families are not seen as strangers or temporary residents, but are regarded as regular members of these communities. Service members are routinely seen in camouflage fatigues at local stores and restaurants, and vehicles bearing Department of Defense stickers are a part of everyday life in these cities. Every person interviewed by the study team either had personal experience in the military (often at JBLM), or was directly related to or otherwise acquainted with someone stationed at JBLM. In support of this observation, both Lakewood and Lacey have statues in prominent locations that pay tribute to service members and their families.

In 2009, Lakewood was awarded a grant from the Department of Defense Office of Economic Adjustment (DOD-OEA) to conduct a regional study to identify and prepare for the impacts of the merging of Fort Lewis and McChord Air Force Base that had begun a few years earlier under BRAC. That effort led to the creation of the South Sound Military and Communities Partnership (SSMCP), which was established within the Lakewood City Department of Economic Development and now operates under the City Manager's Office. The SSMCP serves to foster communication, planning, and collaboration between JBLM and regional communities. The SSMCP coordinated the regional impact study and released thefindings to the public in the 2010 JBLM Growth Coordination Plan.[8] The study identified

[7] Air Force personnel were also deployed from JBLM during this time period but those data were not available to the research team.
[8] See http://www.jblm-growth.com/plan.

portions of the region that could anticipate the greatest impact of growth from JBLM, and recommendations were generated to address the following core needs:

- System of planning, coordination, and collaboration between local communities and JBLM
- Housing (low-cost rentals and privately owned)*
- Education and child care*
- Transportation and traffic*
- Land use (regional planning)
- Public safety
- Community infrastructure (e.g., utilities)
- Physical and behavioral health services*
- Social services

* These items represent community domains with multiple-deployment-related effects identified both in the JBLM Growth Coordination Plan and during the site visit.

Although the SSMCP regional study and resulting growth plan were intended to identify a broad scale of community needs related to growth at JBLM, lessons learned from the needs assessment and the resulting action plans have helped to mitigate the impacts of multiple deployments on this region.

## EFFECTS OF MULTIPLE DEPLOYMENTS ON THE COMMUNITIES

Interviewees did not attribute recent economic changes to multiple deployments, but did report numerous behavioral health issues that they believed to be tied to this deployment pattern. Contributing to this perception were several recent violent events committed by service members from JBLM. Although numerous formal and informal services and supports are available in the community, interviewees indicated the need for a more comprehensive community-based behavioral health system. The current system capacity, they said, was insufficient to meet the current needs of service members and their families, and interviewees anticipated these challenges to persist well after the drawdown of troops in Afghanistan.

### Economic Impact

Multiple deployments of service members from JBLM do not appear to have had large-scale direct effects on general commerce and consumer demand, employment, and the housing markets in Lakewood and Lacey.

#### General Commerce and Consumer Demand

Multiple deployments do not appear to have had a major impact on commerce and demand for consumer goods and services in Lakewood and Lacey. Expansion of businesses in these cities is ongoing, but seems to be related more to the general population growth at JBLM than to the deployment and return of service members. Local businesses around Lakewood did experience an increase in demand in 2010 after the return of the two Stryker brigades, which, in turn, brought an increase in city tax revenues for the third and fourth quarters of 2010 and the first quarter of 2011. Officials in both cities also mentioned that, upon returning from deployment, younger soldiers (those in their twenties) tend to make high-dollar purchases, such as expensive vehicles and recreational equipment. Younger soldiers who do not have family in the area usually need to purchase civilian clothing and furniture and find a place to live if they are unable to stay on base. Interviewees, however, did not describe a purchasing pattern reflecting multiple deployments among service members.

Lakewood's public website describes the city as having about 1,100 businesses.[9] Discussions with a variety of interviewees in the city, including staff from the Department of Economic Development, suggested that Lakewood receives a great deal of daily business from active duty personnel, family members, and affiliated persons working at JBLM. Several of the main entry gates are located on the Lakewood side of the base, making this city the closest location for those seeking meals and other resources (e.g., department stores) off base. This was confirmed by the study team's personal observations while in town. It was not unusual to enter a local restaurant at lunchtime and see at least half of the patrons dressed in camouflage fatigues.

Lacey, which is a few minutes' drive from JBLM, has a variety of newly built shopping areas, restaurants, and hotels, especially near I-5 exits. Business appeared to be steady around town and seemed to be concentrated in the morning and late afternoon/evening during weekdays and throughout the day on the weekends.

**Employment**

According to interviewees, multiple deployments from JBLM have had some impact on employment in this region. Some employers, they said, have had to deal with staff turnover when spouses of deployed service members leave the area. They reported that this has been more of a problem for specially trained and/or certified employees, such as nurses and teachers, because they are difficult to replace. Some employers reportedly have been reluctant to hire spouses of service members out of concern that they may stay only for a short time and need to be replaced. One employer said

> You have the issue of military spouses getting work. They're probably not going to be here more than 2 or 3 years; employers here know that and I think that impacts the spouse's ability to get good, long-term employment.

In addition, a couple of interviewees said they have heard comments from community members, including a few local employers, about a reluctance to hire service members who have separated from the military because employers have concerns about these veterans' emotional stability. Some interviewees wondered if the message about this bias might be reaching service members, given that some retired soldiers have not been listing their military service on job applications.

---

[9] See www.cityoflakewood.us.

## Housing

Seventy-two percent of JBLM active military and their family members live off base in local communities, mostly in Lacey, Lakewood, and Tacoma. During interviews with staff from the SSMCP and Lakewood city government, the study team learned that some family members leave Lakewood to stay with relatives while their service members are deployed. Although a precise number was not given, one official commented that "it feels like 50%." An example was given by a city official who is a regularly attending member of a local church located close to JBLM; he said that the church experienced a 50% drop in attendance after family members moved away during a deployment. In Lacey, such departures are reportedly less common. Lacey government officials reported that not only do family members tend to stay in Lacey during the service members' deployment, but often other family/supports arrive in Lacey to stay with them.

Interviews with officials from Lakewood city government and a focus group conducted with 13 regional real estate agents suggested that the multiple deployments have created a mindset among service members that has had a negative impact on the local housing market. For decades, service members had been purchasing homes in the region because they expected to be stationed at JBLM for a few years. Even if deployed, many expected to return to JBLM and live in the area for a while. In recent years, however, home sales have declined, particularly around Lakewood, and increasing numbers of families stationed at JBLM have turned to renting. Local real estate agents believed the switch from ownership to renting has been related to a few factors:

- Service members are no longer secure in knowing how long they will be stationed at JBLM. The current trend has been for service members to be based at JBLM for only a few years before being transferred to another base. Sometimes orders for transfer come during deployment, in which case family members may need to move before the service member returns. This has made it difficult, and impractical in some instances, for service members to purchase a home and "commit" to a community.
- Younger service members seem to choose Lakewood for residency given its proximity to the base, and this age group tends to represent a "renting" population.
- Renting has become a more desirable option for service members whose spouses may move out of the area during the deployment.
- When some service members get orders to move to a new base, they need to sell their homes quickly and sometimes take a financial loss on the sale. This type of financial loss may affect a service member's credit score, which, if too low, could interfere with the individual's security clearance.

Data from the *2011 Community Needs Survey* support interviewees' reports of a decline in home buying and an increase in rentals in the area. The survey indicates that approximately 60% of active duty service members who live off base rent. Staff from Lakewood's Department of Economic Development reported that the decrease in home ownership has led to a decrease in the use of home-related services, such as lawn care, construction, and the like. During the realtors' focus group, one interviewee said that every home sale results in an additional $60,000 in spending in the local economy of Lakewood; the decline in sales, this individual believed, has thus had an effect on local revenues. Further research indicates that this figure more accurately reflects new home construction and that in Washington State, a typical home sale yields up to $42,500 in a combination of income generated from real estate activities, consumer purchases such as furniture and remodeling, and a "multiplier effect" of spending on local restaurants, sporting events, and so forth.[10]

The realtors' comments notwithstanding, it cannot be ruled out that some of the changes in home ownership in this region are related not to service members' deployment experiences, but to the economic downturn of the last few years. Additional research would need to be conducted in order to determine how much deployment experiences have figured into service members' decisions.

**Transportation**

The most frequently mentioned issue that interviewees of all types tended to tie to the deployments from JBLM had to do with increased traffic in the area. This was most evident in the summer of 2010 when about 10,000 service members returned to JBLM (followed by any family members that had left temporarily) and joined daily commuter traffic on I-5. Lakewood and the SSMCP have been working on securing DOD/Office of Economic Adjustment (DOD-OEA) grants and funding from the Washington State Department of Transportation to upgrade the roads because traffic is expected to increase over time. A Lacey official described how the multiple deployments negatively affect traffic in his city[11]:

> When [service members are deployed], family stays here. . . . A great deal of time other members of the family come up . . . and they stay here for a while and they bring in other cars during that 9-month period when the military component is gone. So that has a major impact on our roadways, on our corridor.

Officials in these communities noted that they continue to work with JBLM and officials in Washington to figure out ways to alleviate the transportation stresses caused by multiple deployments.

**Information and Communication**

Lakewood government officials and the school districts have good channels of communication with JBLM. Lacey community leaders receive military information more informally, as do local residents. They rely on public media, personal communications with people they know who work at JBLM, and online information to learn about JBLM activities and resources.

---

[10] Economic Impact of Real Estate Activity: Washington. National Association of Realtors Research, February 2012. Available at http://www.realtor.org/sites/default/files/reports/2012/economic-impact-real-estate-activity-washington-2012-02.pdf.

[11] This same official also indicated that despite the adverse effects of the traffic increases, incoming family members have helped the local economy generally: "We would like to say we also are enhanced somewhat with the additional monies they bring in to spend in our communities and we reap the sales taxes and other fees and taxes they pay while they're here."

**Public Discussion of Deployment-Related Issues**

During interviews, the team asked respondents how information about the deployments and demobilizations are communicated in the region and how residents learn about available resources. Respondents in the "general public" said they "formally" learn about the deployments from local TV and print media, but often obtain information informally from relatives or acquaintances assigned to JBLM. Although the personal and family challenges related to multiple deployments, such as mental health disorders and family stress, were mentioned in a variety of community contexts and during the course of several interviews, several interviewees, including the police, indicated relatively poor communication about services available for managing deployment-related disorders, such as PTSD.

**Communication Between JBLM and City Government**

Lakewood's government officials are kept apprised of deployment schedules through the SSMCP's ongoing planning partnership with JBLM. In addition, the city's Department of Social Services facilitates the Lakewood Community Collaboration, a community organization that includes representatives from numerous social service agencies who meet quarterly. A military representative from Army Community Services (ACS) is invited and often attends.

In contrast to Lakewood, Lacey government officials said they tend to learn about deployments the same way as the general public, that is, through the media or personal contacts affiliated with JBLM. The only group indicating it had a *formal* system of communication to learn about the deployment schedule was the Clover Park School District (CPSD), which operates the schools around Lakewood and on JBLM. Details about this communication effort are described in the next section of the report. Law enforcement officials noted a strong relationship with their counterparts at JBLM, but said they learn about deployments and demobilizations through "word of mouth."

**Communication Between JBLM and Local Law Enforcement**

The relationship with, access to, and communication between local law enforcement and JBLM seemed to differ by city. Lakewood police described an "excellent relationship with JBLM," well-established formal connections with the military police, and an ability to always be in communication with JBLM as needed. All incidents involving a service member are immediately directed to officials at JBLM and "all staff know how to contact the provost marshal or MP [military police unit] on base." A JBLM liaison officer is stationed at the Lakewood police station every weekend, specifically to deal with any service member who becomes involved in police-related activity. Lacey police described a different relationship. Although they are part of a law-enforcement breakfast group in South County that is attended by the JBLM provost marshal, this venue does not result in regular communication between the city and JBLM or a way to address arrests involving service members. Information about troop deployment and return cycles are learned informally (e.g., through personal contacts and acquaintances on base) by the Lacey police; there is no formal notice for the city of when to expect deployment-related changes.

### Information Sources for Military Families

JBLM has extensive information about military-sponsored services available to military members and their families, including a downloadable orientation document. Family Readiness Groups (FRGs) appear to be available to all military members and their families and can be an important source of information and support, especially for the nondeployed spouse. There was evidence of some informal networks, such as Facebook pages for South Sound military spouses, and the team learned of some efforts within the community to reach out to military families. Yet except for the YMCA, which offers programs for military families, identifying or connecting with these programs during the site visit proved difficult. Armed Forces Day, held on base and open to the public, had virtually no community-based (off-base) resources advertised to military families except for the Veterans of Foreign Wars (VFW) and the American Legion. There was no outward evidence of support groups, for example, and there were no faith-based organizations, social services, mental health, or child care organizations present at this event. Yet one of the most important services mentioned by every person interviewed was the need for behavioral and mental health information, education, and counseling related to multiple deployments. Services to meet the mental health needs of service members and their families were described as not readily available and with long waiting lists. Yet the few nonmilitary organizations at the event included only mortgage services, Internet-based educational programs for college degrees, and chiropractors.

## Community Health

In discussions about the effects of multiple deployments on community health, interviewees focused on the spillover effects in school of deployment-related stress experienced by children and their parents. They also discussed perceptions that service members who have been deployed multiple times are returning home with PTSD and a concomitant propensity for violence.

### Children's Issues

School district representatives said that some children from military families, especially those of elementary age, have exhibited behavioral problems. They discussed issues they see their students from military families confronting, such as dealing with the culture that comes with living on base, dealing with one or both parents being deployed, having to move and being uprooted every few years, and experiencing the loss of family members. They described these children and their parents as experiencing periods of readjustment both when a parent deploys and when the parent returns. Interviewees described school-age children with a deployed parent as often having difficulty with anger management and dealing with feelings of loss. They also said some children seem to internalize their feelings about the deployed parent and worry about the parent who has stayed home and who must assume new responsibilities and the role of a single parent.

Interviewees from the school districts and community programs also talked about the challenges that many families face when service members return home. This relearning and change of roles when the service member returns can be just as stressful as when that parent deployed, as described by one community interviewee:

One parent described how her children thought their Dad was coming back. They thought he would be the same person, laugh the same way, act the same way to them, but he is a different person now.

School representatives and community program staff also described seeing an increase of "belligerent" behavior from parents in military families toward school and program staff in the past few years. The interviewees said they assume the behavior comes from parents who are dealing with the stress of single parenting during multiple deployments and then reconnecting and reestablishing the family roles when the service member returns. This has been especially challenging for families in which there is only a short period of time between deployments. Said one program staff member:

> They (service members) don't have enough time to shut it off (state of constant vigilance needed for combat situations) before they go out again.

The school systems have responded to their students' needs by making mental health supports more available and finding ways to honor military families through special events (see the Community Competence section). Many school representatives suggested that mental health counseling was a significant need for children from military families, especially those with deployed parents.

**Service Members' Behaviors**

Interviews with law enforcement officers offered a mixed picture of service member behaviors that affect the community and are possibly related to multiple deployments. Lacey officers reported that in recent years the city has been experiencing an increase in domestic violence calls, as well as an increase in arrests of service members driving while intoxicated. In the past few years, they said, officers in this city have been encountering negative attitudes toward law enforcement from some of the service members:

> The other thing we've noticed . . . the military members who are arrested have an *extremely* different view of the police department. . . . It's markedly different and it's only been in the past 4 to 5 years that we've seen the change, but it's a *radical* change. It's a disrespect for law enforcement, just a complete and utter disrespect. We're lower than potato peelers and privates to them. Whereas before that it was "Sir, yes, Officer"—it was very formal 4 or 5 years ago, now it's "You're not my chain of command, expletive, expletive, expletive." That's pretty routinely what we're running into now. I don't know what exactly changed to fuel that, but something changed. It's very noticeable.

In addition, Lacey police reported encountering increasing numbers of service members who, while under arrest, have said doctors told them that their diagnosis of PTSD "excused them" from being charged with any crime.

In contrast, the Lakewood Police were not able to identify differences in service members' behavior from any other time in the past 25 years. While they did describe encountering incidents of after-hours disorderly conduct from service members, no tie was made to the deployment cycles or population increases at JBLM. In fact, Lakewood police described these incidents as "business as usual."

Numerous interviewees in both cities spoke about relatively recent, local incidents of serious, negative behavior involving service members that reached the media. There were at least two instances of attempted suicide by service members: one that necessitated response by a SWAT team, and a second incident that involved the fatal shooting of a service member who had a gun pointed at police. They also cited two recent hostage situations involving active duty service members, one of whom was an officer. Interviewees described these events as being sensationalized in the press, which has added to an increasing perceived association between local crime and PTSD. Members of the Lacey Police Department suggested that a component should be integrated into local police training so that they can be better prepared to understand issues related to combat and stresses felt by returning service members.

Hospital representatives also reported seeing an increase in patients with PTSD symptoms and "special needs" instructions, such as to not slam doors, enter quietly, and so forth, related to PTSD. Although no data were provided, representatives of the health care system described seeing increased smoking and use of alcohol and more obesity, on top of PTSD and traumatic brain injuries, among service members and that the incidence of these health issues was higher upon return from deployments. They expressed concern that these trends will have significant public health effects that the community will have to absorb for years to come.

## Community Competence

Interviewees described a wide array of services and supports available for service members and their families. These include various school-based services for military youth and numerous formal services and supports for service members dealing with either physical or emotional injuries related to multiple deployments. Despite the variety of resources, community members expressed the need for additional services to a demand they perceived to be increasing.

### Education

Community representatives from both Lakewood and Lacey described having relatively large populations of students from military families (military dependent children) in some of their schools. Site visit interviews focused primarily on the Clover Park School District (CPSD) because it runs all of the schools on JBLM. Out of 25 elementary schools in the CPSD, 6 operate on base, with a population of 90% or more military dependent children in attendance. Two additional schools are located very close to the base and also have high numbers of military dependent children. In other elementary schools in this district, about 15% of the students are from military families. All secondary schools in the district are located off base, and in three of them military dependent children make up 50% to 75% of the population. Recognition of the military presence in the CPSD was noticeable. The CPSD administrative offices are located in one local school and had "Welcome Home" posters developed by the city of Lakewood in the student services building. CPSD also had a picture of a service member in uniform in its most recent annual report.

As noted previously, the school district was the only agency interviewed during the site visit that appeared to receive any direct communication about deployment cycles. The CPSD interfaces with a military liaison at JBLM who attends school board meetings and provides teacher training on military life and issues affecting military dependent children. CPSD representatives also noted that the superintendent meets monthly with the garrison commander. Communication has been more frequent in the past 2 years as the district prepares to rebuild five of the six schools located on base. Yet despite the open lines of communication, the SSMCP report indicated that regional schools are affected negatively by multiple deployments that result in either overburdened or underused classrooms; the report also indicated that district schools receive short notice of population changes that will affect staffing and budgets.[12] Families in these districts tend to be "mobile"; interviewees cited a 50% mobility rate of students, the majority of which is attributable to military moves. School district administrators described this constant transition of students as having a negative impact on the schools and the children themselves, who may be relocated in the middle of a school year.

CPSD has several programs to help students in their districts cope with impacts from the deployments and other issues associated with a military presence in the area. In the CPSD, schools located on base, in partnership with JBLM, can access a school-based mental health program that provides psychiatric care to all students in the schools if requested. The administration of this program is being piloted through CPSD, which is the second district in the country to use it.[13] The schools also have access to licensed social workers and other licensed/credentialed master's-level or Ph.D.-level practitioners through Military Family Life Consultants (MFLCs), who provide outreach to students and their families needing mental health and other support services (e.g., formal counseling sessions or referrals to other resources). CPSD has also benefited by receiving several Department of Defense Education Activity (DoDEA) grants, one for academic support and professional development and another for providing school-based mental health counselors in three of the secondary schools off base that have high military-dependent student populations. At the time of the site visit, this grant program was in its second year and was cited as very successful. The counselors' presence in the schools was described as providing support either informally, by talking in the hallway, or by formal counseling sessions with children and family members, or both. At the time of the site visit, the CPSD also was waiting to hear about an award of a $2.5 million grant to fund mental health services.

The North Thurston Public School (NTPS) district, which serves Lacey, also has programs in place to support the estimated 20% of the district's student population who are from military families. For example, NTPS secured a DoDEA grant to provide children in 6 of their 13 elementary schools with positive behavioral social and emotional supports. These include support groups for children with parents who have been deployed to allow them an opportunity to share with other children who are in similar situation at home. These lunch-time groups have engaged parents, including nondeployed spouses, to share what it is like to adjust to being the only parent

[12] See the Joint Base Lewis-McChord Growth Coordination Plan (December 2010), available at www.jblm-growth.com.
[13] The program has been modeled after a successful program administered in on-base schools in Hawaii.

at home. Returning service members also attend and share what it was like to be separated from the family. Other activities sponsored by the NTPS include participating in the creation of special floats to honor children from military families in the local town parade and provide them with "bracelets" that help instill a sense of pride in their service member parents.

The school programs are supplemented by community programs that offer support to children and their parents. Discussions with staff from community programs such as the Boys and Girls Club, the Kiwanis Club, and the YMCA suggest that these and other local programs recognize the unique stressors that military families have been experiencing from the deployments.

**Physical and Mental Health Care Services**

By observation, the region appears to have numerous physical health providers available to serve active duty military, veterans, and their family members. In addition to Madigan Army Medical Center and hospitals in both Lakewood and Lacey, there are several community health centers in Pierce County. Almost all community members spoke highly of Madigan Army Medical Center and cited its reputation and level of care as major reasons that active duty service members request JBLM as their last posting. Indeed, it is only one of three designated Level 2 trauma centers in the entire United States Army Medical Command. One of the barriers to accessing care, however, is that the military-connected population is increasingly dispersed throughout the region and Madigan Army Medical Center is located on an old section of highway not designed to accommodate the current volume of traffic. Recently, the SSMCP was awarded nearly $6 million to reconfigure a bridge and highway interchange closest to the hospital to decrease travel time and increase safety and increase use of the facility. In a similar vein, Lacey residents were described as regarding services on base as "North of the river" or "over the bridge" and therefore inaccessible.

Both Lakewood and Lacey host many urgent care centers, physician offices, and other medical service providers, but it was challenging to identify or contact a representative from the health care system who could speak to issues in the region and provide an overview. This observation was validated by a representative of the health care system who described health care in the region as "fragmented" and "lacking coordination," especially with respect to care for military families. On base, multiple deployments have resulted in increased turnover of case managers whose job is to facilitate referrals to community providers. When a case manager is deployed, any collaborative relationships that the manager had established in the community are lost because the case manager's replacement has no history of working with the community "outside the gate."

Within the region, access to health care by service members and their family members was described as increasingly problematic because of a serious lack of primary care providers who accept TRICARE health insurance. Although "on paper" it appeared that many providers will take the insurance, "in reality" most providers are at their capacity and are closed to new TRICARE patients. In addition, interviewees said there was a serious shortage of primary care providers overall in the region to care for the increasing population, much of it military affiliated. Interviewees described how some providers will provide limited care to military families out of a “feeling of obligation” or as their “patriotic duty,” and there is a project that engages providers in donating services on a short-term basis. Project Access, started in 2009, is a network of physicians and other ancillary providers in both Thurston and Pierce counties who voluntarily donate health care to people without health insurance or to those who meet poverty criteria. Interviewees indicated almost critical shortages of behavioral and mental health care, and the SSMCP described serious shortages of dental care, indicating that dental health care is not affordable and a major concern among military families.

Although hospital representatives did not describe a major influx of patients or emergency room (ER) visits during deployment and return cycles, one of their suggestions was to be better informed of these cycles so that they could be better prepared for *possible* increases in ER visits. Several interviewees mentioned that service members and their family members will access the local ER because of its proximity to their homes, and many interviewees described how service members and their families will seek drug and alcohol treatment and/or mental health care off base and pay out of pocket so that they are not reported in the military system as needing or receiving these services. In the words of one interviewee:

> If you are an officer or an officer’s wife, you don’t want to be seen walking in to the building where everyone knows it is where the mental health providers are. For enlisted, you don’t want to be seen as showing any weakness.

The high rate of PTSD subsequent to multiple deployments has had a significant impact on off-base availability of licensed mental health practitioners (e.g., LCSW-C, psychologists, and psychiatrists) in this area. Reportedly, JBLM has been heavily recruiting these practitioners from off-base facilities around the region, offering salaries that exceed what many off-base providers can afford to pay. And because of the salary differential, off-base providers then have a hard time replacing staff members who have left to work at JBLM. This reportedly has resulted in a staffing shortage in community provider agencies and a reduced availability of behavioral health services in the civilian sector.

## Social Capital

### Support Networks

The region overall appears to show ongoing support for service members and their families. Lakewood has had a military presence for more than a hundred years, and Lacey appears to have welcomed military families to join its community. Community programs in these cities, such as the Boys and Girls Club, the YMCA, and the Kiwanis Club, are among many that offer programs and activities for military families. Many of the informal supports that are available around JBLM seem to be generated from and operate at the “grassroots” level and tend to be referred by word of mouth around the region. One military spouse who is also a social service provider commented on the informal support networks:

> I am part of a wives group on Facebook. . . . I have noticed recently a lot of questions from wives about how others get through and handle deployments . . . as well as how to handle some of the changes they notice in their husbands when they return. It seems that

wives are reaching out more to others that have experienced deployments rather than seek help from . . . Military Family Life Consultants.

The team learned about several support programs during the site visit, including the following:

**Project New Hope Military Family Retreats.** This program was developed in 2008 in Minnesota and then started in Washington State with the support of the local Lions Club. It sponsors free retreats targeting military families who have experienced multiple deployments and are experiencing high stress personally and within their families, or both, including mental health concerns and PTSD. The program aims to "facilitate the re-integration of veterans and active duty combat veterans back into their family and community environs."[14] Professional counseling is available at the retreat.

**The Pet Brigade** (www.thepetbrigade.com). This program helps coordinate foster care and other boarding services for pets of service members who are getting ready to be deployed from JBLM. A similar program, Concern for Animals, provides low cost/free veterinary care and helps find homes for animals that have been abandoned by service members who have been deployed.

**YMCA.** The Lakewood YMCA offers a variety of activities for military families: "Parents Night Out" gives nondeployed spouses time to work out or enjoy recreational activities at the YMCA while staff watch their children. "Oxygen for Your Relationship" is a program designed to help couples who have experienced deployment separation to reconnect.

**Kiwanis Club.** During the interviews with members of the local chapter, the team learned about several different activities and events that this group sponsors for local children, including those with parents who have been deployed. Among these events are gift donations and donation trees (pick a family name from the tree and buy their wish list) during the holidays, camps, and various seasonal recreational events (e.g., fishing, swimming, hiking).

**VA Hospital golf course.** The local VA hospital funded the modification of a local 18-hole golf course to enable service members who became disabled during deployment to play the course.

**The Association of the United States Army (AUSA).** AUSA has a local chapter in both Lakewood and Lacey. The chapters enlist the support of local businesses to fund services such as care packages for the troops, holiday dinners for military families, bon voyage and welcome home rallies for deploying and returning service members, packages for returning service members who are single, financial grants to JBLM charities, and recreational events.

**Women of Valor, Princess Warrior Group.** This is a support group for female service members who had been sexually assaulted during their military service.

---

[14] See http://www.projectnewhopewa.com/ and http://www.projectnewhopewa.com/about.html.

Both social service and city representatives mentioned that the local emergency food network and other food banks in the region are other community resources used by military families. Meeting the housing needs for service members recently released from duty, primarily young families or single men, was described as challenging, and neither Lakewood nor Lacey has a homeless shelter. Housing assistance is most commonly provided by a private program in Tacoma, the Associated Ministries, which provides referrals to emergency, transitional, and permanent housing as well as some rental and utility assistance.

### Faith Community

Most interviewees in this region had word-of-mouth knowledge about local churches that conduct support activities for deploying service members and their families. But despite its efforts, the study team was not able to secure an interview with any of these groups to learn the specifics of their programs. And a discussion with a minister who runs a shelter in the county similarly revealed no specific details about any churches near JBLM that provide supports explicitly for service members and their families. Thus, although support programs may be available to service members and their families through faith-based organizations, referral to such programs may occur on a case-by-case basis rather than through broad publicity.

## SUMMARY

### What Is Working

This region has already put into operation certain elements that seem to have helped local communities support service members and their families, as well as the community as whole, during the current deployments.

- The work supported by the South Sound Military and Communities Partnership (SSMCP) has given this region a head start in identifying and preparing for impacts from the expected increase in population at JBLM and, in turn, any associated impacts from deployments from the base. Surveys sponsored by the SSMCP have provided vital information about community needs and demographic characteristics of service members, which is facilitating community planning efforts. The SSMCP enables JBLM leadership to participate in the coordination and implementation of planning efforts for the City of Lakewood and other parts of the region and keeps the Lakewood government in the loop about changes and activities planned for the base.
- Military liaisons, where they exist in these communities (e.g., schools, Lakewood Police Department), have been instrumental in keeping the community systems they are involved with informed about activities and changes affiliated with JBLM.
- Local schools have been identifying needs and organizing supports to meet the mental health needs of students living on and off base. They have been coordinating these efforts with JBLM and seeking grant funds to maintain these support programs throughout the deployment cycle.

- There appear to be a multitude of grassroots programs in the region that are designed to offer support and services to military families. Staff in these programs appear to be well aware of the unique stressors and needs facing military families in the region.
- The general attitude toward service members and their family members in these communities is one of acceptance. Members of these communities, whether affiliated with the military or not, do not treat service members as outsiders and have been willing to offer support and honor these men and women for their service.

### Needs and Challenges

- Emergency services and health care providers reported not having good communication channels with JBLM. As a result, they described not feeling sufficiently prepared to deal with the needs of service members and their families who are dealing with the stresses of multiple deployments.
- Although there are many grassroots programs in the region that offer supports for service members and their families, learning about such programs seems to come by talking to the right person at the right time. There remains no central point of contact for obtaining information about these important programs.
- Lakewood Police have access to a military liaison; however, other local police departments, such as Lacey's, do not. The Lacey police have been seeking training from JBLM to better understand the stressors that service members are facing and be prepared to deal with them.
- Local mental health providers have been hearing from clients and co-professionals that JBLM has been encouraging service members and their family members to seek services on base. Some service members and their families prefer to go to off-base providers and will even pay in cash to keep their need for such services "off the radar screen." Off-base providers are concerned that there is fast becoming an insufficient supply of licensed and certified off-base providers because JBLM has been recruiting these professionals to work on base. They are also concerned that JBLM is not meeting the demand for mental health services—they hear of long waiting lists and lengthy times between appointments.

### Suggestions from the Community

- Various interview sources saw a need for public education about what PTSD is and what it isn't to help minimize the growing stigma that returning service members are facing.
- Local law enforcement suggested that information about PTSD be integrated into police training so that officers can be better prepared to understand what actions might trigger a negative response in service members.
- Local law enforcement also suggested that service members should be briefed on local laws when they arrive at JBLM so that they are not surprised by the legal consequences of certain crimes (e.g., a DUI charge results in automatic arrest and their car being towed).

- Staff from community support programs (formal and informal) would like to see a central point of contact for referral and information dissemination to help the public become more aware of the different programs that are available for service members and their families.
- School representatives said there is a need for mental health counseling for children in military families.

# Georgetown, South Carolina

Case Study Report

# Impacts of Multiple Deployments: Georgetown, South Carolina

## OVERVIEW

This report summarizes findings from the study team's ethnographic site visit (June 17–22, 2012) to Georgetown, South Carolina. Overall, the study team did not find that the two deployments by the local National Guard unit had any effects—positive or negative—on the local community as a whole. Data supporting this finding are presented in the pages that follow, including information obtained from interviewees about the local economy, school system, and the community at large. Although the team does not discount the possibility that the community was largely unaffected by these events, we also present several possible explanations for this result.

## GEOGRAPHIC ORIENTATION

### Community: Georgetown, South Carolina

Georgetown (population 9,000[1]) is situated on the coast of South Carolina, 35 miles south of Myrtle Beach and 60 miles north of Charleston. It is located on the Winyah Bay in South Carolina's Low County, the tidal region along the coast that has a rich and distinctive cultural heritage. Throughout much of its history, African Americans have represented the greatest proportion of area residents, and still do so today: In 2010, 56% of the town's citizens were African American, 36% were white, and 5% self-identified as Hispanic. Georgetown is the county seat of Georgetown County, which includes several small unincorporated communities and the major cities of Andrews, Murrells Inlet, and Pawley's Island. The National Guard unit of interest—the 1st Battalion of the 178th Field Artillery—has its headquarters at the National Guard Armory in Georgetown, but also includes armories in Andrews, Manning (Clarendon County), Clinton (Laurens County), and

**Data Sources**

- National Guard members
- National Guard family members
- Mayors
- Chamber of Commerce
- Greater Georgetown Business Association
- Georgetown County School District staff
- Social service organizations
- VFW and the American Legion
- VFW Ladies Auxiliary
- United Way
- Family Readiness Group leader
- Georgetown emergency services personnel (fire and police)
- Andrews Police Department
- Georgetown County Sherriff's Office
- Georgetown Hospital
- Georgetown County Mental Health
- *Georgetown Times* (newspaper)
- Secondary sources (newspaper articles, videos, town/county websites)
- Ethnographic observation

[1] See http://quickfacts.census.gov/qfd/states/45/4528870.html.

Hemingway (Williamsburg County). For the purposes of the site visit, the study team focused primarily on the community of Georgetown.[2]

Even to the casual observer, it is clear that Georgetown's history has shaped its present: Thanks to the nutrient-rich soils in this area, early 18th century plantation owners amassed enormous wealth through the cultivation and export of indigo. To get their products to market more quickly, the town became the official port of South Carolina in 1732 and for many years ranked as the third largest port in the country. This piece of Georgetown's history is reflected in its many stately pre–Revolutionary War homes, historic markers dedicated to the Winyah Indigo Society, and countless businesses around town that have incorporated "indigo" into their names (e.g., Indigo Vision Center, Indigo Physical Therapy). The area also played a significant role in the American Revolution: Two Georgetown residents (Thomas Lynch, Sr. and Jr.) were signers of the Declaration of Independence, and a third resident, Francis "Swamp Fox" Marion, became (in)famous for his use of guerrilla tactics against the British. Revolutionary War markers can be found throughout town, and in homage to their fearless predecessor, the local National Guard unit is named the "Swamp Fox Unit."

By the end of the war, the agricultural focus of the region had changed—indigo had begun to be cultivated in other, easily accessed regions of the world, thus reducing the profitability of the crop. Rice, which was readily grown in the tidal region, became the next source of wealth. By 1840 Georgetown County alone was producing almost half of the entire rice crop in the United States. This crop's importance to the region can be learned about in the Rice Museum, which is located along historic Front Street downtown. Predictably, the Civil War and Reconstruction brought about significant changes to the area. With the abolition of slavery, large-scale cultivation of rice was no longer possible and the area settled into a long period of economic downturn. At least two legacies of the Reconstruction era remain: African Americans, who historically greatly outnumbered white settlers, represent the majority of the current population, and Georgetown has never recovered its earlier economic prosperity and prominence.

This period of history notwithstanding, there are certain companies in the area that remain strong: International Paper, for example, operates a mill in Georgetown that has over 600 employees; the local steel mill, currently owned by Luxembourg-based Acelor-Mittal, is down from its height of 1,200 workers, but still employs approximately 300 area residents; and there are numerous power generation plants in the county that residents said offer job opportunities. Also, Georgetown business leaders continue to promote tourism in the area, highlighting both the excellent recreational fishing opportunities in the bay and regional rivers, as well as the town's rich history. In addition to several museums in town (e.g., Rice Museum, Georgetown History Museum, and a soon-to-open Maritime Museum), local entrepreneurs have created excellent

[2] The study team made numerous efforts before the site visit to set up appointments with individuals in Andrews, all to no avail. The one appointment that was made was canceled by the interviewee; and on-site efforts to talk with city officials proved limited, at best. For reference, Andrews is located about 19 miles to the northwest of Georgetown, away from the coastal traffic. Numerous interviewees said they were saddened by that town's loss of industry over the years. A drive down the main thoroughfare fully supported their concerns, as storefront after storefront sat empty and quiet. Census data suggest a slight decline in residents over the last 10 years: In 2000, the town had 3,068 residents; by 2010, this number had dropped by 6.7%, to 2,800. As in Georgetown, the majority of residents self-identify as African American (65%), 30% are white, and 4% are Hispanic. These data can be found at http://www.city-data.com/city/Andrews-South-Carolina.html.

dining and shopping opportunities in the town's Historic Waterfront district. The downtown area appeared busy, and business was relatively brisk during the study team's visit.

These new opportunities notwithstanding, interviewees expressed the opinion that job options are limited in the region and that incomes are low. As of 2009, median household income in Georgetown was $29,831, compared with a statewide median of $42,442 and a national median of $50,221. In the same year, the median per capita income in Georgetown in 2009 was $17,383, far lower than South Carolina's median ($31,653) and the national median ($38,846). Household income in Georgetown differed greatly by race, with whites bringing in $22,808 and African Americans at roughly half that amount ($11,958).[3] As of May 2012, the unemployment rate throughout Georgetown County stood at 9.5%.[4] These data support interviewees' assertions that the National Guard offers many local residents an important way to supplement their income through monthly drills, and bring in more household income while deployed.

**Military Installation: South Carolina National Guard Unit**

Georgetown Armory is the headquarters of the 1st Battalion 178th Field Artillery Unit of the South Carolina National Guard. The unit consists of several hundred (500+) National Guard members from armories throughout South Carolina, but the local communities of Georgetown, Andrews, Manning, Clinton, and Hemmingway are also strongly represented. Interviewees estimated approximately 200 unit members are "local," with roughly 100 to 120 based inGeorgetown and another 80 or so residing in Andrews.[5] Murrells Inlet and Pawley's Island also contributed citizens to the unit, but reportedly not in such large numbers.

The battalion's history is as old as Georgetown's, for it helped to defend South Carolina against the British. The unit primarily served as a home guard through the Civil War, but its composition changed markedly for a two-decade period during Reconstruction. At this time, ex-Confederate soldiers were not permitted to serve in the state militia; thus, the unit included only African Americans. By the end of the 19th century, however, several Reconstruction-era laws were rescinded; the unit was racially integrated by the turn of the 20th century. Today, interviewees said, the unit has roughly equal numbers of African Americans and whites.

Although the 1/178th was deployed to battle and served admirably in both World Wars, after the Second World War it served in its more traditional role, that is, providing support for civic unrest or during local emergencies (e.g., Hurricane Hugo in 1989). In June 2004, however, as the war in Iraq was intensifying, the unit was put on alert for deployment to that combat theater. Interviewees reported that the orders, which came quickly,[6] caught the entire community by surprise:

---

[3] Georgetown 2009 data obtained at http://www.city-data.com/city/Georgetown-South-Carolina.html. National household income data for 2009 were obtained at http://www.census.gov/prod/2010pubs/acsbr09-2.pdf. National and South Carolina per capita income for 2009 obtained at http://bber.unm.edu/econ/us-pci.htm.

[4] See http://eascinc.com/unemployment_rate.html.

[5] Interviewees gave the study team significantly different numbers about how many members deployed with the unit each time and, of those, how many were from Georgetown County. Our working assumption is that most local Guard members deployed each time; the team is awaiting confirmation on that number from the Georgetown armory.

[6] The adverse effects on the community of this short notice are discussed later in this report.

> It was the Saturday of drill we got the alert and then by the Monday it became official. It was that fast, it was head-spinning. [Guard member]

> The first time it was 6 weeks, "Hey, you're going." And 6 weeks later they were gone. [Family member]

Guardsmen said that after arriving in Iraq they conducted convoy security operations, logging some 5 million miles while transporting goods and people between the Iraq and Kuwait borders. The first deployment lasted 15 months, and, despite driving over heavily IED-seeded roads, interviewees reported only minor casualties (i.e., one serious IED wound and no deaths).

The second deployment was to Afghanistan in 2010. This time, soldiers were given notice of the deployment a year in advance. This second deployment lasted about 9 months and consisted of mixed assignments, such as supporting Provincial Reconstruction Teams (PRTs) and providing various security forces around the country. The unit had two members (both from Pennsylvania) killed during the second deployment, but interviewees said that most other casualties were minor. They also noted that it was difficult to generalize about posttraumatic stress disorder (PTSD) within the unit following this second deployment because unit members were assigned such different tasks from one another. While one service member served on a NATO air base, they said, others were in the countryside conducting counter-insurgency missions. Exposure to combat and the potential for PTSD thus varied greatly among unit members.

Although the 1/178th traditionally has been a "home-town unit," members said that after the first deployment, the makeup of the unit changed:

> When I got in [over a decade ago], everybody lived within 35 to 40 miles away from [the Georgetown] Armory. Now . . . we've got guys coming from Florence . . . we've got kids coming from Columbia . . . we've got people that live out of state. . . . But when I first got in, it was, you know we had 120 people from the unit and 20 of those people live somewhere else [but] the other 100 were from this area. They were born and raised in Georgetown. . . . The entire communications section either worked at the power plant or International Paper or the steel mill. Every one of them. And those guys have all retired. In the meantime, we get new kids—"Hey I'm from New Hampshire, I'm going to Coastal Carolina [University] and I'm going to join the Guard to help pay for college." So he has no real ties here, he's got no family here. It's different.

Interviewees said the second deployment did not result in a similar wave of retirements. Although the unit itself was deployed to combat twice in a 6-year period, some unit members continue to volunteer for "individual deployments," that is, signing up with another South Carolina unit that is set to deploy, in an effort to bolster the family's income. One individual interviewed by the study team, for example, was about to leave for his third deployment and said his sole objective in volunteering was to bring in additional money that could support him and his wife during their retirement. In addition, interviewees believed that individuals could be *ordered* to the combat theater if they had skills that were needed in another deploying unit.

Thus, in assessing the community effects of the National Guard deployments, it is important to realize that the 1/178th has been deployed twice in support of the OIF/OEF engagements. But numerous unit members have deployed additional times—some voluntarily, some involuntarily—to Iraq, Afghanistan, or to other regions of the world where American troops are maintaining a strong presence (e.g., Kosovo, Kuwait). Although the study team focused primarily on the effects of the two unitwide deployments, it is important to bear in mind that some interviewees had been affected by the absence of a family member or employee for additional periods of time.

### Relationship Between Community and National Guard

The Georgetown community presented itself as very supportive of its National Guard unit. Everyone with whom the study team spoke knew there was a local unit, could direct the team to the armory's location, and knew that the unit had been deployed more than once. Not everyone personally knew of someone in the National Guard, but many did. In fact, some interviewees began an interview saying, "I don't really know anything about the Guard," but after talking with the team for a few minutes, thought of one or two people they know—or that their friends or family know—who had been deployed.

Regardless of the degree of personal connectedness, Georgetown residents who spoke with the study team said that Guardsmen are family, friends, and neighbors who make up the everyday fabric of the community. Residents also knew that the unit's primary mission historically has been to defend their hometown and that these are the men who help save their homes and families during a natural disaster. The presence of these citizen soldiers has two implications. First, community members said they are not always thinking of "John Smith" as a National Guard member; rather, they think of him as the person he is and the role he serves in the day-to-day community (e.g., police officer, school staff). In some respects, then, an individual's role in the National Guard may go unnoticed on a regular basis. Yet because the National Guard's original role has been hometown defense, when a need arises, the community rallies. One interviewee spoke of the "quiet visibility" of the National Guard:

> This [Georgetown] group is almost nonexistent . . . from my point of view. I don't see them, like visible. They are low key. They are down at the armory doing their thing or they are out wherever they are being sent to take care of firefighting or whatever. Very low key. But if ever it comes in that something needs to be done, then the community is right there with them. Nobody steps back.

A second interviewee echoed this perspective:

> Our National Guard is really a hometown defense. If you erect fundraisers for the National Guard for a project, everybody in the community jumps in. There is no issue on that. We've done a golf tournament, the fundraiser for the school kids, I have had several things that have been like immediate and the money has just poured in, just from the community. Andrews is the same way. They are smaller, closer. Their group is really tight over there.

Guard members noted that even with the composition of the unit changing over time, from town members to people from outside of the area, "90% of the community has been supportive regardless of the makeup." They attributed this support to the fact that lifelong residents of Georgetown have seen a parent, grandparent, uncle, cousin, or friend in the unit at some point, and thus unit composition hardly matters: "The unit as a whole has always been a local thing, something for the community to support, even if you don't know the people being deployed." One interviewee summed up local attitudes when she said, "The community, in my opinion, has always been behind the National Guard troops. We have our favorite word—'our' unit."

## EFFECTS OF MULTIPLE DEPLOYMENTS ON THE COMMUNITY

### Economic Impact

#### Effects of Deployments on the Economy

Data collected during the site visit suggests that the multiple deployments have had little noticeable effect on the local economy. Only one source suggested a potential economic loss to the community resulting from the deployments, specifically, a loss of the hotel and restaurant income the city would otherwise receive if Guard members were home and coming to Georgetown once a month for drill. The team did not hear a similar concern expressed by any other interviewees, but it is possible that in a small town like Georgetown, even this once-a-month decline would be noticed by local businesses.

Employers also did not recount any major negative effects from the deployments. For the most part, employers said, the numbers were small and they simply redistributed the individuals' duties among the remaining staff members. Interviewees reported no disruptions to any of the major businesses in the area, such as International Paper or the steel mill. One interviewee said, "Nobody shuts down because the Guard guys go, other than the armory."

The idea of a "small number," however, is relative to the size of the business. Although the hospital, which reportedly employs more than 2,000 individuals, might be able to absorb the absence of a couple of staff, small businesses had more difficulties. One interviewee provided the following example:

> We had one guy—he was a chiropractor. He had his own practice. He had to shut his practice down to go on deployment—for both deployments. He referred his clients over to another chiropractor who [he] has a friendly relationship with. [His patients] continued to get treatment and he got back and flipped his sign—"Yes, we're open"—and said, "Hey, I'm back." And [his patients] came right back to him.

Most employers described the deployments as, at worst, "disruptive" and "creating turmoil" for the workers left behind. For example, the Fire Department reported the strain of having to promote another member of the department *twice* to fill the gap of the deployed soldier, only to demote that same person each time the soldier returned home:

> He's probably the one who got affected the most. Because he moved up for a year, came back down, moved up for, I think, 9 months, and then back down again.

In addition, employers reported that Guard members are participating in many more trainings since the deployments began and compared with their once-a-month and 2-week summer drills in the past. Employers said they cannot replace these individuals for such a short amount of time, which leaves other employees to pick up the extra work and less time off for those workers who are not in the Guard:

> We're not going to start saying, "You're fired because you're doing this." But it creates operational issues for us. When he [goes to] training for a month or two, I don't have time to promote someone back and forth for a month. If he's gone for a year, we can do that. [But] what it also does for us, it limits the people allowed to take off other times. Because if he's gone, my shift is already down and I let two more people off, then I have to hire overtime to come back in and fill in.

Soldiers returning to some of the positions, such as fire fighters, were said by interviewees to need additional time for retraining so that they can be brought back up to speed on any new protocols, group dynamics, or any training they may have missed:

> He has a big learning curve to get back . . . it takes a couple of months to get him back up to where we feel comfortable, so that people [he works with] feel comfortable. [Emergency services worker]

Employers also mentioned that as a result of changes to the Family and Medical Leave Act, spouses can take up to 12 weeks of leave during a calendar year to attend military-related events (e.g., training, meetings, support groups, and dinners for Guard members or their families). Spouses can also use this time to take care of their children or attend to other responsibilities they may have taken on while their spouse was away. One employer said it is "fortunate" he doesn't have more than one Guard or family member on staff, and a similar sentiment was expressed by others. The impacts have been small, but only because the number of Guard members deployed has been small. Some employers said that if that number had been greater, even by one, the impact on their businesses would have been much more severe.

**Effects of the Economy on Deployments**

Although the deployments per se reportedly had no large-scale effects on the local economy, respondents did indicate the reverse, namely, that the *economy* had effects on *deployments*. Few job opportunities in the area, when combined with extraordinarily low wages, make deployments a win-win for Guard members and businesses alike. Guard members said that during deployment, some members end up earning twice as much as they would be making in their regular Georgetown jobs. In addition, they said, although not common, a couple of individuals received not only their military pay while deployed, but also their salaries for their civilian jobs, giving them nearly three times their normal salary for the time they were deployed. One individual said, "[That Guard member] is making a lot of money. That's getting forwarded into local business . . . paying off his debt." Although not on a grand scale, deployments were said by interviewees to have increased cash flow for many families, as well as for the local economy.

The earning potential associated with the deployments has had other effects. Interviewees said that the potential for high earnings has led many members of the National Guard and the Individual Ready Reserve to either volunteer for additional deployments or take positions with military contractors, such as Blackwater. Blackwater positions were said to be particularly attractive for members of local law enforcement, who reportedly could earn as much as five times their annual salary for a year's service in Iraq or Afghanistan. Interviewees said that the former chief of police in Andrews left for such an opportunity, as did three officers with the Georgetown Police Department, two from the Georgetown Fire Department, and nearly 15 Sheriff's Office deputies. A representative from the Sheriff's Office said these departures have created more turnover in the department's workforce than the National Guard deployments did, not simply because of the numbers but because even when they return home after a year, many individuals decide to return to the combat theater because they have gotten used to living on the higher salary.

In addition to the appeal of extra money, interviewees said individuals may voluntarily redeploy because they miss the excitement and adrenaline associated with combat activities. Emergency medical services (EMS) personnel offered the following observations:

> It's kind of "The Hurt Locker" mentality. You feel like you're a part of something, something bigger than you. And then you come back and they've got to answer a dog call down on Front Street or, you know, shoplifting at Wal-Mart. And you say, "Man, I could be where it's at." [EMS provider 1]

> It's not the same because it's not the same level. Like he said, dog call, shoplifting call, my guy's going to install a smoke detector at Mrs. Smith's house at 3 o'clock in the morning, or help little Johnny across the street here for the school guard or going to a car fire or car wreck, there is nothing to it. As opposed to dodging bullets or looking for roadside bombers or some of these other things . . . and even when we do have the big call, a shooting call, or a large structure fire, that's only short lived, then it's over, versus the constant [adrenaline] pumping the whole time while you're there. [EMS provider 2]

Interviewees suggested that the experiential and financial opportunities the wars have created for local residents have led some individuals to voluntarily deploy several times, and those deployments, in turn, have had an adverse effect on their business operations.

## INFORMATION AND COMMUNICATION

### Communication About Deployments

Interviewees consistently said that word-of-mouth is the primary channel through which information flows, a not-unexpected finding in a small, close-knit community. In many cases, such as when a community need arises, that channel functions quickly and efficiently:

> If it ever comes in that something needs to be done [for the Guard unit], then the community is right behind it. Nobody steps back from that. Just go to one Council Meeting, say what's gonna happen, before you know it, whoever they're having breakfast with downtown . . . the old men sit there, and all you gotta do is tell 'em once and the whole street knows. . . . They're like the fathers in this little city here, and if there's issues going on, every business knows about it because they'll be talking fast and personal to 'em. [Community member]

But when dealing with a large bureaucratic organization such as the U.S. military, word-of-mouth has not always been sufficient. As noted previously, the first deployment occurred so quickly that informal communication channels were not able to keep up. One newspaper reporter said that prior to the first deployment he had been hearing rumors within the community about the possibility and wanted to confirm those stories with the state headquarters in Columbia. "We wanted simply to let folks know, 'Hey, there's going to be a deployment in 5 months or whatever,' because these are our relatives, our neighbors, our friends, [and] our church members." Yet efforts to obtain official information about the rumored event proved "challenging." This interviewee described the irony of trying to get the "official word" to support information that was already widely known throughout the community. "It's going to be common knowledge amongst the community, so why not [give us information]?"

Beyond getting the formal notice, the communication challenges associated with the first deployment had real effects within the community. First, interviewees said, because of the lack of information, the towns were not prepared to give their community members an appropriate send-off to war:

> The first deployment, nobody knew about it, nobody understood it. The send-off was very, very small. Some people didn't even know it was happening. [Family member]

> The first time it was so fast and the public affairs people at State HQ were in denial. "No, this unit's not going anywhere." Because of operational security, they didn't want to spill the beans too much until, "Hey, the buses are at the armory, you guys [in the community] get together and do a parade for them going out." [Guard member]

In addition, the Family Readiness Groups (FRGs), a key resource for spouses of deployed service members, had neither the experience nor adequate time to prepare for the first deployment:

> Our first deployment, there really wasn't a good FRG system in place . . . because it was

> so quick—we got FRGs in the units, we've had them for years, but . . . it was always maybe once a year they'd get together to talk about the Christmas dinner or a springtime family day, something like that. So it was pretty much a nonexistent FRG really. We found out when we deployed to Iraq and you had some people that they volunteered, "Ok, I'll be the FRG leader or whatever" . . . but they had really no idea of how to do it. They were just there to get everybody together. [Guard member 1]

> And it may have been that way because our people just didn't know, we had no exposure to it. [Guard member 2]

Although communication challenges existed before and throughout the first deployment, interviewees consistently stated that "lessons learned" from the first deployment helped improve information flow for the second one. For example, a much greater proportion of the community was involved in the send-off for the soldiers as they left for Afghanistan on the second deployment than when they left for Iraq:

> There was a lot more local preparation. . . . It was much more involved. . . . They actually hired their Guard people full-time that were here locally to prepare for leaving the second time. So it was a whole different approach to how they were leaving. . . . Supposedly that was learned from the first deployment. [Reporter]

> The coming and going for Afghanistan was vastly more superior and more heartfelt and everything else than Iraq. [For Iraq], it was just a little cluster of families at whatever armory you were leaving from. [For the second deployment], coming out of Georgetown all the way out past Andrews, both sides of the road, traffic was lined up, flags, and honking, and fire truck with the ladder out and a flag over it. . . . We also had a local motorcycle crew of guys, the American Legion Riders . . . they escorted us out with a little motorcycle motorcade on the way going out to the airport. [Guard member 1]

Interviewees also described the FRG as having gone through some positive changes as a result of lessons learned:

> The Family Readiness Group . . . learned some things that would be better to do when the second deployment came around. And it seemed like they were better organized. . . . They have been sharing information with us, if they have a family activity—a yard sale or whatever—to raise funds. . . . Not that there were lots and lots of those, but we knew about more of them and they did more of them for the second deployment. [Reporter]

> Following [the Iraq deployment], I think the State, the Guard, realized, "Wait, we need to get something going here where we actually train these volunteers to kind of know what to do at an FRG meeting and to anticipate what questions are going to be asked and how to answer them." And so they put together basically a training program for the volunteers. . . . At the end of it, you've got an FRG leader who has contacts across the state [and] has a list of resources. [Guard member]

Despite the establishment of more formal communication patterns in these areas, community members said communication challenges persist in several critical domains. During a focus group with school faculty and staff, for example, an administrator said she had not noticed any effects on her students and, before coming to the group, had asked her guidance counselors what, if any, problems they had seen. "They really could not think of very many kids who were affected." When the moderator offered, "So no news is good news?" the administrator responded:

> I don't know if that's the case or not because there may be some things we need to put in to place so we can find out if there *are* some issues. We don't have anything like that going on.

Others in the group said that although an organization[7] had come into town during the second deployment and offered to set up a communication plan with the district, "that never happened." As a result, participants said schools would have only learned about students with deployed parents through word of mouth:

> The [guidance counselors] wouldn't have known unless the parent contacted them. [Participant 1]
>
> And personal history, if you knew that parent had contacted you about something as a teacher or if you were a principal. [Participant 2]

One participant added:

> It would have been good if [staff] could have known and the guidance counselor could've checked in on [the children] to give them that added level of support.

Employers found themselves in a similar position to school staff and also indicated the need for more formal communication from Guard leaders instead of having to rely on word of mouth:

> You'll start to get a rumbling. . . . "The rumor is there's going to be a deployment." So you start to get the rumor that it's happening. And usually these guys will go to Guard duty one weekend and find out that it's becoming real. [*How much notice do you have?*] Six months out you start hearing the rumors. [EMS provider 1]
>
> As it becomes closer, the employees will start talking about it because they talk among themselves. And probably 2 to 3 months out it becomes pretty much knowledge that it's going to happen. [EMS provider 2]

According to the Uniformed Services Employment and Reemployment Rights Act (USERRA), employees are instructed to show their employers the letters they receive from the National Guard saying that their units are being deployed. The National Guard is not responsible for alerting employers. Employers the team talked to said they did see these letters, but they would have liked some type of official announcement as early as possible so they could put plans in place. One individual, frustrated with the disruptions caused by trainings, added, "I would just

[7] No participants were certain of the name of the group.

like to know if these are all mandatory or my staff member is volunteering to go." A human resources director for one company said he believed he has to keep the individual's position open, regardless of whether the National Guard member's deployment was voluntary or involuntary. And, according to USERRA, both voluntary and involuntary service in support of National Guard unit deployments confer job protections if the law's criteria are met by service members. Clearly, however, some employers in Georgetown felt they had insufficient information about these pending disruptions and the legal protections regarding deployed service members' jobs. As noted earlier, more formal communications with the National Guard might help alleviate some of the related stresses.

**Communication About Available Resources**

As discussed in the next section, formal resources for National Guard members, their families, or other community members affected by multiple deployments appeared to be in relatively short supply. Interviewees described a mental health service delivery system that is lean, at best, and most Department of Veterans Affairs (VA) services are located elsewhere (e.g., in Myrtle Beach or Charleston). But for those services and supports that are available locally, communication appears compromised. One example stood out for the study team. In preparation for the visit, the team had identified through the Internet a VA center in Georgetown and had endeavored to get in touch with the contact person, but with no success. During an interview on-site with a community member whose husband helps link veterans with medical services, the team heard that the local VA center was closed. The woman said her husband had been driving people all the way to Myrtle Beach to complete the paperwork necessary to qualify for services.

Team members accepted the woman's account as an explanation for the inability to contact anyone at the clinic, but were confused by the apparent currency of the clinic's Internet site. Early one afternoon the team tried to locate the facility and found the building at the address listed on the Internet. The building, however, did seem closed: No cars were parked out front, and the American flag was noticeably absent. One team member walked up to the door and, seeing no lights on in the facility, returned to the car and started to drive away. Another team member asked if she had actually tried to open the door and, not having done so, she returned to the building and found the door unlocked. At the sound of the door opening, a staff member came out and the study team member told her the community rumor that the facility had closed. The woman replied, "We're not closed. We just moved from the old County Building back in March."

It was unclear how information about the move had been conveyed to the veterans' community, but it was clear why rumors persisted of the facility's closure: The team had already spotted the old County Building, a one-story modular building on the north side of town that clearly was undergoing a complete rehabilitation. Its parking lot was surrounded by construction vehicles, and men in hardhats were seen coming in and out of all sections of the building. Yet the new location did not appear to be open, either. During subsequent drives past the facility, the team saw few cars in the parking lot and no raised American flag. In a community that relies heavily on interpersonal communication, outward appearances can easily misinform.

## Community Health

Although the team heard a few stories of individuals struggling from the deployments, there did not appear to be any large-scale adverse effects on community health. Most reported that "everything is okay" and there was nothing stated during the interviews or observed by the site visit team to suggest otherwise. If there are health issues because of the deployments, they likely exist at the individual or family level and do not appear to be affecting the larger community.

### Physical Health

The deployments did not result in any deaths, and the team heard reports of only one major injury during the first deployment (an IED tore into a unit member's arm, but interviewees reported that "he is fully recovered"). Although two unit members were killed during the second deployment, neither individual was "local." Any other casualties from that deployment were reported as "minor injuries." Thus, it was not surprising that when interviewees were asked about community effects of the deployments, they had difficulty naming any effects, much less physical ones. Study team members did not make any observations that countered citizens' perspectives in this regard; for example, they did not see young service members in wheelchairs.

### Mental/Behavioral Health

The study team asked numerous interviewees if they had concerns about National Guard members' returning home with PTSD, traumatic brain injury, or other mental health issues. Most interviewees reported they had not heard of any significant problems among unit members. And interviews with employees of the County Mental Health Office, as well as with individuals from social service agencies such as the Family Justice Center and the Center Against Spousal Abuse (CASA) similarly suggested that mental and behavioral health issues related to the deployments were minimal and well within the realm of what was to be expected after emerging from a combat zone. In fact, one unit member said that "everyone comes back with PTSD," an attitude that he believed to be widely shared and that made seeking behavioral health supports more palatable to members of the unit. Unit members and their spouses also noted that after the second deployment, there was an increased focus placed on behavioral and mental health by the State Headquarters of the National Guard. Specific activities associated with reintegration included having the National Guard members work on reconnecting with spouses and friends, as well as learning how to watch for warning signs of possible suicidal behavior in their fellow soldiers.

The very few cases described to the study team of National Guard members who suffered from one or more serious behavioral health issues were not specific. It was also not clear whether these cases were a result of multiple deployments, or of just being deployed in general. In addition, because of overlapping social networks, the study team began to surmise that the various cases described by interviewees might, in fact, be the same one or two instances.

Although no one described any community-level behavioral health effects from the deployments, several interviews said that because the second deployment was fairly recent, they would not be surprised to see problems emerge in a couple of years. At present, the study team believes, the community appears to be lacking adequate resources to meet the mental health needs of Guard members and their families should the onset of problems be delayed.

**Children's Health**

Interviewees did not describe any noticeable stresses the deployments placed on children or any problems that have been observed as a result of the multiple deployments. Family members said their children often were sad and confused about the father[8] being deployed, butno one described any cumulative adverse effects from the multiple deployments. In some cases, particularly for the younger soldiers who have been through two or more deployments, their children were very young (infants) during the first deployment or not even born yet. In these cases, certainly, any behavioral health issues cannot be directly attributed to the fact that the father was deployed twice. One Guard member said that his child was in his early teens during the second deployment; the second deployment wasn't easier per se, he said, but his son was at an age where he was better able to understand what was going on.

As noted earlier, school staff did not report any issues with children whose parents had deployed. As mentioned, however, the lack of communication between Guard leaders and the schools may have prevented teachers or faculty from recognizing which children might be experiencing deployment-related distress.

**Substance Abuse/Domestic Violence Rates**

Interviewees consistently reported no rise in alcohol or drug use in Georgetown as a result of the multiple deployments. The study team was told that drug-related crime is a significant problem within the city, but that officers did not see returning service members engaged in any of these activities.

The team also spoke with representatives of two social services agencies devoted to family issues, and neither believed the deployments have had any effect on local domestic violence rates. There were a couple of cases described by interviewees in which an individual who had returned from a deployment appeared to have behavioral health issues that contributed to domestic violence, but they reported these to be isolated instances within the community. Law enforcement representatives similarly reported no increase in emergency calls related to domestic issues.

## Community Competence

As suggested elsewhere in this report, formal services related to the stresses of multiple deployments—in particular, mental health services—are in limited supply in Georgetown and surrounding communities. Discussion with a provider at the County Mental Health facility revealed the extent of the problem:

- In a need to cut some of its low-revenue services, she said the hospital shut down its inpatient psychiatric unit a couple of years earlier. Currently, individuals experiencing

[8] Reportedly there are no women in the 1/178th.

a psychiatric crisis can be taken to the hospital, but will be held in the emergency room (sometimes for a couple of days, she said) until an inpatient bed can be found elsewhere (e.g., in Myrtle Beach or Charleston).

- She also said that because so few residents have adequate insurance or the financial resources to pay for private health care, there were very few private mental health practitioners in the area. Those who are available are based in Pawley's Island or Murrell's Inlet, and both locations, she believed, would necessitate a substantial drive (at least 15 miles one way to Pawley's) and thus a significant expenditure on gasoline.
- She reported there is one full-time psychiatrist working for the county and several "temporary" psychiatrists who rotate through the facility. The county does provide some telepsychiatry services, but patients must come into the Georgetown building to be video linked to a physician and must otherwise be eligible for county-funded services.
- As a result of budget cuts throughout the state, the provider said that there are strict eligibility criteria for county-funded mental health services. Individuals who have PTSD, for example, must also be diagnosed with another major psychiatric disorder (co-occurring depression, schizophrenia, anxiety, or bipolar disorder) before they are eligible to receive services.

Consistent with what the team heard from other interviewees, this provider said service members or their families who are eligible for VA services are referred to either the VA hospital in Charleston or the VA clinic in Myrtle Beach. Because both locations are about a 1-hour drive from Georgetown, it is likely that individuals would have to take time off from work to receive care.

Although the Georgetown National Guard unit was fortunate in having survived two deployments to a combat theater with only one local casualty (an injury, not a death), the team wondered how a community so lacking in behavioral health resources would have handled things had one or more National Guard members been killed in action. Interviewees from law enforcement, the fire department, and even the schools noted that they have critical incident response[9] capabilities that can be put into place on a moment's notice; but services for dealing with the day-to-day stresses of deployments do not appear to be readily available to residents of Georgetown and the surrounding rural communities. Moreover, it did not appear to the study team that sufficient services were available for those few individuals mentioned by respondents who reportedly had struggled after returning from deployment.

[9] School staff said the school district does not use this term, but has a plan in place for helping students and teachers cope with similar situations, e.g., death of a student.

## Social Capital

The ties binding members of this community together create what appears to be a strong and effective informal support system. The team heard about many types of informal supports. As noted earlier, several interviewees spoke of the area's long history of "patriotism" and "support for the military" and how that history lives on through the area's continued support for its citizen soldiers. This was further enhanced by the National Guard's role of helping the local community deal with the effects of a natural disaster. In short, interviewees said the National Guard takes care of the community and the favor is returned by the community supporting the Guard. That support, they suggested, bolstered the emotional health of the Guard members and their families.

Also, interviewees regularly pointed out the role of churches in providing supports such as financial assistance and pastoral counseling. Although no interfaith or multicongregational efforts were noted, the study team was told often that if a need is present, a church will take care of members of its own congregation.[10] Similarly, employers in the emergency services arena described their units as a "family" and said that when members of the unit are deployed, theymake sure to invite these individuals' spouses and children to any unit social events (e.g., Christmas parties, summer picnics).

In addition, the National Guard members were said to provide each other with mutual support; one family member said she understands the importance of the once-a-month "weekends with the boys" in helping her husband cope with any residual effects of the deployments. Although some spouses might resent these events, this family member believed the trainings provided her husband with invaluable peer support and a safe place to talk through any deployment-related issues.

Finally, the team heard that extended families are themselves a critical form of informal support. For example, the team spoke by telephone with a National Guard member who was about to leave on his third deployment and asked where his wife finds support during his extended absences. He described a social geography of support, noting that his wife's sister lives next door on one side of their home, her brother lives next door on the other side, one of his relative lives directly across the street from their home, and a second relative of his lives next to that individual. "She has plenty of support when I'm gone," he laughed. One interviewee, a relative newcomer to the area, said she was envious of her neighbors who could say to each other, "Well, when your grandmother went to grade school with my grandmother. . . ." The roots are deep and the interrelationships are strong.

## SUMMARY

In most respects, the study team found little indication that the multiple deployments of the local National Guard unit or of its members had any major adverse effects on the community.

---

[10] The study team did hear one counter-example from a woman whose son had been deployed three times. She said she had wanted to send a care package to him during one deployment and asked her pastor for financial assistance in mailing the package. Her request was refused, she said, and it ultimately cost her more than $50 to send the package overseas. She explained the pastor's refusal as being rooted in greed, saying the church is always asking its members for donations, but then it is unwilling to provide support when members of the congregation express a need.

Interviewees noted no large-scale impacts on the economic health of the area; no one could detail any broad, community-level experience with National Guard members' returning from combat with PTSD or other theater-related challenges; school staff had difficulty recalling any major impacts within the district, either in terms of student distress or having to compensate for the large-scale loss of faculty or staff. Some interviewees recounted stories about "one person I know. . . ." (e.g., a colleague, family member, or acquaintance), but the greater Georgetown community appears to have been largely unaffected by the deployment experiences.

At some level, the lack of apparent community-level effects is not surprising. The team's understanding is that about 200 local unit members deployed each time and suffered few physical casualties across the two deployments. Further, some observers might argue that because this was a National Guard unit rather than a regular active duty unit, it had not deployed to the worst of the combat theaters and the lack of community effects is consistent with a less severe level of combat experience.

The study team does not discount that as a possible explanation, but, in keeping with good social science practice, cannot rule out other competing, but plausible, explanations. First, it is possible that interviewees could describe no major effects because they themselves had not heard of anything happening among their friends and neighbors. This would be consistent with the large body of sociological literature on Southern culture that notes, in particular, the cultural importance of keeping one's "personal business" private. Interviewees did describe a couple of individuals and their families who, they believed, had experienced difficulties as a result of the deployments, but they also indicated that if a family were struggling, that struggle might be shared only within the family or with their church pastors.

Second, and in keeping with this value, it is also possible that community members were reluctant to share the community's "personal business" with strangers. In point of fact, the study team was told more than once that some community members' reticence might be because the study team was from the North. The team is hesitant to embrace that explanation because it would be hard for so many interviewees, with such different backgrounds, to so consistently "keep up appearances." Nevertheless, it cannot be ruled out.

Third, and importantly, the team would be remiss not to discuss the possible role of race and race relations in the findings. Georgetown, like many towns in the Deep South, remains largely segregated along racial lines; and if the economy is driving some individual deployments, income disparities by race (as noted earlier in the report) could have a differential effect on which unit members volunteer for additional deployments. Although the team made numerous efforts to establish connections with the African American community, those efforts were largely unsuccessful. A few contacts obtained through staff at the hotel yielded brief, on-site telephone interviews, but the team did not establish enough credible connections to determine if the African American community was affected differently by the multiple deployments. This is an important limitation of this report that the reader should bear in mind when considering the implications of the site visit findings.

Finally, the reader should consider the importance of the long-standing social ties within the community and the strength of these deeply rooted informal networks (e.g., families, neighbors, coworkers, faith community). While social scientists may have slightly over-romanticized life in small towns or villages, there is little question that "community," in its purely sociological sense, is a powerful force that can bolster a group of individuals through the toughest of times. The study team surmises that Georgetown's sense of community may have served as a protective factor to both deployed National Guard members and their families alike.

Any or all of these explanations may be valid; additional, longer term research would need to be conducted, however, to determine which factors are most relevant to the study team's finding of a negligible effect of multiple deployments on the community.

## Challenges

Community members noted a couple of challenges they faced during the deployments and supports they believe could be put in place should the unit be deployed again to a combat area. Formal communication between the community and National Guard leadership was described by numerous interviewees as "complicated" and "problematic." In most instances, the "rumor mill" worked faster than official reports from National Guard leaders, leaving many residents uncertain about which rumor they heard was closest to the truth. As a result, the community was described as being unprepared to appropriately send its citizens off to their first combat deployment and to provide support for the family members who remained behind. Although respondents said communications improved between the first and second deployments, they believe there is continued room for improvement.

A second area of potential need is the formal mental health service delivery system. According to interviewee descriptions, it appears to be lean: Interviewees reported no inpatient mental health beds in town, few private-pay mental health practitioners (such as psychologists), and only one full-time psychiatrist. In addition, the team was told that severe state budget cuts had resulted in strict eligibility requirements for county mental health services. Any individual service members struggling with the effects of their deployments likely are going outside of the area to get the professional supports they need. And although interviewees did not describe any large-scale negative behavioral health effects from the deployments, concern was expressed that the presentation of symptoms may still happen. If so, the area does not appear to have the service capacity to meet a large-scale emerging need.

## Community Suggestions

The primary suggestion from community members was for improved communication with National Guard leaders. Areas specifically mentioned included the more timely flow of information to local media outlets (e.g., the *Georgetown Times*) and the development of a mechanism to keep school district personnel, particularly principals and guidance counselors, apprised of which children may be experiencing distress because a parent is deployed.

The need for a more robust mental health system was *not mentioned by interviewees*, but is noted by the study team as a possible service gap. The informal support networks are strong and may have mitigated many adverse effects of multiple deployments on service members, their families, and the community; but these networks may not be strong enough to deal with significant behavioral health challenges. Consideration might be given to ways in which individuals with more pressing issues could receive the services they need closer to home.

# Little Falls, Minnesota

## Case Study Report

# Impacts of Multiple Deployments: Little Falls, Minnesota

## OVERVIEW

This report contains summary findings from Westat's ethnographic case study of Little Falls, Minnesota. The study goal was to assess how the Little Falls community has been affected by military deployments to Operation Iraqi Freedom (OIF) and Operation Enduring Freedom (OEF) from neighboring Camp Ripley, a 53,000-acre training facility run by the Minnesota National Guard. Data were collected through telephone interviews and a site visit to Little Falls (July 8–11, 2012). Because the National Guard units that deploy from Camp Ripley include members from various communities, it is difficult to pinpoint the impact of multiple deployments on Little Falls. Interviewees described challenges in the community that include limited economic opportunities, insufficient mental health resources for families throughout the deployment cycle, and a need for more timely mental health screenings for National Guard members postdeployment. Little Falls has a strong, organized group of leaders working to develop and enhance services for National Guard members and families, but collective reliance on individuals and small organizations has contributed to compassion fatigue among individuals doing the most.

**Data Sources**

- Mayor
- City government employees (i.e., convention and visitors bureau)
- County government employees (i.e., sheriff and veterans service, social service, public health employees)
- Community service organizations
- Behavioral and mental health organizations
- Hospital employees
- Community members
- Churches
- Local businesses
- Camp Ripley command and key staff
- Family Readiness Group leaders
- Observation
- Secondary sources (e.g., news articles, Internet videos, survey results provided by respondents)

## GEOGRAPHIC ORIENTATION

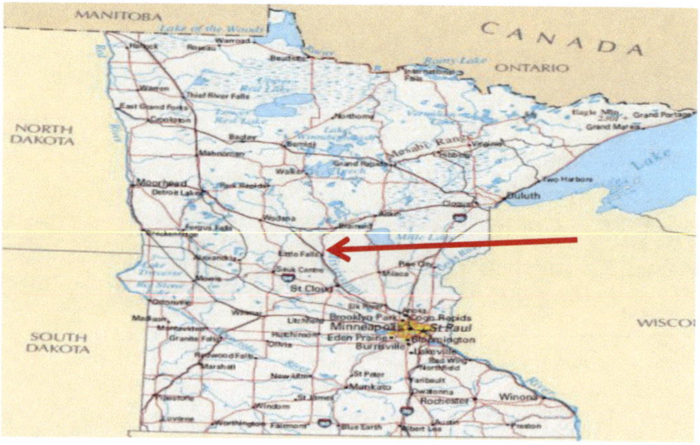


### Community: Little Falls, Minnesota

Little Falls is a small city (population of 8,427) in central Minnesota, approximately 100 miles northwest of Minneapolis. Its origins are traced to 1848, making Little Falls one of the oldest communities in Minnesota. Early development was prompted by a sawmill and a set of dams, built and rebuilt, on the Mississippi River. The sawmill and logging facilitated the construction of Fort Ripley, a frontier outpost located on land that is now part of Camp Ripley. Thus, ties between Little Falls and the military are as old as the town itself. The current Camp Ripley installation opened in 1931.

> Camp Ripley has been a military base around Little Falls since the creation of this community. It is there and it is a part of our lives and that's just the way it is. [Mayor]

These days, Little Falls is home to—as one interviewee describes it—"a good mix" of tourism, industry, and farming. Camp Ripley employs approximately 1,000 civilians and active duty soldiers, making it the largest local employer. Many residents also find jobs in local government because Little Falls is the county seat of Morrison County. Other notable employers include a hospital, Larson Boats, a snowplow manufacturer, and a direct mail company. Surrounding rural farmland, especially south of town, supports mostly corn and soy bean crops. Less than 40 miles to the north is the Brainerd Lakes region, which attracts hunters, fishermen, and outdoorsmen from across the state. Anyone walking through downtown Little Falls in the summertime is likely to see passenger trucks towing boats, all-terrain vehicles, personal watercraft, or campers. According to the 2010 U.S. Census, most of the population of Little Falls is white (96%), as is surrounding Morrison County (98%).

Unemployment and jobs are important concerns among locals, although unemployment rates are well below the current national unemployment rate, which is above 8%. Residents noted that Morrison County and neighboring counties in central Minnesota have historically had higher levels of unemployment than elsewhere in the state. One hosptial staff member said, "We are still one of the 10th to 12th poorest counties in the state, despite having Camp Ripley. It's just always been that way." Residents also noted that there were fewer good jobs in the community because of recent downsizing of Larson Boats and the closing of Crestliner, another large boat manufacturer.[1] However, as of May 2012, the unemployment rate in Morrison County was 5.7% and had been on the decline, no longer noticeably different from the average 5.6% unemployment rate in Minnesota.[2]

Alcohol and substance abuse were also of general concern to the community. Participants widely regarded alcohol as "an issue in Morrison County," and sources at the local hospital observed that alcohol-related deaths were "significantly up" in 2012. Substance abuse among teens, particularly heroin and methamphetamine, was also noted as a public concern by hospital sources.

## Military Installation Orientation: Minnesota National Guard

Approximately 13,000 soldiers and airmen serve in the Minnesota National Guard, making it the fifth largest National Guard, even though Minnesota is the 26th most populous state.[3] The National Guard's mission statement declares that under the "new normal" they have three separate missions: federal, state, and community. In times of war, Minnesota National Guard soldiers and airmen can be called into federal active service with the president of the

---

[1] See http://www.startribune.com/sports/outdoors/84191752.html.

[2] Federal Reserve Economic Data (FRED). See http://research.stlouisfed.org.

[3] Minnesota National Guard 101 http://www.minnesotanationalguard.org/aboutus/assets/Guard101.ppt.

United States as commander in chief. They can also be used by the governor to assist the state during disasters and other state emergencies. Finally, National Guard units are expected to contribute to their communities through participation in the workforce and educational institutions and by performing community service.[4]

The geographic orientations of people who serve in the units are loosely coupled with the location of the unit. Although a National Guard unit is based out of a town, only a subset of the unit includes town residents. Sources familiar with the National Guard told us it is not uncommon for members of the Minnesota National Guard to drive 3 hours for their monthly drill. A source at Camp Ripley explained that people may sign with different National Guard units across the state for promotion and career advancement. Because individuals may augment and deploy with other units depending on their skill set or military occupational speciality (MOS), deployments can also occur separately from unit affiliation.

### A History of Deployment

The Minnesota National Guard has a history of deploying units under their federal mission, going back to Bosnia in the 1990s. Relevant to the site visit study, the Minnesota National Guard has had multiple deployments under OIF and OEF—as of 2011, approximately 8,000 soldiers have deployed to Iraq.[5] The Minnesota National Guard has also contended with long deployments. Between 2005 and 2007, the Minnesota 34th Infantry based out of Camp Ripley was "extended indefinitely," ultimately to a 22-month deployment, the longest deployment of any infantry unit since World War II.[6]

### Military Installation: Camp Ripley

Camp Ripley's main entrance is 8 miles north of Little Falls. Camp Ripley was a mobilization station for troops during World War II and Korea and reached its current 53,000-acre size in the early 1960s. Camp Ripley now serves as a regional training center and is home to three armories and several units of the Minnesota Army National Guard, most notably the 1st Brigade Combat Team, 34th "Red Bull" Infantry Division. It employs approximately 1,000 full-time civilian and military staff.

As an installation of the Minnesota National Guard, Camp Ripley is state—not federal—property, and it shares its resources with several other state services. It has been the host for the Minnesota State Patrol Academy since 1996 and also supports training for the Minnesota Department of Public Safety, Minnesota Department of Natural Resources, and the Minnesota Department of Transportation.[7]

---

[4] Minnesota National Guard: Vision, Mission and Values; available at http://www.minnesotanationalguard.org/tagscorner/assets/091026_Vision_Mission_and_Values.pdf.

[5] Minnesota National Guard Annual Report 2011; available at: http://www.minnesotanationalguard.org/aboutus/assets/2011_Annual_Report.pdf.

[6] "Pentagon has committed to paying bonuses to 2,500 Minnesota National Guard soldiers"; available at http://www.minnesotanationalguard.org/press_room/e-zine/articles/index.php?item=2440.

[7] Minnesota National Guard Annual Report 2011; available at http://www.minnesotanationalguard.org/aboutus/assets/2011_Annual_Report.pdf.

Camp Ripley's use as a military training center has expanded over the last few years. Annual National Guard training, which used to occur only in the summer months, has been extended to February, and community members noted that the installation is in use for "8 to 9 months."[8] Camp Ripley now provides training for active duty military and National Guard units from many states. During the site visit, the team observed units from the Illinois National Guard. Because of the cold Minnesota winters, Camp Ripley also hosts international troops for training, including a long-standing partnership with the Norwegian Army.

**Relationship Between Community and Base**

Community members described Camp Ripley as "a good neighbor" and felt that Little Falls and Camp Ripley had a "strong relationship" and a "partnership." They pointed out that the base is the largest employer in the community and is an "important economic factor in Morrison County."

Community members said that Camp Ripley hosts community events, such as activities for the schools, the Boy Scouts, and veterans. Moreover, the base is open to the public. Team members noted that the military museum on base was widely publicized in the community. In addition, participants mentioned the Camp Ripley/Veterans State Trail, which is being planned on Camp Ripley's western borders. When completed, it will be a paved public trail for cyclists and motorized vehicles, part of a larger network of biking trails that extend the length of the Mississippi River.[9]

Roots between the community and Camp Ripley, which many intervieweess seemed to describe interchangably with the National Guard as a whole, are also personal. Participants explained that most families in Little Falls have some connection to Camp Ripley, either through a family member who works there or someone who is in the National Guard. Sources in the local schools noted that "there is hardly a kid that walks through our school that doesn't know someone that's in the miliary, either their next door neighbor, their uncle, their aunt, their brother, their sister, their mom, their dad."

Community residents describe Little Falls as a "military friendly" town. Shows of support for the troops and veterans are quite visible. At the intersection of Broadway and First, the main intersection in town, the American National Bank proudly displays a "We Support Our Troops" banner. Nearby, the Veterans Memorial honors Morrison County residents who have died in service (only one OIF casualty in Morrison County). To cross the Mississippi river, one takes the Memorial Bridge, a Works Project Administration construction "dedicated to all veterans who have honorably served our country." The bridge is lined with flags from each of the five branches of the military, a gift from the Little Falls American Legion in 2011.[10] The local Wal-Mart displays a "wall of fame" of employees who have deployed. One community member supported the team's observations, noting that the deployments "drew the community so close. . . . Everybody is involved in something to say thank you."

[8] See also http://m.brainerddispatch.com/news/2012-04-03/thunder-camp-ripley-looks-forward-busy-summer.
[9] See also http://www.crvtrail.com.
[10] See also http://www.cityoflittlefalls.com/cityuploads/M%2002-07-11%20REGULAR.pdf.

In Little Falls, team members repeatedly heard that "everyone wants to help, they just aren't sure how." Under the surface, however, cracks were beginning to show. Because of the length of the conflicts and the length of some of the deployments, many community members were noticing compassion fatigue. One interviewee, for example, noted a sharp decline in partcipation in the Beyond the Yellow Ribbon program; over a year ago, he said, there were 32 members; that number had dwindled to 4 at the most recent meeting. The study team also heard that fewer businesses offer discounts to the military than they used to, and the team both heard and observed that, if they are offered, businesses do not seem to be advertising them prominently. Another community member felt that the military was not as appreciative of the community's "heroic" efforts as it had once been. As a result, he said, the communities were beginning to focus on other local populations in need of assistance.

## EFFECTS OF DEPLOYMENT ON THE COMMUNITY

### Economic Impact

Multiple deployments per se have not had a strong overall economic impact on the community, but some individual employers have had deployment-related problems.

#### Commerce

Overall, the team observed minimal economic impact on Little Falls from multiple deployments. Because the National Guard units include members from throughout the state, it was not uncommon for only a handful of Little Falls residents to deploy at any given time. Residents felt these numbers were too low to present any economic impact at a community level. One city official said, though, that Camp Ripley has a *positive* economic impact because the base brought soldiers and contractors into the community, who in turn brought revenue into the community's restaurants and shops, "millions of dollars . . . *hundreds* of millions of dollars."

#### Housing

The housing market in Little Falls appears to be stable. One leader said that houses are on the market for only short periods of time because of new staff moving into the area to work at Camp Ripley. Driving through the community, the study team did not see many "For Sale" signs and noted only a handful of new, small-scale housing developments. Unlike in other communities in this study where active duty military relocate every few years, most National Guard members the study team spoke with had lived in Little Falls for many years, if not their whole lives. When they deployed, their families remained in the community.

#### Employment

Similarly, the overall labor supply has been unaffected by deployments. There was a general perception that unemployment was high and the community generally lacked a sufficient supply of jobs. In Little Falls, several residents believed that service members often signed up (and re-upped) for deployments because it was a job and paid well. Interviewees expressed concern that in the long term the drawdown of troops would return more service members without jobs to the community. Officers at Camp Ripley mentioned a recent Minnesota National Guard survey that identified unemployment as the leading concern among members. A January 2012 survey of the 1st Brigade Combat Team during a 1-year deployment in Kuwait (for which the Brigade Support Batallion is headquartered at Camp Ripley) showed that nearly 19% would be unemployed when they returned home and 44% were concerned about their employment.[11]

Though unemployment was a leading concern, some interviewees questioned service members' desire to find a job in the short term. For example, a recent job fair held at the community college, promoted heavily at Camp Ripley, was underattended by veterans and service members. One contributer described veterans' attendance as, "very disappointing given all the work that went into preparing this event." Community members provided different explanations for why the event was so poorly attended. One felt there was a "breakdown in communication" between the command leadership and soldiers in making service members aware of the event. Another believed that many service members on base that day did not see the value of attending because they live in distant communities or were not in the job market at the time: "I live in Rochester, why would I go to a job fair in Little Falls?"

**Impacts on Individual Employers**

Although there appear to be negligible overall community-level effects, several community members said the multiple deployments were taking a toll on individual businesses. They pointed out that employers struggled if the business was small (e.g., one or two people) or if the person that deployed held a unique skill set that was not easily replaceable:

> I think with . . . small companies, like with two soldiers, you know, they're scraping by anyway and the two soldiers get deployed. Well, the company closes. We had a family that ran a cement company . . . he got deployed and nobody knew what to do and they ended up losing that big business. I [own a small business]. If I had gotten deployed I may as well just shut the doors 'cause who's gonna run it? Who's gonna know how to order? It's tough, it's really tough, especially in a small town because it's a lot of small businesses. . . . I would say a lot of small companies are closing their doors because of deployments. [Community member]

> As a manager . . . I know the difficult part is trying to cover for somebody when it's a temporary deployment. It's not forever and we have to keep their position open. That's really difficult. . . . We all felt it when Dr. [surgeon] was gone. You're holding this spot and trying to fill it, but that's hard for anybody filling it because they know it's not permanent, and you really don't know for sure when they will come back, if they are going to be *able* to come back. . . . [Hospital employee]

Hospital staff also pointed out that the loss of a key staff member for an extended period of time can potentially result in lost revenues for the facility, particularly if other staff are stretched too thin to cover the deployed individual's workload.

---

[11] See http://www.minnesotanationalguard.org/units/unit_template.php?unit=134bc and http://www.minnesotanationalguard.org/generallyspeaking/120304_ERT_in_Kuwait.pdf.

## Information and Communication

Leaders in the community were generally satisfied with Camp Ripley's efforts to communicate with them, although two local residents said the base could do more to inform citizens of when soldiers are returning from deployment and provide more details about base activities open to the public.

### Information on Deployments

Generally, community members said they believe issues around deployments are openly discussed. They felt that information about deployments was in the newspapers,[12] and people were turning out to welcome troops home. Some community members, though, felt that they were not always aware of the details regarding deployments, such as when and where to welcome a returning unit, particularly one with a small number of local residents.

> When they came home, they wanted to get the soldiers back to their families as quickly as possible, and to the nearest armory to their home. I think that created a lot of heartaches and issues with the families because you build this up in your mind when they're gone and you want them to have this huge welcome home. My daughter got dropped off at the St. Cloud armory [and there was] maybe a handful of people there. They weren't escorted in. . . . My husband's unit, they returned at 11:30 at night. I will hand it to Little Falls. There were fire trucks, there were police, there was Sheriff's Department and everything. They escorted them all the way out to camp, lights and sirens going all the way. It was midnight. . . . My husband and daughter have both said they feel like they were just dropped back in and supposed to be able to pick up. It's hard for them not having that huge welcome home. [School employee]

Similarly, although events at Camp Ripley have been promoted in the local papers, it may not always be clear whether the events are for service members, their families, or the public.

> When they do have events, it would be helpful if they'd say that the public was invited . . . if the public was encouraged to attend I think they would. A lot of times I think people don't know: "Is this [just] a veterans and family thing? Am I kind of stepping into it [by] not being one of them?" . . . I think the public wants to support them, but sometimes they're supporting them by *not* stepping in. . . . "Is it a family thing or is that something we should go to?" So that's something they could do better . . . just having that outreach for people who care. [Community member]

The Family Assistance Center (FAC) also pointed out that not all family members have a good understanding of what the service member is doing while they are deployed. With the absence of information, they worry and jump to the worst conclusions because of stories they may have heard in the media. Community members stressed the importance of providing

---

[12] News in Little Falls is provided by two local newspapers (the weekly *Morrison County Record* and the daily *Brainerd Dispatch*), Little Falls Radio (KLTF AM 960, WYRQ FM 92.1, and KFML FM 94.1), and *Lakeland News,* a nightly local news broadcast on Lakeland Public Television. Events and stories regarding Camp Ripley were regularly covered by these news outlets.

additional education to family members who may not have a long-standing relationship with the military.

### Information About Services

Information about services and supports for military families often travels through gatekeepers. In particular, the FAC at Camp Ripley offers resources, referrals, and support to service members across branches and military family members, and the Veterans Service Officer (VSO) in Morrison County assists veterans, such as helping them access Department of Veterans Affairs (VA) benefits. The FAC liaison and VSO were visible and widely known in the community for working with service members, and in nearly every interview, team members were asked if they had spoken with them. Beyond the Yellow Ribbon, a statewide organization started by a few small cities that has spread through local communities, also seeks to connect service members with resources in their areas. FACs, VSOs, and the efforts of Little Falls to be designated as a Yellow Ribbon community are discussed later in this report.

## Community Health

Mental and behavioral health concerns dwarfed discussions of other health issues expressed in most interviews, but were difficult for most interviewees to link specifically to deployments. Even counselors with knowledge of which community members had deployed were resistant to connecting mental health issues to multiple deployments. Alcohol use, which was said to be a problem in the region, was reported by two persons to be greater after deployment "when they have been without for so long," with a potential to increase with multiple deployments. The absence of an inpatient mental health unit in the community and limited access to psychiatric care was expressed as a challenge. Several interviewees said that another particular challenge was that National Guard members fail to report health problems, including mental health issues and back injuries, to maintain their deployment status.

> I see a lot of folks who their livelihood depends on their availability to stay in the Guard. . . . Where else will they go in the area where they can get secure employment that has fringe benefits? It pays well, compared to a lot of private sector jobs. . . . I've dealt with folks that have come back saying "I tweaked my back [but] I don't want to say things about it because I don't want to jeopardize my future and my family's future. . . . Where am I going to go to get a job to pay my mortgage payment and help my kids through school?" . . . A lot of folks minimize the disabilities they've had simply because they're protecting themselves and their families for that employment purpose. [County government employee]

### Family and Children's Issues

Among the concerns that community members voiced about multiple deployments, concerns about children were prevalent. Stressors for children of deployed families are seen as an unmet need that community members did not know how to address.

A variety of respondents reported that bonding was difficult for the youngest children, who might not recognize a parent returning from deployment even if they had seen them on the computer screen during video chats. Similarly, most interviewees perceive that older children and adolescents, as one leader put it, "are acting out . . . with anger, misbehaving," but gave few ways in which this manifests itself. Conversely, two school employees told us that the National Guard kids are not the ones acting out. One said, "Most kids of dads who are deployed don't want to add to the stress. They don't get in trouble. I haven't seen any adverse effects." One person emphasized the importance of keeping children active in sports, Scouts, and other organized activities. Another described the Boys and Girls Club, which opened locally in the last few years, as busy and an important addition to the community.

A few interviewees explained that addressing children's mental health predeployment could prevent some problems. One said that "a counselor that drops by the house to see how it's going" during and after deployment could help children to process their feelings.

> That would be helpful. . . . I think probably weekly or every other week, a little extra. Maybe a little counseling that looks like a visit to a kid, versus somebody that's telling me what to do. Just chit chat with a couple of folks that might give them ideas, maybe do a little extra education stuff with them when they're in that 5-6-7-8 years old. Because at that point, I don't even think they know how to process their feelings. [City government employee]

Opinions on the benefits of Skype communication between family members were mixed. Several interviewees said it was a good way for a very young child to connect with and recognize a parent when they return from deployment. However, one National Guard member said that his roommate during deployment often started his day badly with his wife's complaints about what was going on at home.

A county employee told us that the state of "might deploy" is stressful for the entire family. When deployment orders come in, additional training time—as much as a year—is required predeployment, and postdeployment events at bases around the country before returning home also take time away from the family. The stress takes its toll on the family. One member of the health community told us, "I feel the tension sometimes" between a returning soldier and spouse and said that couples struggle with how to manage the house when one parent has made decisions in the other's absence. Although several interviewees reported that deployments cause an increase in divorce, a few explained that the dissolution of those marriages is caused by weak relationship foundations rather than by deployment. They told us that if a couple gets married too quickly, weeks before being deployed, or, as one person described, via videocast, the relationship is more likely to fail.

**Behavioral Health Issues**

Many community members reported substance abuse and suicidal thoughts as problems among National Guard members, but it is difficult to link them specifically to deployments. As noted in the description of formal supports, alcohol use is common in the community generally. Two interviewees who work closely with activated National Guard members indicated that drinking increases with deployments and is worse after multiple deployments. Similarly, drug abuse is a problem in the community. Team members were told that local civilians use marijuana, crystal methamphetamine, and heroin, but service members are tested monthly, so, as one counselor reported, they stick to "pills and alcohol."

Suicide is a local concern, but has always been a concern. A few interviewees recalled a suicide at Camp Ripley a few years ago during annual training, as well as calls about suicidal ideation both at Ripley and in the community. National Guard suicides are evident in the press, but may not link directly to the community. When asked by the study team whether the suicides could be linked to mulitple deployments, interviewees said it was difficult to connect these instances to deployments.

Also, as discussed earlier, unaddressed mental health issues will put an extra burden on civilian health care providers in the future. As noted, the small emergency facility in Little Falls can quickly reach capacity if the ER is holding a patient with acute mental health needs who requires a locked room and law enforcement presence.

**Physical Health Issues**

Back pain was the most commonly mentioned physical health issue stemming from multiple deployments, though most interviewees did not discuss physical health issues. The prevalent concern was about what one interviewee termed the "young immortals"—National Guard members who want to remain deployable and therefore fail to report injuries (that may make them eligible later) for a VA disability claim. One counselor who works with veterans voiced concern for the future of OIF/OEF soldiers:

> That 25-year-old limping around with the knee, now it's no problem. . . . By the time he's 35, he can't get out of his own vehicle. We have to get these folks aware. I hear "Well, there's a lot of guys that are worse off than me, I don't want to jeopardize . . . my ringing in the ears isn't that serious." That's all well and good when you're younger, but when you get to that retirement age, where is your health insurance going to be and you're not VA eligible anymore because you didn't file a claim for disability?

Conversely, two interviewees who had deployed previously mentioned their own service-related back injuries as their reason for leaving military service.

As with mental health issues, unaddressed physical health issues may put an extra burden on civilian health care providers or go untreated. As one source knowledgeable about the National Guard pointed out, service-related disabilities are not covered by employer health care. With only a 5-year statute of limitations to file VA claims, Nation Guard members may be left without VA-covered care for a lingering injury.

**Health Issues and Law Enforcement**

The perception from law enforcement is that there has been no appreciable increase in DUI or suicides among the National Guard as a result of deployments, although statistics among the general population might indicate an increase. Community members were mixed in their perceptions of the impact of multiple deployments on law enforcement, particularly the issue of domestic violence. A law enforcement informant told us, "I haven't seen it," but representatives of a human service organization believe that domestic violence increases with deployments.

## Community Competence

Several services are available to support service members and their families at Camp Ripley (during training and the deployment cycle), through the VA, and in the civilian community in Little Falls and Morrison County. There were no obvious gaps in formal health care supports for activated service members or veterans with a service-connected disability, though several of the supports that were said to be most valued are less than 5 years old. Moreover, team members were told about barriers to seeking services, including young National Guard members who do not report injuries in order to "remain deployable," a stigma related to National Guard members' seeking mental health assistance, resentful service members and spouses who want nothing to do with the military, and civilian unfamiliarity with the specific services available. Interviewees reported gaps in services for military families.

### Behavioral and Mental Health Services

Interviewees almost uniformly identified local mental and behavioral health as the biggest deployment-related challenge for all age groups in their community. Financial management skills were also mentioned as a stressor for service members who deploy.

Mental health issues are beginning to be addressed with an approach that was described in an interview as evolving, primarily through nonprofit Northern Pines, which provides a range of mental health education, counseling, and psychiatry across six counties. Northern Pines is the mental health contractor supporting children in Little Falls community schools, as well as individuals training at Camp Ripley. According to interviews and documents available online, a Northern Pines employee who is an OIF/OEF Army veteran identified the need and garnered support from the executive director to provide services for veterans and families.[13] Family eligibility has evolved to offer sliding-scale services, and "families" is now defined as spouses, children, and parents of deployed soldiers or veterans. Several respondents reported that the program has worked closely with the National Guard in the last few years to provide outreach and support at reintegration events, as well as responding to emergency mental health calls at Camp Ripley. The veterans program is run by a part-time coordinator and full-time VISTA national service program volunteer committed from Fall 2011 through 2013, and one interviewee reported that they are bringing another veteran counselor on board in August 2012. One mental health professional, however, said these services are still underused by eligible community members.

Several interviewees explained that a Mobile Crisis Outreach (MCO) and stabilization team serves the six counties through Northern Pines.[14] In addition to responding to acute mental health needs in hospital emergency rooms, homes, and law enforcement facilities, the MCO team

---

[13] See also http://www.npmh.org/Veterans%20Service/NPVSMP%20Brochure2.pdf.
[14] See also http://www.npmh.org/mobile-crisis-outreach.html.

has been called to Camp Ripley "on occasion . . . anyone in need is never turned away from here." The value of MCO to Ripley, which includes a counselor with military experience, came up in several interviews and one person said, "We wouldn't survive without them." Another interviewee described several instances when the team was called to Camp Ripley and successfully identified issues of addiction and suicidal ideation.[15]

Several interviewees mentioned the contributions of Lutheran Social Service (LSS), a Minnesota not-for-profit organization, in providing services for veterans. LSS C.O.R.E. (Case Management, Outreach, Referral and Education) is a statewide program for military, veterans, and family members. A few interviewees emphasized the value of the program's financial counseling. LSS C.O.R.E. also provides telephone mental health counseling and referrals. One person the study team spoke with, however, said that some community leaders described challenges in providing referrals to local resources, which are discussed in the following pages.

**Physical Health Services**

St. Gabriel's Hospital is located in Little Falls. It provides full-service care, and underwent significant renovation in 2007, expanding patient care facilities. The hospital is the first place many local area residents arrive after being injured or if they experience a mental health crisis bceause it has the only emergency room (ER) in the area. They see occasional traffic in the ER from Camp Ripley related to the county's MCO efforts. A hospital worker explained that with an eight-bed ER, the community's resources are insufficient to address the most acute psychiatric needs. She went on to explain the value of the crisis team and mediating the security hazards posed by treating people in crisis in the ER:

> It can take hours and hours to find a place to place someone that needs placement. They end up at the far corners of the state. . . . There is a safety problem both for them and for staff, in your small critical access hospitals, which is all Morrison County has, and surrounding us. We don't have behavioral health units. We don't have psychiatrists. . . . When you've got somebody in a locked room and you're supposed to be watching them all the time with a sheriff outside guarding them. That wouldn't happen if we didn't have the crisis team there. We still have eight other rooms that are full, plus people in the waiting room. [Hospital employee]

**Military and VA Supports**

The National Guard and VA reportedly provide the first line of support to activated National Guard members and their families through the FAC and other services at Camp Ripley, FRGs, the VA clinic in Brainerd, and the expanded VA campus in St. Cloud. The mayor in Little Falls commented, "I would say they handle it among themselves."

Formal events during predeployment, at demobilization, and at 30/60/90-day reintegration events were described by various respondents as important supports. At these large events, National Guard members are reportedly provided with information about benefits, asked

[15] See also Brunswick, M. (2012, January 29). Anti-suicide program for military runs low. *StarTribune*. Available at http://www.startribune.com/local/130949523.html.

individually about service-connected injuries, enrolled in the VA Health Care System (with "80 to 90 percent enrollment in Minnesota" according to one military leader), and provided with contact information to access a range of services. Local providers, including the Morrison County VSO and Northern Pines veterans program, told us that they participate in these events. For example, the VSO speaks with returning soldiers individually to identify any service-connected injury or disability, including mental health issues that may be presenting, and help them complete VA paperwork. There was general agreement that many of the mental health issues the counselors see postdeployment with veterans and families present at or after a 1-year "honeymoon period." One National Guard member informally mentioned a new 1-year reintegration event, but this does not appear to be a statewide program.

Both military-affiliated and civilian interiewees unanimously identified the FAC at Camp Ripley as a primary support for addressing stressors around the deployment cycle. Several of them described how counselors listen to stories of individual challenges, follow up on concerned phone calls from neighbors, and connect service members and their families to needed services. For example, the FAC provides assistance to National Guard families with financial issues by contacting community volunteers to shovel snow and by giving them grocery cards from the community or firewood from Camp Ripley. Several interviewees told us that the FAC proactively offered consistent individual outreach to those who *might* be struggling, and counselors told us that they are on call 24 hours a day. One source close to the Camp Ripley FAC told us:

> Some of [the veterans served] you had to seek out. Maybe their neighbors would call and say, "I know he's been out of work and his unemployment stopped from deployment. They have no groceries and I'm getting worried about them." I would call them up and say something like, "I'm calling everybody that was deployed. . . . How are things going?" They always say, "It's going great." "Oh really? Are you working yet?" "No." "Well how are you feeding your family and paying your bills?" "Well that's an issue." Then they start talking about it and pretty soon we're paying their rent and their electric. You can't wait for them to come in, because most of them won't. They've still got that military pride. [Community member]

Interviewees identified FRGs as a support, but the effects are mediated because members of deployed units come from broad geographic areas. One FRG leader said the geographic distance "is hard. You send emails to these people, but very seldom will they travel 100 miles to attend a 2- or 3-hour FRG meeting. . . . We did make phone calls from time to time too, but most of the time you do not put a name and a face together." In part because soldiers attach and reattach to multiple units, FRGs were said to be less active or even "dormant" when the unit was not deployed. In addition, two women service members said their husbands were unlikely to participate in FRG activities. Several National Guard members and spouses described the challenges and said the primary contacts used for support are the FACs.

Military OneSource was mentioned in passing in a few interviews as a resource during deployment, but its utility was limited for National Guard members and families before and after activation. In addition, two interviewees asked how you would counsel a child over the phone.

Several persons the team spoke with said that the St. Cloud VA Health Center has expanded services to meet the growing demand, including adding a women's health clinic and increasing the number of mental health care providers to "almost 30." Both veterans and service providers in Little Falls said the St. Cloud VA was doing a good job. As one service provider in the community said, "I can't say enough positive things about St. Cloud VA, one of the best because it's got the small-town flavor. At the Minneapolis one, you never see the same person twice. Locally, I think we're doing well." Although improved, services for veterans are still reportedly stretched. In addition, team members were told that, although veterans are legally entitled to time off of work for health care, they may be laid off if they regularly miss work for appointments.

TRICARE was mentioned as the only health insurance some National Guard members could obtain for their families. However, one provider said that "there have been huge issues around TRICARE and behavioral health reimbursement" and the paperwork is "a nightmare." But another provider was more positive, saying, "On the medical side, it doesn't take as long as it once did."

**Other County Services**

Several interviewees referred us to the Morrison County VSO, who helps those who were deployed to the OEF/OIF theaters to navigate the bureaucracy of the VA and access physical and mental health benefits after deployment. Although the VSO is state mandated, several interviewees told us that the supports provided by the Morrison County VSO are exceptional. These include presentations and brief one-on-one sessions during reintegration events, as well as assisting returning soldiers in filling out VA paperwork, reviewing VA decision letters, and helping with appeals as needed. The office provides counseling, assistance in obtaining benefits for any service-connected disability, and transportation in the Veterans Van once a week to the St. Cloud VA Health Center. At a time when other counties were downsizing their VSOs, the Morrison County Commission reportedly approved expanded staffing to include a veterans service case aide and provided more private office space in the county office building to increase confidentiality for veterans seeking help and offer more support than counties with larger veteran populations. As a result, in addition to serving OEF/OIF veterans and other veterans in Morrison County, two interviewees told the team that the office is now contacted by veterans from other counties for assistance.

**Beyond the Yellow Ribbon of Morrison County**

Beyond the Yellow Ribbon (BTYR) is a Minnesota program to link military members and their families to informal programs and supports in the community.[16] The Morrison County effort, which several interviewees said is in process, has 12 subcommittees to address how to connect individuals with services across domains in what one committee member called "single touch." Many interviewees described it as an important way for community members to show support and said it will be strong when in place. Yet there were questions from a few community members regarding the value of BTYR to National Guard members and their families; currently there are significant overlaps with FAC, which is the major point of referral; and one resident

[16] See http://www.beyondtheyellowribbon.org/yellow-ribbon-community-campaign.

who was very familiar with the resources at Camp Ripley described the services provided by theBTYR as "vague."

The Military Family Care Initiative, created by then-Minnesota First Lady Mary Pawlenty and mentioned by a few community members, has been incorporated into BTYR.[17]One National Guard member said she had used the program to locate services. She contacted a Lions Club group in St. Cloud while she was deployed; they sent a group of volunteers to spend a day chopping wood for her family.

Gaining BTYR status involves identifying and connecting leaders in key areas, including city/civic/military, public safety/judicial, and businesses/employers.[18] Although team members were told that the action plans have not been completed by the various committees, several interviewees reported increasingly systematic efforts to ensure that businesses are military friendly—for example, offering a discount to individuals with military identification and joining Employer Support of the National Guard and Reserve (ESGR). ESGR businesses receive tools to locate returning service members and a tax credit for participating. One small business owner in town showed us a statement of support that she had signed a few hours before.

## Social Capital

Virtually all community members the team spoke with identified Little Falls as a small town with a "neighborly" culture, and informal supports appeared to be strong.

### Small Town Relationships

Team members heard from a variety of sources that extended families live in the region, everyone knows everyone, families help families, and neighbors help neighbors in need. The community also appeared to be receptive to newcomers.[19] Several residents who had relocated from elsewhere in Minnesota to work at Camp Ripley described informal supports they had received that the team viewed as comparable to the supports described by those whose families had been there for generations. Interviewees commonly offered the examples of shoveling snow or taking care of children without pay. One interviewee described a variety of informal supports provided to her husband and children while she was deployed:

> [What] he did have was a friend at Ripley who provided childcare at Ripley. . . . My girlfriend's family took my girls for free on weekends. . . . That was huge. [My husband] would get to drop them off on Friday, pick up on Sunday, mow the grass, do whatever . . . I have a church that's very nice. While I was gone, someone picked up my child and brought her to school for a year, back and forth to daycare. So I think it's individual help. [City government employee]

One downside of the reliance on informal supports, according to several interviewees, was that National Guard members and their families do not always ask for help when they need

---

[17] See https://www.militaryfamilies.state.mn.us/about.php.
[18] See http://www.beyondtheyellowribbon.org/images/stories/PDF/YRRP_Min_Requirements_and_Best_Practices-City.pdf.
[19] During the site visit, team members did not encounter anyone who was not originally from Minnesota.

it. Virtually all interviewees told us that people want to help, but a few stated that "they don't know how," and another explained that needs must be identified by the individual or someone close. Local families were described as "proud," and people may refuse help or be angry if help is provided without a request. However, interviews with residents indicated that even if someone does not ask for or refuses help, formal services, such as those from Northern Pines and the FAC are sometimes engaged by a call from a neighbor. One service provider recommended asking specific questions—for example: "Do you need anything? 'No.' Do you need your gutter cleaned? 'Well, yes.'"

**Extensions of Formal Supports**

Several of the individuals who provide formal deployment cycle support were identified by interviewees as the go-to people to address the impact of multiple OIF/OEF deployments on Little Falls. This round-the-clock availability was also described in several interviews as a community stressor leading to "burn out" among the staff of the key programs. One community member described the continuing late-night calls she receives to drive a drunk National Guard member home after return from deployment. She went on to say:

> Even though I've quit my job, I'm still doing it, kind of. I'm still out there and helping. . . . Families still call me, because I've been doing it for so long, to ask questions about retirement, "What if I get deployed again? How do I go about getting into the VA?" So I answer questions like that. If you go to the fair and things somebody is always stopping you and asking what can I do about that. Hopefully I can help them. If I can't, I can't, and I send them to the Family Assistance Center then . . . I'm probably always going to do that. [Community member]

Another resident told us about how serving local veterans presents a personal challenge:

> I had an episode a couple of months ago. I went to the grocery store after work and one of these guys—not OIF/OEF ers—bumped into him in a parking lot, he's chewing on my ass all the way into the grocery store, bitching about the VA . . . what kind of compensation is that . . . I told him to call me in the morning, I can't do a damned thing about it at the grocery store. I give him the slip. He must have had a mission, because there I am going through checkout and he's waiting to chew on me all the way out to the car. After a while that gets more than a little old. [County government employee]

**Faith Community**

The faith community does not appear to play a central role in addressing the impacts of multiple deployments in Little Falls. Churches were mentioned in only a few interviews, and military support was not evident on church websites. A church employee described a clergy forum at the St. Cloud VA to address issues they might see in their membership related to deployments, as well as available VA services. One community member described a church that assembled decks of playing cards for deploying soldiers; another mentioned sending care packages. Otherwise, the help provided from the faith community was described as "individual" by several community members.

## SUMMARY

As one interviewee told us: "People make the difference." Though formal structures are slowly coming into place, Little Falls is a small town that still relies heavily on its people to support its community members.

### What's Working

In Little Falls, residents are the souce of many of its strengths in assisting active duty and activated National Guard members and families during deployment and reintegration. Such supports are often personal and occur on a case-by-case basis. Interviewees also praised strong leadership in the community for improving and expanding organized supports to assist military members and veterans and their familites, including those who have experienced multiple deployments. They spoke positively about the following efforts:

- The Veterans Service Office in Morrison County: This office helps veterans and National Guard members navigate the bureaucracy of the VA after deployment. Both the Morrison County office space and staff were expanded to meet growing needs.
- Northern Pines: With the increased the need for mental health services for veterans, service members, and their families, the leadership at Northern Pines has been extremely responsive, supporting half of the costs for the expansion under the organization's overhead. One of the services provided by Northern Pines is the Mobile Crisis Outreach (MCO) program, a partnership among six counties that is meeting a need on base and in the community for soldiers that go into crisis or are suicidal or have suicidal thoughts. The program also provides needed security in hospital emergency rooms, providing staff to separate the patient from others seeking care at the ER.
- Beyond the Yellow Ribbon: Though still in development in Little Falls, many community leaders believe this program holds promise for offering a one-stop shop to connect service members with community resources. Because it is a joint effort between the community and the National Guard, it has the potential to organize community capacity, thereby reducing burden on key liaisons and preventing burnout. Other community leaders were less enthusiastic, however, and were waiting to see how the BTYR program distinguishes itself from other, extant community efforts.
- Good working relationship between Little Falls and Camp Ripley: Solid communications between the base and the town were believed to have helped mitigate the effects of multiple deployments on Little Falls.

### Community Needs

Community members raised several concerns related to deployments, with some concerns focused on current needs but others addessing potential longer-term needs:

- Several community members raised concerns about the long-term mental well-being of service members and the future services they will need. National Guard members the study team spoke with believe the 30/60/90-day postdeployment screenings are valuable, but both those members and mental health professionals pointed out that mental health issues may arise later than 90 days—sometimes 12 to 18 months after they return from deployment.
- Two interviewees close to the National Guard were concerned that people are falling through the cracks. One described the challenge that exists when National Guard members want to remain deployable and do not seek needed services. If they do not report military-related injuries or health problems on a timely basis, they will not be eligible for VA disability claims later when their problems worsen and may affect their employability.
- Some mental health professionals interviewed by the study team indicated that postdeployment mental health screenings available to National Guard members are not as effective as they could be. One interviewee observed that these screenings are not as consistent as those available to Army soldiers. They said that mental health screening questions during the 30/60/90-day reintegration events were asked by VSOs, who might be great at referring service members to appropriate clinicians, but who generally are not trained in mental health issues and interventions. Unless service members self-report, they said, the responsibility is on the chain of command (especially the first sergeant) to identify symptoms of depression or posttraumatic stress and encourage service members to seek help.
- Most community members the team spoke with think there are insufficient mental and behavioral health supports for children in military families. Community members frequently had trouble articulating what the needs are, except to say "children act up." But some members we spoke with observed anger among teenagers. Others were concerned about behavioral responses among elementary school-aged children, for example, ages 6 to 8.
- Community members also observed a general lack of formal supports for military families. Team members were told that the FRG model is not always a reliable support for families of the deployed because members of the National Guard units are geographically dispersed. Military spouses we spoke with were as likely to turn to the FAC as to their FRG leader. Moreover, there were no support groups in Little Falls. Northern Pines observed that when they attempted to set up groups on post, the main interest was from the spouses. However, the timing and location of the groups was not conducive to attendance by families or spouses.
- With the impending drawdown in troops, local community members pointed to the long-term need for economic opportunities for returning service members. Without jobs, these community members felt that behavioral and mental health problems would escalate.

- Some interviewees pointed to the need for supports for the supporters. Although the dedicated individuals that make up the fabric of Little Falls are unquestionably a strength, the emotional nature of the work takes a toll. One mental health professional said, "Everyone who works with the veterans burns out." Supporters themselves have sought counseling to deal with the stress of working with service members and veterans.
- Though many community members were satisfied with Camp Ripley's efforts to engage the community, a few raised questions about how effectively Camp Ripley communicated details about events, such as job fairs and welcome home activities for returning troops. Others said that, even though Camp Ripley publicized base events in the local newspaper, it was not always clear whether these events were for the public or military families only.

**Suggestions from the Community**

The community offered the following suggestions for possible improvements or next steps that may help address the needs associated with multiple deployments:

- The military should add a mental health screening beyond 90 days because mental health issues may surface later on.
- Providers of mental health supports should increase the number of mental health professionals with military experience. Interviewees said it is the shared experience that increases credibility and makes service members more willing to confide in a mental health professional: One OIF/OEF veteran who provides mental health services said, "We'll send a professional out there. They'll talk for 2 hours and will get almost nothing. I go out there for 10 minutes, they ask me where I served, I tell them. Boom, we have all the information we need."
- Children with parents who are deployed should receive counseling. Rather than formal counseling, the visit could be an informal check-in. One participant suggested play therapy for toddlers, and another participant suggested a "chat" to help children process their feelings.
- There should be more education for the business community on mental health issues among service members. This type of outreach, such as a seminar or a forum, would help educate employers on what symptoms or issues to look for in service members they employed and how they could assist service members in reintegration efforts.
- More entrepreneurship supports should be provided in order to improve jobs in the region. As National Guard members reintegrate into the community, they may aspire to open their own businesses. Businees leaders said entrepreneurship supports would help the National Guard members to understand how to start and manage a small business.

# F

# SAMPLE OF GOVERNMENT DATA AND DATABASES

This description of data and databases covers a small sample of the data that the committee attempted to secure. In some cases, the committee was successful in obtaining data; in most cases, however, it was not. In its effort to conduct analyses that would provide information pertinent to its charge but not available in the literature, the committee had hoped to link data from these databases with the Defense Manpower Data Center (DMDC) data that it received on all those deployed. The committee provides here a brief explanation of some of those data and databases.

## SELECTED DEPARTMENT OF DEFENSE DATA AND DATABASES

### Defense Manpower Data Center

Since 1974, the DMDC has maintained an archive of Department of Defense (DOD) data, including all branches and components (active duty, reserve, and guard) of military personnel, manpower, training, and financial data. Data have been collected on over 42 million persons connected to DOD, and they have been followed through their military life (accession, service, separation, and retirement). The DMDC combines data from numerous programs (such as the Defense Enrollment Eligibility Reporting System [DEERS]) and personnel files (for active duty, reserve, guard, retired military personnel, contractors, and civilians) and data from many other sources (such as the Department of Veterans Affairs [VA], the Social Security Administration [SSA], and Medicare) to allow reporting of entitlements, benefits, and readiness; for personnel identification, validation, and authentication; and for decision-support purposes. (https://www.dmdc.osd.mil/appj/dwp/index.jsp)

### Postdeployment Health Assessment and Postdeployment Health Reassessment

The Postdeployment Health Assessment (PDHA) is a self-conducted health screen for examining physical and mental health outcomes associated with deployment. It is meant to be completed in the theater of operation before redeployment, ideally within 5 days but not more than 30 days before departure from theater. The PDHA is also to be completed by all reserve-component personnel activated to active-duty status for more than 30 days in support of any contingency operation. (https://g1arng.army.pentagon.mil/programs/pdha/pages/default.aspx)

The Postdeployment Health Reassessment (PDHRA) is a self-conducted health screen for examining physical and mental health outcomes associated with deployment that is conducted 90–180 days after deployment and is required for all service members and reserve-component personnel who deployed outside the continental United States for 30 days or more. (https://g1arng.army.pentagon.mil/programs/pdha/pages/default.aspx)

**Survey of Spouses**

On May 10, 2010, DOD launched the Military Family Life Project, the first large-scale, longitudinal DOD-wide survey to assess quality-of-life issues that might affect military families during and after deployments. Invitations to participate in the online survey—starting May 10, 2010, and available for 3 months—were mailed to 100,000 military spouses and 40,000 married service members in all services selected at random. Spouses were encouraged to complete the survey online quickly, and those who did not respond were sent a paper copy of the survey. Spouses were to be contacted again for a follow-up survey in the following year. The survey is voluntary and confidential.
(http://www.militaryhomefront.dod.mil/MOS/f?p=MHF:DETAIL1:0::::SID,COHE:20.60.0.0.0.0.0.0.0,256706)

The DMDC has conducted longitudinal surveys of active-duty and reserve military spouses to determine how DOD can support military families better and assess the attitudes and opinions of the military community pertaining to a wide array of personal issues. The Survey of Active Duty Spouses is administered to spouses of active Army, Navy, Marine Corps, and Air Force members who have served for at least 6 months and below flag rank. The 2006 survey was conducted from November 21, 2005, to June 1, 2006, and had a 32.7% response rate. The 2008 survey was conducted from March 14 to August 4, 2008, and had a 28% weighted response rate. Data pertaining to background information, permanent change-of-station moves, spouse deployment, deployment effects on children, use of Military OneSource, education and employment, financial and health well-being, and feeling about military life were collected. (DMDC. 2006 Survey of Active-Duty Spouses: Administration, Datasets, and Codebook. Report No. 2006-034. March 2007. Available at:
http://www.dod.mil/pubs/foi/Personnel_and_Personnel_Readiness/Personnel/DMDC_2006-034.pdf)

(DMDC. 2006 Survey of Active Duty Spouses: Financial Well-Being and Spouse Employment Survey Note. Note No. 2008-005.
http://www.military.com/spouse/fs/0,,fs_SpouseSurvey,00.html?ESRC=mscc.n)

(The survey is also conducted among spouses of reserve component personnel. http://www.allmilitary.com/board/viewtopic.php?id=24752; limitations of the survey may be found at http://afs.sagepub.com/content/early/2010/01/19/0095327X09358652.abstract)

**TRICARE**

TRICARE is the DOD's collective health care program that provides health benefits for military personnel, military retirees, their dependents, and activated members of the guard and reserves. Services may be provided through managed care providers directly in DOD facilities, which include 44 inpatient hospitals and medical centers and 291 ambulatory care clinics in the United States, or through the purchased care system, which includes 379,233 network individual providers (for primary care, behavioral health, and specialty care) and 3,146 TRICARE network acute care hospitals (Department of Defense, 2011; Merlis, 2012). There is also a fee-for-service option for care administered by civilian providers who are not part of the network (Deployment Health Clinical Center, 2012).

To enroll in a TRICARE plan, service members, their families, and retirees must first establish eligibility through DEERS. Active-duty and retired service members, including National Guard and reserve members activated for at least 30 days, are automatically registered in DEERS, but individual service members are responsible for registering their family members, updating their status, and ensuring that their information is current and correct (TRICARE Management Activity, 2009). Active duty service members, including members of the reserve components activated for at least 30 days, automatically enroll in TRICARE Prime[1] at no cost.

DEERS contains data on all service members and family members who are eligible for TRICARE coverage. Family members must be entered by the service member, and people are responsible for updating their information in the database. (http://tricare.mil/mybenefit/home/overview/Eligibility/DEERS)

The Military Health System Data Repository (MDR), maintained by the Defense Health Service, is the centralized repository for DOD health-system data to capture, integrate, validate, and distribute health data in DOD health care networks. (http://health.mil/Libraries/OCIO_Documents/MDR_Fact_Sheet.pdf)

Included in the MDR are the Standard Inpatient Data Record (SIDR) and the Standard Ambulatory Data Record (SADR), which are generated by the Composite Health Care System (CHCS). CHCS contains data on direct care in each DOD medical treatment facility (MTF). For example, patient registration, appointments and scheduling, patient administration, nursing, pharmacy, laboratory, radiology, and dietetics information and services are recorded. CHCS aids in patient administration, billing and accounting, and workload assignment tasks and allows medical-records tracking and quality assurance.

(DHIMS. CHCS factsheet. http://dhims.health.mil/docs/factsheets/factsheet-CHCS.pdf)

The SIDR contains information pertaining to inpatient services for military health system beneficiaries in each MTF and contains details on patient stay, diagnoses, procedures, bed days, treatment facility, and personal data.

(DHSS. Interface Control Document Describing the Standard Inpatient Data Record [SIDR] Data Exchange to MDR Mod 2. ICD-1300-3110-06. Sept 16, 2010)

The SADR includes direct care outpatient-service data on each MTF or clinic. Patient information, provider, diagnoses, treatments, and insurance information are included.

(DHSS. Interface Control Document Describing the PID Enhanced SADR Data Exchange from ADM Mod 3. ICD-1300-3310-04. May 29, 2008).

---

[1] TRICARE Prime is a managed care option offering.

# SELECTED DEPARTMENT OF VETERANS AFFAIRS DATA AND DATABASES

## Assistant Deputy Under Secretary for Health Monthly Enrollment File

The Veterans Health Administration (VHA) Assistant Deputy Under Secretary for Health (ADUSH) Monthly Enrollment File (the Enrollment File) is a compilation of national statistics on VHA expenditures, enrollment, and patients. It is also used to develop statistical models for forecasting enrollment and expenditures and for policy analyses. Numerous files provide data for the VHA ADUSH Monthly Enrollment File.
(http://www.virec.research.va.gov/RUGs/RUG-ADUSH-EF-FY99-06-ER.pdf)

## Patient Treatment File and Outpatient Care File

The Patient Treatment File (PTF) is an automated system for recording and tracking inpatient care received in VA and non-VA medical facilities (at VA's expense). The PTF provides an abstract of inpatient activity (hospital care), diagnoses, procedures, and surgeries performed from the time of admission to the time of discharge from inpatient care.
(https://www1.va.gov/vhapublications/ViewPublication.asp?pub_ID=1650)

The Outpatient Care File is a file of outpatient visits and ambulatory care. Clinical encounters are characterized by a "stop code," a three-digit code that corresponds to a location where care was provided.
(http://www.herc.research.va.gov/files/RPRT_8.pdf)

## Decision Support System

The Decision Support System (DSS) generates estimates of the cost of inpatient hospital stays and outpatient health care encounters. The DSS consists of a set of programs that use relational databases to provide cost and other information. VA notes that the DSS allows measurement of quality of care, clinical outcomes, and financial impact and assists in reporting, analysis, budgeting, and modeling of care and costs. DSS data are available in the form of National Data Extracts, SAS datasets of selected DSS fields by fiscal year, and DSS production databases, and contains facility-level cost and clinical data.
(http://www.herc.research.va.gov/data/dss.asp)

## Medical SAS Datasets

The Medical SAS Datasets contain inpatient and outpatient information. Medical SAS Datasets contain national, patient-level, and administrative data on VHA care extracted from the National Patient Care Database (NPCD, a relational database) by fiscal year. Inpatient data are from the PTFs. (http://www.virec.research.va.gov/MedSAS/Overview.htm)

## National Patient Care Database

The NPCD is a relational database, updated daily, of VHA clinical information. It contains patient information, service information (including date and time, provider, and location), diagnoses and procedures, patient's primary care provider, and some patient-status

information, such as exposure to Agent Orange.
(http://www.virec.research.va.gov/NPCD/Overview.htm)

The committee had hoped to access numerous additional databases, including the Pharmacy Benefits Management Database (a national database of information on all prescriptions dispensed in the VHA System beginning with fiscal year 1999) and the VHA Vital Status File (which contains information for determining the vital status of veterans who enrolled in or received care from the VHA or received benefits from the Veterans Benefits Administration).

## VETERANS BENEFITS ADMINISTRATION DATA SOURCES

### Compensation and Pension Disability Information

The National Center for Veterans Analysis and Statistics collects, validates, and analyzes data pertaining to veterans and VA benefits and programs. Data collected, analyzed, and reported include demographic and socioeconomic data, use of and expenditures for VA programs (health care, home loans, education benefits, and compensation and pension), and data from the National Survey of Veterans (including data on education, employment, home loans, insurance, and demographics). (http://www.va.gov/vetdata/index.asp)

### Veterans Service Network

The VETSNET (new version of the Compensation and Pension [C&P] file) Veterans Service Network Corporate Mini Master File consists of selected fields from the Veterans Benefits Administration (VBA) Corporate Database. Updated monthly, the VETSNET Corporate Mini Master File contains a selected subset of VBA fields of information on compensation and benefits to veterans or their beneficiaries. Current and terminated benefits are included. This data file is to replace the C&P Mini File (a data extract of the legacy Benefits Delivery Network containing data only on current benefits).
(http://www.virec.research.va.gov/VETSNET/Overview.htm)

### Beneficiary Identification Records Locator System

The VBA database containing VA beneficiaries since 1973 is known as the Beneficiary Identification Records Locator System (BIRLS). BIRLS contains records of beneficiaries, including survivors of veterans who applied for death benefits.
(https://www.va.gov/vetdata/Glossary.asp)

The BIRLS Death File is an extract of the BIRLS database that contains death information (but not cause of death) on deceased veterans; it is updated monthly. Death information is gathered from VHA hospitals, the VA National Cemetery Administration, and family members' applications to VBA for death benefits.
(http://www.virec.research.va.gov/BIRLS/Overview.htm)

## OTHER DATASETS OF INTEREST

The committee had hoped to link data from the datasets below to the DMDC data to gain a full appreciation of the deployed population and so that it could examine employment and earnings, cause of death, criminal statistics, and whether veterans deployed to Operation Enduring Freedom or Operation Iraqi Freedom or their family members had applied for Medicaid:

- SSA files.
- National Death Index.
- National Crime Information Center files maintained by the Federal Bureau of Investigation.
- Centers for Medicare & Medicaid Services.

## REFERENCES

Department of Defense. 2011. *Evaluation of the TRICARE program.* Washington, DC: Department of Defense.

Deployment Health Clinical Center. 2012. *DOD and VA Federal Healthcare Services.* http://www.pdhealth.mil/hss/healthcare_services.asp#mhs (accessed September 25, 2012).

Merlis, M. 2012. *The future of health care for military personnel and veterans.* Washington, DC: Academy Health.

TRICARE Management Activity. 2009. *Evaluation of the TRICARE program, FY 2009 report to Congress.* Washington, DC: Department of Defense.